FOOD ALLERGY

Commissioning Editor: *Sue Hodgson*
Development Editor: *Sven Pinczewski*
Editorial Assistant: *John Leonard*
Project Manager: *Vinod Kumar Iyyappan*
Design: *Kirsteen Wright*
Illustration Manager: *Merlyn Harvey*
Illustrator: *Robert Britton*
Marketing Managers (UK/USA): *Gaynor Jones/Abigail Swartz*

FOOD ALLERGY

John M. James, MD
Colorado Allergy and Asthma Centers, P.C.
Private Clinical Practice
Fort Collins, CO, USA

Wesley Burks, MD
Professor and Chief
Pediatric Allergy and Immunology
Duke University Medical Center
Durham, NC, USA

Philippe Eigenmann, MD
Head, Pediatric Allergy Unit
Department of Child and Adolescent
University Hospitals of Geneva
Geneva, Switzerland

ELSEVIER
SAUNDERS
Edinburgh   London   New York   Oxford   Philadelphia   St Louis
Sydney   Toronto   2012

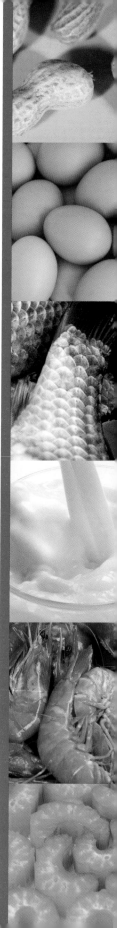

SAUNDERS is an imprint of Elsevier Inc.

WD
310
F686
2012

Notices

Knowledge and best practice in this field are constantly changing. As new research and experience broaden our understanding, changes in research methods, professional practices, or medical treatment may become necessary. Practitioners and researchers must always rely on their own experience and knowledge in evaluating and using any information, methods, compounds, or experiments described herein. In using such information or methods they should be mindful of their own safety and the safety of others, including parties for whom they have a professional responsibility.

With respect to any drug or pharmaceutical products identified, readers are advised to check the most current information provided (i) on procedures featured or (ii) by the manufacturer of each product to be administered, to verify the recommended dose or formula, the method and duration of administration, and contraindications. It is the responsibility of practitioners, relying on their own experience and knowledge of their patients, to make diagnoses, to determine dosages and the best treatment for each individual patient, and to take all appropriate safety precautions.

To the fullest extent of the law, neither the Publisher nor the authors, contributors, or editors, assume any liability for any injury and/or damage to persons or property as a matter of products liability, negligence or otherwise, or from any use or operation of any methods, products, instructions, or ideas contained in the material herein.

British Library Cataloguing in Publication Data
Food allergy.
1. Food allergy.
I. James, John. II. Burks, Wesley. III. Eigenmann, Philippe.
616.9′75-dc22

ISBN-13: 9781437719925

Library of Congress Cataloging in Publication Data
A catalog record for this book is available from the Library of Congress

Printed in China
Last digit is the print number: 9 8 7 6 5 4 3 2 1

Contents

Preface   vii

List of Contributors   ix

Acknowledgments   xiii

1   Overview of Mucosal Immunity and Development of Oral Tolerance   1
     Corinne Keet and Robert Wood

2   Food Antigens   15
     E. N. Clare Mills, Philip E. Johnson, and Yuri Alexeev

3   The Epidemiology of Food Allergy   33
     Katrina J. Allen and Jennifer J. Koplin

4   Clinical Overview of Adverse Reactions to Foods   49
     John M. Kelso

5   Atopic Dermatitis and Food Allergy   61
     Tamara T. Perry, Debra D. Becton, and Stacie M. Jones

6   Food-induced Urticaria and Angioedema   75
     Julia Rodriguez and Jesús F. Crespo

7   Pollen–Food Syndrome   83
     Antonella Muraro and Cristiana Alonzi

8   The Respiratory Tract and Food Allergy   99
     John M. James

9   Food-induced Anaphylaxis and Food Associated Exercise-induced Anaphylaxis   113
     Motohiro Ebisawa

10   Eosinophilic Gastroenteropathies (Eosinophilic Esophagitis, Eosinophilic
     Gastroenteritis and Eosinophilic Colitis)   129
     Dan Atkins and Glenn T. Furuta

11   Food Protein-induced Enterocolitis Syndrome, Food Protein-induced Enteropathy,
     Proctocolitis, and Infantile Colic   143
     Stephanie Ann Leonard and Anna Nowak-Węgrzyn

12   Approach to the Clinical Diagnosis of Food Allergy   165
     Jonathan O'B. Hourihane

13   In Vivo and In Vitro Diagnostic Methods in the Evaluation of Food Allergy   175
     S. Allan Bock

14   Oral Food Challenge Procedures   185
     Gideon Lack, George Du Toit and Mary Feeney

15   Management of Food Allergy and Development of an Anaphylaxis
     Treatment Plan   205
     Jacqueline Wassenberg and Philippe Eigenmann

16   Patient Education and Empowerment   219
     Kim Mudd and Robert Wood

17   Future Therapies for Food Allergies   235
     Anna Nowak-Węgrzyn and Hugh A. Sampson

18   Natural History and Prevention of Food Allergy   251
     Scott H. Sicherer and Atsuo Urisu

19   Diets and Nutrition: Cross-reacting Food Allergens   265
     Vicki McWilliam

20   Diagnostic and Therapeutic Dilemmas: Adverse Reactions to Food Additives,
     Pharmacologic Food Reactions, Psychological Considerations Related to
     Food Ingestion   285
     John O. Warner

Index   297

We take great pride in presenting an exciting new textbook entitled *Food Allergy: Practical Clinical Approaches to Diagnosis and Management*. Our main goal was to create a practical, relevant and clinically-based resource for food allergy and related adverse reactions to foods. The specific target audience was allergy specialists, medical residents and fellows-in-training, general pediatricians, family physicians, nutritionists and other health professionals with an interest in this important topic. Our hope was that the individual chapters in this textbook would provide the reader with ready access to pertinent information. The chapters have been specifically templated with boxed key points, clinical pearls and case studies to help illustrate key teaching points. In addition, an accompanying web-based version of this textbook will be available to all readers via secure access, with searchable text, images for download to use in presentation and links to other online resources.

Food allergy is an important public health problem that affects children and adults and appears to be increasing in prevalence. The impact of food allergy in the community is commonly underestimated. Besides the few patients with potentially life-threatening reactions to trace amounts of foods, there are large numbers of patients on eviction diets based on unclear diagnosis. Also because patients frequently confuse nonallergic food reactions, such as food intolerance, with food allergies, there is an unfounded belief among the public that food allergy prevalence is higher than the reality. The medical care team works in the chasm between the public perception and scientific reality of food allergy. The rapid growth in knowledge in this clinical area has been staggering and continues to be gratifying as reflected in the topics covered in this textbook. While there is no current cure for food allergy (i.e. the disease can only be managed by allergen avoidance or treatment of symptoms), there are exciting new developments in potential new therapies. Topics addressed in this textbook include mucosal immunity and oral tolerance, basic science of food antigens, epidemiology, diagnosis and management of food allergy, GI tract and food allergy, natural history, as well as the management of food allergy and anaphylaxis. Hopefully, this textbook will help to identify key gaps in the current scientific knowledge to be addressed through future research, but also supply to the primary care provider clear guidelines on how to address a patient with suspected food allergy.

The development and creation of this new textbook on food allergy would not have been possible without the expert assistance of our contributing authors, as well as the excellent guidance and editorial assistance from the expert staff at Elsevier Ltd. We certainly hope that the reader will find this resource to be useful and practical in dealing with patients with food allergy and other adverse reactions to foods.

John M. James MD
Wesley Burks MD
and
Philippe Eigenmann MD

Yuri Alexeev, PhD
Project Scientist
Institute of Food Research
Norwich
UK

Katrina J. Allen, MBBS, BMedSc, FRACP, PhD
Associate Professor
Paediatric Gastroenterologist/Allergist
Department of Paediatrics
University of Melbourne Royal Children's Hospital
Group Leader
Gut and Liver Research Group
Infection, Immunity & Environment
Murdoch Children's Research Institute
The Royal Children's Hospital
Parkville, VIC
Australia

Cristiana Alonzi, MD
Assistant Professor
Food Allergy Referral Centre
Department of Pediatrics
Padua General University Hospital
Padua
Italy

Dan Atkins, MD
Professor of Pediatrics
National Jewish Health
Associate Professor of Pediatrics
University of Colorado Medical School
Denver, CO
USA

Debra D. Becton, MD
Assistant Professor of Pediatrics
University of Arkansas for Medical Sciences
Arkansas Children's Hospital
Little Rock, AR
USA

S. Allan Bock, MD
Research Affiliate
Department of Pediatrics
National Jewish Health
Department of Pediatrics
University of Colorado Denver
Denver, CO
USA

Jesús F. Crespo, MD, PhD
Allergy Specialist
Servicio de Alergia
Hospital Universitario 12 de Octubre
Instituto de Investigación Hospital 12 de Octubre
Madrid
Spain

George Du Toit, MBBCh, MSc, FCP, FRCPCH
Consultant in Paediatric Allergy
King's College London
The Medical Research Council and Asthma UK
Centre in Allergic Mechanisms of Asthma
Division of Asthma, Allergy and Lung Biology
Guy's and St Thomas' National Health Service
Foundation Trust
London
UK

Motohiro Ebisawa, MD, PhD
Department of Allergy
Clinical Research Center for Allergology and
Rheumatology
Sagamihara National Hospital
Sagamihara, Kanagawa
Japan

Philippe Eigenmann, MD
Head, Pediatric Allergy Unit
Department of Child and Adolescent
University Hospitals of Geneva
Geneva
Switzerland

Mary Feeney, MSc, RD
Clinical Research Dietitian
King's College London and
Guy's and St Thomas' National Health Service
Foundation Trust
London
UK

Glenn T. Furuta, MD
Professor of Pediatrics
University of Colorado Denver School of Medicine
Department of Pediatrics
Digestive Health Institute, Section of Pediatric
Gastroenterology, Hepatology and Nutrition
Director, Gastrointestinal Eosinophilic Diseases
Program
The Children's Hospital
National Jewish Health
Denver, CO
USA

Jonathan O'B. Hourihane, DM, FRCPI
Professor and Head of Department
Paediatrics and Child Health
University College Cork
Cork
Ireland

John M. James, MD
Colorado Allergy and Asthma Centers, P.C.
Private Clinical Practice
Fort Collins, CO
USA

Philip E. Johnson, BSc(Hons), PhD
Postdoctoral Research Scientist
Institute of Food Research
Norwich
UK

Stacie M. Jones, MD
Professor of Pediatrics
Chief, Allergy and Immunology
Dr. and Mrs. Leeman King Chair in Pediatric
Allergy
University of Arkansas for Medical Sciences
Arkansas Children's Hospital
Little Rock, AR
USA

Corinne Keet, MD, MS
Assistant Professor of Pediatrics
Johns Hopkins School of Medicine
Baltimore, MD
USA

John M. Kelso, MD
Division of Allergy, Asthma and Immunology
Scripps Clinic
San Diego, CA
USA

Jennifer J. Koplin, BSc
Murdoch Children's Research Institute
Royal Children's Hospital
Parkville, VIC
Australia

Gideon Lack, MBBCH (Oxon), MA (Oxon), FRCPCH
Professor of Paediatric Allergy
King's College London
The Medical Research Council and Asthma UK
Centre in Allergic Mechanisms of Asthma
Division of Asthma, Allergy and Lung Biology
Guy's and St Thomas' National Health Service
Foundation Trust
London
UK

Stephanie Ann Leonard, MD
Fellow
Jaffe Food Allergy Institute
Department of Pediatrics
Division of Allergy and Immunology
Mount Sinai School of Medicine
New York, NY
USA

Vicki McWilliam, BSci MND APD
Clinical Specialist Dietitian, APD
Department of Allergy and Immunology
Royal Children's Hospital
Melbourne
Australia

E. N. Clare Mills, BSc PhD
Programme Leader
Institute of Food Research
Norwich
UK

Kim Mudd, RN, MSN, CCRP
Research Nurse/Program Coordinator
Johns Hopkins Division of Pediatric Allergy/
Immunology
Johns Hopkins Hospital
Baltimore, MD
USA

Antonella Muraro, MD, PhD
Head
Food Allergy Referral Centre Veneto Region
Department of Pediatrics
Padua General University Hospital
Padua
Italy

Anna Nowak-Wegrzyn, MD
Associate Professor of Pediatrics
Jaffe Food Allergy Institute
Department of Pediatrics
Division of Allergy and Immunology
Mount Sinai School of Medicine
New York, NY
USA

Tamara T. Perry, MD
Assistant Professor
Arkansas Children's Hospital Research Institute
College of Medicine
Department of Pediatrics
University of Arkansas for Medical Sciences
Little Rock, AR
USA

Julia Rodriguez, MD, PhD
Allergy Specialist
Head of the Allergy Service/Division
Servicio de Alergia
Hospital Universitario 12 de Octubre
Instituto de Investigación Hospital 12 de Octubre
Madrid
Spain

Hugh A. Sampson, MD
Professor of Pediatrics
Jaffe Food Allergy Institute
Division of Pediatric Allergy and Immunology
Mount Sinai School of Medicine
New York, NY
USA

Scott H. Sicherer, MD
Professor of Pediatrics
Jaffe Food Allergy Institute
Mount Sinai School of Medicine
New York, NY
USA

Atsuo Urisu, MD, PhD
Professor
Department of Pediatrics
Fujita Health University
The Second Teaching Hospital
Nagoya
Japan

John O. Warner, MD, FRCP, FRCPCH, FMed Sci
Professor of Paediatrics and Head of Department,
Imperial College
Director of Research, Women and Children's
Clinical Programme Group
Imperial College Healthcare NHS Trust
St. Mary's Campus
London
UK

Jacqueline Wassenberg, MD
Chief Resident
Division of Allergology and Immunology
Department of Pediatrics
University Hospitals of Lausanne
Lausanne
Switzerland

Robert Wood, MD
Professor of Pediatrics and International Health
Johns Hopkins School of Medicine
Baltimore, MD
USA

Acknowledgments

There are so many individuals who have helped shape my career in medicine and my on-going professional development as a clinical specialist in Allergy, Asthma and Immunology. These include my clinic staff, fellow staff physicians and partners and most importantly, my patients who have taught me so many valuable lessons. In addition, I certainly could not have completed this textbook without the expert assistance of my co-editors, Dr. Wesley Burks and Dr. Philippe Eigenmann and the staff at Elsevier. Finally, special acknowledgments should be made to my father, Dr. David James, who provided my initial inspiration to choose a career in medicine, Dr. Hugh Sampson, who was my clinical/research mentor during my fellowship training at Johns Hopkins University in Baltimore, Dr. Wesley Burks, who was my first division chief at the Univeristy of Arkansas for Medical Sciences in Little Rock, AR and to my wife, Kristie, and my two children, Dylan and Maddie, who all have always supported me along my journey.

John James MD

I would like to thank the many patients and families with food allergy who have allowed me to learn from them. Also, I want to thank the many mentors who helped guide and direct me, Dr. Rebecca Buckley, Dr. Hugh Sampson, Dr. Jerry Winklestein and Dr. Hank Herrod; the advice they have given me has been invaluable. Additionally I want to acknowledge my co-editors, Dr. John James and Dr. Philippe Eigenmann, without whom this project would not have been nearly as much fun. Lastly and most importantly I want to thank my family, my wife, Jan, and our children Chris, Sarah and Collin for constant support and encouragement.

Wesley Burks MD

I would like to thank the clinical staff and the research team at the University Children's Hospital who ease the many tasks of our daily work, also allowing activities such as editing a book, broadly seeding knowledge on food allergy into the medical community. As in daily clinical practice or in research activities, this book would not have been possible without efficient and nice team work. My thanks go to Dr. John James and Dr. Wesley Burks, the colleagues contributing the chapters, and the team at Elsevier. All the knowledge shared in this book would not have been possible without education, and this gives me the opportunity to thank among many mentors, Dr. Hubert Varonier who helped me to get on the tracks of pediatric allergy, and Dr. Hugh Sampson whose support and education has been invaluable. Finally, my wife Chantal and our children Alexandra and Oleg supported me in all ways in my professional activities, many thanks to them.

Philippe Eigenmann MD

CHAPTER 1

Overview of Mucosal Immunity and Development of Oral Tolerance

Corinne Keet and Robert Wood

KEY CONCEPTS

- The GI mucosa is the major immunologic site of contact between the body and the external world.
- The manner in which immune cells encounter antigen determines the subsequent immunologic response.

- Oral tolerance is a complicated process, probably proceeding by several overlapping mechanisms.
- Many factors, including developmental stage, microbial exposures, diet and genetics, influence the balance between allergy and tolerance.

Introduction

The mucosa is the principal site for the immune system's interaction with the outside environment. Unlike the skin, which is characterized by many layers of stratified epithelium, the intestinal mucosa is lined with a single layer of columnar epithelium. Almost two tons of food travel past this thin barrier each year. More than one trillion bacteria representing about 500 distinct species live in contact with it. The vast majority of these bacteria are non-pathogenic commensals, but pathogens lurk in this diverse antigenic stew, and even the commensal bacteria have the potential to cause harm if not kept in check. The mucosal immune system performs the essential job of policing this boundary and distinguishing friend from foe.

Not only must the mucosal immune system determine the local response to an antigen, but, as the primary site of antigenic contact for the body, it also plays a central role in directing the systemic response to antigens. Oral tolerance – the modulation of the

immune response to orally administered antigens – is a fundamental task of the mucosal immune system. In general, as befits the ratio of benign to pathogenic antigens it encounters, the default response of the mucosal immune system is tolerance. The tendency to tolerize to fed antigen can even be used to overcome already developed systemic sensitization, something known and exploited long before the specific cells comprising the immune system were identified. Yet, despite the general bias toward tolerance, the mucosal immune system is capable of producing protective responses to pathogens. This response is controlled by recognition of inherent characteristics of the antigen, or contextual cues such as tissue damage. In general, the immune system is remarkably skilled at responding properly to the antigens it encounters. Failures, albeit uncommon, can be very serious. Food allergy is a prime example of the failure of oral tolerance.

How the mucosal immune system determines when to sound the alarm and when to remain silent is the focus of this chapter. In it, we examine the normal response to food proteins, how that response can go awry, and the factors that tip the balance.

Structure and function

The primary role of the GI tract is to absorb food and liquid and eliminate waste. To achieve this goal, the surface of the tract is both enormous (100 m²) and extremely thin. The lumen of the intestinal tract provides a hospitable environment for bacteria that help break down foods into absorbable nutrients. However, the thinness of the barrier between external and internal creates a grave danger. It is not just nutrients, but toxins, pathogenic bacteria, viruses and parasites that are kept out by a single cell layer only. Breaks in this thin barrier create a risk of systemic infection. The complex task of protecting this border involves both non-specific and highly targeted techniques.

Chemical defenses

Protection begins with chemical and physical measures that keep some of the potentially harmful antigens (both food and microbial) from contact with the mucosal immune system and thus from generating an inflammatory response. Although the intestinal lumen is one of the most microbiologically dense environments in the world, bacteria and large antigens are actually maintained at some distance from the epithelial cells that line the GI tract. This is accomplished by a rich glycocalyx mucin layer (the mucus), which is produced by specialized intestinal epithelial cells. Antimicrobial peptides are caught in the mucous layer in a concentration gradient that provides a zone of relative sterility immediately proximal to the epithelial layer. In mouse models, deficiency of either the mucins or the antimicrobial peptides results in chronic inflammation. In humans, mutations causing abnormal production of the antimicrobial peptides are associated with the autoimmune syndrome Crohn's disease.[1,2] Whether dysfunction in the mucous layer or antimicrobial peptides play a role in the development of food allergy is an area yet to be explored.

What is known is that the enzymatic degradation of food proteins is a first line of protection against allergic sensitization, and that defects in digestion

of food antigens contribute to allergy. Many food proteins never get a chance to cause the systemic immune responses characteristic of allergy because they are labile and are denatured by the acidic contents of the stomach. Allergens tend to be proteins that are resistant to this degradation, and thus capable of reaching immune cells to cause sensitization and reaction. For example, β-lactoglobulin and Ara h2, some of the relevant allergens for milk and peanut allergy, respectively, are not denatured by the conditions of the GI tract. Other potential allergens, such as the birch homologs found in many fruits, are easily broken down: although they can induce oral symptoms in cross-reactive individuals, they do not typically initiate sensitization by themselves. Several studies have lent evidence to the importance of the normal enzymatic processes in preventing allergy by showing that antacids impair oral tolerance in both animals and humans. Further, in mice, encapsulation of potentially allergenic foods facilitated allergy by allowing intact allergen to be present in the small intestine.[3]

The fact that most proteins are broken down by acid and enzymes may help explain why most foods tend not to be allergens, but it does not explain why allergy to stable proteins remains relatively rare. Peanut, for example, contains several proteins that are not degraded, yet only about 1% of the US population is allergic to it, despite near universal exposure. Clearly, other factors come into play after the digestive processes of the stomach.

Trafficking of antigen across the epithelium

Proteins that are not degraded by enzymatic processes can come into contact with the immune system in a number of ways. Transport across the epithelium is both active and passive, occurring both in the spaces between the cells and across them (Fig. 1.1).

The high-volume route for fluid is via the paracellular spaces, and the overall permeability of the mucosa is regulated by tight junctions that seal the space between epithelial cells. The leakiness of these junctions is subject to a variety of factors, including cytokines, medications and nutritional status. Permeability varies along the GI tract, and even within a short area, as the pores of the villi allow passage of larger solutes than those of the

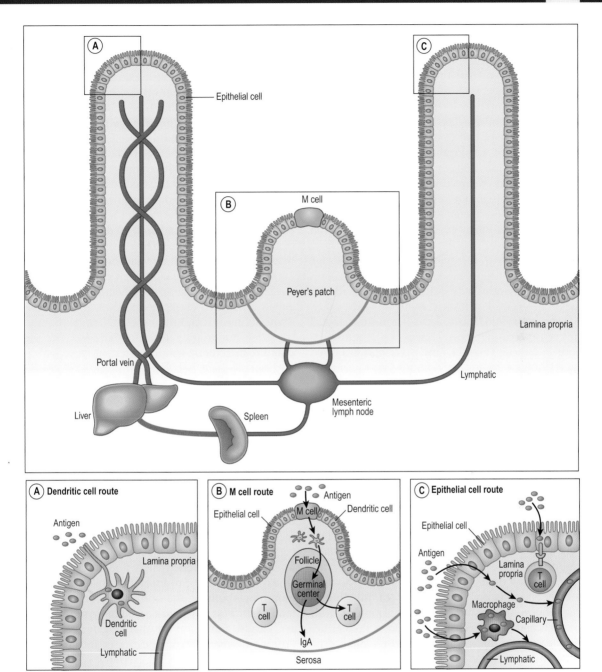

Figure 1.1 Antigen sampling in the gut. (A) Dendritic cells sample antigen directly by extending processes into the lumen. (B) Antigen taken up by M cells travels to the underlying Peyer's patches. (C) Antigen can cross the epithelium for transport to antigen-presenting cells, T cells, or into the lymphatic circulation. Reproduced with permission from: Chehade M, Mayer L. Oral tolerance and its relation to food hypersensitivities. J Allergy Clin Immunol 2005; 115: 3–12.

crypt.[2,4] Cytokines associated with both autoimmune and allergic disease disrupt barrier function and increase permeability.[5] Children with food allergy have been shown to have increased intestinal permeability, both at a time when they are regularly consuming the relevant allergen and after a long period of avoidance.[6,7] Other evidence for the importance of barrier function in allergy is the high rate of new sensitization in people taking the anti-rejection medicine tacrolimus, which causes mucosal barrier dysfunction. Although tacrolimus has other effects on the immune system, the high rate of new food allergies after solid organ transplantation is thought to be due its effects on mucosal integrity.[5]

In addition to the paracellular route, several alternative transport systems actively carry proteins, electrolytes, fatty acids and sugars across cells. Specialized modified epithelial cells called M (or microfold) cells act as non-professional antigen-presenting cells. These cells stud the follicle-associated epithelium overlying specialized collections of immune cells called Peyer's patches. They express receptors that recognize microbial patterns and aid in the endocytosis and transfer of antigen to the basal surface of the epithelium. This is especially important for bacteria, but may also be relevant for food allergens.[4]

Other non-specialized columnar epithelial cells form vesicle-like structures that allow transport of dietary proteins across cells. The formation of these vesicle-like structures seems to be dependent on MHC class II binding, but transocytosis can also occur via binding of antigen to IgA, IgE, and IgG. Transport via IgE may be especially important in the acute allergic response and in the amplification of allergy.[4] In contrast, secretory IgA, which accounts for the majority of the immunoglobulin produced by the body, complexes with antigen and facilitates transport across the epithelium to antigen-presenting cells, with a tolerogenic outcome.

A final method of antigen transport involves direct sampling of the luminal contents by extensions of antigen-presenting cells. Dendritic cells found in the lamina propria form their own tight junctions with intestinal epithelial cells and can project directly into the intestinal lumen. These projections increase when invasive bacteria are present, and sampling via this route seems to be especially important for the transport of commensal and invasive bacteria.[4]

Initial contact with the mucosal immune system

Once the antigen has been captured by dendritic cells, either by direct sampling or after processing through epithelial cells, the fate of the immune response depends on the interaction between dendritic cells and naive CD4+ T cells. Of the professional antigen cells associated with the gut, dendritic cells are the most important. They are found throughout the mucosal-associated lymph tissue and comprise a large class of phenotypically and functionally diverse cells. Subspecialization of these cells is thought to depend on their derivation (some develop from lymphoid precursors and some from myeloid precursors), their maturity, and environmental cues. This interaction can occur in specialized aggregations of antigen-presenting cells, T cells and B cells, such as Peyer's patches, in the loose aggregations of lymphocytes in the lamina propria, or, most importantly for food antigens, in the draining mesenteric lymph nodes.

Although there is communication between the mucosal and systemic immune systems, contact that is essential for both protective immune responses and oral tolerance, there is significant compartmentalization of responses at the mucosal level. The mesenteric lymph nodes act as a 'firewall', keeping the systemic immune system ignorant of much of the local immune response. In animals whose mesenteric lymph nodes have been removed, massive splenomegaly and lymphadenopathy develop in response to typical exposure to commensal organisms. In fact, much of the interaction with commensal organisms never even reaches the level of the mesenteric lymph nodes. IgA+ B cells, which collectively produce the majority of the immunoglobulin in the body, are activated at the level of the Peyer's patches and lamina propria and act locally. Induction of this IgA response can proceed normally in mice deficient in mesenteric lymph nodes. Although the response to commensals happens largely at the level of the Peyer's patches and lamina propria, for food antigens it seems that the mesenteric lymph nodes are key for the active response that constitutes oral tolerance. Mice without Peyer's patches develop oral tolerance normally, but those without mesenteric lymph nodes cannot. For food antigens, it seems that the typical path is for dendritic cells in the lamina propria to traffic to the mesenteric lymph nodes for presentation to CD4+ cells.[7,8]

Different experimental models have shown somewhat different kinetics of traffic to mesenteric lymph nodes after oral antigen. However, within days after exposure, dendritic cells carry orally fed antigen to the mesenteric lymph nodes and cause T-cell proliferation. T cells stimulated in this way then travel back to the mucosa and to the systemic lymph nodes.[9]

Once captured and processed, antigen presented by dendritic cells can cause several distinct immune responses. It is this interaction that determines whether allergy or oral tolerance develops.

What is oral tolerance?

Before we can begin to discuss what factors influence the development of oral tolerance, we must discuss what is meant by oral tolerance. There is disagreement at a fundamental level about how oral tolerance to foods develops. Not only are the specific mechanisms of oral tolerance imperfectly understood, but also the overall paradigm. Here we explore different theories about the development of oral tolerance.

Immune deviation

Starting in the 1980s, with work from Coffman and Mosmann, researchers began to describe distinct subsets of CD4+ T cells that were characterized by distinctive cytokine milieus and resulting disease or protective states.[10] A central paradigm in immunology for the past two decades has been this division of effector CD4+ T cells into Th1 and Th2 cells, both responsible for different mechanisms of clearing infection and both causing different pathological states when overactive. The cytokines that Th1 cells secrete (such as IFN-γ) activate macrophages and facilitate clearance of intracellular pathogens. In contrast, Th2 cells produce cytokines that promote class switching and affinity maturation of B cells, and signal mast cells and eosinophils to activate and proliferate. Th2 responses are important for clearance of extracellular parasites.

Allergy is dominated by the Th2 response and is characterized by IgE production, eosinophilia, mast cell activation, and, in some cases, tissue fibrosis. For many years it has been posited that the central defect in allergy is an imbalance between Th1 and Th2 responses. This model, although an oversimplification, has proved helpful in identifying factors that promote allergy. In the original model naive T-helper cells were stimulated by dendritic cells to develop either as Th1 or Th2 cells. Cytokines necessary and sufficient for Th1 polarization include IL-12 and INF-γ, but the mechanisms of Th2 differentiation have remained elusive. Two cytokines, IL-4 and IL-13, play a role, but are not essential for the development of high numbers of Th2 cells in the mouse model. Until recently, a leading hypothesis was that Th2 differentiation is the default response that occurs in the absence of Th1-directing signals. The theory of Th2 as a default has appeal because it harmonizes nicely with the so called 'hygiene hypothesis', in which inadequate infectious stimuli create the conditions for allergy. If Th2 deviation were the default, allergic responses would naturally develop in the absence of Th1 driving infectious stimuli. Recent work, however, suggests that Th2 differentiation requires other signals, including OX40L from dendritic cells, but that the signals essential for Th1 differentiation are stronger and predominate if present.[11]

Despite the compelling qualities of this theory, it is now clear that the reality is much more complicated. Although allergy is characterized by a Th2 response, an increasing body of evidence calls into question whether it is simply the balance between Th1 and Th2 responses that lies at the crux of the problem of allergy. Epidemiologic studies do not consistently show a reciprocal relationship between incidence of Th1 imbalance (i.e. autoimmunity) and Th2 imbalance.[12] Adoptive transfer of Th1 cells in mice cannot control Th2-induced lung inflammation.[13] A recent study showed that allergic subjects had low-level Th1-type cytokine responses to allergenic stimulation that matched the non-allergenic responses but were simply overwhelmed by the massive Th2 cytokine response.[14] Most importantly, other types of CD4 cells important in the control of both allergy and autoimmunity have been identified.

Regulatory T cells

The existence of T cells with suppressive capacity was first recognized in the 1980s. Initially, centrally derived T-regulatory cells were identified. These cells are important in regulating autoimmunity and are generated in the thymus, in a process of T-cell selection that has been compared to Goldilocks' sampling of the bears' oatmeal. T cells with too strong an attraction to self antigens are deleted, as

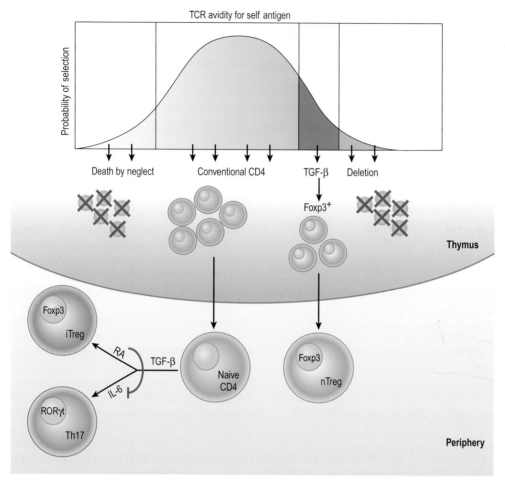

Figure 1.2 The development of regulatory T cells. In the thymus, avidity of the T-cell receptor for self antigen determines the fate of the T cell. In the periphery, naive Foxp3– CD4+ T cells can develop into FoxP3+ T-regulatory cells or Th17 cells, depending on the cytokine milieu. Reproduced with permission from: Mucida D, Park Y, Cheroutre H. From the diet to the nucleus: vitamin A and TGF-beta join efforts at the mucosal interface of the intestine. Semin Immunol 2009; 21: 14–21.

are those that do not bind well at all, and thus will not be effective antigen presenters. The majority of the remaining cells bind 'just right' at a moderate level and are destined to become effector T cells, but a subset that binds to self antigens more strongly persists and becomes suppressive T cells (Fig. 1.2).[15] A transcription factor, FOXP3, is essential for the suppressive nature of these cells and has served to identify them. The importance of these cells in autoimmune disease has been amply demonstrated, both in animal models – autoimmune disease can be induced by depletion of these cells – and in natural human diseases. Children with IPEX (immune dysregulation, polyendocrinopathy,

enteropathy, X-linked) syndrome have mutations in the FOXP3 gene leading to absent or abnormal levels of regulatory T cells. These children have early and severe autoimmune gastrointestinal and endocrine disease. Bone-marrow transplant that replaces the T-regulatory cells successfully reverses the disease.

Children with IPEX also have food allergy and eczema, demonstrating a failure of tolerance to antigens that are not present in the thymus. More recently, the importance of peripherally generated T-regulatory cells has become clear. As with the centrally generated T-regulatory cells, FoxP3 marks these cells (called iTregs), although other related subsets of suppressor T cells generated in the periphery do not express Fox P3. T-regulatory cells are preferentially induced in the mesenteric lymph nodes, where the cytokine TGF-β is a key mediator of T-cell differentiation. In the past decade, it has been determined that T-regulatory cells and a newly described T-cell subset, Th17 cells, develop reciprocally under the influence of TGF-β. A cytokine, IL-6, drives differentiation to Th17 cells, whereas a metabolite of vitamin A, retinoic acid, was recently discovered to inhibit Th17 differentiation and promote T-regulatory development in the presence of TGF-β.[16] Vitamin A, which is not produced by the human body, is converted to its active form, retinoic acid, by epithelial cells and dendritic cells. The fact that generation of suppressor cells is dependent on an orally derived factor that is converted to an active form by the intestinal epithelium may help explain how the gut is maintained as a tolerogenic site.[17]

Peripherally generated T-regulatory cells have a multitude of effects on other immune cells. Through the action of secreted cytokines, such as IL-10 and TGF-β, they act on B cells, reducing IgE production and inducing the blocking antibody IgG4; on Th1 and Th2 cells, suppressing their inflammatory activities; and on dendritic cells, inducing them to produce IL-10 and further stimulate the development of regulatory T cells. In addition, they have direct interaction with mast cells through cell surface ligands (Fig. 1.3). In sum, they control both Th1- and Th2-mediated inflammatory responses.[18]

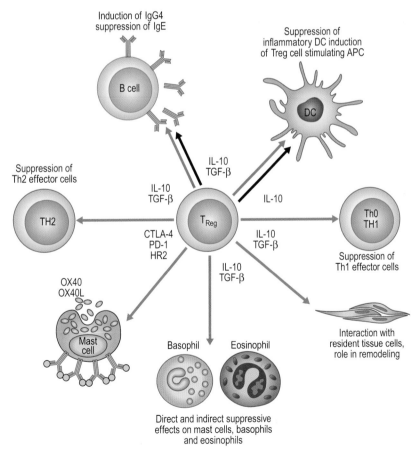

Figure 1.3 T-regulatory cells have direct and indirect effects on many different types of effector cells. Suppressive cytokines include interleukin-10 (IL-10) and transforming growth factor-β (TGF-β). Another mechanism of suppression is by cell–cell contact via OX40-OX40ligand (red arrows: suppression; black arrows: induction). Reproduced with permission from: Akdis M. Immune tolerance in allergy. Curr Opin Immunol 2009; 21: 700–7.

Antigen-specific peripherally induced T cells are essential for oral tolerance. Oral tolerance proceeds normally in mice lacking centrally derived T-regulatory cells, but fails in mice unable to induce regulatory cells peripherally.[16] In humans, T-regulatory cell function has been implicated in both IgE- and non-IgE mediated food allergy. Children with active non-IgE mediated milk allergy had lower T-regulatory cells than controls in one study, whereas another, also of non-IgE mediated milk allergy, showed that T-regulatory function was associated with outgrowing the disease. In IgE-mediated milk allergy, increased numbers of T-regulatory cells were found in children with a milder phenotype who were better able to tolerate cooked milk than those with a more severe phenotype who reacted to cooked milk.[6]

T-regulatory cells seem also to be important for the effectiveness of allergen-specific immunotherapy. Oral and sublingual immunotherapies (reviewed in Chapter 17) have emerged as a very promising treatment for food allergy. Although the precise mechanisms by which they work are not yet known, an increase in FOXP3+ T-regulatory cells was found in the initial stages of peanut immunotherapy, with a return to baseline by 2 years on therapy.[6]

Th17 cells, which develop reciprocally with T-regulatory cells, promote inflammatory responses at the gut and seem to be especially important for protection against infection.[19] Deficiency of Th17 cells, as in Job's syndrome (also known as hyper-IgE syndrome), is characterized by abnormal responses to infectious stimuli, as well as very high levels of IgE. However, despite these high levels, specific sensitization is less common and the causes of high IgE in this syndrome are not clear.[20] Th17 cells do seem to be important in certain types of asthma that are less atopic, but whether they have a role in either prevention or promotion of food allergy has not been determined.

Other methods of tolerance

Other mechanisms of oral tolerance overlap with those discussed above. For control of self-reactivity, besides deviation and responsiveness to suppression, T cells have other mechanisms that allow them to be switched off or killed. In general, activation of the cell in the absence of co-stimulatory signals results in anergy. Anergy refers to a T-cell state where proliferation to antigen on rechallenge is impaired, but can be reversed with sufficient quantities of the T-cell growth cytokine IL-2. Blockage of co-stimulatory receptors can induce anergy, as can other methods of TCR cross-linking without co-stimulation, such as stimulation with soluble peptides. Deletion is a related process, and can follow anergy.

Several studies have shown that anergy and deletion can be important in oral tolerance to food antigens. In a key paper, Chen and colleagues[21] found that high doses of a model antigen caused initial activation of T cells followed by apoptosis of antigen-specific T cells. Low doses led to increases in what we now know to be regulatory T cells. Similarly, Gregerson et al.,[22] in a model of autoimmune uveoretinitis, found that low doses of fed antigen caused suppressive mechanisms to kick in, and that transfer of lymphocytes from treated animals transferred suppression to untreated animals. At higher doses, anergy was the predominant mechanism, and this could not be transferred to a naive animal.

Anergy, apoptosis and suppressive mechanisms are not mutually exclusive and have been shown to work simultaneously.[23,24] In all likelihood, the normal response to food proteins involves a combination of immune deviation, regulatory factors and anergy/deletion of reactive clones. It makes sense that something as important as oral tolerance would have highly redundant mechanisms.

Factors that influence the development of oral tolerance versus allergy

Factors both intrinsic to the individual and related to environmental exposures influence the development of allergy. Those that have been identified so far include age, microbial exposures, genetics, nutritional factors, and dose and route of antigen.

Developmental stage

The neonatal GI tract differs from the adult tract in significant ways, including the robustness of physical and chemical barriers, the composition of the microbial flora, and the maturity of the gut-associated immune system. Overall, these differences predispose the infant to the development of allergy, although the precise developmental window of risk and the optimal strategy to prevent allergy in infants are among the most contentious areas in the field of allergy.

Part of the difficulty of resolving these controversies lies in the inadequacy of the animal models. Both human and rodent neonates have increased intestinal permeability compared to their adult counterparts. However, in humans, the transition from the highly permeable fetal gut to a more mature gut barrier occurs in the first few days of life, compared to more than a month in rats.[25]

One well-studied area is the difference in gastric pH and pancreatic enzyme output between infants and adults. With their immature barriers to regurgitation of caustic gastric contents, infants secrete much less acid into the stomach and have decreased pancreatic enzyme output, and do not reach adult levels of pH for the first few years of life.[25] As discussed above, acidic and enzymatic digestion is a first-line defense preventing some potentially sensitizing proteins from reaching relevant immune cells. Combined with somewhat increased intestinal permeability, this increases the chances of intact allergen crossing the epithelial border.

Once across the epithelial border, the immune system that the antigen encounters is very different in neonates than in adults. Both cellular and humoral branches of the immune system are immature. Total numbers of dendritic cells are lower, as is their ability to respond to co-stimulatory factors that typically elicit a Th1-type response. Further, CD4+ T cells are themselves highly skewed in a Th2 direction in the neonate, and have poor production of IL-12, a cytokine involved in Th1 responses. The inability to mount Th1 responses but ability to mount Th2 responses leads to an environment where potential autoimmunity or reactivity to maternal antigens is dampened, responses to microbial insults are deficient, and allergic responses are relatively favored.[26]

The fetal and neonatal immune system is also characterized by varying levels of T-regulatory cell function. At the time of birth, T-regulatory cells are found less frequently in cord blood than in adult blood, and those found have less efficient suppressive function after stimulation.[28] However, there is some evidence that, at least in mice, neonatal T cells have a propensity to develop into T-regulatory cells.[27] Given the uniquely stressful experience of birth, one could question whether what is found in cord blood is a valid reflection of the intrinsic qualities of the neonate. Regardless, the T-regulatory cell compartment is one area where neonatal and adult responses vary considerably, with important implications for the development of allergy.

The humoral immune system is also immature in the infant. Immaturity of the humoral immune system is at least partially compensated for by unique features of breast milk. Breast milk contains large amounts of secretory IgA and some IgG. Maternally supplied IgA substitutes for the infant's relative lack, complexing with dietary proteins and promoting non-inflammatory responses.[25] IgG found in breast milk plays a similar role, with added nuances. Neonates express a receptor for IgG in their intestinal epithelium (the FcRn receptor). This allows for active transport of IgG from breast milk into the neonatal circulation. In addition to absorbing maternal antibody to be used in fighting infections, the FcRn receptor can also transport intact antigen complexed with IgG directly from the lumen to lamina propria dendritic cells, contributing to oral tolerance. In mice, antigen complexed to IgG in breast milk has been shown to induce antigen-specific T-regulatory cells in a manner independent of the other ingredients in breast milk. Interestingly, this was enhanced in mothers who were sensitized to the allergen.[29]

Other components of breast milk are important in oral tolerance. Pro-forms of the tolerogenic cytokine TGF-β are abundant in breast milk. They are thought to be physiologically active after exposure to the acidic gastric environment, and epidemiologic work in humans suggests that higher levels are associated with protection from atopic disease.[30,31]

Despite these pro-tolerogenic features, the presence of allergen in breast milk does not always lead to oral tolerance. Allergens are found both free and complexed to antibody in breast milk, and infants can become sensitized to proteins encountered in breast milk and react to them. Complicating the picture further, maternally ingested or inhaled allergens have also been found in the placenta, although whether this allergen is transferred to the fetal circulation remains unclear. Studies in mice have shown variation in the results of prenatal exposure by the dose of antigen. Mice whose mothers had low doses of prenatal exposure to a model allergen developed tolerance to that allergen. With higher doses there was transient inhibition of IgE production upon challenge, but after the immediate neonatal period the mice had increased susceptibility to the development of allergy to that allergen.[32]

Whether sensitization or oral tolerance to these antigens occurs probably depends on a complex interaction between the non-allergen components of breast milk, infant factors, and the dose and timing of the allergen.

Route of exposure

Some have suggested that the primary route of sensitization leading to food allergy is via the skin. In this model, oral exposure is almost always tolerogenic. Allergy happens when the skin encounters potentially allergenic foods prior to oral contact. Eczema, which creates breaks in the skin and an inflammatory backdrop, predisposes to allergic sensitization. Evidence supporting this model includes the fact that mice can be sensitized via low-dose skin exposure, some epidemiologic evidence tying peanut oil-containing lotions to peanut allergy, and the differences in immune responses induced by antigen-presenting cells in the skin and in the gut. However, this theory has not been conclusively proven.[33]

Microbial influences

The most compelling theory for the wide variation in incidence in allergic disease remains the so called 'hygiene hypothesis'. In general terms, this theory posits that the decreased burden of infection, especially childhood infections, characteristic of the western lifestyle does not adequately stimulate the developing immune system into a non-allergic phenotype. The beauty – and the limitation – of this theory is that it is sufficiently broad to encompass a wide range of theoretical mechanisms by which infection might prevent allergy, including Th1 skewing and induction of T-regulatory cells, and that it does not specify what infections are actually essential.

Epidemiologic evidence supporting the hypothesis includes the fact that allergy is more common in developed than in developing countries, in city than in farming communities, in children who do not attend daycare, and in older siblings than in younger siblings, especially younger siblings in large families. A thorough analysis of farming communities in Europe identified unpasteurized milk and the presence of multiple species of farm animals living under the same roof as key protective factors of the rural life. In other populations, markers for parasitic infections, such as Schistosoma, are associated with reduced rates of allergy. In addition, differences in the microbial content of drinking water have been linked to the disparate rates of atopic disease found in genetically similar populations of people living on different sides of the Finnish/Russian border. Similar epidemiologic studies also associate infection with protection from autoimmune disease.[34]

Evidence tying actual differences in gut flora to allergy has been mixed, with some finding that allergic children have different colonization patterns, and others failing to replicate the result. Birth by Caesarean section, which does not expose the infant to the normal maternal vaginal and fecal flora, has been associated with alterations in the infant's fecal flora. In one study,[35] Caesarean delivery was associated with an increased risk of wheezing, although this was not replicated in another study. Methodological problems with how gut flora were analyzed may be a part of the confusion, as the relevant bacteria may be hard to culture.

In rodent models, intestinal colonization is essential for normal development of the immune system and for the ability to induce oral tolerance. Recent work has identified certain bacterial components as being essential for the development of the normal gut immune system.[36] Specific mechanisms for prevention of allergy by infection are still being worked out. In humans, the mechanisms have been most carefully explored in prospective studies of children growing up on European farms. In these studies, several mechanisms of protection from allergy were identified, including upregulation of Toll-like receptors (TLRS), increased T-regulatory cell function and alterations in prenatal serum cytokine levels.[37–39] Prenatal farm exposure has been identified as particularly protective for the development of allergy. Whether the prenatal exposure is mediated by colonization of the infant, epigenetic changes passed from mother to child, or by so far unidentified features of the intrauterine environment, is unknown.

Nutritional factors

Nutritional factors are one way in which the prenatal environment or early life could modify the risk for allergic disease. Because diet has changed so rapidly in developed countries over the last half century, nutritional factors are candidates to explain the rapid increase in allergic disease and the geographic variation in disease. The Mediterranean diet in general during pregnancy has been associated with protection from respiratory allergy and wheeze in children.[40] It has been suggested that an important difference between more 'westernized' diets and the Mediterranean diet is the presence of different isoforms of vitamin E found in cooking oils. D-α-tocopherol, found in olive oil and sunflower oil, has anti-inflammatory effects by reducing cell adhesion molecules on epithelial cells. D-γ-tocopherol, the predominant isoform of vitamin E found in vegetable oils in westernized diets, has opposite effects on epithelial cells.[41] The effects of these isoforms on food allergy have not been adequately explored.

Another dietary factor that may have a role in protection from allergy is polyunsaturated fatty acids (such as those found in fish oil). In a randomized placebo-controlled study, supplementation with omega-3 polyunsaturated fatty acids during pregnancy and breastfeeding was associated with lower sensitization to food proteins and eczema.[42] Epidemiologic studies have found similar results, although not uniformly.[43]

Besides fatty acids, vitamin D is also found in fish oil. Vitamin D levels vary significantly within westernized populations. Vitamin D is found in the diet, both naturally in foods such as fatty fish and in fortified dairy products, and is also produced by the skin with exposure to sun. Populations living at very northern or southern latitudes, as is the case in most developed countries, are at risk for deficiency. Vitamin D is a steroid hormone with pleotropic effects. Its many effects on the immune system can vary by dose. To innate cells, it promotes the production of antimicrobial peptides, while also downregulating some TLRs. The effects on Th1 cells include downregulation of IFN-γ at the gene level. Effects on Th2 cells depend on the dose, with very high or low levels associated with increased Th2 deviation. Overall, T-regulatory cells are upregulated. Epidemiologic studies of the relationship between vitamin D supplementation and allergy or wheeze have found mixed results, and have typically been very susceptible to recall bias. Several recent population studies have linked latitude and season of birth with acute food allergy episodes, implicating lack of sun exposure in the pathogenesis of food allergy. Studies that prospectively assess the relationship between vitamin D and development of allergy are under way.[44,45]

Vitamin A, which has a clear role in the development of oral tolerance, is found in sufficient amounts in almost all western diets. Blood levels are tightly controlled, and so although vitamin A may be necessary for the development of oral tolerance, differences in intake may not be an important risk factor for food allergy. Whether variations in intake relate to the development of oral tolerance has not been explored.

The role of folic acid in allergy and asthma is another area of intense study, although its specific role in oral tolerance has not been determined. The interest in folic acid is driven by its potential role in the modification of DNA expression through epigenetics, and by the fact that folic acid intake has changed markedly in the past two decades. Epigenetics refers to heritable changes in gene expression that are not due to changes in the underlying DNA sequence. The major mechanism of epigenetic change is through changes in methylation of DNA. Folic acid, which is a methyl donor, was added to all grain products in the US in 1998 by FDA mandate. In 2008, Hollingsworth et al.[46] showed in a mouse model that maternal supplementation with folate led to suppression of a gene known to be important for the balance between Th1 and Th2 skewing, among other effects. In contrast, in a cross-sectional epidemiologic study, Matsui and Matsui[47] found an inverse relationship between folic acid levels and total IgE, atopy and wheeze. The role of folic acid in allergy and airway disease remains highly controversial.

Genetics

A family history of food allergy in particular, and atopy in general, is a major risk factor for the development of food allergy. Teasing apart the role of environment and genetics in failures of oral tolerance has been complicated by the lack of uniform definitions for food allergy, and by the probability that what we call food allergy actually comprises several distinct phenotypes. Further, as has been demonstrated best for asthma, it is likely that gene–environment interactions mandate precise determinations of environmental factors when trying to determine the role of genetics (and vice versa). For example, in studies of asthma, a genetic variant in the receptor for lipopolysaccharide (a bacterial product important in stimulating innate immune responses) is protective at high levels of endotoxin (such as might be found on a farm), but increases the risk of asthma when levels of endotoxin are low.[48] Exposure to both microbial products and allergens probably modifies whatever genetic risk factors there are for food allergy.

However, no matter how it is defined, and under what environmental conditions, it is clear that there is a large genetic component to food allergy. For example, a British study found that a child with a peanut-allergic sibling had a five times increased risk of peanut allergy than the general population. Depending on how food allergy is defined, and on the population studied, the heritability of specific food allergies has been estimated to be 15–80%.[48] Despite the clear heritability of food allergy, it is not yet clear which genes are most important for the normal development of oral tolerance. The genes that most obviously cause food allergy when mutated, such as FOXP3, in which food allergy is part of a larger syndrome, are probably only responsible for a fraction of the overall burden of disease.

Candidate genes that have been explored with varying levels of success include those for antigen presentation, cytokines, and intracellular signaling. Human leukocyte antigens, which determine the antigenic epitopes presented to the immune system, were early targets for study. Although initial studies showed an association with certain food allergies, repeat studies did not replicate those results. Two genes known to be involved in Th2 differentiation, SPINK5 (serine protease inhibitor Karzal type 5) and the gene for IL-13, have shown association with food allergy in preliminary studies. Studies of two other genes that would be logical to be involved, the gene for the receptor for lipopolysaccharide, discussed above, and the gene for IL-10 (which is important in T-regulatory cell development), have found inconsistent results. Larger studies are under way to try to further elucidate the genetic factors important in the normal development of food tolerance.[48]

In summary, the balance between oral tolerance and allergy is influenced by a complicated array of factors, including genetic susceptibility, microbial exposure, dietary factors, and the route, dose and timing of allergen exposure. Environmental influences begin in the womb, and perhaps before, and are modified by the mother's genetics and own allergic history. So far we have only scratched the surface of this field.

Opportunities for prevention

With the steep rise in allergy in general, and food allergy in particular, the need for interventions that might prevent allergy has become more imperative.

However, implementing a successful preventive strategy is like threading a narrow needle: any intervention can have unintended consequences. So far, preventive strategies have focused most heavily on the timing of antigen exposure, with some attention to trying to alter the gut flora and to non-allergen related dietary factors.

The history of recommendations about the timing of allergen exposure serves as a cautionary tale about the dangers of making policy for populations without clear evidence. Although previous AAP recommendations suggested that pregnant and lactating women with a family history of allergy avoid peanuts and tree nuts, and possibly eggs, fish and milk, more recent reviews of the literature have concluded that there is no good evidence that maternal avoidance is beneficial. Indeed, small interventional studies have suggested that maternal avoidance is not risk-free, and that maternal egg and milk avoidance can be harmful nutritionally. The most recent advisory statement by the AAP retracts the previous recommendation, stating instead that there are not enough data to make any recommendation.[49]

The best time to introduce allergens directly to the infant is even more contentious. Previous recommendations were that at-risk children avoid cows' milk until their first birthday, egg until the second, and peanut, tree nuts and fish until the third. In the decade since those recommendations were made in the US and the UK, the incidence of food allergy has continued to grow rapidly, and prominent allergists are questioning whether more harm than good is being done by avoiding allergens early in life. Some tentative epidemiologic evidence supports the notion that early introduction could be helpful. Evidence includes the low rate of peanut allergy in Israel, where peanuts are eaten early, compared to the high rate in genetically similar populations in the UK, where peanuts typically are not eaten early. A large interventional study of early peanut introduction in children with eczema or egg allergy currently under way in the UK will hopefully shed light on this question. In the meantime, pediatricians, allergists and parents are left without clear guidance about when to start highly allergenic foods.

Probiotics for the prevention of allergy are another area where initial high promises have not been met. Given the data for the importance of gut microbiota in the development of the intestinal immune response, it would make sense that one could alter the microbial contents with beneficial results. Prebiotics, which contain elements that stimulate specific bacterial growth, and probiotics, which contain the bacteria themselves, have been used in many small studies for the prevention and treatment of allergic disease. In sum, the studies suggest a small beneficial effect for the prevention of atopic dermatitis, but no benefit for the treatment of established disease or for the prevention of other atopic conditions. Larger, well-designed studies are required before probiotics can be confidently recommended.[50]

Other dietary factors are promising, although they have not yet been fully evaluated. As discussed above, the single randomized controlled study of fish oil found some protection from food allergy, but this needs to be replicated. It is not yet clear whether an increase or reduction in vitamin D and folic acid would be the best intervention for prevention of food allergy. Well-designed prospective epidemiologic studies are the first necessary step to sort this out.

Conclusions

Oral tolerance is a complex, active process that occurs in the gut-associated immune system. Although the precise mechanisms have not been completely elucidated, regulatory T cells seem to be essential for its development and maintenance. Other, overlapping mechanisms, including immune deviation, anergy and deletion, also play a role. Many factors affect the balance between allergy and oral tolerance. They include genetic variations, the dose, timing and route of antigen exposure, the microbial milieu, and probably other dietary factors. This field is still young, and much remains to be done to identify the mechanisms of allergic sensitization. Because of the complexity of the system, some things will not be known until interventional studies in humans are carried out.

References

1. Sansonetti PJ, Medzhitov R. Learning tolerance while fighting ignorance. Cell 2009;138:416–20.
2. Turner JR. Intestinal mucosal barrier function in health and disease. Nat Rev Immunol 2009;9:799–809.
3. Untersmayr E, Jensen-Jarolim E. The role of protein digestibility and antacids on food allergy outcomes. J Allergy Clin Immunol 2008;121:1301–8; quiz 9–10.
4. Menard S, Cerf-Bensussan N, Heyman M. Multiple facets of intestinal permeability and epithelial handling of dietary antigens. Mucosal Immunol 2010;3:247–59.
5. Groschwitz KR, Hogan SP. Intestinal barrier function: molecular regulation and disease pathogenesis. J Allergy Clin Immunol 2009;124:3–20; quiz 1–2.
6. Scurlock AM, Vickery BP, Hourihane JO, Burks AW. Pediatric food allergy and mucosal tolerance. Mucosal Immunol 2010;3:345–54.
7. Berin MC, Mayer L. Immunophysiology of experimental food allergy. Mucosal Immunol 2009;2:24–32.
8. Chehade M, Mayer L. Oral tolerance and its relation to food hypersensitivities. J Allergy Clin Immunol 2005;115:3–12; quiz 3.
9. Macpherson AJ, Slack E, Geuking MB, et al. The mucosal firewalls against commensal intestinal microbes. Semin Immunopathol 2009;31:145–9.
10. Zhu J, Paul WE. Heterogeneity and plasticity of T helper cells. Cell Res 2010;20:4–12.
11. Liu YJ. Thymic stromal lymphopoietin and OX40 ligand pathway in the initiation of dendritic cell-mediated allergic inflammation. J Allergy Clin Immunol 2007;120:238–44; quiz 45–6.
12. Jarnicki AG, Tsuji T, Thomas WR. Inhibition of mucosal and systemic T(h)2-type immune responses by intranasal peptides containing a dominant T cell epitope of the allergen Der p 1. Int Immunol 2001;13:1223–31.
13. Neurath MF, Finotto S, Glimcher LH. The role of Th1/Th2 polarization in mucosal immunity. Nat Med 2002;8:567–73.
14. Prussin C, Lee J, Foster B. Eosinophilic gastrointestinal disease and peanut allergy are alternatively associated with IL-5+ and IL-5(-) T(H)2 responses. J Allergy Clin Immunol 2009;124:1326–32 e6.
15. Yun TJ, Bevan MJ. The Goldilocks conditions applied to T cell development. Nat Immunol 2001;2:13–4.
16. Mucida D, Park Y, Cheroutre H. From the diet to the nucleus: vitamin A and TGF-beta join efforts at the mucosal interface of the intestine. Semin Immunol 2009;21:14–21.
17. Strober W. Vitamin A rewrites the ABCs of oral tolerance. Mucosal Immunol 2008;1:92–5.
18. Akdis M. Immune tolerance in allergy. Curr Opin Immunol 2009;21:700–7.
19. Weaver CT, Hatton RD. Interplay between the TH17 and TReg cell lineages: a (co-)evolutionary perspective. Nat Rev Immunol 2009;9:883–9.
20. Milner JD, Brenchley JM, Laurence A, et al. Impaired T(H)17 cell differentiation in subjects with autosomal dominant hyper-IgE syndrome. Nature 2008;452: 773–6.
21. Chen Y, Inobe J, Marks R, et al. Peripheral deletion of antigen-reactive T cells in oral tolerance. Nature 1995; 376:177–80.
22. Gregerson DS, Obritsch WF, Donoso LA. Oral tolerance in experimental autoimmune uveoretinitis. Distinct mechanisms of resistance are induced by low dose vs high dose feeding protocols. J Immunol 1993;151: 5751–61.

23. Perruche S, Zhang P, Liu Y, et al. CD3-specific antibody-induced immune tolerance involves transforming growth factor-beta from phagocytes digesting apoptotic T cells. Nat Med 2008;14:528–35.

24. Sun JB, Czerkinsky C, Holmgren J. Sublingual 'oral tolerance' induction with antigen conjugated to cholera toxin B subunit generates regulatory T cells that induce apoptosis and depletion of effector T cells. Scand J Immunol 2007;66:278–86.

25. Verhasselt V. Oral tolerance in neonates: from basics to potential prevention of allergic disease. Mucosal Immunol 2010;3:326–33.

26. Zaghouani H, Hoeman CM, Adkins B. Neonatal immunity: faulty T-helpers and the shortcomings of dendritic cells. Trends Immunol 2009;30:585–91.

27. Wang G, Miyahara Y, Guo Z, et al. 'Default' generation of neonatal regulatory T cells. J Immunol 2010;185: 71–8.

28. Schaub B, Liu J, Schleich I, et al. Impairment of T helper and T regulatory cell responses at birth. Allergy 2008;63:1438–47.

29. Mosconi E, Rekima A, Seitz-Polski B, et al. Breast milk immune complexes are potent inducers of oral tolerance in neonates and prevent asthma development. Mucosal Immunol 2010;3:461–74.

30. Nakao A. The role and potential use of oral transforming growth factor-beta in the prevention of infant allergy. Clin Exp Allergy 2010;40:725–30.

31. Oddy WH, Rosales F. A systematic review of the importance of milk TGF-beta on immunological outcomes in the infant and young child. Pediatr Allergy Immunol 2010;21:47–59.

32. Fusaro AE, de Brito CA, Taniguchi EF, et al. Balance between early life tolerance and sensitization in allergy: dependence on the timing and intensity of prenatal and postnatal allergen exposure of the mother. Immunology 2009;128:e541–50.

33. Lack G. Epidemiologic risks for food allergy. J Allergy Clin Immunol 2008;121:1331–6.

34. Okada H, Kuhn C, Feillet H, et al. The 'hygiene hypothesis' for autoimmune and allergic diseases: an update. Clin Exp Immunol 2010;160:1–9.

35. Guarner F. Hygiene, microbial diversity and immune regulation. Curr Opin Gastroenterol 2007;23:667–72.

36. Round JL, Mazmanian SK. The gut microbiota shapes intestinal immune responses during health and disease. Nat Rev Immunol 2009;9:313–23.

37. Ege MJ, Herzum I, Buchele G, et al. Prenatal exposure to a farm environment modifies atopic sensitization at birth. J Allergy Clin Immunol 2008;122:407–12, 12 e1–4.

38. Schaub B, Liu J, Hoppler S, et al. Maternal farm exposure modulates neonatal immune mechanisms through regulatory T cells. J Allergy Clin Immunol 2009;123:774–82 e5.

39. Pfefferle PI, Buchele G, Blumer N, et al. Cord blood cytokines are modulated by maternal farming activities and consumption of farm dairy products during pregnancy: the PASTURE Study. J Allergy Clin Immunol 2010;125:108–15 e1–3.

40. Chatzi L, Torrent M, Romieu I, et al. Mediterranean diet in pregnancy is protective for wheeze and atopy in childhood. Thorax 2008;63:507–13.

41. Berdnikovs S, Abdala-Valencia H, McCary C, et al. Isoforms of vitamin E have opposing immunoregulatory functions during inflammation by regulating leukocyte recruitment. J Immunol 2009;182:4395–405.

42. Furuhjelm C, Warstedt K, Larsson J, et al. Fish oil supplementation in pregnancy and lactation may decrease the risk of infant allergy. Acta Paediatr 2009;98:1461–7.

43. Robison R, Kumar R. The effect of prenatal and postnatal dietary exposures on childhood development of atopic disease. Curr Opin Allergy Clin Immunol 2010;10:139–44.

44. Dimeloe S, Nanzer A, Ryanna K, et al. Regulatory T cells, inflammation and the allergic response-The role of glucocorticoids and Vitamin D. J Steroid Biochem Mol Biol 2010;120:86–95.

45. Vassallo MF, Banerji A, Rudders SA, et al. Season of birth and food-induced anaphylaxis in Boston. Allergy 2010;65:1492–3.

46. Hollingsworth JW, Maruoka S, Boon K, et al. In utero supplementation with methyl donors enhances allergic airway disease in mice. J Clin Invest 2008;118:3462–9.

47. Matsui EC, Matsui W. Higher serum folate levels are associated with a lower risk of atopy and wheeze. J Allergy Clin Immunol 2009;123:1253–9 e2.

48. Hong X, Tsai HJ, Wang X. Genetics of food allergy. Curr Opin Pediatr 2009;21:770–6.

49. Greer FR, Sicherer SH, Burks AW. Effects of early nutritional interventions on the development of atopic disease in infants and children: the role of maternal dietary restriction, breastfeeding, timing of introduction of complementary foods, and hydrolyzed formulas. Pediatrics 2008;121:183–91.

50. Johannsen H, Prescott SL. Practical prebiotics, probiotics and synbiotics for allergists: how useful are they? Clin Exp Allergy 2009;39:1801–14.

CHAPTER 2

Food Antigens

E. N. Clare Mills, Philip E. Johnson, Yuri Alexeev

Introduction

The immune system possesses remarkable flexibility in the number of ways in which it works to protect the body from hazards, including infective microorganisms, viruses and parasites, employing both cellular agents to remove and inactivate hazards, as well as molecules, notably immunoglobulins (Igs), which form part of the humoral defense system. Igs are synthesized in a number of different forms, or isotypes, and have been classified on a structural, physicochemical and functional basis including IgA, IgG (of which there are a number of subtypes identified in humans, including IgG_1 and IgG_4), IgM and IgE. All are characterized by an antibody-binding site generated to bind specifically to 'non-self' molecules, which are generally known as antigens. These include molecules found in microbial pathogens, parasites, environmental agents such as pollen and dietary proteins. Albeit not exclusively so, antigens tend almost entirely to be proteinaceous in nature, although some carbohydrate moieties can be recognized, and the lipopolysaccharide antigens of microbes are particularly effective elicitors of humoral immune responses.

However, in the allergic condition classified as a type I hypersensitivity reaction, the antibody repertoire to selected environmental antigens is altered, the body synthesizing larger quantities of the antibody isotype normally produced in response to parasitic infections, IgE. The molecules recognized by IgE are frequently termed allergens and, if polyvalent in nature, they may be able to cross-link mast-cell-bound IgE and in so doing trigger mediator release, the inflammatory mediators then going on to trigger tissues responses which are manifested as allergic symptoms in an allergic reaction.

The sites that an antibody recognizes on its cognate antigen have been termed epitopes and can be classified into two different types. The first of these have been termed continuous or linear epitopes and are where antibody recognition is based almost entirely on the amino acid sequence, with very little effect of conformation. In general such antibodies can bind well to short linear peptides of 10–15 residues in length that correspond to the epitope sequence in the parent protein. They also often recognize both native folded and unfolded antigens well. A second type of epitope has been termed conformational and is where the secondary, tertiary and quaternary structural elements of a protein antigen bring together sometimes quite distant regions of the polypeptide chain. In general, antibody binding to such epitopes is disrupted when proteins unfold, and it can be difficult to map such epitopes using linear peptides as they do not resemble the structural epitopes brought about by the folded nature of the antigen. Structural studies have indicated that antibody binding to proteins involves a surface area of 650–900 Å^2, contacts outside the immediate epitope area being important in binding although they may not determine antibody specificity. Such definitions are in some ways arbitrary, and it may be in some instances that several linear epitopes could come together to form a conformational epitope.

Allergens have been defined by the International Union of Immunological Societies as being molecules that must induce IgE-mediated (atopic) allergy in humans with a prevalence of IgE reactivity above 5%. Although it does not carry any connotation of allergenic potency, an allergen is termed as being major if it is recognized by IgE from at least 50% of a cohort of allergic individuals, otherwise it is known as minor. Allergens are given a designation based on the Latin name of the species from which they originate and composed of the first three letters of the genus, followed by the first letter of the species and finishing with an Arabic number. Thus, an allergen from *Mallus domesticus* (apple) is prefaced Mal d followed by a number, which is largely determined by the order in which allergens are identified. The numbers are common to all homologous allergens (also known as isoallergens) in a given species, which are defined on the basis of having a similar molecular mass, an identical biological function, if known, e.g. enzymatic action, and >67% identity of amino acid sequences. For those species where the first three letters of a genus and the first letter of a species are identical, the second letter of the species is also used.

Many proteins are post-translationally modified with glycans and such structures can bind IgE, glycan-reactive IgE being found in between 16% and 55% of food-allergic patients. These are best characterized for the asparagine-linked carbohydrate moieties (*N*-glycans), with $\alpha(1-3)$ fucose and $\beta(1-2)$ xylose representing the major cross-reactive carbohydrate determinants (CCDs), which are found in many plant food and pollen allergens but are distinct to mammalian *N*-glycans. However, there is debate about whether IgE to CCDs has biological significance, and whether it can result in clinically significant allergic symptoms. This is probably because such glycans tend not to be polyvalent, and consequently are unable to trigger cross-linking of IgE receptors, the IgE binding may be of low IgE affinity, and the presence of blocking antibodies may downregulate the allergic response. *O*-linked glycans are also found in plant proteins, albeit less frequently than *N*-glycans. There is evidence that single β-arabinosyl residues linked to

hydroxyproline residues are important in determining the IgE-binding activity of an allergen from mugwort pollen known as Art v 1, although *O*-linked glycans have yet to be described in food allergens.

In the process of describing the active agents involved in food allergies a large number of allergens have now been identified with the greatest diversity existing for plant food allergens, perhaps reflecting the diversity of plant-derived foods that humans consume. They include nuts, seeds, grains, and a variety of fresh fruits and vegetables. Although it appears that individuals can be allergic to any of a vast number of foods, it appears that the majority of allergies are triggered by a more restricted selection, and that the allergens triggering those reactions belong to a restricted number and type of protein. This observation has led to certain restricted numbers of foods being termed the 'Big 8' which includes milk, eggs, fish, crustacean shellfish, tree nuts, peanuts, wheat and soybean. Other important allergenic foods or food groups have emerged, some of which, along with the 'Big 8' must be labeled on manufactured foods in certain countries and regions of the world to allow allergic consumers to avoid them. These include molluscan shellfish, mustard, celery (root celery or celeriac) and lupin. This review will focus on the structural attributes and common properties of allergens and then describe in more detail the allergens found in more commonly important allergenic foods.

Common properties and structural attributes of food allergens

The last 10–15 years have seen an explosion in the number of allergenic proteins described from a vast array of foods, which has allowed the application of various bioinformatic tools to classify them according to their structure and function into protein families. Some years ago this was undertaken for both plant and animal food allergens, together with pollen allergens. This analysis has demonstrated that the majority of allergens in each of these groups fell into around three to 12 families, the remaining allergens belonging to around 14–23 families comprising one to three allergens in each. Thus, around 65% of plant food allergens belonged to just four protein families, known as the prolamin, cupin, Bet v 1 and profilin superfamilies, whereas animal-derived food allergens fall into just three main families, namely the tropomyosins, EF-hand

and caseins. A summary of the major and several of the minor allergen families is given below.

Animal food allergen families

Tropomyosins (Fig. 2.1)

Tropomyosins are contractile proteins which, together with the other proteins actin and myosin, function to regulate contraction in both muscle and non-muscle cells and are ubiquitous in animal cells. They comprise a repetitive sequence of heptapeptide repeats that spontaneously form two strands of α-helix which then assemble into two-stranded coiled coils. These monomers then assemble into head-to-tail polymers along the length of an actin filament. These are the major allergens of two invertebrate groups, Crustacea and Mollusca, which include the food group commonly known as shellfish. They have been identified as both food and inhalant allergens, being characterized as allergens in dust mite and cockroach, and consequently have been termed invertebrate pan-allergens. IgE-epitope mapping has shown that sequences unique to invertebrate tropomyosins, located in the C-terminal region of the protein, play an important role in their allergenic potential. Their lack of homology between vertebrates and invertebrates means there is no cross-reactivity between IgE from shellfish-allergic individuals and animal muscle tropomyosins.

Parvalbumins (Fig. 2.2)

Parvalbumins represent the second-largest animal food allergen family and are abundant in the white muscle of many fish species, where they have a role regulating free intracellular calcium levels, which are important for muscle fiber relaxation. They are ubiquitous in animals and have been classified into two different types, α and β, which possess distinct evolutionary lineages but are structurally very similar. In general it is the β-parvalbumins that are allergenic. Structurally they are characterized by a calcium-binding motif found in many proteins, known as an EF-hand, which comprises a 12 amino

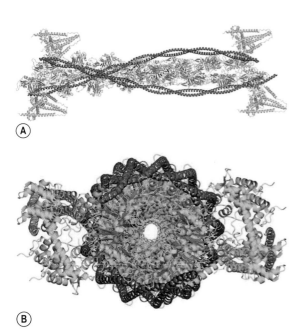

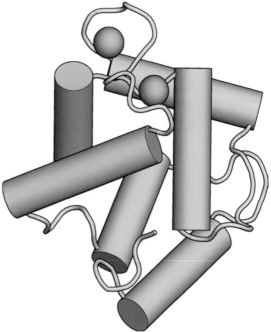

Figure 2.1 Three-dimensional structure of tropomyosin in insect flight muscle (PDB code 2W4U) and example of a tropomyosin from an invertebrate which is typical of the allergenic tropomyosins found in crustaceans and molluscs. (a) A view along tropomyosin chains; (b) a cross-sectional view. Tropomyosin is shown in red. Other proteins are troponin and actin. α-Helices and loops are shown in cyan and yellow, respectively.

Figure 2.2 Three-dimensional structure of calcium-liganded carp parvalbumin (PDB code 4CPV, Cyp c 1). Parvalbumin has two calcium-binding sites which have the same structural motif formed by an α-helix linked to a second α-helix by a 12-residue loop around the calcium cation. Calcium cations are shown as green spheres. α-Helices are shown in cyan cylinders and loops are shown in yellow.

acid loop flanked on either side by a 12 residue stretch of α-helix. Parvalbumins possess three EF-hand motifs, two of which bind calcium, and consequently, as with many other proteins with integral metal ions, the loss of calcium causes a change in protein conformation which is associated with a loss of IgE-binding capacity. Recently a sarcoplasmic calcium-binding protein has been identified as an allergen in pacific white shrimp *Litopenaeus vannamei* called Lit v 4.0101, allergenic homologs of which can be found in other crustacean species such as lobster. This protein also possesses an E-F-hand motif and is thought to be an invertebrate parvalbumin, as it also functions as a calcium-buffering protein in invertebrate muscle.

Caseins (Fig. 2.3)

The major protein in milk is a fraction known as casein which comprises a heterogeneous mixture of structurally mobile proteins known α_{s1}-, α_{s2}- and β-caseins, although the α_{s2}-casein gene is not expressed in humans. These proteins possess clusters of phosphoserine and/or phosphothreonine residues which bind calcium, forming a shell around amorphous calcium phosphate to form microstructures called nanoclusters. This ability allows calcium to reach levels in milk that exceed the solubility limit of calcium phosphate. The α_{s1}-, α_{s2}- and β-caseins assemble into large macromolecular structures known as casein micelles,

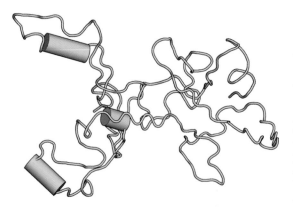

Figure 2.3 Modeled three-dimensional structure of bovine β-casein (Bos d 8). α-Helices and loops are shown in cyan and yellow, respectively. Structure reference: Beta-Casein variant A structure: T. F. Kumosinski, E. M. Brown, and H. M. Farrell, Jr., Three-Dimensional Molecular Modeling of Bovine Caseins: An Energy-Minimized Beta-Casein Structure (1993) Journal of Dairy Science, 76: 931–45.

which are stabilized by a polypeptide chain known as κ-casein. The α- and β-caseins are related to the secretory calcium-binding phosphoprotein family together with proteins involved in mineralization and salivary proteins, whereas κ-caseins may be distantly related to fibrinogen γ-chain. There is considerable similarity in the caseins from different mammalian milks used for human consumption, which explains their IgE cross-reactivity.

Minor animal food allergen families

There are several less well represented animal food allergen families which encompass ligand-binding proteins that function as carriers, enzymes and protease inhibitors. One of the types of carrier molecule is known as the lipocalin family, a group of diverse proteins that share about 20% sequence identity but have a conserved three-dimensional structure. They are characterized by a central tunnel which can often accommodate a diversity of lipophilic ligands, and are thought to function as carriers of odorants, steroids, lipids and pheromones, among others. The majority of lipocalin allergens are respiratory, having been identified as the major allergens in rodent urine, animal dander and saliva, as well as in insects such as cockroaches, although the only lipocalin that acts as a food allergen is the cows' milk allergen, β-lactoglobulin. Another carrier protein family are the transferrins, eukaryotic sulfur-rich iron-binding glycoproteins which function in vivo to control the level of free iron in biological fluids.

Another minor family is the glycoside hydrolase family 22 clan of the *O*-glycosyl hydrolase superfamily to which lysozyme type C and α-lactalbumins belong, being structurally homologous despite having very different functions, α-lactalbumin being involved in lactose synthesis in milk, whereas lysozyme acts as a glycohydrolase, cleaving bacterial peptidoglycans. Furthermore, α-lactalbumin, unlike hen's egg lysozyme, binds calcium. A second minor allergen family comprising enzymes are the arginine kinases, which have been identified as allergens in invertebrates. They belong to a family of structurally and functionally related ATP:guanido phosphotransferases that reversibly catalyze the transfer of phosphate between ATP and various phosphogens.

Two different types of protease inhibitor families are also allergenic. These include the serpins, a class of serine protease inhibitors of which some family members have lost their inhibitory activity.

A second type are the Kazal inhibitors, which also inhibit serine proteases and can contain between 1 and 7 Kazal-type inhibitor repeats.

Plant food allergen families

Prolamins (Fig. 2.4)

The prolamin superfamily was initially identified on the basis of a conserved pattern of cysteine residues found in the sulfur-rich seed storage prolamins, the α-amylase/trypsin inhibitors of monocotyledonous cereal seeds, and the 2S storage albumins. Subsequently other low molecular weight allergenic proteins have been identified as belonging to this superfamily, including soybean hydrophobic protein, non-specific lipid transfer proteins and α-globulins. The conserved cysteine skeleton comprises a core of eight cysteine residues that includes a characteristic Cys–Cys and Cys–X–Cys motif (X representing any other residue). Two additional cysteine residues are found in the alpha-amylase/trypsin inhibitors. Apart from the seed storage prolamins, which are characterized by the insertion of an extensive repetitive domain, members of this superfamily share a common three-dimensional structure. This comprises a bundle of four α-helices stabilized by disulfide

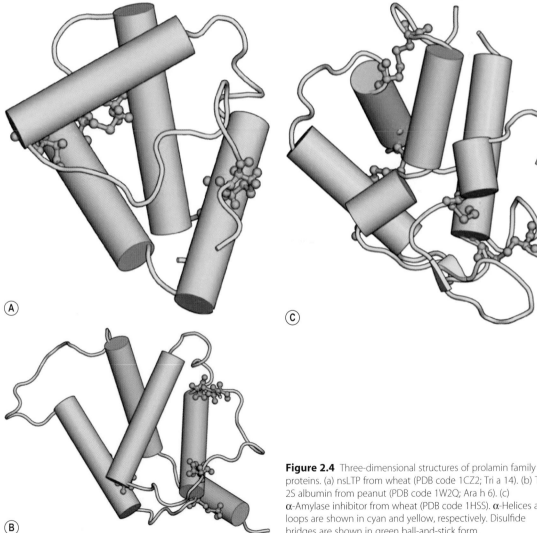

(A)

(B)

(C)

Figure 2.4 Three-dimensional structures of prolamin family proteins. (a) nsLTP from wheat (PDB code 1CZ2; Tri a 14). (b) The 2S albumin from peanut (PDB code 1W2Q; Ara h 6). (c) α-Amylase inhibitor from wheat (PDB code 1HSS). α-Helices and loops are shown in cyan and yellow, respectively. Disulfide bridges are shown in green ball-and-stick form.

bonds which are arranged in such a way as to create a lipid-binding tunnel in the nsLTPs which is collapsed in the 2S albumin structures. It is also responsible for maintaining the three-dimensional structure of many of these proteins even after heating, which is associated with their retaining their allergenic properties after cooking and may contribute to their resistance to proteolysis.

2S albumins

A major class of seed storage proteins, the 2S albumins are usually synthesized in the seed as single chains of 10–15 kDa which may be post-translationally processed to give small and large subunits which usually remain joined by disulfide bonds. The type of this processing depends on the plant species,those in sunflower being single-chain albumins and those in Brazil nut being two-chain albumins. They can act as both occupational (sensitizing through inhalation of dusts) and food allergens.

Lipid transfer proteins

The name of these proteins derives from the fact they were originally identified in plants because of their ability to transfer lipids in vitro, but their actual biological function in plants is unclear. Because their expression is regulated by abiotic stress, belonging to pathogenesis-related protein group 14, they may have a role in plant protection. They are located in the outer epidermal tissues of plants, such as the peel of peach or apple fruits, and this, together with their lipid-binding characteristics, has led to the suggestion they are involved in transporting cutin and suberin monomers to the outer tissues of plants, where they polymerize to form the outer waxy layers. They have been termed pan-allergens and are the most widely distributed type of prolamin, being found in a variety of plant organs including seeds, fruit and vegetative tissues. Thus, in addition to being identified in many different fruits and seeds, they have also been characterized as allergens in the pollen of several plant species such as olive and Parietaria judaica as well as inhalant allergens involved in occupational allergies to dusts such as wheat flour in Baker's asthma. The IgE cross-reactivity of LTPs from the *Rosaceae* fruits has been demonstrated and related to conservation of their surface structure but to date such cross-reactivity has not been demonstrated between pollen and food allergens. Certainly allergy involving peach LTP Pru p 3, has been demonstrated to be independent of pollen LTP sensitization and is associated with much higher levels of peach Pru p 3 specific IgE, implying it is the primary sensitizing agent involved in this food allergy.

Seed storage prolamins

The cysteine skeleton and α-helical structure generally characteristic of the prolamin superfamily has been disrupted in the seed storage prolamins as a consequence of the insertion of a repetitive domain rich in the amino acids proline and glutamine. This repetitive domain dominates their physicochemical properties of the seed storage prolamins and is thought to adopt a loose spiral structure formed from a dynamic ensemble of unfolded and secondary structures comprising overlapping β-turns or poly-L-proline II structures. They are the major seed storage proteins of the related cereals wheat, barley and rye, those from wheat being able to form large disulfide-linked polymers that comprise the viscoelastic protein fraction known as gluten. These proteins are characteristically insoluble in dilute salt solutions, either in the native state or after reduction of interchain disulfide bonds, being instead soluble in aqueous alcohols.

Bifunctional inhibitors

This group of allergens are restricted to cereals, individual subunits acting as inhibitors of trypsin (and sometimes other proteinases), α-amylases from insects (including pests) or both,leading to their being termed bifunctional. These proteins can have a role as allergens in occupational allergies to wheat flour, such as baker's asthma, or in food sensitizing via the gastrointestinal tract. They were initially identified in extracts made with mixtures of chloroform and water and are often called CM proteins, but are also soluble in water, dilute salt solutions or mixtures of alcohol and water.

Bet v 1 homologs (see Fig. 2.7)

A very important group of allergens are those that are homologous to the major birch pollen allergen Bet v 1. A β-barrel protein that can bind plant steroids in a central tunnel, Bet v 1 and its homologs belong to family 10 of the pathogenesis-related proteins and may have a role in plant protection, acting as a steroid carrier, although this has not been confirmed. The conservation of both primary structure (amino acid sequence) and the molecular surfaces of Bet v 1 and its homologs explains the cross-reactivity of IgE and hence the widespread cross-reactive allergies to fresh fruits and vegetables frequently observed in individuals with birch pollen allergy. Two classical examples are the allergies to fruits, such as apple, and nuts, notably hazelnut. In both instances individuals tend to have allergy to birch pollen and suffer from oral allergy syndrome on consumption of fresh apple or hazelnuts which is associated with the presence of IgE specific for the Bet v 1 homologues found in these foods, known as Mal d 1 and Cor a 1 respectively.

Cupins (Fig. 2.5)

A functionally diverse protein superfamily, the cupins have probably evolved from a prokaryotic

ancestor and are found in microbes and plants but not animals. They are characterized by a β-barrel structure from which their name is derived, 'cupin' meaning barrel in Latin. Using this basic structural motif, a diverse range of biological functions have been derived, including sporulation proteins in fungi, sucrose-binding activities and enzymatic activities found in germins, where manganese is bound in the center of the barrel. In flowering plants the cupin barrel has been duplicated to give the bi-cupins, which include the 7S and 11S seed storage globulins. The 11S globulins, sometimes termed legumins, are hexameric proteins of ~300–450 kDa. Each subunit is synthesized in the seed as a single chain of ~60 kDa, which is post-translationally processed to give rise to acidic (~40 kDa) and basic (~20 kDa) chains, linked by a single disulfide bond, and are rarely, if ever, glycosylated. The 7/8S globulins, also termed vicilins, are somewhat simpler, comprising three subunits of ~40–80 kDa, but typically about 50 kDa.

Minor plant food allergen families

As with animal food allergens there are a number of minor families. One of the most important of these are the profilins (Fig. 2.6), a group of

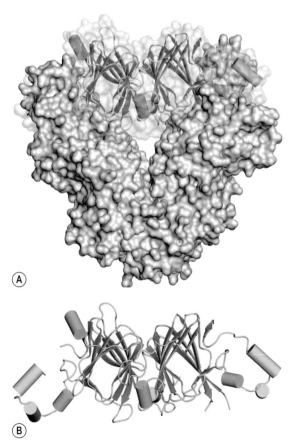

(A)

(B)

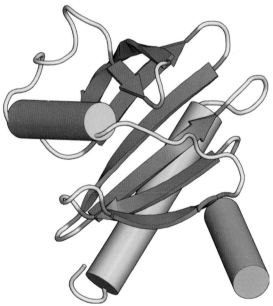

Figure 2.5 Three-dimensional structure of native soybean β-conglycinin trimer (PDB code 1IPK; Gly m 5). (a) The structure consists of three chains, A, B and D. Chains are shown in space-filling representation; (b) chain B is shown in cartoon mode. α-Helices are shown as cyan cylinders. β-Pleated sheets and loops are shown in magenta and yellow, respectively.

Figure 2.6 Three-dimensional structure of birch profilin (PDB code 1CQA, Bet v 2). α-Helices are shown as cyan cylinders. Single β-pleated sheets and loops are shown in magenta and yellow, respectively.

allergens involved in the pollen–fruit allergy syndrome. Cytosolic proteins found in all eukaryotic cells, profilins are thought to regulate actin polymerization by binding to monomeric actin and a number of other proteins. However, only profilins found in plants, where they are highly conserved, have been described as allergens. As a consequence, profilin-specific IgE cross-reacts with homologs from virtually every plant source, and sensitization to these allergens has been considered a risk factor for multiple pollen allergies and pollen-associated food allergy. However, the clinical relevance of plant food profilin-specific IgE is still under debate.

Many of the remaining minor plant food allergen families have a role in protecting plants from pests and pathogens. Two types of enzyme family have been described as plant food allergens, including the glycoside hydrolase family 19 proteins known as class I chitinases, which are involved in latex-food allergies, and the cysteine (C1) papain-like proteases. Plant class I chitinases degrade chitin, a major structural component of the exoskeleton of insects and of the cell walls of many pathogenic fungi, and hence have a role in protecting plants against pests and pathogens. They possess an N-terminal domain that is structurally homologous with hevein, a major latex allergen, which is thought to bind chitin. As a consequence of this homology, class I chitinases from fruits such as avocado, banana and chestnut have been identified as major allergens that cross-react with IgE specific to the latex allergen Hev b 6.02. The 43-residue polypeptide chain of hevein-like domains contains four disulfide bonds, to which they owe their stability, and because of their widespread occurrence in plants have been termed pan-allergens. The cysteine proteases, to which fruit allergens belong, notably in kiwi, were originally characterized by having a cysteine residue as part of their catalytic site, although some members may have lost the capacity to act as proteases, a notable example being the soybean P34 protein, in which a glycine has replaced the active site cysteine residue.

Other minor plant food allergen families include the Kunitz/bovine pancreatic trypsin inhibitors and some lectins. The Kunitz inhibitors are active against serine, thiol, aspartic and subtilisin proteases, and in plants they probably play a role in defense against pests and pathogens. They belong to a superfamily of structurally related proteins which share no sequence similarity and which

includes such diverse proteins as interleukin (IL)-1 proteins, heparin-binding growth factors (HBGF) and histactophilin. The thaumatin-like proteins (TLPs) are structurally similar to the intensely sweet-tasting protein thaumatin found in the fruits of the West African rainforest shrub *Thaumatococcus daniellii*. They are also involved in plant protection, belonging to the PR-5 family of proteins.

Common properties and predicting allergens

What does the classification of allergens into protein families tell us? Great efforts have been made to use bioinformatic methods to predict what makes some proteins allergens and not others, especially to support the allergenic risk assessment process for allergens in novel foods and genetically modified organisms destined for food use. However, it is not yet possible to predict allergenic activity in proteins, and it is clear that membership of one of a limited number of protein families is not in itself sufficient to determine allergenic activity. However, proteins from the same family often share common properties conferred by the structural features of that particular family. It seems that several factors contribute to determining whether a given atopic individual will become sensitized to a given individual. These include the genetic make-up and atopic tendencies of the exposed individual and factors such as the abundance of an allergen in a food, its structure, and the biochemical and physicochemical properties of the allergen. These include a protein's 'stability', reflecting its ability to either retain or regain its original native three-dimensional structure following treatments such as cooking, and to resist attack by proteases, such as those encountered in the gastrointestinal tract. Such stability has the potential to be modified by ligands, such as lipids and metal ions. Other factors, such as interaction with membranes, the ability to aggregate, or the presence of repetitive structures, may also influence allergenic potential. It may also be that, although glycans are not so important in triggering allergic reactions in individuals once sensitized, they may play a role in effecting sensitization in the first place. However, an understanding of structural relationships and common properties does help to explain many of the cross-reactive allergies observed and the common responses of many different types of food allergy to processes such as cooking. The following sections give a summary of the current knowledge of allergens in the major allergenic foods identified to date.

Animal food allergens

Cows' milk

Cows' milk is an important allergenic food in early childhood, allergies in adults being rare. Allergens that have been identified include proteins found in both whey and curd fractions. Major whey allergens include β-lactoglobulin (Bos d 5), the only lipocalin that acts as a food allergen. An 18.4 kDa protein with a lipocalin β-barrel structure, it has a ligand-binding tunnel which can bind a variety of lipophilic molecules, including retinoic acid and fatty acids such as palmitate. It is stabilized by two intramolecular disulfide bonds together with a single free cysteine residue. The other whey protein allergen is α-lactalbumin (Bos d 4), a calcium-binding protein that belongs to the glycoside hydrolase family 22 clan. It has a superimposable three-dimensional structure with the egg allergen lysozyme. A 14.2 kDa calcium-binding protein, α-lactalbumin is stabilized by four disulfide bridges and has a role in regulating lactose synthase. Its three-dimensional structure is primarily α-helical in nature, with some 3_{10} helix and β-sheet the parts of the polypeptide which form the calcium-binding site being the most ordered (less mobile, more rigid) part of the protein structure.

In addition to the whey proteins, the major allergens of cows' milk are the caseins (Bos d 8), a heterogeneous mixture of proteins called α_{s1}-, α_{s2}- and β-caseins which are produced by a polymorphic multigene family and undergo post-translational proteolysis and phosphorylation. Other minor allergens identified in milk include the iron-binding protein lactoferrin, serum albumin (Bos d 6) and immunoglobulin (Bos d 7). IgE cross-reactivity studies in a group of cows' milk-allergic infants showed that although all but 10% had serum IgE against α_{s2}-casein, only around half recognized α_{s1}-casein, and only a small proportion (15%) had IgE against β-casein. The high level of homology (e.g. >90%) between whey proteins and caseins from different mammalian species explains the extensive IgE cross-reactivity observed between the milks of cow, sheep and goat, individuals with cows' milk allergy generally reacting when undergoing oral challenge with goats' milk; allergies to goats' or

sheep's milk have been emerging, although the IgE reactivity seems to be limited to the casein fraction. Reduced IgE cross-reactivity has been observed with mares' milk proteins, such that some individuals with cows' milk allergy can tolerate mares' milk, and there are indications that camels' milk also has a reduced IgE cross-reactivity compared with cow's milk. Such observations have led to the suggestion that milk from mammals such as horse, donkey and camel might have some utility as a substitute for cows' milk suitable for consumption by cows milk allergic individuals, be used in selected cases of cows' milk allergy, once they have been processed to make them suitable for consumption by human infants.

Food processing procedures can result in further modification of cows' milk proteins, with pasteurization resulting in β-lactoglobulin becoming covalently attached to casein micelles and thermal treatments, in particular spray drying, resulting in extensive lactosylation. Thus, the allergenic activity of β-lactoglobulin has been found to increase 100-fold following heating in the presence of lactose, whereas severe thermal processing, such as baking, appears to reduce the allergenicity of milk compared to less severe heat treatments. Both whey proteins form thermally induced aggregated structures and at high protein concentrations form gelled networks, whereas caseins can have a tendency to aggregate. Both α-lactalbumin and the caseins are highly susceptible to digestion by pepsin, being rapidly degraded. In the case of α-lactalbumin this may relate to the pH-labile nature of the allergen, which unfolds at low pH, whereas the caseins, as mobile proteins, are excellent substrates for pepsin. These properties contrast with those of β-lactoglobulin, which is resistant to pepsin at physiological concentrations and is digested only slowly by the duodenal endoproteases trypsin and chymotrypsin. Processing may modify their susceptibility to digestion, and although thermal denaturation enhances the digestability of β-lactoglobulin it does not affect the susceptibility of caseins to digestion. However, interaction with other food components and food matrices can have unexpected effects. Thus, adsorption to oil droplets increases the susceptibility of β-lactoglobulin to pepsinolysis, whereas adsorption of β-casein results in certain fragments being protected from pepsinolysis, including regions spanning known IgE epitopes. Such effects of processing may underlie the differences in clinical reactivity of baked milk foods, compared to less extensively thermally processed milk products.

Egg

A second important allergenic food of infancy and childhood is egg, for which a number of allergens have been identified. These include the dominant hen's egg-white allergen Gal d 1, the extensively glycosylated Kazal inhibitor (comprising three Kazal-like inhibitory domains) known as ovomucoid, and the serpin serine protease inhibitor ovalbumin, Gal d 3. It is ovomucoid that is responsible for the viscous properties of egg white, whereas ovalbumin accounts for more than half the protein in egg white. Gal d 1 comprises three tandem domains (Gal d 1.1, Gal d 1.2, Gal d 1.3) stabilized by intradomain disulfide bonds, the Gal d 1.1 and Gal d 1.2 domains possessing two carbohydrate chains each, whereas around only half the Gal d 1.3 domains are glycosylated. Such extensive glycosylation acts to stabilize the protein against proteolysis. Two other proteins are minor allergens which are also homologs of cows' milk allergens. One is lysozyme, also known as Gal d 4, a glycosidase belonging to the glycoside hydrolase family 22 clan of the O-glycosyl hydrolase superfamily, and is homologous to cows' milk α-lactalbumin (Bos d 4). A second is the sulfur-rich iron-binding glycoprotein ovotransferrin, which is homologous to the cows' milk allergen lactoferrin. Although the major egg allergens are found in egg white, there are indications that certain yolk proteins may also act as allergens. Thus, the egg yolk protein α-livetin has been designated the allergen Gal d 5, and recently the vitellogenin-1 precursor has been identified as a minor allergen and termed Gal d 6.

It has been shown that the egg white allergen ovomucoid becomes disulfide linked to the gluten proteins during baking, with a concomitant reduction in the allergenic activity of soluble extracts. These effects are apparent even following kneading. During storage of eggs ovalbumin is transformed into a more thermostable form known as S-ovalbumin, which denatures at 88° rather than the 80°C characteristic of the native protein. The conversion involves conformational changes rather than proteolysis and is the result of elevation of the egg's pH, with typically about 80% of the ovalbumin being converted into the S form on storage at 20°C for a month. Nothing is known about the impact of such changes on the allergenicity of this protein. Both ovalbumin and ovomucoid can be readily digested by pepsin, but it appears that peptide fragments of ovomucoid can retain their IgE-binding capacity, albeit in a patient-dependent manner. It maybe that those individuals likely to retain their egg allergy beyond childhood show IgE reactivity towards digestion-resistant fragments, whereas those who outgrow their allergy have IgE responses only to the intact protein. Ovalbumin and lyoszyme are often used as fining agents in wine production, but evidence to date suggests they lose their allergenic activity when used in this way.

Fish

One of the first fish allergens to be described was the allergenic parvalbumin of cod, Gad c 1, but a number have now been identified in many different fish species and can therefore be considered to be the pan-allergens in fish. Clinical cross-reactivity to multiple fish in individuals with allergy based on the major fish allergen parvalbumin is a common observation. This can be explained by the structural similarity of the parvalbumins from various fish species, although their lower levels in the dark muscle of some fish species, such as tuna, may mean they are less problematic allergens in such types of fish. Similarly, the cross-reactivity of fish and frog muscle in fish-allergic individuals can be explained by the structural similarities between their parvalbumins, although intriguingly one of the allergens in frog is an α-parvalbumin.

One of the first records in the literature of processing affecting allergenicity is the report of Prausnitz on the sensitivity of Kustner towards cooked, but not raw, fish. However, it has rarely been reported in the literature that food processing increases allergenic activity. In general it seems that fish allergens are stable to cooking procedures, the parvalbumins being generally resistant to heat and proteolysis. A likely explanation for this observation is that the E-F-hand structure of parvalbumin, whilst unfolding at elevated temperatures is able to refold on cooling, providing calcium is still present, thus regaining its native, IgE-reactive conformation. Such thermostability undoubtedly contributes to the ability of this major fish allergen to retain its allergenic properties after cooking, although the severe heat treatment does have an effect, the IgE-binding activity of canned fish having been estimated to be 100–200 times lower than that of boiled fish. Thermal treatment of fish results in the formation of parvalbumin oligomers, which are generally associated with a loss of IgE-binding capacity, whereas processes such as smoking appear to potentially increase allergenicity and may result in the formation of novel allergens.

Molluscan and crustacean Shellfish

Members of a family of closely related proteins present in muscle and non-muscle cells, tropomyosins are major seafood allergens found in various species of Crustacea, including shrimp, crab and lobster, as well as Mollusca, such as abalone, mussels, squid and octopus. First characterized as allergens in shrimp, tropomyosins are now acknowledged to be invertebrate pan-allergens. To date, all allergenic tropomyosins have been confined to vertebrates and invertebrates and are highly homologous to non-allergenic forms from invertebrate species, sequence differences being confined to the first two residues of the IgE epitope in the C-terminal portion of the protein, which is crucial for IgE binding. The uniqueness of this region to invertebrate tropomyosins explains the lack of IgE cross-reactivity between shellfish and animal muscle tropomyosins. Recently efforts to exploit this similarity in order to graft 'allergenic' invertebrate tropomyosin epitopes onto the human tropomyosin scaffold have shown that conformational epitopes play a major role in the allergenicity of tropomyosin, which cannot be identified using short synthetic peptides. The extensive homologies between allergenic tropomyosins result in IgE cross-reactivity, individuals sensitized to tropomyosin from one particular crustacean species often showing IgE cross-reactivity, which is often (although not always) accompanied by clinical allergy to many crustacean species. However, such extensive cross-reactivity is less clear with regard to mollusc reactivity, which may be restricted to cross-sensitization. The field of crustacean and molluscan shellfish allergies is made complex by the diverse range of shellfish species that humans consume, which are often described using broad terms such as "shrimp" or "seafood". It is important to make distinctions between crustacean and molluscan shellfish but further research is needed to gain the evidence currently lacking to further classify crustacean shellfish allergies on the basis of, for example, allergens from fresh- or marine species or differences in IgE reactivity to the fast- compared to slow-muscle tropomyosins. A minor group of allergens identified in shrimp are the

arginine kinases, which have also been identified as cross-reactive allergens in the Indian meal moth, king prawn, lobster and mussel. Other shrimp allergens include a sarcoplasmic calcium-binding protein, triosephosphate isomerase (TIM), and several contractile proteins including myosin light chains, troponin C and troponin I. The proteins appear to be generally heat stable, their allergenicity being unaltered by boiling. Tropomyosins have been detected in the cooking water, but in general there have been few studies on the impact of cooking on shellfish and crustacean allergenicity.

Plant food allergens

Fresh fruits and vegetables

Many allergens in fresh fruits and vegetables are related to inhalant allergens, particularly those found in birch pollen and latex. It is thought that individuals initially become sensitized to the inhalant allergens in pollen and latex and subsequently develop allergies to a variety of fresh fruits, vegetables, nuts and seeds, because the close structural resemblance of inhalant allergens and their homologs in foods allows IgE developed to the inhalant allergens to bind (or cross-react) with homologs found in foods. In addition, it appears that some fruit and vegetable allergens can sensitize individuals directly.

A large number of allergenic homologs of Bet v 1 have been identified in a variety of fruits and vegetables involved in pollen–fruit cross-reactive allergies, with perhaps the most important including the Rosacea fruits such as apple (Mal d 1), cherry (Pru av 1) and peach (Pru p 1). They have also been identified as allergens in emerging allergenic foods, such as kiwi fruit (Act d 8) and exotic fruits such as jackfruit and Sharon fruit. In addition, allergenic Bet v 1 homologs have also been identified in vegetables, notably celery (Api g 1) and carrot (Dau c 1) (Fig. 2.7). A second group of IgE-cross-reactive allergens originally identified in connection with birch pollen allergy are the profilins, and as with Bet v 1, a wide range of homologs of the allergenic profiling in birch and other allergenic pollens have been identified in a variety of fruits and vegetables. Many of the foods that contain allergenic Bet v 1 homologs also contain allergenic profilins. There have been concerns that although profilins can sensitize individuals, the resulting IgE

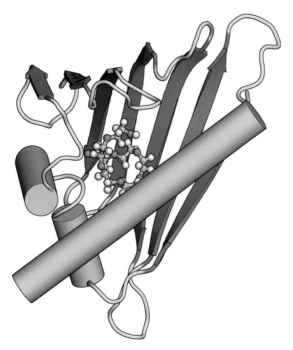

Figure 2.7 Three-dimensional structure of major carrot allergen Dau c 1 from the Bet v 1 family of allergens (PDB code 2WQL). The structure is complexed with polyethylene glycol oligomer. α-Helices are shown as cyan cylinders. Single β-pleated sheets and loops are shown in magenta and yellow, respectively.

lacks biological activity and does not play a role in the development of allergic reactions, but this does not seem to be a general rule and in certain patients they may be able to trigger an allergic reaction.

Another type of allergy to fresh fruits and vegetables found in Europe appears to be generally confined to the Mediterranean area and does not seem to be associated with prior sensitization to other agents such as pollen. Unlike the birch pollen allergies it tends to be manifested with much more severe, even life-threatening allergic reactions and involves a different group of allergens, known as the non-specific lipid transfer proteins (LTPs). These have emerged as important allergens because of their role in causing severe allergies to peach (Pru p 3), and subsequently have been termed pan-allergens, with cross-reactive homologs having been found in other fruits such as apple (Mal d 3) and grape (Vit v 1), together with vegetables such as asparagus, cabbage (Bra o 3) and lettuce. It is not clear whether peach is the initial sensitizing allergen and that other allergies to fruits develop as a

consequence of IgE-cross-reactivity, in a manner akin to the development of Bet v 1 -related allergies (see above); whether each different type of LTP is able to sensitize via the gastrointestinal tract; or whether there is a 'missing' inhalant allergen, such as another LTP in pollen.

A third group of relevant fruit allergens are those involved in the latex–fruit cross-reactive allergy syndrome, which include the class I chitinases. Several allergens have been described from a variety of plant foods, including avocado (Pers a 1), banana (Mus p 1.2) and chestnut (Cas s 1). Other allergens involved in IgE cross-reactive allergies between foods and latex include patatin, a storage protein from potato that has also been shown to be cross-reactive with the latex allergen Hev b 7, along with other proteins from avocado and banana. Efforts to reduce the burden of latex allergy by, for example, reducing the use of powdered latex gloves by health professionals in particular, may ultimately reduce the prevalence of such latex-related food allergies, although this will need verifying in future.

An increasingly important allergenic fruit is kiwi, which contains several representatives of minor plant food allergen families, including a thaumatin-like protein (TLP, Act d 2), and a thiol protease, actinidin (Act c 1), together with allergens such as kiwellin. Other less widely found fruit and vegetable allergens include germin-like proteins, which have been identified as allergens in bell pepper and orange pips (Cit s 1) and for which the N-linked glycans have been found to be important for IgE binding. Fruit seed storage proteins corresponding to the 7S and 11S seed storage globulins have also been identified as allergens in tomato. Another type of allergen identified in celery root is the flavin adenine dinucleotide (FAD)-containing oxidase (Api g 5), a 53–57 kDa protein which is extensively glycosylated, posesses cross-reactive glycans and, albeit able to bind IgE, does not seem to be able to stimulate histamine release.

As the major allergens are pathogenesis-related proteins, their level of expression changes in plants in response to abiotic stress and pathogen attack, and changes during the process of fruit ripening and post-harvest storage. Thus, the levels of LTP allergens in fruit such as apple (Mal d 3) tend to be higher in freshly picked fruit but decrease during storage, whereas the levels of Bet v 1 homologs (Mal d 1) tend to be lower in freshly picked apples and to increase following modified-atmosphere storage for several months. Processing also affects the allergenic properties of allergens in fruits and vegetables in different ways, and it seems that different fruit tissues may respond in different fashions. Thus, for allergens such as Bet v 1 homologs, for which the IgE-binding sites are generally conformational in nature, processing procedures that denature this protein generally result in a loss of IgE reactivity, and this is particularly true of fresh fruits, although the allergenic Bet v 1 homolog from celeriac seems to retain its allergenic activity after thermal processing. The Bet v 1 homologs also tend to be labile to gastrointestinal digestion, although there are suggestions that whereas IgE epitopes may be destroyed, the short peptides resulting from gastrointestinal digestion maybe able to act as T-cell epitopes and hence may modulate immune responses, even if not involved in elicitation.

In contrast, allergens from the prolamin superfamily appear to be both resistant to thermal processing procedures and highly resistant to gastric and duodenal digestion. Notable among these are the LTPs, which are generally highly resistant to both gastric and duodenal proteases, and it seems likely that they survive digestion in a virtually intact form, a property that has been associated with their allergenic potency. They also resist thermal denaturation, often refolding on cooling, and have been found in fermented foods and beverages such as beer (where they make an important contribution to foam stability) and wines, although combinations of low pH and heating may be sufficient to denature the protein. Similarly, TLPs appear to be stable to thermal processing, being found even in highly processed products such as wine, and being highly resistant to simulated gastrointestinal digestion. Thus the allergenic TLP from kiwi fruit is highly resistant to simulated gastrointestinal proteolysis, and the stability of TLPs to food processing is shown by the presence of allergenic grape TLPs surviving the vinification process and being found in wine. It is likely that the rigidity of the protein scaffold introduced by intramolecular disulfide bonds is responsible for the stability of allergens such as LTPs, and TLPs are probably reponsible for their stability to proteolysis. Similarly, the intramolecular disulfide bonds in the chitin-binding domain class I chitinases may confer stability, although the allergenic homolog from avocado, Pers a 1, is extensively degraded when subjected to simulated gastric fluid digestion. However, the resulting peptides, particularly those corresponding to the hevein-like domain, were clearly reactive both in vitro and in vivo.

Tree nuts and seeds

The major allergens of tree nuts and seeds include other members of the prolamin superfamily, the 2S albumins and the cupin seed globulins, both of which often function as a protein store in the seed. 2S albumins have been identified as important allergens in nuts, including walnut allergen (Jug r 1), almond, Brazil nut (Ber e 1), hazelnut and pistachio (Pis v 1) and in seeds such as oriental and yellow mustard (Bra j 1) and (Sin a 1), Ses i 1 and 2 from sesame, and the 2S albumin from sunflower seeds (SFA-8). These allergens seem to be highly potent and may well dominate allergic responses to many nuts and seeds. In addition to the 2S albumins, a second major group of allergens found in nuts and seeds are the 11S and 7S seed storage globulins that belong to the cupin superfamily. Seed storage protein allergens have been described in a variety of nuts and seeds, with both 11S and 7S seed storage globulins having been reported as allergens in hazelnut (Cor a 11 [7S globulin] and Cor a 9 [11S globulin]), cashew nut (Ana o 1 and Ana o 2) pistachio (Pis v 2 and Pis v 3), walnut (Jug r 2 and Jug r 4), and sesame seed (Ses i 1, Ses i 6). The 11S globulins have also been shown to be allergens in almond, also known as almond major protein (AMP) and mustard (Sin a 2). The close botanical relatedness of species such as cashew and pistachio and the high levels of homology between the major allergens in these tree nuts explain the cross-reactive nature of allergies to these nuts. There are suggestions that conformational epitopes exist in these proteins, which are also responsible for IgE cross-reactivity between allergens from species where homologies are weaker. However, it is difficult to distinguish between polysensitization and cross-reactivity.

In addition to the pollen–fruit cross-reactive allergy syndromes, it is emerging that Bet v 1 homologs in various nuts and seeds can cause similar allergies. These have been especially well documented for hazelnut, where an isoform, Cor a 1.04, has been identified which resembles Bet v 1 more closely than the allergenic Bet v 1 homolog from hazelnut pollen (Cor a 1.01). There are also reports of LTPs found in nuts and seeds triggering allergies similar to those observed in fruits such as peach, including LTP allergens from walnut (Jug r

3) and hazelnut (Cor a 8), the latter having recently been shown to be an allergen in a population from Northern Europe.

Another group of potentially important allergens that have been identified in the last few years are the oleosins, a group of proteins associated with oil bodies, where they play an important role in packaging and stabilizing the oil droplet surface, having a portion of the protein structure buried in the oil phase and a second domain on the aqueous facing surface. These have been identified as allergens in sesame and hazelnut. The effects of cooking and food processing tend to mirror those observed for fruit and legume allergies, with, in general, cooking reducing the reactivity of Bet v 1 type allergens but having much less of an effect on allergens from the prolamin superfamily, such as LTPs and 2S albumins.

Legumes, including peanut

Many of the allergen types found in other plant foods have also been identified in allergenic legumes. They include allergenic homologs of the cupins, with both the 7S and 11S seed storage globulins having been identified in peanut, and are known as Ara h 1 (conarachin) and Ara h 3 (arachin), respectively. Ara h 1 is N-glycosylated during synthesis in the peanut seed and is recognized by IgE from individuals with glycan-reactive IgE, but it is thought that this is not clinically significant in eliciting an allergic reaction. Although generally thought to be less of a problematic allergenic food than peanut, similar allergens are found in soybean, with the 7S globulin β-conglycinin and 11S globulin glycinin being termed allergens Gly m 5 and 6, and appearing to be markers of more severe allergy to soybean, although in this study the majority of individuals with soybean allergy also had allergy to peanut.

The most potent allergen in peanuts is the prolamin superfamily 2S albumin, Ara h 2, 6 and 7, respectively. Intriguingly, although 2S albumins are found in soybean, they do not appear to be major allergens in this legume. Allergenic seed storage proteins have been identified as allergens in lentil (Len c 1) and pea (Pis s 1), which can be cross-reactive with peanut. Such cross-reactivity is particularly problematic with lupin, with both the 7S and the 11S seed storage globulins, known as β-conglutin and α-conglutin, respectively, having been identified as allergens, lupin β-conglutin (Lup an 1) having been designated the major allergen.

Both proteins have significant homology to the peanut allergens Ara h 1 and Ara h ¾, explaining the clinical cross-reactivity observed between these two legumes.

Bet v 1 homologs and profilins involved in the cross-reactive pollen syndromes have been identified in a number of legumes, the most important being the peanut Bet v 1 homologs known as Ara h 8, along with peanut profiling. The Bet v 1 homolog from soybean, known as Gly m 4, albeit more generally associated with mild symptoms, can occasionally be associated with particularly severe reactions, the differences in potency possibly being explained in part, at least, by the extent of food processing.

Other allergens identified in peanut include an oleosin and a lectin, peanut agglutinin. Several other soybean allergens have been described including a Kunitz trypsin inhibitor and a member of the cysteine protease family, the 34 kD so-called oil body-associated protein, known as Gly m 1, and Glym Bd 30 k. Another soybean allergen which is of relevance in countries such as Japan is the 23 kDa protein known as Gly m 28 k, which is glycosylated and contains important IgE-reactive glycans also found in a derived 23 kDa peptide.

In general, the vicilin-like and legumin-like seed globulins both exhibit a high degree of thermostability, requiring temperatures in excess of 70°C for denaturation. The globulins have a high propensity to form large aggregates on heating, which is widely exploited in legume food ingredients such as flours and isolates, to generate a diverse range of foods. These aggregated protein structures appear to a large degree to retain, their native secondary structures. The allergenic 2S albumin allergens are even more thermostable than the globulin allergens. A consequence of so many thermostable allergens is that legumes retain their allergenicity after cooking, and it appears that, for peanut at least, modification by sugars to produce Maillard adducts may even enhance the allergenic potential of peanut allergens. However, processes such as boiling result in the loss of globulins from peanuts and lentils into the cooking water, and may in part account for observations that boiled peanuts appear less allergenic than their roasted counterparts.

Despite such thermostability, the 7S globulins are highly susceptible to pepsinolysis, although several lower molecular weight polypeptides seem to persist following digestion of the peanut 7S globulin allergen Ara h 1, and there is evidence they still possess IgE-binding sites following proteolysis. Similarly, in vitro simulated gastrointestinal digestion results in rapid and almost complete degradation of the protein to relatively small polypeptides, although these retain their allergenic properties. There are indications that the peptides do not remain monomeric but can assemble into larger structures, and it may be that this propensity to aggregate is responsible for the protein retaining its allergenic properties even when hydrolyzed. In contrast, the 2S albumins, like the structurally related LTPs, are relatively resistant to simulated gastrointestinal proteolysis. Such factors may account for the allergenic potency of these prolamin superfamily members.

Cereals

In addition to triggering the gluten-induced enteropathy celiac disease, wheat and other cereals can trigger IgE-mediated allergies, although the condition is as widespread as allergies to foods such as egg and peanut, despite a public perception that wheat allergy is prominent. Cereals, and in particular wheat, can trigger allergic conditions such as atopic dermatitis and exercise-induced anaphylaxis (EIA), where patients only experience an allergic reaction on exercising within a certain interval after eating a problem food.

The main seed storage proteins of cereals, known as seed storage prolamins, are highly heterogeneous, and in wheat comprise a mixture of 60–100 polypeptides. They have the relic of the conserved disulfide skeleton of the prolamin superfamily into which a repetitive domain of variable length, composed largely of glutamine and proline residues, has been inserted. The proteins are characteristically soluble in aqueous alcohols and include two major fractions, the monomeric gliadins soluble in dilute acetic acid or 70% (v/v) ethanol, and polymeric glutenins, which require the presence of reducing agent and 25% propanol for solubility. This lack of solubility in dilute salt solutions, such as those commonly used in clinical diagnostics, makes the diagnosis of wheat and cereal allergies more complicated and may mean that such allergies go undiagnosed or even missed. A number of prolamin allergens have been described, including the monomeric γ-, α- and ω-5 gliadins and the polymeric high molecular weight and low molecular weight subunits of glutenin. Of these, the ω-5 gliadin has been described as being a marker for more severe exercise-induced allergic reactions to wheat. As well as the poorly soluble seed storage prolamins, the water- and salt-soluble albumins and globulins can also act as allergens, notably other members of the prolamin superfamily. Thus, several different forms of the cereal trypsin/α-amylase family have been identified as inhalant and food allergens in wheat and other cereal foods such as rice. Furthermore, the LTPs have been described as allergens in foods such as maize, spelt and wheat (Tri a 14).

Cooking appears to affect the allergenicity of all the cereal allergens, and it has been suggested that baking may be essential for the allergenicity of cereal prolamins with indications being that IgE binding proteins in cereals resist digestion to a greater extent after baking. There do appear to be differences in the responsiveness of allergens to cooking by the same protein from different plant species. Thus, wheat LTP unfolds at a slightly lower temperature than maize LTP (60° as opposed to 75°C), and cooking reduces the IgE-binding capacity of wheat LTP in some patients and not others. In contrast, maize LTP appears highly resistant, its allergenic activity being unaffected by cooking, like that of the α-amylase inhibitors. It is interesting to note that barley LTP, which is structurally closer to wheat than maize LTP, unfolds following extensive heating such as is employed in wort boiling, but that on cooling a proportion remains irreversibly denatured, the remainder refolding to the native structure. This may explain why some individuals react to LTP remaining in beer after brewing, where it probably plays an important role in foam stabilization.

Allergens in diagnosis and treatment of food allergies

Currently the gold standard for diagnosis of food allergy remains double blind placebo controlled food challenge, although frequently diagnosis is performed based on clinical history together with food specific serum IgE and/or a positive skin prick test. Whilst easier to perform these tests currently only assess whether an individual is sensitised (i.e. have food specific IgE) but it is known that many of these individuals do not necessarily express a clinical reaction on exposure to the food they are sensitised to – often in up to 50% of cases. One way of improving the specificity and sensitivity of in vitro diagnostics, such as serum IgE tests, maybe to use individual purified allergens rather than relying on crude food extracts. This has given rise to the term component resolved diagnosis, with purified authenticated allergens being used either in classical formats, such as the ImmunoCAP, or more recently using microarray technology where minute quantities of individual allergens are spotted onto a solid support – often a glass slide. Such "chip" based diagnostics have advantages in using relatively small volumes of serum but provide a much more complex readout for the clinician to understand. For example, given the IgE cross-reactivity of allergenic parvalbumins from many fish species, is it sufficient to test only for IgE towards one representative parvalbumin molecule such as Gad c 1? Similarly could a representative shellfish allergen, such as the tropomyosin allergen Pen a 1 provide diagnosis for all crustacean shellfish allergies? There are indications that sensitisation to tropomyosin is an effective marker of shrimp allergy and may offer superior diagnostic efficiency compared to total shrimp IgE and skin testing. However, whether tropomyosin from one shrimp species can be used as a diagnostic marker for allergy to either all crustacean species and/or molluscan shellfish allergy, remains to be proven. It is also emerging that the peanut 2S albumin allergens Ara h 2 and Ara h 6 are important indicators of clinical allergy to peanut. The patterns of reactivity to particular molecules can show a geographic distribution and has been well characterised for allergies to fruit such as apple for which Bet v 1 homologue sensitisation appears to dominate in Northern Europe whilst LTP sensitisation being more relevant in the Mediterranean area. This may mean that component resolved approaches need to take account of such factors, and whilst sensitisation to the LTP allergen from peach, Pru p 3, is highly likely to have a diagnostic utility in Mediterranean populations, its usefulness remains to be established in other populations where the relationship between sensitisation to LTP and clinical allergy remains to be defined. Thus, component resolved approaches have great potential to improve diagnosis of allergy but are in their infancy and require further validation to assess the robustness and utility in different populations.

In addition to improving the sensitivity and specificity of *in vitro* diagnostics for food allergy, our greater knowledge of allergens is also being used to improve the treatment of food allergy. Currently the major treatment for food allergy involves individuals avoiding their problem food, and for those with a history of severe allergies, they are equipped with rescue medication in case of accidental exposure. As a consequence of societies increasing reliance on prepackaged and processed foods, allergenic ingredients may not always been apparent, making reading of food labels a way of life for food allergic consumers. However, these strategies can fail, and as a result food allergy is a significant cause of anaphylaxis, one of the main causes of emergency admissions to hospital, and which can result in fatalities. To date the most effective treatment which comes closest to a cure is allergen-specific immunotherapy (SIT) but it has not been successfully applied to food allergy because anaphylactic side-effects are too numerous and severe. One strategy which is now being applied to improve the utility of SIT for food allergy is modify the allergen in such way that its decreased IgE-binding capacity, and hence its potency to elicit and allergic reaction, is significantly, reduced. Through a knowledge of the molecular basis of allergenic activity allergenic molecules are being redesigned to retain their immunological activity at the level of the T-cell (and hence retain their capacity to desensitise and individual) whilst reducing adverse reactions by modiying their IgE-epitopes. Some examples where this has been attempted are the humanization of the tropomyosin from shrimp, known as Pen a 1 and produce mutant fish parvalbumin molecules which are hypoallergenic yet may retain their ability to desensitise.

Conclusion

The last decade has seen a rapid increase in our knowledge of the molecules in foods that cause and trigger allergic reactions. They appear to be restricted to a small number of protein families, but we still do not understand why certain protein and protein scaffolds dominate the landscape of allergen structures. Indications are that the relationships between protein structure and allergenicity are very subtle, and for food proteins are further complicated by relatively poorly understood processing-induced changes. Such effects may modulate the allergenicity of food proteins, and may either reduce or increase the allergenic activity of individual molecules, different protein structures responding in different ways. Investigating the factors that modulate the allergenicity of proteins is a research challenge for the coming years, and will require studies on allergen structure and properties to be linked with studies in animal models and clinical research. This is important if we are to realize the potential of new diagnostic approaches, such as component resolved diagnosis, as well as identifying processing strategies and novel processing techniques that may reduce the allergenicity of foods. It will also require clinicians and allied health professionals to have a deeper knowledge of the impact food-processing procedures may have on the allergenicity of foods, and the molecules responsible for them. Such knowledge will enable health professionals to provide patients with the knowledge they need to avoid problems foods effectively.

Bibliography

General references about allergens and allergen structure

Breiteneder H, Mills ENC. Molecular properties of food allergens. J Allergy Clin Immunol 2005;115:14–23; quiz 24.

Radauer C, Bublin M, Wagner S, et al. Allergens are distributed into few protein families and possess a restricted number of biochemical functions. J Allergy Clin Immunol 2008;121(4):847–52.

Chapman MD, Pomés A, Breiteneder H, et al. Nomenclature and structural biology of allergens. J Allergy Clin Immunol 2007;119(2):414–20.

EFSA Panel on Genetically Modified Organisms (GMO). Scientific Opinion on the assessment of allergenicity of GM plants and microorganisms and derived food and feed. EFSA Journal 2010;8(7):1700. [168 pp.]. doi:10.2903/j.efsa.2010.1700.

Salcedo G, Sánchez-Monge R, Barber D, et al. Plant non-specific lipid transfer proteins: an interface between plant defence and human allergy. Biochim Biophys Acta 2007;1771(6):781–91.

Mills EN, Jenkins J, Marigheto N, et al. Allergens of the cupin superfamily. Biochem Soc Trans 2002;30(Pt 6):925–9.

Fötisch K, Vieths S. N- and O-linked oligosaccharides of allergenic glycoproteins. Glycoconj J 2001;18:373–90.

Effects of food processing on allergens

Mills ENC, Sancho AI, Rigby NM, et al. Impact of food processing on the structural and allergenic properties of food allergens. Mol Nutr Food Res 2009;53(8): 963–9.

Maleki SJ, Hurlburt BK. Structural and functional alterations in major peanut allergens caused by thermal processing. J AOAC Int 2004;87(6):1475–9.

Nowak-Wegrzyn A, Fiocchi A. Rare, medium, or well done? The effect of heating and food matrix on food protein allergenicity. Curr Opin Allergy Clin Immunol 2009; 9(3):234–7.

Animal food allergens
Cow's milk:

Wal JM. Structure and function of milk allergens. Allergy 2001;56(Suppl 67):35–8.

Egg:

Mine Y, Yang M. Recent advances in the understanding of egg allergens: basic, industrial, and clinical perspectives. J Agric Food Chem 2008;56(13): 4874–900.

Fish and Shellfish:

Lopata AL, Lehrer SB. New insights into seafood allergy. Curr Opin Allergy Clin Immunol 2009;9(3):270–7.

Lopata AL, O'Hehir RE, Lehrer SB. Shellfish allergy. Clin Exp Allergy 2010;(6):850–8.

Taylor SL. Molluscan shellfish allergy. Adv Food Nutr Res 2008;54:139–77.

Plant food allergens
Fresh fruits and vegetables:

Egger M, Mutschlechner S, Wopfner N, et al. Pollen-food syndromes associated with weed pollinosis: an update from the molecular point of view. Allergy 2006;61(4): 461–76.

Fernández-Rivas M, Benito C, González-Mancebo E, et al. Allergies to fruits and vegetables. Pediatr Allergy Immunol 2008;19(8):675–81.

Peanut, Soybean and other legumes

L'Hocine L, Boye JI. Allergenicity of soybean: new developments in identification of allergenic proteins, cross-reactivities and hypoallergenization technologies. Crit Rev Food Sci Nutr 2007;47(2):127–43.

Tree nuts:

Roux KH, Teuber SS, Sathe SK. Tree nut allergens. Int Arch Allergy Immunol 2003;131(4):234–44.

Wheat:

Battais F, Richard C, Jacquenet S, et al. Wheat grain allergies: an update on wheat allergens. Eur Ann Allergy Clin Immunol 2008;40(3):67–76.

Tatham AS, Shewry PR. Allergens to wheat and related cereals. Clin Exp Allergy 2008;38(11):1712–26.

Allergens in diagnosis and treatment of food allergies

Sommergruber K, Mills ENC, Vieths S. Coordinated and standardized production, purification and characterization of natural and recombinant food allergens to establish a food allergen library. Mol Nutr Food Res 2008;52(S2):S159–S165.

Asero R, Ballmer-Weber BK, Beyer K, et al. IgE-mediated food allergy diagnosis: Current status and new perspectives. Mol Nutr Food Res 2007 Jan;51(1): 135–47.

Sastre J. Molecular diagnosis in allergy. Clin Exp Allergy 2010;40(10):1442–60.

Valenta R, Linhart B, Swoboda I, et al. Recombinant allergens for allergen-specific immunotherapy: 10 years anniversary of immunotherapy with recombinant allergens. Allergy 2011 Feb 26. doi: 10.1111/ j.1398-9995.2011.02565.x

Further reading

Mills ENC, Shewry PR, editors. Plant Food Allergens. Oxford: Blackwells; 2003. p. 219.

Mills ENC, Wichers H, Hoffman-Sommergruber, K, editors. Managing Allergens in Foods. Cambridge UK: Woodhead Publishing; 2007. p. 315.

CHAPTER 3

The Epidemiology of Food Allergy

Katrina J. Allen and Jennifer J. Koplin

KEY CONCEPTS

- Food allergy is on the increase in developed countries, although good-quality prevalence data are lacking.
- Factors contributing to the epidemic appear to be related to the modern lifestyle but as yet are poorly understood.
- The population prevalence of the four most common IgE-mediated food allergies in infancy and childhood by challenge-proven outcomes are approximately: cows' milk (2–3%), egg (1–2%), peanut (1–2%) and tree nuts (<1%), although there is marked heterogeneity in the quality of studies to date.
- The incidence of food allergy-related anaphylaxis, the most severe consequence of food allergy, is rising particularly in the under 4-year age group.
- There is little information about the population prevalence of challenge-proven non-IgE-mediated food allergies.
- Future epidemiological studies should address previous study design deficiencies. For prevalence estimates, population-representational sampling frames should be employed. Appropriate adjustment for potential confounding factors such as family and personal history of allergy, and as genetic markers become available, genetic predisposition, will be critical to understanding risk factors for the development of food allergy.

Introduction

Childhood food allergy is an evolving public health problem that appears to have risen rapidly in industrialized countries.[1] Despite an increasing number of studies mounted to investigate the rise of both allergic disease in general and food allergy in particular, the cause of the epidemic of food allergy remains elusive.

It is estimated that about a quarter of the population will have an adverse reaction to food (of which food allergy is just one type) during their lifetime,[2] most of which will occur during infancy and early childhood. An estimated 10–15% of children report symptoms of food allergy, although the prevalence of IgE-mediated food allergies (i.e. symptoms of food allergy in the context of a positive skin prick test) is reported to be lower, at approximately 6–8% in children under 3 years and 3–4 % of the adult population.[3] By contrast, not much is known about the prevalence of non-IgE-mediated food allergies, although both eosinophilic esophagitis and celiac disease have been documented to be increasing.[4,5]

There has been a significant increase in public awareness of food allergies, with broad media attention, owing to the concerning increase in the prevalence of both food allergy and its most serious manifestation, anaphylaxis. However, some medical practitioners remain skeptical about the role of food allergies in a number of clinical syndromes, such as atopic dermatitis, colic and gastroesophageal reflux in infancy, despite an increasing body of evidence that food allergy can contribute to these conditions.[6]

How do we define and measure food allergy?

As outlined in Chapter 4, food allergy is defined as an abnormal immunologic response to food proteins resulting in an adverse clinical reaction, and can be broadly divided in to two types: those that are mediated by food-specific immunoglobulin class E (IgE) antibodies and those that are not. Of the two, much more is known about IgE-mediated than non-IgE-mediated food allergy. More than 90% of IgE-mediated food allergies in children are caused by just eight food items: cows' milk, soy, hen's egg, peanuts, tree nuts, wheat, fish and shellfish. Most children with cows' milk and egg allergy develop tolerance by late childhood, but allergies to peanut, sesame seeds and tree nuts are more persistent, with less than 20% developing tolerance.[7] As a result, cows' milk and egg allergies are uncommon in adults and allergies to peanuts, tree nuts, fish and shellfish predominate.

There have been many studies in the past few decades suggesting that food allergy is over-reported by individuals.[8] There are many reasons for this. Symptoms of food intolerance may be mistaken for food-allergic symptoms, or poorly defined symptom complexes such as recurrent abdominal pain, chronic fatigue or attention deficit hyperactivity disorder may be attributed to allergic reactions to food even where there is no evidence to support such contentions. Furthermore, although there are well-described diagnostic criteria for IgE-mediated food allergies (i.e. evidence of an acute allergic reaction, either through history or food challenge, in the context of positive IgE antibodies to the food in question), non-IgE-mediated food allergies can be difficult to accurately diagnose and depend for the most part on elimination–rechallenge sequences performed in the home environment. As such, any study on the prevalence of food allergy needs to be contextualized by the outcome used to define the condition. Table 3.1 outlines the strengths and limitations of various study methodologies employed to measure prevalence.

Ideally, studies of the prevalence of IgE-mediated food allergy use double-blind placebo-controlled

Table 3.1 Strengths and weaknesses of various study design and outcome methodology for the assessment of food allergy prevalence

Outcome	Strengths	Limitations
DBPCFC	'gold standard' for diagnosis	Expensive, time-consuming, risk of anaphylaxis in allergic individuals, usually has fairly low compliance rate
Open food challenges	Less time-consuming, likely to have improved compliance rates compared with DBPCFC	Difficult to confirm whether delayed or subjective symptoms are due to food ingestion without the use of a placebo arm
	Likely to be accurate for detecting immediate objective symptoms of allergy	Risk of anaphylaxis in allergic individuals
Self or parent-report alone	Inexpensive, no risk of adverse reaction in the allergic individual, expect high compliance rates	Known over-reporting of allergy by individuals
		Individuals can be allergic to a food even in the absence of previous overt exposure to that food – no information on food allergy for these individuals
Food-specific IgE antibodies (SPT or blood test)	Blood test poses no risk of allergic reaction even in highly allergic individuals	Using low threshold to define sensitivity – will overestimate proportion with true allergy
	SPT relatively non-invasive	Using high threshold to define sensitivity – will miss some allergic individuals with lower levels
Self- or parent-report + food-specific IgE antibodies	Improved accuracy compared with report of symptoms or food-specific IgE antibodies alone	Possible to have detectable levels of IgE antibodies in the absence of previous overt exposure to a food – unclear whether these individuals would react on ingestion

food challenges (DBPCFC) – the gold standard for the diagnosis of IgE-mediated food allergy. Because this procedure is expensive, time-consuming, poses a small risk of food challenge induced-anaphylaxis to the individual and generally has low compliance rates among study participants, a number of alternative methods have been used in epidemiological studies. These include open food challenges without the use of a placebo arm, and self- or parent-reporting of acute (and usually objective) allergic symptoms, sometimes combined with measurement of levels of IgE specific to food allergens. Open food challenges pose the same level of risk as DBPCFC but are less time-consuming and therefore might achieve better compliance, but are best limited to studies of younger study participants (e.g. less than 2 years of age) as patient-reported subjective symptoms are not likely to compromise the challenge outcome. Both self-reported and parent-reported food allergies are likely to overestimate true food allergy.

Although a number of publications have described in detail the methodology of food challenge protocols, it is rather surprising that without exception none have clearly delineated beforehand which particular symptoms constitute a positive versus a negative challenge. Although most protocols state that a positive challenge is demonstrated by evidence of an immediate reaction consistent with IgE-mediated food allergy such as urticaria, angioedema or anaphylaxis, none recommend how to interpret more subjective symptoms such as abdominal pain or nausea, or the more ubiquitous and less clearly defined sign of an eczema flare. Nor are there published guidelines regarding the interpretation of a small number of transient urticarias during a challenge. As such, challenge-proven outcomes, albeit the gold standard, may also be limited by interpretative differences between studies.

CLINICAL CASE

An 11-year-old girl was first diagnosed with peanut allergy at the age of 2 years following an acute allergic reaction to a bite of a peanut butter sandwich. Within minutes of ingestion she developed facial angioedema and generalized urticaria, which resolved spontaneously over the next several hours. She was referred to an allergist for assessment, where a history was obtained and confirmation of an IgE-mediated peanut allergy was made in the context of a large positive skin prick test wheal 15 mm in size (and a negative saline control). The child had concurrent asthma and was prescribed an adrenaline

(epinephrine) autoinjector, with advice about allergen avoidance and a demonstration about how and when to use adrenaline. She was monitored every 1–2 years with serial skin prick tests. At ages 3, 5 and 7 years her SPT remained elevated above 8 mm. However, at age 9 her SPT was 6 mm and at 11 it had fallen to 4 mm. She had not had any accidental ingestion reactions to peanut since her initial diagnosis. At the age of 11, when her SPT was 4 mm, an oral food challenge was recommended which was DBPCFC. The girl developed nausea and mouth tingling with the second dose of the placebo arm, but then went on to successfully tolerate the allergen arm and is now tolerant to peanuts.

A further limitation of even the small number of studies that have conducted formal graded food challenges is that they have not addressed the question of whether study participants are representative of the population from which they were sampled. The generalizability of their results may therefore be poor. Although many cohort studies are plagued by low participation, one problem which is particular to studies of allergy is the tendency for families at high risk of disease to be over-represented among participants. The extent to which this type of selection bias may affect results is rarely formally assessed, although recent cohort studies of food allergy have begun to address this using short questionnaires to assess the prevalence of risk factors for allergy among those who do not wish to undergo testing for food allergy.[9]

Owing to the difficulties associated with performing large-scale studies of challenge-proven food allergy, many population-based prevalence studies have relied on the indirect marker of food-specific IgE-antibodies. Methods used to detect the presence of IgE specific to food allergens include skin prick testing (SPT) or in vitro measurement of food allergen-specific IgE using the CAP-fluoroenzyme immunoassay (CAP-FEIA) or radioallergosorbent test (RAST). For these three methods, individuals are declared to have tested positive if the size of the wheal (SPT) or measured IgE level (CAP-FEIA or RAST) exceeds a prespecified threshold. Such individuals are said to be 'sensitized' to the food being studied, but confirmation of food allergy at least requires symptomatic ingestion of the food. However, at least 50% of individuals with a positive SPT have confirmed food allergy by formal food challenge, and if higher cut-off wheal sizes are used it is possible to increase the proportion of those above the threshold wheal size with food allergy to >95%.[10] Similar positive predictive values for serological food-specific IgE antibodies have also been published.[11]

Even the most severe consequence of food allergy, anaphylaxis, is limited by varying opinions on what constitutes anaphylaxis. Although variations in definition may not significantly affect clinical care, problems arise when attempting to determine the population prevalence of this condition. Several classification systems have been used; however, a recent consensus document has defined anaphylaxis as a 'serious allergic reaction that is rapid in onset and may cause death', and proposed diagnostic criteria for use in clinical care.[12] According to these criteria, a diagnosis of anaphylaxis can be made if there is involvement of the respiratory or cardiovascular systems during an allergic reaction; or if a less severe reaction occurs in the setting of previously diagnosed allergy and likely exposure to the relevant allergen.

What is the current prevalence of food allergy?

Because of the difficulties in measuring food allergy, discussed above, the true prevalence has been difficult to establish. Existing studies of the incidence, prevalence and natural history of food allergy are difficult to compare owing to inconsistencies and deficiencies in study design and variations in the definition of food allergy. Although over 170 foods have been reported to cause IgE-mediated reactions, most prevalence studies have focused only on the eight most common food allergens, as these account for more than 90% of presentations to allergists.

Rona et al.[8] assessed data from 51 publications and provided separate analyses for the prevalence of food allergy for five common foods (cows' milk, hen's egg, peanut, fish and shellfish), stratified by whether the studies were in adults or children. The investigators report a pooled overall prevalence of self-reported food allergy (Fig. 3.1a) for adults and children of 13% and 12%, respectively, to any of these five foods. However, pooled results are far lower (about 3%) when food allergy is defined as either sensitization alone, sensitization with symptoms (Fig. 3.1b), or positive double-blind, placebo-controlled food challenge (Fig. 3.1c). This difference between reported food allergy and food allergy assessed by objective measures confirms that such allergies are over-reported by patients, and that objective measurements are necessary to establish a true food allergy diagnosis.

CLINICAL CASE

A 2-year-old boy presented with intermittent constipation that commenced at around 12 months of age when he was converted from cows' milk formula to fresh cows' milk. He had been exclusively breastfed until 6 months of age, at which point he was started on solids and weaned on to cows' milk formula. He had not had colic, reflux, constipation or other gastrointestinal symptoms in the first 12 months of life. Further questioning elicited that he had developed an acute episode of fever and vomiting around 12 months of age, and the constipation had developed within days of that episode. The patient's mother had recently started the child on soy milk, with little change in bowel habit. Upon presentation to the allergist a history was elicited that suggested that the constipation was highly unlikely to be related to cows' milk allergy. A skin prick test to cows' milk was negative, and 1 month of stool softeners was prescribed plus a cows' milk-free diet. The parents were then advised to cease the stool softener and reintroduce cows' milk into the diet, and to return for review if the constipation recurred. The parents telephoned to inform the allergist that the child's constipation had resolved and not recurred when milk was reintroduced.

Two recent cohort studies from the UK and Denmark reported that the foods most often responsible for symptoms of food allergy in infants and young children were egg, cows' milk and peanuts. In the Danish study, the prevalence of egg and milk allergy both reached a peak at around 18 months of age, at 2.4% and 1.0% for egg and milk, respectively, with around 20% becoming tolerant to egg by 3 years and 100% becoming tolerant to milk by 6 years of age.[13] In a recent Australian study, the prevalence of challenge-proven peanut allergy at 1 year of age was 3%, sesame allergy 0.8% and raw egg allergy 8.9%.[14]

Both prevalence figures and the spectrum of food allergens appear to vary considerably between geographical regions, and are thought to reflect variations in diet between different cultures. Alternatively, some of the differences in food allergy prevalence between regions may be explained by either genetic variation across populations or variations in exposure to environmental factors, such as sunlight (i.e. related to vitamin D levels) or factors related to the hygiene hypothesis (as discussed below).

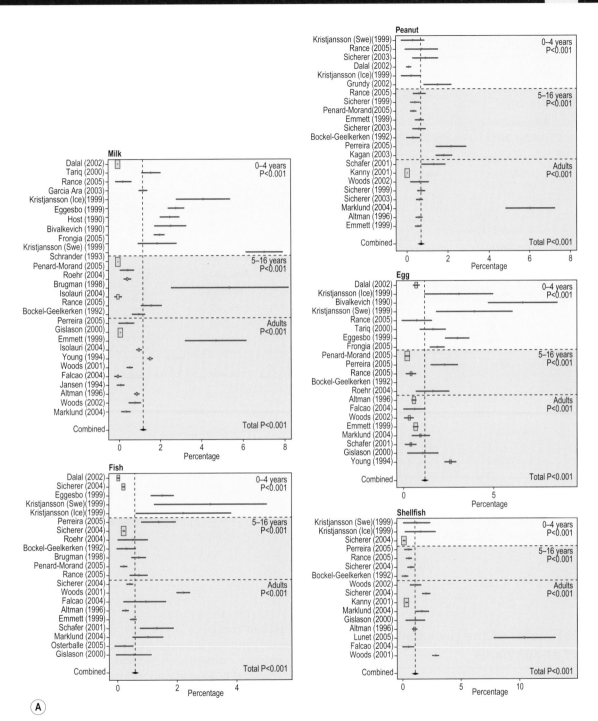

Figure 3.1 Population prevalence of (A) self-reported hypersensitivity to specific foods: peanut, cows' milk, eggs, fish and shellfish, stratified by age; (B) symptomatic food allergy in the context of a positive skin prick test or serological IgE to any food, fish, shellfish, peanuts, cows' milk and egg stratified by age and; (C) the prevalence of challenge-proven allergy to any food, fish, cows' milk, egg. P values indicate level of heterogeneity by age group and total. Reprinted with permission from: Rona RJ, Keil T, Summers C, et al. The prevalence of food allergy: A meta-analysis. J Allergy Clin Immunol 2007; 120: 638–46.

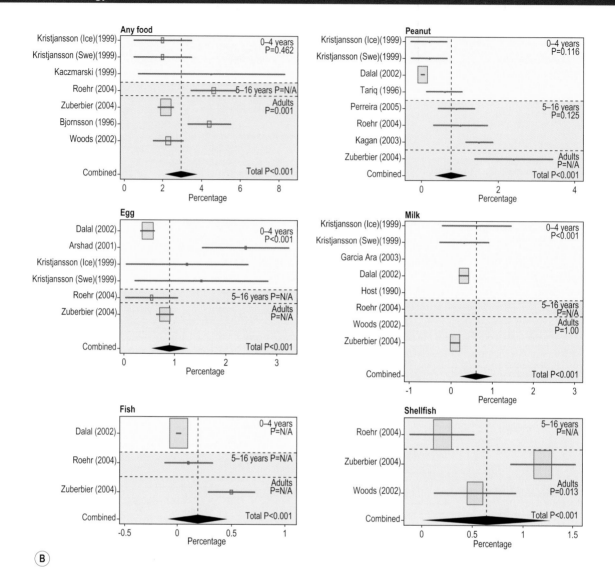

Figure 3.1 *Continued*

Estimates of the prevalence of anaphylaxis

Food allergy is the leading cause of anaphylaxis treated in hospital emergency departments in Western Europe and the United States. The epidemiology of anaphylaxis has recently been reviewed.[15] In the United States, food allergy alone appears to account for approximately 30 000 anaphylactic reactions, 2000 hospitalizations, and an estimated 200 deaths each year. The population prevalence of anaphylaxis has been difficult to quantify owing to

a lack of consensus on the definition of anaphylaxis, analysis of different sample populations (e.g. emergency department presentations, hospital admissions, general practitioner presentations, specialist allergist presentations), and the use of varying methodologies for data collection.

Population studies have estimated the incidence or prevalence of anaphylaxis in Western countries to be in the range of 8–50 per 100 000 person-years, with a lifetime prevalence of 0.05–2.0%. Reported population prevalence rates vary internationally, with studies from the US reporting 49.8 per 100 000 person-years, the UK 8.4 per 100 000 person-years,

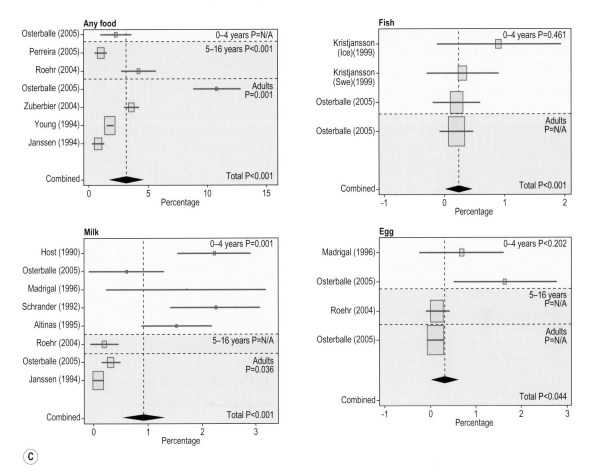

Figure 3.1 *Continued*

and Australia 13 per 100 000 person-years. However, the variation in prevalence rates may reflect differences in sample populations, data collection methods and definitions of anaphylaxis rather than true differences in anaphylaxis rates between countries, as the UK prevalence estimate was derived from a GP database, the US incidence rate was determined from a population cohort in Minnesota, and the Australian minimum incidence of anaphylaxis in the population was estimated based on the number of anaphylaxis cases presenting to an allergy specialist in a captured population. Disparate prevalence rates have also been found in separate studies from the same country, with a second US study reporting a much lower prevalence of anaphylaxis of 10.5 per 100 000 person-years for children and adolescents enrolled at a health maintenance organization.

Anaphylaxis admissions data from national database systems in the UK and Australia revealed a population prevalence of 3.6 per 100 000 (2003/2004) and 8.0 per 100 000 (2004/2005), respectively. The varying prevalence between the two countries may be due to underlying differences in the prevalence of food allergy in general, or more simply to a difference in coding practices between the two types of medical system. Using a statewide administrative database, the rate of anaphylaxis admissions for New Yorkers aged 0–20 years was 4.2 per 100 000. However, these admissions figures are likely to underestimate the true population prevalence of anaphylaxis, as not all presentations will result in hospital admission, and misclassification of the presenting disorder in hospital settings may occur. A review of National Electronic Injury Surveillance System data from 34 participating emergency departments over a 2-month period in 2003 found that 57% of likely anaphylactic events were not assigned an ED diagnosis of anaphylaxis.

Epidemiology of fatal anaphylaxis

Data from national mortality reporting systems in the UK and Australia estimate the prevalence of anaphylaxis fatalities from all causes to be 0.33 deaths per year per million population in the UK,[16] with a higher rate in Australia of 0.64 deaths per year per million population.[17] Fatal episodes of anaphylaxis in the UK were reported to be due to food/possible food in 31% of cases, with the remainder due to medication (44%), insect sting (23%) and other (4%). In contrast, only 6% of anaphylaxis deaths in the Australian study were due to food, with the majority of deaths due to medication/probable medication (57%) and insect sting (18%).

For food anaphylaxis, admissions peaked in males under 5 years of age, whereas deaths occurred predominantly in females aged between 10 and 35 years. Risk factors for a poor outcome from an episode of food-related anaphylaxis include age (risk is highest in adolescents and young adults), peanut or tree nut allergy, coexisting and poorly controlled asthma, posture (failure to be kept in the supine position), lack of access to self-injectable adrenaline, and failure to administer adrenaline in a timely manner. Although never formally investigated, hypothetical reasons for poorer outcomes in the adolescent and young adult age group include increased risk-taking behaviors, issues of transition from parental locus of control, failure to adequately educate young people about the risks of anaphylaxis at the time that they are taking increased responsibility for their own health, and finally an increased prevalence of both asthma and poorly managed asthma in these age groups compared to those under 5 years of age.

Role of race and gender in food allergy

Although gender disparities in the prevalence of some allergic disorders, including allergic asthma, have been well described, the relationship between gender and food allergy is less clear.[18] The relationship between gender and allergy appears to vary by age, with studies of allergic asthma showing that in childhood males are more often affected, whereas in adults the reverse is true. Studies of gender and food allergy are limited, and few have used oral food challenges as the outcome. Of the data that are available, it appears that females are more likely than males to report food allergy in adulthood. Findings in childhood are less clear, with some studies of peanut sensitization and allergy finding a male predominance whereas others found no gender differences.

Similarly, racial/ethnic differences in asthma prevalence have also been well described, although so far there have been very few studies investigating the influence of ethnicity on the likelihood of developing food allergy. One UK study found that non-Caucasian infants were overrepresented in a pediatric food allergy clinic compared to general pediatric clinics.[19] In the US, the 2007 National Health Interview Survey found that non-Hispanic children had higher rates of reported food allergy than Hispanic children.[20]

Is the incidence of food allergy increasing?

The prevalence of IgE-mediated food allergies appears to be increasing in industrialized countries following the previously documented rise in prevalence of other atopic conditions such as asthma, eczema and allergic rhinitis. The paucity of earlier studies on prevalence has precluded a clear evidence base for a rise in food allergy, although there is circumstantial evidence to suggest that it has occurred since the early 1990s.

Recent studies have tried to confirm anecdotal evidence of an increased incidence of peanut allergy. In a UK study, Grundy et al.[21] found an increase in reported peanut allergy from 0.5% to 1.5% in two sequential early childhood cohorts from the same geographic area, surveyed 6 years apart. However, the difference did not reach statistical significance, perhaps due to lack of numbers, or because the number of years between measurement points may have been insufficient to demonstrate an increase in allergy.

Between two United States-wide phone surveys, the prevalence of self-reported peanut and/or tree nut allergy increased from 0.6% to 1.2% between 1997 and 2002 among children, though no change was observed for adults.[1] In a more recent Canadian study, the prevalence of peanut allergy was found to be stable between 2000–2002 (1.63%, 95% CI 1.30–2.02%) and 2005–2007 (1.50%, 95% CI 1.16–1.92%).[22,23] A systematic review by Chafen et al.[24] concluded that it is unclear whether there has been a real rise in food allergy over the last few decades, and estimated that the current prevalence of food allergy in the US, Europe and Australia could be as low as 1% or as high as 10%. Reliable surveillance of allergy prevalence within populations will be required to measure any future increases.

Hospital records have been examined in an attempt to assess the prevalence of more serious allergic reactions. Poulos and colleagues[25] found a continuous increase in the rates of hospital admission for angioedema (3.0% per year), urticaria (5.7% per year), and, importantly, anaphylaxis (8.8% per year), over a 10-year period from 1993. A fivefold increase in food-induced anaphylaxis among children under 5 years was a notable finding, and parallels the findings of population-based prevalence studies.

What is the cause of the rise in incidence of IgE-mediated food allergy?

The reasons for the presumed increase in food allergy prevalence are not known, but the short period over which the increase has occurred suggests that genetic factors alone cannot be causative, as changes to the genome occur at an evolutionary pace. Environmental factors must therefore be central, although these may be mediated through epigenetic modification (as discussed below). It appears that these environmental factors are linked to the 'modern lifestyle', as food allergy is more common in developed than developing countries, and migrants appear to acquire the incident risk of allergy of their adopted country. Although environmental factors, including those associated with the hygiene hypothesis, as well as dietary factors have been found to be associated with the development of eczema and atopy, it is not clear whether these also play a role in the development of food allergy.[26] As well as the factors associated with other atopic diseases, it is likely that there are some food allergy-specific risk factors. These might include change in methods of food preparation, increased use of antacids and proton pump inhibitors, use of medicinal creams containing food allergens, and the later introduction of allergenic foods into the diet of infants.

The 'hygiene' hypothesis

Multiple environmental factors associated with the hygiene hypothesis (i.e., the hypothesis that early exposure to microbial antigens promotes healthy immune development and reduces the risk of developing allergies) have been linked to allergic outcomes such as asthma or allergic sensitization. These include cesarean section delivery, companion animal ownership, exposure to other children (either siblings or through childcare attendance), and exposure to farm animals or domestic pets (Fig. 3.2).

The impact of gastrointestinal flora composition

The composition of the gastrointestinal flora in infancy is affected by various factors, but as the fetal intestine is sterile the initial colonizing events in the infant are likely to be highly important in governing the type of commensal bacteria present in the first few days of life, and possibly longer. The initial colonizing event is likely to be influenced by mode of delivery, with infants delivered by cesarean section having less contact with maternal flora, which acts as a source of intestinal bacteria for the newborn. It has been hypothesized that differences in colonization might lead to an increased risk of allergy among infants born by cesarean section. It is possible that commensal bacteria in the gastrointestinal tract may exert an immunomodulatory effect that leads to tolerance to both the commensal bacteria themselves and also to ingested food allergens. A recent systematic review of the literature identified only two studies that examined the relationship between mode of delivery and food allergy, and a further two used sensitization as the outcome.[27] Of the studies that examined food allergy, one found an increase among infants born by cesarean section only if there was a maternal history of allergy, whereas the second found no difference in food allergy according to mode of delivery. Further studies using objectively confirmed food allergy as the outcome are required to determine whether delivery by cesarean section increases the risk of food allergy.

The 'old friends' hypothesis

Following the initial colonizing events at birth, the infant immune system continues to be exposed to stimulus not only from the commensal bacteria in

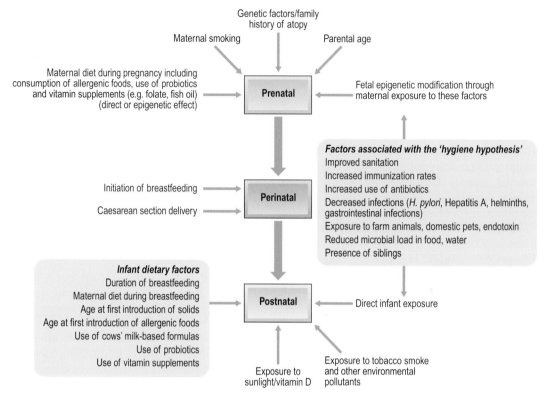

Figure 3.2 Factors potentially associated with risk of IgE-mediated food allergy.

the gastrointestinal tract but also from external sources. The 'old friends' hypothesis states that the immune system evolved at a time of constant exposure to certain organisms in the environment, such as helminths and environmental saprophytes found in food and water. These organisms needed to be tolerated, either because they were harmless and ubiquitous (environmental saprophytes) or because mounting an immune response would damage the host (some helminths). It is thought that continued exposure to these organisms might have caused downregulation of the immune response not only to these organisms but also to self-antigens (autoimmunity) and food allergens (food allergy), possibly through the induction of regulatory T cells. Reduced exposure to these groups of organisms in the modern environment could therefore potentially explain the increase in allergic diseases and autoimmunity.

Other factors associated with a 'modern lifestyle' include myriad changes to our level of public health, including improved sanitation, secure water supplies (with associated decreased prevalence of *Helicobacter pylori* infection), widespread use of antibiotics and increasing rates of immunization, reduced helminthic infestation, improved food quality (and presumably less microbial load in the food chain) as well as generally improved nutrition and associated obesity (Fig. 3.2). These factors might work individually or in concert to cause a failure in the development of oral immune tolerance in the first year of life, when IgE-mediated food allergy is most likely to develop.

These factors have all come into play some time in the last half of the 20th century, and yet the rise in food allergy prevalence appears in the context of the early part of the 21st century. There is strong evidence that environmental exposures play a key role in activating or silencing genes by altering DNA and histone methylation, histone acetylation and chromatin structure. These 'epigenetic' modifications determine the degree of DNA compaction and accessibility for gene transcription. If the hygiene hypothesis is found to be central to the rise of both atopy in general and food allergy more specifically, this effect might be expressed through a delayed generational effect and the impact of maternal epigenetic modification on fetal priming of the immune system. There are now many elegant animal models showing how environmental changes at critical times during development (both in utero and postnatally) can profoundly alter the phenotype of genetically identical animals through epigenetic modification.[28] These effects are currently under investigation in a number of centers throughout the world.

Other changes to the gastrointestinal milieu

The allergenicity of some food allergens is reduced or eliminated when subject to acid pH levels equivalent to those found in the human stomach (pH 1.5–3.0). Untersmayr and colleagues[29] hypothesized that the widespread use of anti-ulcer mediation in the last 20–30 years may have contributed to an increasing prevalence of food allergy. In a study of adult patients they found that 3 months of anti-ulcer therapy resulted in an increase in food-specific IgE in 25% of all treated patients, and there was a boost of pre-existing food-specific IgE in 10%. They concluded that the relative risk for the increase of an IgE response to food allergens after only 3 months of treatment was 10.5. In newborns, the intragastric pH ranges from 6.0 to 8.0. After birth there is a burst of acid secretion, resulting in transient adult gastric pH levels (pH 1.0–3.0) for 24–48 hours. However, after these first days of life gastric acid production remains low and adult pH levels in the stomach are not reached again until the average age of 2 years. It has been suggested that the widespread and increasing use of agents such as proton pump inhibitors in infants with 'colic' in Western populations (for presumed gastroesophageal reflux) may be one of the significant contributory factors of the 'modern lifestyle' resulting in an increased prevalence of allergies.

Similarly, *H. pylori*-associated atrophic gastritis reduces acid secretion. The infection is usually contracted in the first years of life and tends to persist indefinitely if untreated. At least half of the world's human population has *H. pylori* infection, but rates of infection have fallen dramatically in developed countries over the last 20 years for as yet unidentified reasons. Widespread use of antibiotics, improved public hygiene measures and better water quality may all play a role in its decreasing prevalence, which could coincide with the rising prevalence of food allergy.

Following on from this line of thought, the dramatic change over the last 30 years in the timing of introduction of solids from around 3 months of age to after 6 months (as discussed below) could potentially mediate changes in acid secretion and result in changed allergenicity of foods at a critical window of opportunity.

Evidence for change in the timing of introduction of solids and the impact on food allergy prevalence

Along with changes in food quality and a likely decrease in the microbial content of foods, there has also been a trend to delay the age at which foods are introduced to infants. Whereas in the 1960s infants were typically given solid foods in the first 3 months of life, the 1970s saw the introduction of guidelines recommending delayed introduction of solids until after 4 months of age because of a perceived link between the early introduction of gluten and celiac disease. By the late 1990s, expert bodies began to recommend delaying solids until after 6 months of age, with a further delay in the introduction of allergenic foods such as egg and nuts until at least 2 years of age recommended for infants with a family history of allergy. This did not, however, appear to have the desired effect of reducing the prevalence of food allergy, and in 2008, lack of evidence of a protective effect led to the removal of advice to delay the introduction of any foods beyond 4–6 months of age.

Recently, it has been suggested that delayed introduction of allergenic foods may actually prevent the normal development of tolerance, which occurs when foods are introduced during a 'window of opportunity' in early infancy.[28] This is consistent with the observation that Israeli infants are introduced to peanut at a young age, yet Israeli schoolchildren experience a low prevalence of peanut allergy, whereas the opposite is observed in the UK.[30] Of the studies to date investigating the relationship between timing of introduction of allergenic foods and food allergy, only one has controlled for potential confounding factors such as personal and family history of allergy.[31,32] This study found that infants introduced to cooked egg at 4–6 months of age were less likely to have egg allergy at 1 year of age compared to those introduced to egg later.

Randomized controlled trials of the early introduction of allergenic foods are currently under way to clarify the degree to which such an effect may be found in association with the development of food allergies.

Breastfeeding and food allergy

The relationship between breastfeeding and food allergy is currently not clear. Since randomized controlled trials allocating infants to breastfeeding or not breastfeeding are not ethically feasible, evidence is limited to observational studies which have so far shown conflicting results. Like studies of the timing of introduction of foods, observational studies of breastfeeding and food allergy are limited by the possibility of confounding by a family history of allergy or early signs of atopic disease in the infant. Studies of breastfeeding and food allergy are also complicated by the fact that infants can be exclusively breastfed (without the use of supplementary formulas or other foods) or breastfed with supplementary formulas, in which case the amount of breastfeeding compared with formula may vary between individuals. It has also been hypothesized that breastfeeding at the time when foods are introduced into the infant diet, rather than the duration of breastfeeding alone, may be protective against the development of allergy,[28] although this has yet to be confirmed.

The role of genetics in predisposition to food allergy

There is increasing evidence for a strong genetic component to allergies, and particularly food allergy. Twin studies have shown that the concordance rate for peanut allergy was much higher among monozygotic (64.3%) than dizygotic (6.8%, $p < 0.0001$) twin pairs.[33] A recent study of familial aggregation observed the heritability of common food allergies (sesame, peanut, wheat, milk, egg white, soy, walnut, shrimp, cod fish) to be 15–30%.[34]

Food allergy occurs more frequently in infants with eczema. Recently, eczema has been found to be closely associated with defects in skin barrier permeability and loss of function mutations in the filaggrin (FLG) gene. A number of recent studies have linked null mutations (R501X and 2282del4) in FLG with an increased susceptibility to eczema.[35] Individuals with two null alleles in FLG have been shown to be 4–7 times more likely to have eczema than those without.[36] FLG appears to play an essential role in epithelial integrity: a severe breakdown in the function of the protein produced can result in the skin disorder ichthyosis vulgaris. However, it is not known whether defects of FLG and/or other epithelial barrier functions may act independently to increase the risk of food allergy, and no studies to date have investigated the relationship between food allergy and the FLG null mutations. As the most strongly associated genetic factor currently linked to eczema, it will be important to refute or establish a genetic association of FLG variants with food allergy.

Despite many attempts to investigate risk factors for food allergy, few have yet been identified. This may be because population-based studies have not been able to take into account the fact that food allergy is at least partly genetically determined, as the specific genes that confer susceptibility to food allergy remain unknown. Environmental factors that increase the risk of food allergy may act differently depending on genetic risk, an issue which cannot be completely addressed until genetic risk factors for food allergy are identified.

Food allergy and the 'atopic march'

Atopic diseases such as asthma, allergic rhinoconjunctivitis, eczema and food allergy are closely related. Their manifestations often present in a characteristic sequence that has been named the atopic march. The first signs of atopic diseases are usually food allergies and eczema, which have their greatest incidence during the first 3 years of life. In contrast, IgE-mediated responses to environmental allergens, allergic rhinoconjunctivitis and asthma symptoms mostly develop later in life. Infants who develop early symptoms of allergy, such as sensitization to cows' milk or egg, are also more likely to go on to develop sensitization to environmental allergens and asthma.

Despite the delayed onset between allergen exposure and exacerbation, eczema is often associated with IgE-mediated food allergy, and SPT or food-specific serum IgE testing is helpful in predicting a response to the elimination of cows' milk protein and other food allergens. Infants with early-onset eczema (within the first 6 months) of at least moderate severity have a high incidence of food allergies, in particular to egg and cows' milk.

Non-IgE-mediated food allergies

The most common food associated with non IgE-mediated food allergy syndromes is cows' milk. This may be a function of the fact that infants are most likely to present with non-IgE-mediated syndromes at a time when gastrointestinal mucosal integrity is developing, and cows' milk protein is the most common dietary antigen during the first year of life. It is estimated that cows' milk protein-induced allergy occurs in up to 2% of children under the age of 2 years.[6] Most infants with non-IgE-mediated cows' milk protein allergy develop tolerance by the third year of life. Table 3.2 outlines the defining features that distinguish IgE-mediated from non-IgE-mediated food allergies and their associated syndromes.

Enteropathy resulting from cows' milk is one of the better-understood non-IgE-mediated food

allergies. One prospective cohort study of newborns in Denmark found that the incidence of cows' milk protein (CMP) enteropathy was 2.2% over the first year of life, with a high rate of resolution (97%) by 15 years of age.[37] Reports suggest a rapid rise in the prevalence of eosinophilic esophagitis,[38] a condition that was first linked to food allergy in 1995. Celiac disease is also reported to be increasing in prevalence, although there are some suggestions that improved serological screening studies have increased the case finding for this disease, which has a reported prevalence of 0.5–1.0% of the community[39]. Although symptoms of CMP-induced enteropathy in infancy may be similar to those of celiac disease, the onset often coincides with the dietary introduction of CMP, prior to wheat exposure.

Food allergies appear to play a role in over 90% of children with eosinophilic esophagitis (EE) and up to 40% of infants with symptoms of gastro-esophageal reflux disease (GORD) are thought to have cows' milk allergy.[40] However, there are no clear distinguishing features to identify diet-responsive infants with reflux disease and there is a significant clinical overlap between EE and GORD. Poor response to the use of proton pump inhibitors and more than 15 eosinophils per high-powered field on histology of esophageal biopsies are used to distinguish GORD from EE. Most infants with food-induced GORD or EE usually present within a few weeks of first exposure to the implicated food, with cows' milk most frequently implicated in GORD and cows' milk, soy, wheat, other grains, meat and poultry frequently implicated in EE. The diagnosis of food-induced GORD or EE is made by strict food elimination for a minimum of 2–4 weeks, and subsequent re-challenge.

Table 3.2 Defining features that distinguish IgE-mediated from non-IgE mediated food allergies and their associated syndromes. Modified from Allen KJ, Hill DJ, Heine RG. Food allergy in childhood. Med J Aust. 2006 Oct 2;185(7):394–400.

Class	IgE mediated	Non-IgE mediated
Time to onset of reaction	Immediate <1 hour	Delayed >24 hours
Volume required for reaction	Small (e.g. <10 ml)	Large (e.g. >100 ml)
Symptoms/ syndromes	Urticaria, angioedema, vomiting, anaphylaxis, oral allergy syndrome, eczema	Diarrhoea, eczema, failure to thrive, gastro-oesophageal reflux food protein-induced enteropathy, enterocolitis and proctocolitis, multiple food allergy
Diagnostic procedures	Above signs or symptoms by history or oral food challenge AND positive IgE antibodies (skin prick test or cap-FEIA)	Home based elimination and rechallenge sequence (*no risk of anaphylaxis*)

CLINICAL CASE

A 14-month-old girl was referred for opinion and management of irritability from birth, and vomiting and loose stools with failure to thrive from around 6 months of age. A trial of ranitidine at 2 months of age for possible gastroesophageal reflux disease was unhelpful. She was exclusively breastfed until 6 months of age, and there was no improvement with a partial maternal exclusion of dairy products. Solids were introduced at that time and breast milk was continued until 10 months of age. Soy milk and goats' milk were also tried, with no clear improvement. At 8 months of age she was therefore prescribed an extensively hydrolyzed formula, with improvement in her stool quality but not the vomiting. Family history included maternal celiac disease and atopy, and a sister with eczema. A gastroscopy was undertaken to rule out celiac disease and surprisingly revealed changes consistent with eosinophilic esophagitis. Eosinophils were detected in the following biopsies; 42/high-power field (HPF) upper, 38/HPF mid and 28/HPF in the lower esophagus. There was basal cell proliferation occupying more than 50% of the epithelial thickness, and her stomach and duodenum were normal macroscopically and microscopically. Celiac serology was also negative (IgA 0.77). She subsequently underwent skin prick tests (SPT) which were all negative (cows' milk 0 mm, egg 0 mm, soy 0 mm, wheat 0 mm), but atopy patch testing (APT) was positive for cows' milk protein and soy and negative for egg and wheat. A diet eliminating cows' milk and soy and an amino-acid based formula was started, with subsequent improvement of all symptoms. A follow-up gastroscopy around 12 months later showed a normal esophagus with only 1–2 eosinophils per high-power field detected.

Food protein-induced proctocolitis (an allergic inflammatory process involving the distal colon) usually presents in the first 3 months of life with low-grade rectal bleeding in an otherwise thriving infant, and is the commonest cause of rectal bleeding in infancy after constipation with fissure. Cows' milk protein allergy (CMPA) is the most common cause of proctocolitis, although other food proteins (e.g. soy, rice, wheat) have been implicated.[41] It can occur in breastfed infants, as the antigenic protein β-lactoglobulin has been identified in breast milk.

CLINICAL CASE

A 6-week-old infant who was otherwise thriving presented with low-grade rectal bleeding with no evidence of constipation or a fissure. The infant was fully breastfed and the mother was on an unrestricted diet. The allergist recommended maternal cows' milk avoidance, with some resolution of the bleeding. Additional soy exclusion (with support from an allergy dietitian) resulted in complete remission of the bloody stools. The mother chose to breastfeed until the infant was 12 months of age and delayed the introduction of cows' milk and soy (including solids) until that time. At the 12-month review skin prick testing to cows' milk was negative, and the parents were educated regarding a home-based introduction plan commencing the infant on a daily dose of 5 ml of cows' milk and doubling the dose on a daily basis until a full serving of 200 ml was tolerated, at which time the infant's diet was liberated to all forms of dairy as he remained asymptomatic.

Cows' milk protein allergy in infancy may present with constipation.[42] However, in the absence of clear diagnostic markers there are significant difficulties in making an unequivocal diagnosis of CMP-induced constipation, since there is a wide range of normal stool frequency in infants,[43] and

minor constipation at the time of weaning from breast milk to CMF is relatively common and usually due to non-allergic mechanisms such as the coincidental introduction of solids. Clinical features suggestive of CMP-induced constipation include onset in close relationship to the first dietary introduction of CMP. There is no diagnostic test for CMP-induced constipation, other than CMP elimination for 2–4 weeks followed by re-challenge. Infants with severe constipation require specialist referral to exclude anorectal malformations or Hirschsprung's disease. Increased eosinophils on rectal biopsy support the diagnosis of CMP-induced constipation[44] and management involves strict dietary CMP elimination.

Colic is a multifactorial condition that typically occurs in infants between 3 and 6 weeks, with remission occurring by 4 months of age.[45] The causal relationship between colic and CMPA is controversial, although several trials have demonstrated a significant clinical improvement in response to CMP elimination.[46,47] Persistence of irritability beyond 4 months may suggest an organic etiology, including CMPA. Most infants with colic have no associated atopic disorders, and IgE-based tests for food allergy are not helpful. In infants with diet-responsive colic, colic behavior is mostly reduced within 1 week of dietary modification.

References

1. Sicherer SH, Munoz-Furlong A, Sampson HA. Prevalence of peanut and tree nut allergy in the United States determined by means of a random digit dial telephone survey: a 5-year follow-up study. J Allergy Clin Immunol 2003;112:1203–7.

2. Schafer T, Bohler E, Ruhdorfer S, et al. Epidemiology of food allergy/food intolerance in adults: associations with other manifestations of atopy. Allergy 2001;56:1172–9.

3. Sampson HA. Food allergy – accurately identifying clinical reactivity. Allergy 2005;60(Suppl. 79):19–24.

4. Prasad GA, Alexander JA, Schleck CD, et al. Epidemiology of eosinophilic esophagitis over three decades in Olmsted County, Minnesota. Clin Gastroenterol Hepatol 2009;7:1055–61.

5. Cook B, Oxner R, Chapman B, et al. A thirty-year (1970–1999) study of coeliac disease in the Canterbury region of New Zealand. The New Zealand Medical Journal 2004;117:U772.

6. Allen KJ, Davidson GP, Day AS, et al. Management of cows' milk protein allergy in infants and young children: an expert panel perspective. J Paediatr Child Health 2009;45:481–6.

7. Ho MH, Wong WH, Heine RG, et al. Early clinical predictors of remission of peanut allergy in children. J Allergy Clin Immunol 2008;121:731–6.

8. Rona RJ, Keil T, Summers C, et al. The prevalence of food allergy: A meta-analysis. J Allergy Clin Immunol 2007;120:638–46.

9. Osborne NJ, Koplin JJ, Martin PE, et al. The HealthNuts population-based study of paediatric food allergy: validity, safety and acceptability. Clin Exp Allergy 2010;40:1516–22.

10. Sporik R, Hill DJ, Hosking CS. Specificity of allergen skin testing in predicting positive open food challenges to milk, egg and peanut in children. Clin Exp Allergy 2000;30:1540–6.

11. Celik-Bilgili S, Mehl A, Verstege A, et al. The predictive value of specific immunoglobulin E levels in serum for the outcome of oral food challenges. Clin Exp Allergy 2005;35:268–73.

12. Sampson HA, Munoz-Furlong A, Campbell RL, et al. Second symposium on the definition and management of anaphylaxis: summary report – Second National Institute of Allergy and Infectious Disease/Food Allergy and Anaphylaxis Network symposium. J Allergy Clin Immunol 2006;117:391–7.

13. Eller E, Kjaer HF, Host A, et al. Food allergy and food sensitization in early childhood: results from the DARC cohort. Allergy 2009;64:1023–9.

14. Osborne N, Koplin J, Martin P, et al. Prevalence of challenge-proven IgE-mediated food allergy using population-based sampling and predetermined challenge criteria in infants. J Allergy Clin Immunol 2011;127:668–76.

15. Tang ML, Osborne N, Allen K. Epidemiology of anaphylaxis. Curr Opin Allergy Clin Immunol 2009;9:351–6.

16. Pumphrey R. Anaphylaxis: can we tell who is at risk of a fatal reaction? Curr Opin Allergy Clin Immunol 2004;4:285–90.

17. Liew WK, Williamson E, Tang ML. Anaphylaxis fatalities and admissions in Australia. J Allergy Clin Immunol 2009;123:434–42.

18. Chen W, Mempel M, Schober W, et al. Gender difference, sex hormones, and immediate type hypersensitivity reactions. Allergy 2008;63:1418–27.

19. Dias RP, Summerfield A, Khakoo GA. Food hypersensitivity among Caucasian and non-Caucasian children. Pediatr Allergy Immunol 2008;19:86–9.

20. Branum AM, Lukacs SL. Food allergy among U.S. children: trends in prevalence and hospitalizations. NCHS data brief 2008;1–8.

21. Grundy J, Matthews S, Bateman B, et al. Rising prevalence of allergy to peanut in children: Data from 2 sequential cohorts. J Allergy Clin Immunol 2002;110:784–9.

22. Ben-Shoshan M, Kagan RS, Alizadehfar R, et al. Is the prevalence of peanut allergy increasing? A 5-year follow-up study in children in Montreal. J Allergy Clin Immunol 2009;123:783–8.

23. Sicherer SH, Muñoz-Furlong A, Godbold JH, et al. US prevalence of self-reported peanut, tree nut, and

sesame allergy: 11-year follow-up. J Allergy Clin Immunol 2010 Jun;125(6):1322–6. Epub 2010 May 11.

24. Chafen JJ, Newberry SJ, Riedl MA, et al. Diagnosing and managing common food allergies: a systematic review. JAMA 2010 May 12;303(18):1848–56.

25. Poulos LM, Waters AM, Correll PK, et al. Trends in hospitalizations for anaphylaxis, angioedema, and urticaria in Australia, 1993–1994 to 2004–2005. J Allergy Clin Immunol 2007;120:878–84.

26. Allen KJ, Martin PE. Clinical Aspects of Pediatric Food Allergy and Failed Oral Immune Tolerance. J Clin Gastroenterol 2010;44:391–401.

27. Koplin J, Allen K, Gurrin L, et al. Is caesarean delivery associated with sensitization to food allergens and IgE-mediated food allergy: a systematic review. Pediatr Allergy Immunol 2008;19:682–7.

28. Prescott SL, Smith P, Tang M, et al. The importance of early complementary feeding in the development of oral tolerance: concerns and controversies. Pediatr Allergy Immunol 2008;19:375–80.

29. Untersmayr E, Jensen-Jarolim E. The role of protein digestibility and antacids on food allergy outcomes. J Allergy Clin Immunol 2008 Jun;121(6):1301–8.

30. Du Toit G, Katz Y, Sasieni P, et al. Early consumption of peanuts in infancy is associated with a low prevalence of peanut allergy. J Allergy Clin Immunol 2008;122:984–91.

31. Koplin J, Osborne N, Wake M, et al. Can early introduction of egg prevent egg allergy in infants? A population-based study. J Allergy Clin Immunol 2010;126:807–13.

32. Poole JA, Barriga K, Leung DY, et al. Timing of initial exposure to cereal grains and the risk of wheat allergy. Pediatrics 2006;117:2175–82.

33. Sicherer SH, Furlong TJ, Maes HH, et al. Genetics of peanut allergy: A twin study. J Allergy Clin Immunol 2000;106:53–6.

34. Tsai H-J, Kumar R, Pongracicwz J, et al. Familial aggregation of food allergy and sensitization to food allergens: a family-based study. Clin Exp Allergy 2009;39:101–9.

35. Irvine A. Fleshing out filaggrin phenotypes. J Invest Dermatol 2007;127:504–7.

36. Marenholz I, Nickel R, Rüschendorf F, et al. Filaggrin loss-of-function mutations predispose to phenotypes involved in the atopic march. J Allergy Clin Immunol 2006;118:866–71.

37. Host A, Halken S, Jacobsen HP, et al. Clinical course of cows' milk protein allergy/intolerance and atopic diseases in childhood. Pediatr Allergy Immunol 2002;13(Suppl. 15):23–8.

38. Cherian S, Smith NM, Forbes DA. Rapidly increasing prevalence of eosinophilic oesophagitis in Western Australia. Arch Dis Child 2006;91(12):1000–4.

39. Fasano A, Berti I, Gerarduzzi T, et al. Prevalence of celiac disease in at-risk and not-at-risk groups in the United States: a large multicenter study. Arch Intern Med 2003;163(3):286–92.

40. Iacono G, Carroccio A, Cavataio F, et al. Gastroesophageal reflux and cows' milk allergy in

infants: a prospective study. J Allergy Clin Immunol 1996;97:822–7.

41. Lake AM. Food-induced eosinophilic proctocolitis. J Pediatr Gastroenterol Nutr 2000;30(Suppl.): S58–60.

42. Iacono G, Cavataio F, Montalto G, et al. Intolerance of cows' milk and chronic constipation in children. N Engl J Med 1998;339:1100–4.

43. Tham EB, Nathan R, Davidson GP, et al. Bowel habits of healthy Australian children aged 0–2 years. J Paediatr Child Health 1996;32:504–7.

44. Iacono G, Bonventre S, Scalici C, et al. Food intolerance and chronic constipation: manometry and

histology study. Eur J Gastroenterol Hepatol 2006;18: 143–50.

45. Clifford TJ, Campbell MK, Speechley KN, et al. Sequelae of infant colic: evidence of transient infant distress and absence of lasting effects on maternal mental health. Arch Pediatr Adolesc Med 2002;156:1183–8.

46. Hill DJ, Roy N, Heine RG, et al. Effect of a low-allergen maternal diet on colic among breastfed infants: a randomized, controlled trial. Pediatrics 2005;116:e709–15.

47. Jakobsson I, Lindberg T. Cows' milk proteins cause infantile colic in breast-fed infants: a double-blind crossover study. Pediatrics 1983;71:268–71.

CHAPTER 4

Clinical Overview of Adverse Reactions to Foods

John M. Kelso

Introduction

'Allergy' is the term most often used by patients to describe an adverse reaction attributed to a food. To an allergist, the term implies an IgE-mediated – or at least an immunologically mediated – reaction. Adverse reactions to foods that are not immunologically mediated are best termed 'intolerance'.[1]

This chapter will describe the most common food-related complaints for which patients seek care from an allergist because either the patient or the referring physician believes the reaction to be allergic. There are a host of gastrointestinal disorders, such as gastroesophageal reflux, irritable bowel syndrome and inflammatory bowel disease, where patients may describe symptoms in relation to eating, but these patients are typically referred to gastroenterologists and these conditions will not specifically be considered here.

When a patient presents with a food-related health complaint, the history is paramount and dictates the differential diagnosis, appropriate testing and treatment.[1,2] The physical examination may add some additional information if the patient happens to be seen acutely at the time of a reaction. There are five crucial elements to the history:

1. The suspect(s): What food(s) does the patient believe caused the reaction(s)?
2. Timing: How long from exposure to symptom onset?
3. The nature of the reaction: What are the symptoms?
4. Reproducibility: Has it happened more than once? Does it happen every time?
5. What treatment was administered and what was the response?

IgE-mediated reactions

Urticarial/anaphylactic

Why is it important to determine whether or not a reaction is IgE-mediated? IgE-mediated reactions to foods are potentially life-threatening, and testing and treatment are available. As many as 200 people each year die from such reactions, and most are preventable.[3] A patient may want to avoid onions if they cause heartburn, but if he or she eats some accidentally, the result is discomfort. If a patient is allergic to peanuts, however, the result of an accidental ingestion could be fatal. Knowing whether or not a patient has a food allergy rather than a food intolerance dictates how careful they need to be about avoiding the food. Testing is available to determine whether the patient has IgE antibody specifically directed to the suspect food (see Chapter 13). Non-specific treatment in the form of oral antihistamines and self-injectable epinephrine is available for accidental ingestions for patients with IgE-mediated food allergy, whereas for food intolerance these measures would be unnecessary and unhelpful. Specific treatment in the form of oral desensitization or induction of tolerance will probably become an option in the near future for IgE-mediated food allergy (see Chapter 17), but this would not be expected to help in food intolerance.

Suspect foods

Virtually all reported food allergy deaths have been from one of five foods or food groups: peanuts, tree nuts, fish/shellfish, cows' milk and egg.[4–6] Therefore, patients who are suspicious that one of these foods has caused a reaction are more likely to have IgE-mediated food allergy. Many other foods have been demonstrated to cause such reactions, but they are less likely to do so and less likely to cause life-threatening reactions. Allergens are antigens to which people make specific IgE antibodies. Like most antigens, most allergens are proteins.

Timing

The timing of the reaction is critical. IgE-mediated reactions to food typically begin within minutes to a couple of hours after ingestion.[3] It usually takes only a small amount of the food to cause a reaction, and the reactions generally happen with every exposure. These conditions usually make the diagnosis obvious. Patients who present saying that they think they are allergic to peanuts because they have broken out in hives the last three times they have eaten them are almost certainly allergic to peanuts. On the other hand, patients who present with hives and have no idea what is causing them are very unlikely to turn out to have food allergy as a cause. However, patients are often under the impression that the reaction could be to something they ate the previous day or several days before, or something that they have been eating more of than usual lately, when in fact, if they were allergic to the food, the reaction would have occurred shortly enough after each exposure to make the connection more obvious.

Nature of reaction

The nature of the reaction suggests the likelihood that the reaction is IgE-mediated. IgE-mediated reactions are mast cell-mediated reactions and the symptoms should be consistent with the release of histamine and other mediators from mast cells.[3]

Mast cells are most abundant where we have interface with our environment, namely skin, respiratory tract and gastrointestinal tract. Histamine is also a potent vasodilator, and thus hypotension is another major feature of systemic IgE-mediated allergic reactions. Therefore patients will often describe cutaneous symptoms of flushing, itching, swelling and/or hives. Respiratory complaints can include the symptoms of allergic rhinitis: itchy, watery, red eyes; itchy, runny, stuffy nose; and sneezing. Although such symptoms are typically brought on by exposure to an airborne allergen, once an ingested allergen such as a food has access to the circulation and the allergen attaches to mast-cell-bound IgE in the eyes and nose, the same symptoms result. Pharyngeal complaints can include an itchy or sore throat, or symptoms resulting from laryngopharyngeal edema, such as the sensation of a lump in the throat or difficulty talking, swallowing or breathing. Lower airway symptoms are those of asthma: coughing, wheezing, shortness of breath and chest tightness. Patients who have asthma are more likely to have these symptoms, and such symptoms are more likely to be severe,[5] but even patients with no history of asthma can have the same symptoms as part of an anaphylactic reaction. Gastrointestinal symptoms can include nausea, vomiting, abdominal pain and diarrhea. Symptoms of hypotension are lightheadedness or loss of consciousness. Although it would seem that gastrointestinal symptoms would be the most common manifestation of IgE-mediated food allergy, the most common manifestations are dermatologic, respiratory and cardiovascular.[1] Deaths from anaphylaxis are either due to asphyxia (upper laryngeal edema or severe bronchospasm) or hypotension.[7] Again, pre-existing asthma is an important risk factor for a fatal outcome from an anaphylactic episode.[4,5]

Reproducibility

Most patients assume that one must be born with food allergy and that it persists for a lifetime. Therefore, they believe that if they have eaten a food uneventfully many times in the past that they cannot be allergic to it. In reality, because as with any other IgE-mediated reaction prior exposure is required for sensitization, patients must have had some previous uneventful exposure to become allergic. This previous exposure is most often actually consuming the food, but can also be through less obvious sources, particularly in children. Whenever a lactating mother eats any food, some of that food protein is present in the breast milk for several hours afterwards.[8] Food proteins are present on household surfaces such as countertops and may become airborne, so cutaneous and respiratory exposures may occur.[9] Many foods have immunological cross-reactivity with other foods, and prior exposure may have been to such a food sharing similar proteins.[10] Thus patients may appear to have an allergic reaction on their first exposure to a food, but in fact they have had prior relevant allergen exposure.[8] This prior exposure was sufficient to cause sensitization (i.e. specific IgE antibody production) but not a clinical reaction. Once sensitized, a subsequent exposure to a larger amount causes an allergic reaction.

Once sensitized, an allergic reaction typically occurs with each ingestion. Thus, it is uncommon for patients to react to the ingestion of a food on one occasion but not the next. Similarly, although there may be a dose–response curve where eating more of the food is more likely to cause a reaction or more likely to cause a severe reaction, this is usually not apparent clinically because such a small amount causes an obvious reaction. Therefore it is uncommon for patients with an IgE-mediated food allergy to report that they can tolerate a small portion of a suspect food but not a large portion. Therefore, although it is certainly important to inquire what has happened with the ingestion of the suspect food prior to the ingestion that appeared to have caused a reaction, it is even more helpful to know what has happened with subsequent ingestions. Many patients will have avoided the suspect food after an apparent reaction, but some have not. If the patient can relate that they have consumed the suspect food uneventfully since the apparent reaction, this markedly reduces the likelihood that they are allergic to the food.

There are exceptions to the general rule that, once sensitized, a patient will react to each subsequent exposure to a food. Occasionally some cofactor is required to cause a clinical reaction. These cofactors include exercise, consumption of alcohol and the ingestion of medications known to cause or lower the threshold for mast cell degranulation, such as non-steroidal anti-inflammatory drugs (NSAIDs) or narcotic analgesics.[11–13] Thus, a patient who has made IgE antibodies to a food may still be able to eat that food without reaction. However, if they eat the food and then exercise, or eat the food while taking an NSAID or narcotic, the combination will cause a reaction.

Previous treatment and response to treatment

A final element of the history that can be helpful is determining what treatment was given for previous reactions and whether or not it was helpful. A rash that responded promptly to the administration of an oral antihistamine, or lightheadedness that resolved soon after the administration of epinephrine, would be consistent with the reaction being IgE mediated.

Testing

If the history is consistent with a potentially IgE-mediated reaction, demonstrating the presence of IgE antibody to the food is essential.[1] Although a patient with a classic history is in fact likely to be allergic to the suspect food, testing is required to make a diagnosis. Occasionally an 'obvious' allergic reaction to a food turns out to be a non-IgE-mediated reaction, a coincidence, or an IgE-mediated reaction to another food consumed at the same time. As with all allergy testing, allergy testing for foods should not be done as a screening test, or in the absence of a history or disease that suggests a possible reaction to the food (see Chapter 13).

Skin test vs RAST

There are two methods to look for IgE antibody, skin testing and in-vitro assays of serum for specific IgE antibodies.[1,2] The blood tests are commonly referred to as RASTs (radioallergosorbent tests), although RAST is actually a brand name that has become generic to refer to any of the assays for specific IgE antibody, such as ImmunoCAP, Immulite and Turbo RAST, most of which no longer use radioactive isotopes for detection. Skin tests have the advantage of the results being available quickly, as they are read 15 minutes after placing and can therefore be available at the same visit when the history was taken, whereas RAST results are typically available only days after being drawn and require an additional visit or follow-up phone call to discuss them. RASTs are also typically more expensive. Systemic allergic reactions may rarely occur with skin testing, although vasovagal reactions are just as likely[14] and may also occur with blood drawing. Patients must be off all antihistamines (oral and topical), including medications with antihistaminic activity such as tricyclic antidepressants, for 5–7 days prior to skin testing,[15] whereas these medications do not interfere with RASTs. Skin tests are also generally more sensitive than RASTs, meaning that they are more likely to be positive when IgE antibody is present, although the currently available in vitro assays are nearly as sensitive. In most cases the skin test and RAST results would agree, i.e. both are positive or both are negative. When there is a discrepancy, the majority are a positive skin test and negative RAST, although occasionally the reverse is true.[15]

Positive vs negative

As with any assay, there is some level of result that is considered positive, i.e. distinguishable from background or negative results. For skin prick tests the most commonly used criteria are a 3 mm wheal greater than an appropriate negative control and 10 mm erythema.[1] For RAST assays that quantify specific IgE antibody the cutoff is usually 0.1 or 0.35 kU/L (see Chapter 13).

False positives

Whether detected by skin test or RAST, the presence of IgE antibody does not equate to clinical allergy. As is the case with all IgE-mediated diseases, including allergic rhinitis, allergic asthma and allergic reactions to drugs and stinging insects, not all patients who make IgE antibody to a food will react when they eat that food.[16] The reasons for this phenomenon of clinically irrelevant positive IgE tests are not well characterized. The higher the level of specific IgE antibody to a food, the more likely it is that the patient will react if they eat that food. However, there are patients who have very high levels of IgE to a food yet nonetheless consume it without reaction. Also, although there is a correlation between how much allergic antibody is present and the likelihood of a reaction, there is little correlation between the level of IgE antibody and the severity of that reaction.[2,16] It may be that the particular IgE antibodies that a patient made to a food, albeit few, are nonetheless more likely to cause a reaction because they bind the allergen with greater avidity, or bind more clinically relevant epitopes.

As above, the lower the level of IgE antibody, the less likely the patient is to react, but this correlation is not perfect, i.e. occasional patients with high levels will tolerate the food, whereas occasional patients with low levels have severe reactions. For some foods, a certain level of IgE antibody as measured by RAST or skin test has been correlated with the probability of reacting or not reacting to the food if consumed.[16] These are most often referred to as 'cutoff' values and are better characterized for the probability of reacting to a food, i.e. positive predictive values. For example, if the measured amount of IgE for a certain food is above a certain level, there is a 95% chance that a patient would react if they consumed that food.[2] There are some data on negative predictive values as well, i.e. the probability that the patient will not react to the food. For example, if the measured amount of IgE for a certain food is below a certain level, there is a 95% chance that a patient would not react if they consumed the food.[16] Also, for some foods the levels of IgE antibody that correlates to a 50% chance of reacting to the food have been reported.[17] It is important to realize that there are limits to the generalizability of the use of these cutoff values. Different studies have reported different values, probably because different patient populations and different assay methods were used, but they nonetheless provide a useful guide.

False negatives

Although RAST and skin tests are quite sensitive, they are not perfect. There are patients with a history of food reactions who have negative tests for IgE antibody but nonetheless react when re-exposed to the food. If there is a strong clinical suspicion of an IgE-mediated reaction to a food and a test for IgE antibody is negative, it is important to perform additional testing before concluding that the patient is not allergic. If a patient's skin test result is negative, it may be appropriate to do a RAST, or vice versa. If the skin test with a commercial extract of a food is negative, it may be appropriate to create a crude extract made from the actual food. This is often required in the case of allergy to fruits and vegetables, where many of the allergens are quite labile.[1] For example, a patient who reports itching of the mouth with apple ingestion may well have a negative RAST and skin test with commercial extract, yet have a clearly positive test result when the skin test is performed with the juice from a fresh apple. This is less often the case with the food allergens most likely to cause anaphylaxis, i.e. milk, egg, tree nuts, fish/shellfish and legumes (especially peanut), although occasionally patients with a history of reacting to these foods will react only to a skin test with an extract made from the actual fresh food.

Challenge

The ultimate clinical diagnostic test for food allergy is what happens when the patient consumes the actual food. A patient with a recent history of an allergic reaction to a food and a large positive skin test or highly positive RAST to that food would almost certainly react if they were to eat the food. On the other hand, a patient with a distant history of an allergic reaction to a food and a negative or small positive skin test or low positive RAST to that food might very well not react if they were to eat the food. Patients who can report that they regularly eat a food without reaction are not allergic to that food, irrespective of skin test or RAST results (an exception is atopic dermatitis, as below). Patients who have been trying to avoid a food may nonetheless have accidental ingestions and can report whether or not they reacted. Patients who have successfully avoided the ingestion of a food will not be able to provide this information and at some point may be candidates for an oral challenge under observation. In research settings, these are most often done as double-blind, placebo-controlled food challenges (DBPCFC), whereas in clinical practice they are most often performed as open, oral food challenges.[2] By definition, the challenges have a chance of inducing a life-threatening anaphylactic reaction and must be performed in a setting where there are medical personnel and equipment available to recognize and treat such a reaction should it occur (see Chapter 14).

Natural history

Some food allergies, such as reactions to cows' milk and egg, are commonly 'outgrown', i.e. they resolve spontaneously over a period of time. Others, such as reactions to peanuts, tree nuts, and fish/shellfish are usually lifelong and less likely to be 'outgrown'.[1] There are exceptions, however, as egg or milk allergy occasionally persists into adulthood, and perhaps as many as 20% of toddlers with peanut allergy will outgrow it.[18] Many parents report that their milk- or egg-allergic children react if they eat these foods directly, but tolerate them if they are in baked goods, such as cakes.[19,20] This is presumably because

there is a smaller amount of the protein and/or because it has been cooked at a high temperature for a long time, which may lead to a denaturation of the relevant allergens in these foods. Although this phenomenon has been confirmed by research studies in a majority of milk- and egg-allergic children, it should be noted that in the minority of such children who do not tolerate the foods even in baked goods, their reaction to these baked goods can be severe.[19,20] Although one might wonder whether allowing such exposure in children who tolerate it might delay or prevent their ultimately outgrowing their allergy, studies have indicated that this exposure may actually hasten the resolution of the allergy.[21]

Treatment

The treatment for food allergy is to avoid ingestion of the relevant food allergen and to be prepared to treat an allergic reaction if it occurs following an accidental ingestion.

Avoidance

Patients allergic to a food must be vigilant.[2] They must carefully read packaged food labels and re-read them every time the food is purchased, since the ingredients may have changed even if the overall appearance of the package has not. They must ask questions directly and repeatedly to hosts and food servers about the contents of prepared food. They must make clear that they are asking whether or not a dish contains a food because they have a potentially life-threatening allergy to that food, not simply because they do not care for the taste of the food or wish to avoid it for some other reason (see Chapter 16).

Emergency treatment

Despite these attempts at avoidance, the majority of food allergy deaths occur in patients who knew they were allergic to the food[5] but had an accidental ingestion, usually because the food was 'hidden' in some other food, or a packaged food was contaminated by a food allergen not declared on the label.[22] Therefore, each and every time a food-allergic patient is eating, medications to treat a reaction, namely self-injectable epinephrine and an antihistamine, must be immediately available.[1] If they know they have had such an accidental ingestion they should also take the antihistamine and be prepared to use the self-injectable epinephrine. When to use the self-injectable epinephrine requires some judgment and depends on the nature of previous reactions. Although there are exceptions, most systemic allergic reactions are stereotypic, i.e. the nature and severity of the reaction in the past is likely to be the nature and severity of future reactions.[23] Thus, in a patient who has suffered a truly life-threatening reaction to a food in the past and had an accidental ingestion, the epinephrine should be used even before the onset of any symptoms. On the other hand, in a patient who has never had more than cutaneous reactions with previous ingestions, it may be reasonable to administer the antihistamine and prepare to administer the epinephrine. If at any stage of the reaction, whether the antihistamine has been administered or not, if the patient develops any respiratory symptoms (i.e. not just frank respiratory distress, but any amount of cough, wheeze, shortness of breath or throat swelling or clearing) or any cardiovascular symptoms (i.e. not just frank syncope, but any amount of lightheadedness) or repeated emesis, the epinephrine should be administered. Once the epinephrine has been administered, even if the patient appears to be responding favorably, they should be transported to the nearest emergency department (ED). If the historical or current reaction seems truly life-threatening, it is appropriate to call the emergency medical services (EMS). Although epinephrine is typically very effective in treating anaphylactic reactions, its effect may also be temporary and repeat doses may be required.[24] Consideration can be given to prescribing multiple doses of epinephrine,[24–26] especially if prior reactions have been severe or medical facilities are far away. Reactions may progress to require additional treatment such as oxygen, intravenous fluids, and intubation or tracheotomy. Even if an ED is close by, patients who know they are suffering an allergic reaction to an accidental food ingestion of sufficient severity to warrant the ED visit should administer the epinephrine before going to the ED.

The choice of antihistamine

An antihistamine for use in an acute allergic reaction to a food should have a rapid onset of action. It should also be available in a form convenient for patients to carry with them, since it needs to be immediately available whenever and wherever they are eating. Syrup for small children and rapidly dissolving tablets that can be taken without liquids are best suited for this purpose. Although the number of doses to be used in this circumstance would be expected to be small, an inexpensive generic formulation would also be preferable.

Diphenhydramine has traditionally been the antihistamine of choice for the treatment of acute allergic reactions because of its rapid onset of action, ability to be administered by oral, intravenous and intramuscular routes, availability in capsule, syrup and rapidly dissolving tablet formulations, and its use in published protocols. It is available as an inexpensive generic.

Cetirizine is a reasonable alternative. It has an onset of action as fast as diphenhydramine, and is also available in syrup and rapidly dissolving tablet formulations. It has the advantage of having a longer duration of action and less sedative potential than diphenhydramine. It is also available as an inexpensive generic form.

The choice of self-injectable epinephrine

There are three branded (EpiPen, Twinject and Adrenaclick) and one generic epinephrine autoinjectors currently on the market. Each has advantages and disadvantages.[26] Insurance coverage, cost, ease of carrying (weight and size), ease of use, possible need to carry two doses, and patient preference all must be factored into which device to prescribe. Each EpiPen, Adrenaclick or generic autoinjector delivers one 0.3 mg or 0.15 mg dose (EpiPen Jr.) of epinephrine as an autoinjector. Each Twinject delivers one 0.3 mg or one 0.15 mg dose as an autoinjector and in addition can be dismantled to reveal the syringe; after removal of a collar on the plunger, this syringe with attached needle can be used to administer a second dose of epinephrine in the same milligram quantity as the first dose.

One dose or two

Studies of anaphylactic reactions in general and food-induced anaphylactic reactions in particular suggest that in a sizeable minority of reactions a second dose of epinephrine is required to treat a reaction.[25] It may be appropriate for patients who have suffered severe reactions in the past, or who are further away from emergency medical facilities, to carry two doses of self-injectable epinephrine with them at all times. This can be accomplished by carrying two single autoinjectors or one

Twinject. Although it is more convenient to carry the single Twinject device, the technical aspects of using the second dose from the Twinject might cause some patients to prefer carrying two single autoinjectors.[26]

Oral immunotherapy

Immunotherapy by subcutaneous injection is a well-established and effective treatment for allergic rhinitis, allergic asthma and stinging insect allergy. It is possible that such treatment would be effective for food allergy as well. Studies with peanut injection immunotherapy demonstrated some improvement in the amount of oral peanut ingestion patients could tolerate without reaction, but systemic reactions to the injections were very common and precluded patients from being maintained at an effective maintenance dose.[27] Immunotherapy with altered peanut proteins that are less allergenic but still antigenic is being explored.[28]

Several studies have now shown promise with oral immunotherapy for food allergy.[19-21,29-35] Most of these studies have been with cows' milk and egg, but studies with peanut have also been reported. Although milk and egg allergies are commonly outgrown, for those children who do not outgrow them, they continue to pose the burden of food avoidance and the risk of accidental ingestion. Oral immunotherapy for food, sometimes called specific oral tolerance induction, involves protocols where allergic patients are orally administered a minuscule amount of the food initially, e.g. one drop of a solution made by putting 10 drops of milk in 100 mL of water, and then progressively higher amounts over days to months. Some of the protocols involve administration in an observed setting (clinic or hospital) for the initial doses, or when the dose is increased. Reactions to the food 'doses' can cause systemic reactions, and providers and patients or families need to be prepared to recognize and treat anaphylaxis. Some patients who have completed these protocols have been able to tolerate an unlimited amount of the food, whereas others only tolerate enough to allow them not to react to a small amount of the food, such as might occur in an accidental ingestion. It is unclear whether oral desensitization to food results in permanent desensitization or tolerance, such as might occur to pollen after successful immunotherapy has been discontinued, where intermittent contact with the allergen does not result in symptoms, or whether there is only a temporary desensitization or tolerance, such as occurs with penicillin desensitization, where ongoing exposure to the allergen is required to maintain the desensitized state. Most of the oral food desensitization protocols require daily ingestion of the food. In studies that have achieved successful oral desensitization, where patients are tolerating daily ingestion of the food, some have had the patients avoid the food again for a period of months and then re-challenged them. Some such patients do not react and appear to have achieved a long-term tolerance, whereas others do react and appear to have lost their tolerance (see Chapter 14).[31,33]

Food-dependent, exercise-induced anaphylaxis

As mentioned above, some patients with IgE-mediated food allergy do not react to the ingestion of the food alone, but would react if they ate the food and then subsequently exercised.[11,36] The reason for this is unclear, although it seems possible that the exercise alters the absorption or distribution of the food allergen systemically or renders mast cells more susceptible to degranulation. The foods that have been associated with this phenomenon include the common food allergens (cows' milk, egg, tree nuts, fish/shellfish and legumes, primarily peanut), but have also involved other foods such as wheat or celery. As an exception to the general rule that allergy testing should not be done in the absence of a history of reacting to the food, in the case of food-dependent exercise-induced anaphylaxis the history is not obvious, because when the patient consumes the food without exercise afterward they do not react, and so would not think of themselves as being allergic to the food. Thus, even in the absence of any suspicion of food allergy, patients with a history of exercise-induced anaphylaxis should be tested to all food they eat.[37] If a culprit food is identified, the patient needs to avoid ingesting that food only if they are going to exercise within a few hours afterward. There are some patients with this syndrome who appear to have anaphylaxis if they exercise too soon after eating any food, and they need to avoid eating anything too close to the time of exercising – typically 2–4 hours. All patients with exercise-induced anaphylaxis should be counseled to not exercise alone, to stop exercising at the first sign of a reaction, and to have self-injectable epinephrine available to treat a reaction.

Food allergy causing exacerbation of eczema

About one-third of children with difficult to control eczema have food allergy as an exacerbating factor.[38,39] Unlike urticarial or anaphylactic reactions to foods, when the ingestion of a food exacerbates eczema it may not be obvious because the skin condition is already present.[38] The foods that most often exacerbate eczema are the same as those that cause anaphylaxis (milk, egg, tree nuts, fish/shellfish and legumes, primarily peanut), but other foods can do so as well.[38,39] Thus patients with difficult to control eczema should have skin tests or RASTs for the common food allergens as well as any foods the patient or family suspect of worsening the eczema. Foods that give negative test results are not exacerbating the eczema. The likelihood that a food giving a positive test result is exacerbating the eczema is overall about one-third.[38,39] The size of the skin test or the level of specific IgE antibody on the RAST can be used to determine the chance that a particular food is a factor. Not surprisingly, the higher the test result, the more likely the clinical relevance, with 95% positive and negative predictive value cutoff levels established for some foods, as above.[16] If there is uncertainty that ingestion of a particular food is exacerbating the eczema, it may be appropriate to exclude that food from the diet for a few weeks to see if the eczema improves. If so, the food should continue to be avoided. If not, it can be added back to the diet. There are rare case reports of anaphylaxis when foods have been added back to the diet in this situation, and consideration can be given to doing this under observation.[40]

Pollen-food allergy syndrome (oral allergy syndrome)

Some patients with allergic rhinitis due to grass, tree or weed pollen will report that if they eat certain fresh fruits or vegetables, or occasionally nuts, they get itching in the mouth.[41,42] This pollen–food allergy syndrome has also been known as oral allergy syndrome because the symptoms rarely progress beyond oral itching, although more severe swelling of the tongue or throat or other symptoms of anaphylaxis can develop.[43] Although the pollens and foods are not botanically related, they nonetheless contain common cross-reacting protein allergens. Common examples are ragweed and melons, birch and apple, and mugwort and celery. Thus patients who have been sensitized via the respiratory route to a specific pollen may react when they eat a food containing the same protein. The particular proteins responsible for this phenomenon are quite labile, i.e. easily broken down. This probably explains why the symptoms are usually confined to the mouth, and why the foods can almost invariably be eaten cooked without any reaction. It also probably explains why skin tests with commercial extracts and RASTs with fresh fruits and vegetables are often negative in these patients, but skin tests performed with the juice from the fresh food are positive. Unlike food allergy causing urticarial or anaphylactic reactions, in the case of pollen–food allergy syndrome patients are typically told that they can continue to eat the food if they desire, as long as the symptoms do not go beyond oral itching. Occasionally patients with pollen–food allergy syndrome have more severe, systemic allergic reactions and must completely avoid the food.[42] Given the cross-reactivity between the pollens and foods, there is reason to believe that standard immunotherapy with pollens could, in addition to alleviating allergic rhinitis symptoms, also alleviate the associated food allergy symptoms, and published studies have reported some success with this therapy.[44,45]

Other allergic reactions to foods related to airborne allergens

Some patients who are allergic to natural rubber latex are also allergic to certain foods due to cross-reacting allergens.[46] The food allergies most often associated with latex allergy are banana, avocado, kiwi and chestnut, but many other foods have also been associated.

There are a number of reports of patients who were sensitized to dust mites and then consumed baked goods made with flour contaminated by mites, suffering anaphylactic reactions as a result of ingesting mite allergens.[47–49]

Some nurses with a history of respiratory exposure to psyllium as a result of dispensing psyllium-containing laxatives, have later had anaphylactic reactions when they consumed psyllium-containing breakfast cereals.[50–52]

Eosinophilic esophagitis

In eosinophilic esophagitis, a new or at least newly recognized condition, there is a significant eosinophilic inflammatory response in the esophagus.[53]

The resulting inflammation leads to dysphagia. The condition can develop at any age from infancy to adulthood, and is more common in those with other atopic diseases, i.e. asthma, atopic dermatitis, allergic rhinitis and food allergy. The diagnosis is made by esophagoscopy, which can reveal characteristic gross abnormalities including furrows and rings. The esophagus may also appear normal, and biopsy is essential. The presence of more than 20 eosinophils per high-powered field, particularly in the proximal esophagus, is characteristic. The relationship to food allergy is unclear. An elemental diet is curative, implying that food ingestion is causative.[54] Some investigators have had success eliminating foods to which the patients make IgE antibody, although such patients do not have urticarial or anaphylactic reactions to the foods.[55] Others have empirically eliminated certain highly allergenic food groups, with improvement in the condition. In addition to detecting possible culprit foods by testing for IgE antibody with skin tests or RASTs, additional causative foods have been determined by some researches by patch testing with the foods.[55] In patients in whom food elimination diets are not successful or feasible, treatment with swallowed corticosteroids has been successful.[56] These are not simply oral corticosteroids, but rather corticosteroids intended for inhalation for asthma, which are instead swallowed in a formulation that allows them to coat the esophagus and yet minimize systemic absorption. Finally, in patients whose disease is not responsive to these measures, treatment with anti-IL-5 antibodies (IL-5 activates and prolongs the survival of eosinophils) has been used with some success (see Chapter 10).[57]

Non-IgE-mediated reactions

Lactose intolerance

Perhaps the most common non-IgE-mediated reaction to food is lactose intolerance or lactase deficiency.[58] Human milk contains lactose and human infants produce the enzyme lactase to digest it. Many humans normally undergo a large decline in lactase production after infancy and subsequently develop gastrointestinal symptoms of nausea, cramping, bloating and diarrhea if they consume lactose-containing foods (dairy products). The condition is much more common in Asians and African-Americans, and is probably best thought of as a variation of normal rather than a disease. For patients who are lactose intolerant who wish to consume dairy products, lactase supplementation allows them to do so without symptoms.

Celiac disease

A well-characterized immune- but not IgE-mediated reaction to food is celiac disease (also called gluten-sensitive enteropathy or non-tropical sprue).[59,60] Gluten is a mixture of proteins found in the cereal grains wheat, rye and barley. In wheat, gluten is a mixture of gliadin and glutenin. In some persons with HLA-DQ2 or HLA-DQ8 the ingestion of gluten produces an immune response including IgA antibodies against tissue transglutaminase (TTG). The resulting inflammation in the intestines leads to diarrhea and other gastrointestinal symptoms. Therefore, in patients who report gastrointestinal symptoms in association with the ingestion of wheat, testing for celiac disease should be considered. Serology for IgA anti-TTG antibodies is perhaps the most appropriate test. For the test to be accurate the patient must be consuming gluten and must not be IgA deficient (more common in celiac disease). HLA typing has a very high negative predictive value, i.e. the absence of HLA-DQ2 and HLA-DQ8 virtually excludes the diagnosis, but a very low positive predictive value as most people who have these HLA types do not have celiac disease.

Non-IgE-mediated food protein reactions in infancy

There are a number of food protein-induced illnesses of infancy that are not IgE mediated but which are probably immune mediated (see Chapter 11 for more details). These reactions most often occur to milk protein, but can be caused by other foods as well. Most are outgrown by the age of 1 or 2 years.

Food protein-induced enterocolitis syndrome

Food protein-induced enterocolitis syndrome (FPIES) is a rather dramatic and serious reaction to food proteins[61,62] in which, a couple of hours after food ingestion, infants develop vomiting, diarrhea, hypotension and lethargy. A blood count often reveals a high white count and neutrophilia.

Patients are often evaluated and treated for sepsis. The association to the food may not be recognized at first because of the delay between ingestion and the onset of symptoms. FPIES has been reported in association with milk and soy formulas, as well as solid foods including cereal grains, legumes and meats. Treatment consists of avoiding the suspect foods, which can typically be reintroduced by age 3 without symptoms.

Dietary protein-induced proctitis

Dietary protein-induced proctitis describes blood-tinged stools in otherwise healthy infants caused by ingestion of milk- or soy-based formulas or food proteins in breast milk.[63] There are no confirmatory tests. Suspect foods are eliminated until the blood in the stools resolves. The foods can typically be reintroduced uneventfully at age 1 or 2 years.

Scombroid poisoning

After the ingestion of fish, some persons experience systemic reactions, including flushing, hives, gastrointestinal complaints, dyspnea and hypotension, that seem allergic but which are instead due to scombroid poisoning.[64] The fish are usually of the family Scombridae, which includes tuna and mackerel. Histamine has been demonstrated to be the causative agent: the fish involved contain histidine, which is metabolized to histamine by bacteria in inadequately refrigerated fish.[65] The diagnosis is more likely if others who consumed the same fish had similar symptoms. Skin tests with commercial fish skin test extracts would be negative, whereas a skin test with the suspect fish, if available, would be positive.[66]

IgG food tests

It is quite common for patients to present with laboratory test results for IgG antibodies to foods. These are often performed by alternative medicine practitioners who claim that the foods to which patients make IgG antibodies as demonstrated by these tests are the cause of a whole host of symptoms, not only gastrointestinal complaints, but also fatigue, joint pains and difficulty concentrating. The production of IgG antibodies to foods, however, is a normal immune response.[67] Everyone makes these antibodies and they do not cause adverse reactions. IgG food assays should not be ordered, and patients who have already had them performed should be counseled as above that they are a normal immune response to food, are present in all individuals, and do not cause illness. Patients may have a great deal of psychological and monetary investment in the tests and be skeptical of the notion that they do not mean something. As with any such unconventional testing or treatment, the ultimate goal is for the patient to feel well, and if they feel better not eating a particular food and are still able to have a nutritionally complete and enjoyable diet, then they can certainly do so.

The Food Allergy and Anaphylaxis Network

The Food Allergy and Anaphylaxis Network (FAAN) is an organization of patients and families affected by food allergy. They provide accurate, practical information to those dealing with food allergy – everything from recipes to food recalls for allergen contamination, to how to deal with school, day care, camp etc. – in relation to protecting food-allergic patients from life-threatening reactions. Information can be found at www.foodallergy.org. Patients and families with food allergy should be referred to this valuable resource.

References

1. American College of Allergy, Asthma & Immunology. Food allergy: a practice parameter. Ann Allergy Asthma Immunol 2006;96:S1–68.
2. Sicherer SH, Sampson HA. Food allergy. J Allergy Clin Immunol 2010;125:S116–25.
3. Sampson HA. Anaphylaxis and emergency treatment. Pediatrics 2003;111:1601–8.
4. Yunginger JW, Sweeney KG, Sturner WQ, et al. Fatal food-induced anaphylaxis. JAMA 1988;260:1450–2.
5. Sampson HA, Mendelson L, Rosen JP. Fatal and near-fatal anaphylactic reactions to food in children and adolescents. N Engl J Med 1992;327:380–4.
6. Pumphrey RS. Lessons for management of anaphylaxis from a study of fatal reactions. Clin Exp Allergy 2000;30:1144–50.
7. Pumphrey RS. Fatal posture in anaphylactic shock. J Allergy Clin Immunol 2003;112:451–2.
8. Vadas P, Wai Y, Burks W, et al. Detection of peanut allergens in breast milk of lactating women. JAMA 2001;285:1746–8.
9. Fox AT, Sasieni P, du Toit G, et al. Household peanut consumption as a risk factor for the development of peanut allergy. J Allergy Clin Immunol 2009;123:417–23.

10. Sicherer SH. Clinical implications of cross-reactive food allergens. J Allergy Clin Immunol 2001;108:881–90.

11. Beaudouin E, Renaudin JM, Morisset M, et al. Food-dependent exercise-induced anaphylaxis–update and current data. Eur Ann Allergy Clin Immunol 2006;38:45–51.

12. Alcoceba Borras E, Botey Faraudo E, Gaig Jane P, et al. Alcohol-induced anaphylaxis to grapes. Allergol Immunopathol (Madr) 2007;35:159–61.

13. Harada S, Horikawa T, Ashida M, et al. Aspirin enhances the induction of type I allergic symptoms when combined with food and exercise in patients with food-dependent exercise-induced anaphylaxis. Br J Dermatol 2001;145:336–9.

14. Norrman G, Falth-Magnusson K. Adverse reactions to skin prick testing in children – prevalence and possible risk factors. Pediatr Allergy Immunol 2009;20:273–8.

15. Bernstein IL, Li JT, Bernstein DI, et al. Allergy diagnostic testing: an updated practice parameter. Ann Allergy Asthma Immunol 2008;100:S1–148.

16. Sampson HA, Ho DG. Relationship between food-specific IgE concentrations and the risk of positive food challenges in children and adolescents. J Allergy Clin Immunol 1997;100:444–51.

17. Perry TT, Matsui EC, Kay Conover-Walker M, et al. The relationship of allergen-specific IgE levels and oral food challenge outcome. J Allergy Clin Immunol 2004;114:144–9.

18. Fleischer DM. The natural history of peanut and tree nut allergy. Curr Allergy Asthma Rep 2007;7:175–81.

19. Nowak-Wegrzyn A, Bloom KA, Sicherer SH, et al. Tolerance to extensively heated milk in children with cow's milk allergy. J Allergy Clin Immunol 2008;122:342–7, 7 e1–2.

20. Lemon-Mule H, Sampson HA, Sicherer SH, et al. Immunologic changes in children with egg allergy ingesting extensively heated egg. J Allergy Clin Immunol 2008;122:977–83 e1.

21. Konstantinou GN, Giavi S, Kalobatsou A, et al. Consumption of heat-treated egg by children allergic or sensitized to egg can affect the natural course of egg allergy: hypothesis-generating observations. J Allergy Clin Immunol 2008;122:414–5.

22. Puglisi G, Frieri M. Update on hidden food allergens and food labeling. Allergy Asthma Proc 2007;28:634–9.

23. Reisman RE. Natural history of insect sting allergy: relationship of severity of symptoms of initial sting anaphylaxis to re-sting reactions. J Allergy Clin Immunol 1992;90:335–9.

24. Rudders SA, Banerji A, Corel B, et al. Multicenter Study of Repeat Epinephrine Treatments for Food-Related Anaphylaxis. Pediatrics 2010;125:e711–8.

25. Jarvinen KM, Sicherer SH, Sampson HA, et al. Use of multiple doses of epinephrine in food-induced anaphylaxis in children. J Allergy Clin Immunol 2008;122:133–8.

26. Kelso JM. A second dose of epinephrine for anaphylaxis: how often needed and how to carry. J Allergy Clin Immunol 2006;117:464–5.

27. Nelson HS, Lahr J, Rule R, et al. Treatment of anaphylactic sensitivity to peanuts by immunotherapy with injections of aqueous peanut extract. J Allergy Clin Immunol 1997;99:744–51.

28. Sicherer SH, Sampson HA. Peanut allergy: emerging concepts and approaches for an apparent epidemic. J Allergy Clin Immunol 2007;120:491–503; quiz 4–5.

29. Patriarca G, Nucera E, Roncallo C, et al. Oral desensitizing treatment in food allergy: clinical and immunological results. Aliment Pharmacol Ther 2003;17:459–65.

30. Meglio P, Bartone E, Plantamura M, et al. A protocol for oral desensitization in children with IgE-mediated cow's milk allergy. Allergy 2004;59:980–7.

31. Buchanan AD, Green TD, Jones SM, et al. Egg oral immunotherapy in nonanaphylactic children with egg allergy. J Allergy Clin Immunol 2007;119:199–205.

32. Burks AW, Jones SM. Egg oral immunotherapy in non-anaphylactic children with egg allergy: follow-up. J Allergy Clin Immunol 2008;121:270–1.

33. Staden U, Rolinck-Werninghaus C, Brewe F, et al. Specific oral tolerance induction in food allergy in children: efficacy and clinical patterns of reaction. Allergy 2007;62:1261–9.

34. Longo G, Barbi E, Berti I, et al. Specific oral tolerance induction in children with very severe cow's milk-induced reactions. J Allergy Clin Immunol 2008;121:343–7.

35. Skripak JM, Nash SD, Rowley H, et al. A randomized, double-blind, placebo-controlled study of milk oral immunotherapy for cow's milk allergy. J Allergy Clin Immunol 2008;122:1154–60.

36. Du Toit G. Food-dependent exercise-induced anaphylaxis in childhood. Pediatr Allergy Immunol 2007;18:455–63.

37. Guinnepain MT, Eloit C, Raffard M, et al. Exercise-induced anaphylaxis: useful screening of food sensitization. Ann Allergy Asthma Immunol 1996;77:491–6.

38. Sampson HA. Jerome Glaser lectureship. The role of food allergy and mediator release in atopic dermatitis. J Allergy Clin Immunol 1988;81:635–45.

39. Burks AW, Mallory SB, Williams LW, et al. Atopic dermatitis: clinical relevance of food hypersensitivity reactions. J Pediatr 1988;113:447–51.

40. David TJ. Anaphylactic shock during elimination diets for severe atopic eczema. Arch Dis Child 1984;59:983–6.

41. Mari A, Ballmer-Weber BK, Vieths S. The oral allergy syndrome: improved diagnostic and treatment methods. Curr Opin Allergy Clin Immunol 2005;5:267–73.

42. Kelso JM. Pollen-food allergy syndrome.[comment]. Clinical & Experimental Allergy 2000;30:905–7.

43. Kelso JM. Oral allergy syndrome? J Allergy Clin Immunol 1995;96:275.

44. Kelso JM, Jones RT, Tellez R, et al. Oral allergy syndrome successfully treated with pollen immunotherapy. Ann Allergy Asthma Immunol 1995;74:391–6.

45. Asero R. Effects of birch pollen-specific immunotherapy on apple allergy in birch pollen-hypersensitive patients. Clin Exp Allergy 1998;28:1368–73.

46. Condemi JJ. Allergic reactions to natural rubber latex at home, to rubber products, and to cross-reacting foods. J Allergy Clin Immunol 2002;110:S107–10.

47. Erben AM, Rodriguez JL, McCullough J, et al. Anaphylaxis after ingestion of beignets contaminated with Dermatophagoides farinae. J Allergy Clin Immunol 1993;92:846–9.

48. Blanco C, Quiralte J, Castillo R, et al. Anaphylaxis after ingestion of wheat flour contaminated with mites. J Allergy Clin Immunol 1997;99:308–13.

49. Sanchez-Borges M, Capriles-Hulett A, Fernandez-Caldas E, et al. Mite-contaminated foods as a cause of anaphylaxis. J Allergy Clin Immunol 1997;99:738–43.

50. Lantner RR, Espiritu BR, Zumerchik P, et al. Anaphylaxis following ingestion of a psyllium-containing cereal. JAMA 1990;264:2534–6.

51. James JM, Cooke SK, Barnett A, et al. Anaphylactic reactions to a psyllium-containing cereal. J Allergy Clin Immunol 1991;88:402–8.

52. Freeman GL. Psyllium hypersensitivity. Ann Allergy 1994;73:490–2.

53. Blanchard C, Wang N, Rothenberg ME. Eosinophilic esophagitis: pathogenesis, genetics, and therapy. J Allergy Clin Immunol 2006;118:1054–9.

54. Kelly KJ, Lazenby AJ, Rowe PC, et al. Eosinophilic esophagitis attributed to gastroesophageal reflux: improvement with an amino acid-based formula. Gastroenterology 1995;109:1503–12.

55. Spergel JM, Andrews T, Brown-Whitehorn TF, et al. Treatment of eosinophilic esophagitis with specific food elimination diet directed by a combination of skin prick and patch tests. Ann Allergy Asthma Immunol 2005;95:336–43.

56. Aceves SS, Bastian JF, Newbury RO, et al. Oral viscous budesonide: a potential new therapy for eosinophilic esophagitis in children. Am J Gastroenterol 2007;102:2271–9; quiz 80.

57. Stein ML, Collins MH, Villanueva JM, et al. Anti-IL-5 (mepolizumab) therapy for eosinophilic esophagitis. J Allergy Clin Immunol 2006;118:1312–9.

58. Perino A, Cabras S, Obinu D, et al. Lactose intolerance: a non-allergic disorder often managed by allergologists. Eur Ann Allergy Clin Immunol 2009;41:3–16.

59. Green PH, Jabri B. Coeliac disease. Lancet 2003;362:383–91.

60. van Heel DA, West J. Recent advances in coeliac disease. Gut 2006;55:1037–46.

61. Sicherer SH. Food protein-induced enterocolitis syndrome: case presentations and management lessons. J Allergy Clin Immunol 2005;115:149–56.

62. Mehr S, Kakakios A, Frith K, et al. Food protein-induced enterocolitis syndrome: 16-year experience. Pediatrics 2009;123:e459–64.

63. Ravelli A, Villanacci V, Chiappa S, et al. Dietary protein-induced proctocolitis in childhood. Am J Gastroenterol 2008;103:2605–12.

64. Taylor SL, Stratton JE, Nordlee JA. Histamine poisoning (scombroid fish poisoning): an allergy-like intoxication. J Toxicol Clin Toxicol 1989;27:225–40.

65. Morrow JD, Margolies GR, Rowland J, et al. Evidence that histamine is the causative toxin of scombroid-fish poisoning. N Engl J Med 1991;324:716–20.

66. Kelso JM, Lin FL. Skin testing for scombroid poisoning. Ann Allergy Asthma Immunol 2009;103:447.

67. Keller KM, Burgin-Wolff A, Lippold R, et al. The diagnostic significance of IgG cow's milk protein antibodies re-evaluated. Eur J Pediatr 1996;155:331–7.

CHAPTER 5

Atopic Dermatitis and Food Allergy

Tamara T. Perry, Debra D. Becton and Stacie M. Jones

KEY CONCEPTS

- Atopic dermatitis (AD) is a chronic skin disorder with hallmark features of tissue inflammation and epidermal barrier dysfunction.
- Food allergy is an important trigger for AD.

- 35–40% of infants and young children with moderate to severe AD will have food allergy.
- Food allergy is more likely to be a complicating factor if AD is severe or presents in the first year of life.

Introduction

Atopic dermatitis (AD) is a complex, chronic inflammatory skin disorder that is often associated with food allergy. It is a multifactorial disease linked to a complex interaction between skin barrier function, genetics and environmental factors, including commonly encountered triggers such as allergens, microbes and irritants. As early as the 1890s, the term neurodermatitis was used to describe a chronic, pruritic skin condition seen in patients felt to have a nervous disorder. By the early 1900s, others had noted the occurrence of a similar disorder with asthma and hay fever, and used the term atopy to further describe the combination of these diseases. The term atopic dermatitis was then coined by Wise and Sulzberger[1] in 1933 to more fully describe this skin disorder. Since its earliest description, AD has had as its primary feature intense pruritus triggered by a variety of stimuli. In this chapter, we explore the link between allergic sensitization to specific foods and the condition of AD.

The term 'atopic march' has been coined to describe the natural history and sequential progression of atopic disorders.[2] Atopic dermatitis is often considered the first manifestation of the atopic march, since clinical symptoms of AD often precede the development of other atopic disorders such as allergic rhinitis and asthma. Approximately 60% of children affected by AD will develop symptoms in the first year of life and 85% will do so by age 5. Moreover, as many as 50–80% of children with AD will develop allergic respiratory disease (e.g. asthma and allergic rhinoconjunctivitis) later in life. Because of these strong associations, investigators have explored the role of various allergens, including food allergens, as triggers in the pathogenesis of AD.

Food allergy has been strongly correlated with the development and persistence of AD, especially during infancy and early childhood.[3,4] Also, the skin is the site that is most often involved in food hypersensitivity reactions.[5] In sensitized individuals, food allergen exposure often results in urticaria, itching, and eczematous skin flares. Sensitization and subsequent allergic reactions can occur to any food, but those most commonly associated with AD are milk, egg, soy and peanut. Although allergies to some foods are typically outgrown, others such as peanut or shellfish allergy, may persist and continue to aggravate AD symptoms into late adolescence and adulthood.[3,6–8]

Epidemiology

The prevalence of food allergy in patients with AD varies with the age of the patient and the severity of AD. In a study of 2184 Australian infants, investigators found an association between high levels of food-specific IgE and earlier age of onset of AD and increased disease severity.[9] This group found that AD patients who developed severe disease within the first 3 months of life most commonly had specific IgE to cows' milk, egg and peanut, and were at highest risk for developing food allergy. In another study, investigators noted that in some infants sensitization precedes and predicts the development of AD, whereas in others AD precedes and predicts the development of sensitization. In a meta-analysis on the prevalence of food allergy, Rona and colleagues[10] reported that up to 37% of children with moderate to severe AD had evidence of IgE-mediated allergies to foods. Similarly, in a study of children with AD, Burks et al.[5] diagnosed food allergy in approximately 35% of 165 patients with AD referred to both university allergy and dermatology clinics. Later, Burks and colleagues[5] published findings that 82% of 138 peanut-allergic children seen in an allergy referral clinic had AD. Eigenmann et al.[11] studied 63 unselected children (median age 2.8 years) with moderate to severe AD who were referred to a university dermatologist and reported that 37% of these patients were diagnosed with food allergy after an evaluation that included oral food challenges. Similarly, in a study of more than 250 French children with an established diagnosis of AD, investigators noted that increased severity of AD in the younger patients was correlated with the presence of food allergy.[12]

CLINICAL CASE

AN presented at 9 months of life with symptoms of pruritus, inconsolable crying and sleep disturbance attributed to severe, uncontrolled AD despite topical corticosteroid therapy and emollients. A diagnostic evaluation for food allergy was initiated because of AN's history of urticarial rash with exposure to multiple foods and history of poorly controlled AD. Testing revealed specific sensitivities to multiple foods, including milk (0.56 kU/L), egg (1.14 kU/L), soy (2.15 kU/L), peanut

(20.0 kU/L) and rice (6.38 kU/L). Strict dietary elimination of these foods, along with topical corticosteroids, emollients and antimicrobials for secondary skin infection, led to a dramatic improvement in both skin symptoms and behavior. At 2 years of age, AN's skin symptoms remain controlled on dietary restriction and topical therapies (Fig. 5.1).

To date, studies in adult patients have been limited, and none accurately predict the prevalence or role of foods in AD. In one systematic review of randomized controlled trials to assess the effects of dietary elimination in a mixed group of both children and adults with established AD, investigators concluded that elimination diets were not beneficial in unselected cases.[13] However, there was significant clinical improvement when egg elimination was prescribed for patients with suspected egg allergy. Clearly more work is needed in older adolescent and adult populations to better understand the role of food allergy in AD in these age groups.

Pathogenesis

There are two distinguishing features important to the pathogenesis of AD, cutaneous inflammation and defective epidermal barrier function. Additionally, genetics may play an important role in the pathogenesis of both AD and food allergy.[14] The inflammatory response noted in AD involves both adaptive and innate immunity. The hallmark allergic inflammatory response associated with AD results from antigen-induced changes that include both T-helper cell type 1 (Th1) and type 2 (Th2) profiles of inflammation. Allergen-induced IgE-mediated mast cell activation results in hypersensitivity reactions characterized by tissue infiltration of eosinophils, monocytes and lymphocytes. In acute AD the patterns of cytokine and chemokine expression found in infiltrating lymphocytes are predominantly those of the Th2 type (e.g. IL-4, IL-5 and IL-13).[15,16] Epidermal, myeloid-derived dendritic cells express high-affinity IgE receptors (FcεRI) that bind IgE and which are noted in biopsy tissue from inflamed AD skin. These cells take up and present allergens to Th1, Th2 and T-regulatory cells, all of which are important in AD.[17] In addition, IgE-bearing Langerhans' cells are highly efficient at presenting allergens to T cells, thereby activating a combined Th1/Th2 profile in chronic AD lesions. These findings support a combination of specific IgE antibody, Th1 and Th2 cytokines/chemokines

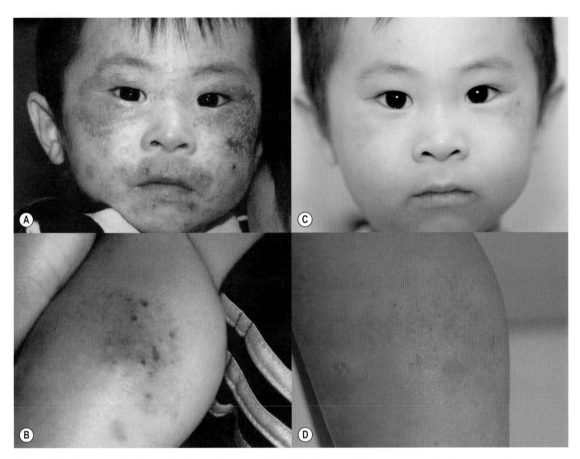

Figure 5.1 AN presented at 9 months of age with severe AD (A, B), behavior problems and sleep disturbance due to intense pruritus. One year later, (C,D) the same patient presented with dramatically improved skin and behavior after elimination of relevant food allergens, topical therapies, antihistamine therapy and a course of antimicrobials for a secondary *S. aureus* skin infection.

in the pathogenesis of AD. The role of food-specific T cells in the pathophysiology of AD has been considered for decades. The atopic patch test (APT) has been used to further evaluate specific allergens and subsequent T-cell activation in affected skin. In some patients who may have a delayed response to foods, investigators hypothesize that the reactions may occur via high-affinity IgE receptors expressed on Langerhans' and dendritic cells, leading to allergen-specific T-cell responses capable of promoting both IgE production and delayed-type hypersensitivity reactions. The APT results demonstrate allergen-specific T-cell infiltration as evidence supporting T-cell involvement in the pathogenesis of AD.[18,19]

Another key feature of AD is defective epidermal barrier function. Important genetic mutations in the epidermal structural protein filaggrin have been

identified as key defects resulting in epidermal barrier dysfunction.[20] These loss-of-function genetic mutations result in decreased epidermal defense mechanisms against allergens and microbes. Filaggrin gene mutations and resultant epidermal barrier dysfunction have been linked to the development, progression and severity of AD, as well as increased susceptibility to skin infections. Epidermal barrier dysfunction may result in increased penetration of allergens through the skin, thereby making the skin a potentially important route by which individuals are sensitized to food and airborne allergens. Fox and colleagues[21] described a dose-dependent association between household peanut exposure and increased risk for the development of peanut allergy. Children with peanut allergy had significantly higher environmental peanut exposure than nonallergic children and high-risk atopic children with egg allergy. This positive relationship between environmental exposure and disease development remained significant after controlling for maternal peanut consumption during pregnancy and lactation. Epidermal barrier dysfunction may also facilitate the ability of viral and bacterial microbes to penetrate the skin, resulting in secondary infections (e.g., chronic/recurrent methicillin-resistant *Staphylococcus aureus* (MRSA), molluscum contagiosum and eczema herpeticum). These infections may further facilitate or enhance the inflammatory response and may serve to further weaken the barrier function, thereby providing a feedback mechanism for chronic disease.

Findings from several studies examining mutations in the filaggrin gene support the genetic link between atopic dermatitis risk and increased propensity to develop other atopic disorders, such as food allergies. In a meta-analysis of 24 studies on filaggrin mutations and atopic dermatitis, as well as 17 studies on asthma, Rodriguez and colleagues[22] concluded that filaggrin gene defects significantly increased the risk of atopic dermatitis diagnosis (odds ratio [OR] 3.12; 95% CI 2.57–3.79), as well as more severe skin disease. Mutations were also found to be significantly associated with the combination of asthma and AD, but not with asthma in the absence of AD. In a German birth cohort of 871 children[23] filaggrin gene mutations had a 100% positive predictive value for the development of asthma among children with atopic dermatitis and early food sensitization. These findings suggest that early genotyping for filaggrin gene defects may identify specific populations at risk – perhaps those with early food sensitization and AD – that might benefit from early interventions aimed to reduce progression of the atopic march.

Although filaggrin gene defects have been implicated as important risk factors for the development and increased severity of AD, it should be noted that the full implications of the filaggrin defects are not completely understood.[20] Not all patients with filaggrin mutations have AD, and similarly not all patients with AD have a known filaggrin gene defect. Also, patients with filaggrin defects have been reported to 'outgrow' symptoms of AD. These observations support the notion that other factors, such as genetics and environmental and dietary exposures, are probably important in clinical manifestations of disease.

Other genetic mutations resulting in clinical disease have provided further insight into the relationship between AD and food allergy. Two disorders provide particularly compelling information. IPEX (immune dysregulation, polyendocrinopathy, enteropathy, X-linked) is a fatal disorder characterized by autoimmune enteropathy, endocrinopathy, severe dermatitis, elevated serum IgE and multiple food allergies. IPEX syndrome results from a gene mutation that affects the FOXP3 protein.[24] FOXP3 (known as the 'master regulator' for T cells) plays a central role in the generation of regulatory T cells that are presumed to be important for the balance between oral tolerance and food allergy development. Similarly, mutations in the serine protease inhibitor Karzal type 5 (SPINK5) gene have been associated with Netherton syndrome, an autosomal recessive disorder characterized by an AD-like rash, associated Th2 skewing and increased IgE levels.[25] Japanese investigators have recently found an association of SPINK5 mutations in children with AD and food allergy. In another investigation, SPINK5 polymorphism was significantly associated with increased disease severity among Japanese children under 10 years with AD and food allergy. Other investigators have found variants in the gene for the proinflammatory cytokine IL-13 in association with early sensitization to foods and total serum IgE levels among a group of 453 children with AD in the Early Treatment of the Atopic Child (ETAC) cohort.[26] Owing to the long-standing historical associations of atopy and AD within families, numerous investigators have identified a population of over 80 genes that have some association with AD. Those implicated often relate to antigen presentation or cell- or antibody-mediated responses, or those involving cell signaling.[14] Little is so far known about gene–environment interactions in AD that may also have important implications in association with food allergy. These genetic studies provide evidence that food allergy and AD are likely to be genetically linked with varying degrees of disease expression within patient populations. Additional genetic studies, in larger and more diverse populations, are in progress to further identify the genetic link between food allergy and AD and will probably provide additional genes of interest.

Clinical features

A variety of allergic and non-allergic triggers are known to aggravate and complicate the condition

Table 5.1 Important triggers of atopic dermatitis

Food allergens	
Milk*	Tree nuts
Eggs*	Fish
Peanuts*	Shellfish
Soy	Wheat
Aeroallergens	
Dust mites	Animal dander
Pollen	Cockroach
Mold	
Microbes	
Bacteria	**Fungi/yeasts**
Staphylococcus aureus	*Pityrosporum ovale*
Streptococcus species	*Pityrosporum obiculare*
	Trichophytan species
	Candida albicans
	Malazassia furfur
Other factors	
Irritants: soaps, detergents, fragrances or fabrics	
Climate or temperature changes	
Psychosocial: anxiety or stress	
*Most common foods in infants and young children with AD.	

of AD (Table 5.1). The role of food allergy in the development or progression of AD has been a topic of debate among clinicians for years, with multiple clinical studies attempting to address the issue. Whether food allergy can aggravate AD is still controversial, owing largely to the fact that signs and symptoms of both food allergy and AD are pleomorphic, and because well-designed clinical trials of food allergen elimination in patients with AD have rarely been performed. In clinical studies, investigators have shown that elimination of the relevant food allergen can lead to improvement in skin symptoms (Fig. 5.1) and that repeat challenges can lead to recurrence of symptoms. Other studies focusing on the immunologic mechanisms have provided evidence supporting the role for food-specific IgE antibodies and T-cell involvement in the disease manifestations of AD. Additionally, several longitudinal studies in high-risk infants have now shown that AD may be delayed or prevented by exclusive breastfeeding, the introduction of hydrolyzed infant formulas or by eliminating highly allergenic foods such as milk and eggs from the diet.[27] Also, recent investigations have reported on the relevance of cutaneous exposure to allergens in the development of food allergy.[21,28]

Clinical evidence supporting the relationship between AD and food allergy

A number of studies have addressed the therapeutic effect of dietary elimination in the treatment of AD. Many of these trials, however, have limitations due to the failure to control for confounding factors such as placebo effect, observer bias, environmental factors and other triggers. In a study of children with AD between the ages of 2 and 8 years, Atherton et al.[29] showed marked improvement in two-thirds of subjects during a double-blind crossover trial of milk and egg exclusion. The study, however, was complicated by high dropout and exclusion rates as well as a lack of control of environmental factors and other triggers of AD. Another study by Juto et al.[30] reported that approximately one-third of AD patients had resolution of their rash, and that half improved on a highly restricted diet. The cumulative results of these studies support the role for foods as triggers in the exacerbation of AD in children. In an early prospective study, Sampson and Scanlon[3] studied 34 children with AD, 17 of whom had food allergy diagnosed by double-blind, placebo-controlled food challenges (DBPCFCs). During 1–4-year follow-up periods, food-allergic patients with appropriate dietary restriction demonstrated significant improvement in their AD compared with the control groups (those without food allergy, or food-allergic patients who did not adhere to dietary restrictions). Lever and colleagues[31] performed a randomized controlled trial of egg elimination in young children with AD and a positive specific IgE test to egg. Fifty-five children were identified by oral food challenge to be egg allergic. There was a significant decrease in the skin area affected and in symptom scores in the children adhering to an egg-avoidance diet compared to the control subjects on no dietary avoidance (percent involvement 21.9–18.9%; symptom score 36.7–33.5).

KF was a 14-month-old with a history of recalcitrant AD. Symptoms of eczematous rash and severe pruritus were not relieved with emollient therapy and twice daily medium-potency topical corticosteroid ointment. Food allergy was suspected and testing led to the diagnosis of egg allergy, with egg-specific IgE of 7.75 kU/L (nl <0.35). Two months after strict egg elimination, KF's AD was well controlled with emollient therapy alone.

Oral food challenges have also been used to demonstrate that food allergens can induce symptoms of rash and pruritus in children with food allergy-related AD. Double-blind placebo-controlled food challenges (DBPCFC) are considered the gold standard for the diagnosis of food allergy, especially in the setting of AD. Several investigative groups have published reports using DBPCFCs to identify causal food proteins that serve as triggers for AD. Multiple studies using oral food challenges have demonstrated a predominance of cutaneous symptoms as manifestation of a positive food challenge.[7,21,32] These studies have shown that cutaneous reactions occurred in 75% of the positive challenges, generally consisting of pruritic, morbilliform or macular eruptions in the predilection sites for AD. Isolated skin symptoms were typically seen in only 30% of the reactions, and gastrointestinal (50%) and respiratory (45%) reactions also occurred. Investigators have also confirmed that a limited number of foods cause clinical symptoms in younger patients with AD (Table 5.2). Milk, eggs and peanuts generally cause more than 75% of the IgE-mediated

Table 5.2 Relevant food allergies in atopic dermatitis according to age

Infants	Children	Older children/adults
Milk	Milk	Peanuts
Eggs	Eggs	Tree nuts
Peanuts	Peanuts	Fish
Soy	Soy	Shellfish
	Wheat	
	Tree nuts	
	Fish	
	Shellfish	

From Sicherer SH, Sampson HA. Food hypersensitivity and atopic dermatitis: pathophysiology, epidemiology, diagnosis, and management. J Allergy Clin Immunol 1999; 104: S114–S122.

reactions. If soy, wheat, fish and tree nuts are added to this list, more than 98% of the foods that cause clinical symptoms will be identified.[4,5,33]

Immunologic evidence supporting the relationship between AD and food allergy

Several studies investigating the immunologic mechanisms of disease have provided support for the role for food-specific IgE antibodies in the pathogenesis of AD. Many patients with AD have elevated concentrations of total IgE and food-specific IgE antibodies. More than 50 years ago, Wilson and Walzer[34] demonstrated that the ingestion of foods would allow antigens to penetrate the gastrointestinal barrier and then be transported in the circulation to IgE-bearing mast cells in the skin. More recent investigations have shown that in children with food-specific IgE antibodies undergoing oral food challenges, positive challenges are accompanied by increases in plasma histamine concentration, elaboration of eosinophil products, and activation of plasma eosinophils.[35-37] Children with AD who were chronically ingesting foods to which they were allergic have been found to have increased spontaneous basophil histamine release (SBHR) from peripheral blood basophils in vitro compared with children without food allergy or normal subjects.[38] After starting the appropriate elimination diet, food-allergic children experienced significant clearing of their skin and a significant fall in their SBHR. Other studies have shown that peripheral blood mononuclear cells from food-allergic patients with high SBHR elaborate specific cytokines termed histamine-releasing factors (HRFs) which activate basophils from food-sensitive – but not food-insensitive – patients. Food allergen-specific T cells have been cloned from normal skin and active skin lesions in patients with AD. In addition, cutaneous lymphocyte-associated antigen (CLA) is a homing molecule that interacts with E-selectin and directs T cells to the skin. One study compared patients with milk-induced AD to control subjects with milk-induced gastrointestinal reactions without AD and with non-atopic controls. Casein-reactive T cells from children with milk-induced AD had a significantly higher expression of CLA than did *Candida albicans*-reactive T cells from the same patients and either casein- or *C. albicans*-reactive T cells from the control groups.[39]

Environmental and dietary exposures important in the development of AD and food allergy

An alternate and emerging paradigm that opposes the traditional model of food allergen sensitization via the ingestion route has been championed by several investigators. This suggests that sensitization to food allergens can occur via cutaneous exposure to antigen owing to poor barrier function in AD skin. Lack and colleagues[28] have confirmed peanut allergy in preschool children with AD and increased exposure to peanut-based skin oils. These observations, along with mouse studies demonstrating that epidermal application of ovalbumin results in the development of eczematous lesions and ovalbumin-specific IgE production, have led Lack to hypothesize that environmental exposure to allergens through the skin of infants' with AD is responsible for allergen sensitivity and allergic disease. As previously noted, this group found a dose-dependent association between peanut exposure in the home and an increased risk for the development of peanut allergy.[21]

CLINICAL CASE

TD was a 15-month-old with a history of mild AD presenting for evaluation of peanut allergy. TD had no known history of peanut ingestion, yet the parents reported two separate incidents of erythema and hives on her cheek within 5 minutes of receiving a kiss from her mother who had recently ingested peanuts. Peanut-specific IgE was 12.5 kU/L. Detailed dietary history confirmed that there was no history of peanut ingestion by TD; however, family members consumed peanut butter on a regular basis.

In addition to these environmental investigations, longitudinal studies have been conducted in general population birth cohorts and cohorts of high-risk infants to determine the role of breastfeeding, maternal diet restriction during pregnancy and lactation, the use of hydrolyzed formulas and delayed food introduction on the development of AD and other atopic diseases.[27] To date, maternal dietary restriction of allergenic foods during pregnancy and lactation has not been shown to significantly affect the development of atopic disease in infants. A recent meta-analysis determined that exclusive breastfeeding during the first 3 months of life is associated with lower incidence rates of AD during childhood in children with a family history of atopy.[40] In two series, infants from atopic families whose mothers excluded eggs, milk and fish from their diets during lactation (prophylaxis group) had significantly less AD and food allergy at 18 months than those whose mothers' diets were unrestricted. Follow-up at 4 years showed that the prophylaxis group had less AD, but there was no difference in food allergy or respiratory allergy.[41,42]

In a comprehensive, prospective randomized allergy prevention trial, Zeiger and colleagues[43,44] compared the benefits of maternal and infant food allergen avoidance on the prevention of allergic disease in infants at high risk for allergic disease during a 7-year longitudinal study. Breastfeeding was encouraged in both prophylaxis (dietary allergen restriction) and control (usual feeding without dietary restriction) groups. Compared to controls, the prevalence of AD and food allergy in the prophylaxis group was reduced in the first 2 years; however, the period prevalence of AD was not significant beyond 2 years. In the German Infant Nutritional Intervention Study (GINI),[45] 2252 healthy term infants were randomized to receive one of four blinded formulas during the first 4 months of life when breastfeeding was insufficient: partially (PHW) or extensively hydrolyzed whey (EHW), extensively hydrolyzed casein (EHC) or cows' milk (CM). The 6-year follow-up study showed a long-term preventive effect of hydrolyzed infant formulas for AD until age 6 years, with the relative risk of a physician diagnosis of AD compared with CM of 0.79 (95% CI, 0.64–0.97) for PHW; 0.92 (95% CI, 0.76–1.11) for EHW; and 0.71 (95% CI, 0.58–0.88) for EHC. Similar findings were noted in a high-risk birth cohort of 120 infants from the Isle of Wight followed for 8 years. Infants in the intervention group (low-allergen diet, hypoallergenic formula and dust mite avoidance) were noted to have less asthma, AD, allergic rhinitis and atopy than those in the control (routine care and feeding) group.

A recent meta-analysis of intervention studies using partially hydrolyzed whey (PHW) formula versus standard cows' milk formula feedings in infants at high-risk for atopy showed an advantage of PHW formula in reducing the risk of AD development during the first 12 months of life. This analysis indicated a 55% decreased risk of AD through 6–12 months among infants who were fed PHW formula.[46] Conversely, several studies in prospective birth cohorts have shown no benefit in delayed dietary introduction of solid foods past 4 months of life on the development of AD, and even note that delayed introduction may be associated with a higher risk of AD.[47]

These studies have led to new recommendations for early nutritional interventions in infants at high risk (defined as one parent or sibling with atopic disease) by the American Academy of Pediatrics (2008),[27] including 1) breastfeeding for the first 4–6 months of life; 2) the use of an extensively hydrolyzed casein (or a partially hydrolyzed whey formula) instead of cows' milk or soy formula when breastfeeding is inadequate during the first 4–6 months of life; and 3) delaying the introduction of solid foods until 4–6 months of age, but not beyond. These recommendations are different from those published by the AAP in 2000, which recommended the delayed introduction of highly allergenic foods in high-risk infants (e.g. peanuts until age 3 years).[48] Currently, there are no general guidelines to address the delayed introduction of allergenic foods for high-risk infants and children who have early manifestations of atopic disease such as food allergy or AD. Recommendations for elimination diets or delayed food introductions for high-risk infants should be determined on an individual basis after consultation and testing by a medical professional trained in the diagnosis and management of food allergies.

Ongoing longitudinal studies may shed further light on the role of food allergy and AD. The NIH-funded Consortium of Food Allergy Research (CoFAR; https://web.emmes.com/study/cofar/) has recently published the baseline characteristics of 512 infants enrolled in a longitudinal observational study of food allergen sensitization and clinical manifestations of food allergy, including the presence of AD.[49] Enrollment criteria for the study included either a positive SPT to egg or milk antigen and either a convincing history of egg or milk allergy or evidence of moderate to severe AD. Allergen sensitization was noted to milk in 78%, egg in 89% and peanut in 69% of subjects at the time of enrollment (ages 3–15 months). Of the subjects, 204 were enrolled based on AD criteria and had never had an acute food-allergic reaction. Lack and colleagues[50] have also suggested a link between food-specific IgE sensitization and cutaneous exposure to antigen through inflamed AD skin lesions and the potential role of early introduction of dietary allergens in reducing atopic manifestations. Similar to findings from the CoFAR group, early results from the LEAP study (Learning Early About Peanut Allergy; www.leapstudy.co.uk) indicate a similar high prevalence of food allergen sensitization associated with AD in early infancy. The LEAP study has enrolled approximately 480 infants with AD and/or egg allergy and will follow them for 5 years in two treatment groups, one avoiding peanuts and the other eating peanuts. These long-term follow-up studies hold promise to provide additional information on the role of food allergy, the timing of food allergen exposure, and environmental and genetic factors that surround the complex issue of food allergy and AD.

Diagnosis

The diagnosis of food allergy in AD may be straightforward in cases with associated signs and symptoms of distinct anaphylaxis. The diagnosis of food allergy in AD, however, is frequently complicated by several factors: the immediate response to the ingestion of causal foods is downregulated with repetitive ingestion, making obvious 'cause-and-effect' relations difficult to establish; other environmental · trigger factors (e.g. inhalant allergens, irritants, microbes) may play a role in the course of disease, often obscuring the effect of dietary changes;[51,52] and specific IgE to multiple allergens is commonly found to many foods, many of which are not associated with clinical symptoms, making a diagnosis based solely on laboratory testing difficult.[53] A combination of history, laboratory assessment and dietary manipulation with oral food challenge is often needed to confirm or refute the diagnosis of food allergy in association with AD (Fig. 5.2).

CLINICAL CASE

CJ was a 4-year-old girl with multiple atopic disorders including severe AD, asthma and various food allergies. Her reactions to foods included both immediate IgE-mediated symptoms after ingestion (urticaria and lower respiratory symptoms) and multiple foods that resulted in AD flare 24–48 hours after ingestion. Her course was complicated by poor nutritional status owing to multiple food restrictions, and IgE testing was positive to all foods, with a total serum IgE 2002 kU/L (0.3–133 kU/L). After a detailed dietary history and oral challenges to foods with a low index of suspicion for reaction, CJ was able to introduce several nutritionally relevant foods to her diet. One year later, her nutritional status and weight gain were appropriate.

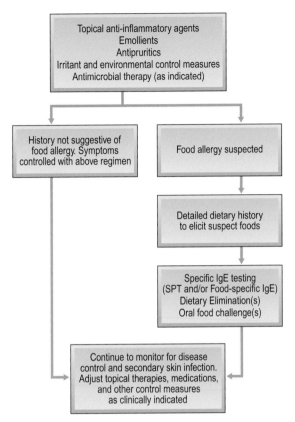

Topical anti-inflammatory agents
Emollients
Antipruritics
Irritant and environmental control measures
Antimicrobial therapy (as indicated)

History not suggestive of food allergy. Symptoms controlled with above regimen

Food allergy suspected

Detailed dietary history to elicit suspect foods

Specific IgE testing (SPT and/or Food-specific IgE) Dietary Elimination(s) Oral food challenge(s)

Continue to monitor for disease control and secondary skin infection. Adjust topical therapies, medications, and other control measures as clinically indicated

Figure 5.2 Treatment algorithm for atopic dermatitis (AD). The majority of patients with AD are adequately controlled with a tailored combination of topical anti-inflammatory medications, anti-pruritic therapy, emollients, and environmental control measures. Selected patients may need antimicrobial treatment for secondary skin infections. Patients with moderate–severe or recalcitrant AD require further investigation to determine the presence of food allergies. Specific IgE testing, dietary elimination and oral food challenges can aid in the accurate diagnosis of clinically relevant food triggers. All patients should be monitored periodically to assess control of symptoms, and medication and dietary modifications made as clinically indicated. (SPT, skin prick testing.)

A careful medical history is essential in the diagnostic evaluation. For breastfed infants a maternal dietary history is essential owing to the passage of food proteins in breast milk to the infant.[27] Selected foods should then be evaluated by testing for specific IgE (e.g. skin prick test [SPT], food-specific IgE immunoassay). A small number of foods account for more than 90% of reactions, and the most common food allergens are listed in Table 5.2.[33,54,55] Food additives have been documented to cause flaring of AD but with a much lower prevalence.[56,57] Emerging evidence suggests that chemical

contaminants in foods (such as oleoresins in fruits, vegetables and spices) or metals or fragrances in foods (such as Balsam of Peru in chocolate or citrus fruits) may cause forms of local or systemic allergic contact dermatitis that may also resemble flares of AD and require food elimination for resolution of symptoms.

As noted in Chapter 13, the diagnosis of food allergy is enhanced by the use of IgE testing to specific foods. In particular, skin prick tests and IgE immunoassays have proved useful, but although helpful, these tests can often be misleading in the setting of concomitant persistent AD. Patients with AD will often have positive SPTs and/or food-specific IgE tests to several members of a botanical family (e.g. cereal grains and grass pollen) or animal species (e.g. milk and beef). These commonly indicate immunologic cross-reactivity but not relevant intrabotanical or intraspecies cross-reactivity of clinical importance. Therefore, the practice of avoiding all foods within a botanical family when one member is suspected of provoking allergic symptoms is generally unwarranted. Rather, the judicious use of specific IgE testing, coupled with clinical history, response to dietary manipulation and possibly oral food challenge, may be needed to make an appropriate diagnosis of food allergy in a patient with AD.[58]

After laboratory studies, the best initial treatment is elimination of the suspected food(s) from the diet, followed by an oral food challenge if indicated. No further testing or food challenges are necessary in cases of severe, acute clinical reactions or anaphylactic reactions associated with food ingestion or exposure (e.g. inhalation or topical), or if dramatic improvement in skin disease occurs with dietary elimination. Because symptoms are chronic in AD and multiple foods may be implicated by specific IgE testing, it is often necessary to perform diagnostic oral food challenges.

Oral food challenges can be invaluable in the appropriate diagnosis and management of patients with AD and possible food allergy.[59] For patients with persistent AD despite optimal topical therapies, oral challenges to major food allergens should be considered when diagnostic testing (food-specific IgE levels and/or SPT) do not correlate with a history of clinical reaction. Oral challenges are also necessary to evaluate the resolution (or the development of natural tolerance) of the specific food allergy and can be performed safely. However, oral challenges are contraindicated when there is a clear recent history of food-induced anaphylaxis. Additionally, patients should be instructed not to perform food challenges of suspect foods at home (or away from medical intervention) because of the potential risk of severe or life-threatening allergic reactions.[60,61]

Management

Despite the fact that investigators have published case reports since the early 1900s of patients whose AD improved after avoiding specific foods, only more recently have larger clinical studies been published to validate the role of food allergy diagnosis and management in the overall management of AD. Despite persistent controversy about the role of food allergy in the pathogenesis of AD, there is now significant laboratory and clinical evidence that would suggest the debate is no longer valid.

The elimination of food proteins can often be difficult, and incomplete elimination of the offending food can lead to confusion and inconclusive results during an open trial of dietary elimination. For example, in a milk-free diet, patients must be instructed not only to avoid all milk products but also to read all food labels to identify 'hidden' sources of cows' milk protein. For example, ingredients such as natural flavoring, caramel flavoring, brown sugar flavoring or margarine may contain milk. Another important issue regarding food restrictions is related to the economic and social impact of dietary elimination.[62,63] Patients avoiding multiple foods may find it difficult to adhere to a diet that eliminates major food groups owing to the cost of allergen-free alternatives, inconvenience, the complexity of dietary needs and taste preferences. Adequate understanding of clinical testing and interpretation of results must be paired with appropriate dietary restrictions – typically only a few foods – to avoid unnecessary dietary restrictions and potential complications.

Care must be taken to ensure that patients on elimination diets have adequate resources, including dietary counseling and education, social support and financial assistance, to best manage their disease. The role of dietary counseling through a registered dietitian cannot be over-emphasized. A registered dietitian cannot only help with counseling regarding dietary avoidance of food allergens, label reading and cross-contact, but can help the patient maintain a healthy, well-balanced diet (e.g., calcium and vitamin D supplementation

during a milk-avoidance diet). The triggers associated with disease pathogenesis and clinical symptoms in patients with AD are vast; however, discerning the role of allergens as a trigger factor, particularly food allergens, early in life is clearly very important. A careful dietary history and appropriate diagnostic testing, coupled with a comprehensive treatment program, can be disease modifying and life altering for patients with AD. Other important aspects of the treatment program, including intense moisturization and hydration, topical anti-inflammatory agents such as corticosteroids or calcineurin inhibitors, irritant avoidance, and antipruritic therapy, are essential to pair with food allergy management for effective, comprehensive therapy (Fig. 5.2).

Natural history

The majority of children outgrow their allergies to milk, eggs, wheat and soy,[3,64] although recent studies have shown that the rate of resolution of some food allergens (e.g. egg and milk) may be slower than previously described (Table 5.3). In one study of the natural history of egg allergy in children followed in a pediatric allergy practice, investigators found that the age distribution of resolution of allergy was 4% by age 4, 12% by age 6, 37% by age 10 and 68% by age 16.[65] The egg-specific IgE level was predictive of allergy outcome and can be used with skin testing to counsel patients on prognosis. In another study, Perry et al.[59] also

Table 5.3 Natural history of food allergy

Food	Median age at diagnosis	Percent expected to develop oral tolerance
Milk	<12 mo	19–75% by age 4 years (79% by age 16 years)
Egg	<12 mo	4–50% by age 4 years (68% by age 16 years)
Soy	<12 mo	25% by age 4 years (69% by age 10 years)
Peanut	14 mo	20% (8% recurrence rate)
Tree Nuts	36 mo	<10%
Fish	>18 years	Not reported

showed that food-specific IgE levels are helpful in determining the likelihood that a child has outgrown their food allergy. Patients allergic to peanuts, tree nuts, fish and shellfish are much less likely to lose their clinical reactivity.[7,66] It does appear, however, that approximately 20% of patients who have a reaction to peanuts early in life may outgrow their sensitivity.[7] Only approximately 9% of patients with tree nut allergy will outgrow their allergy.[8] In one study approximately one-third of children with AD and food allergy lost or outgrew their clinical reactivity over 1–3 years with strict adherence to dietary elimination. Clinical reactivity is lost over time more quickly than the loss of food-specific IgE measured by SPT or serum food-specific IgE testing; therefore, definitive diagnostic testing (i.e. oral food challenges) may be necessary to prevent unwarranted dietary restrictions. The combination of carefully following the history of accidental ingestions coupled with food-specific IgE testing, and oral food challenges when indicated, aids in determining when clinical tolerance is achieved.

Conclusions

In summary, the role of food allergy in the potential development, progression and maintenance of AD is important to consider, especially in infants and young children with refractory disease. As many as 35–40% of such children will have a food allergy complicating their disease, which should be appropriately addressed using the clinical approaches outlined in this chapter. Further investigations are in progress to better refine diagnostic testing in children and adults with suspected food allergy and to better define the role of elimination diets, timing of introduction of allergenic foods, the role of gene–environment interactions, and the relevance of epidermal barrier function in the diagnosis and management of food allergy and atopic dermatitis. Most importantly, clinicians should maintain a high index of suspicion for the potential role of food allergy to best manage their patients with atopic dermatitis.

References

1. Wise F, Sulzberger M. Eczematous eruptions. In: Year Book of Dermatology and Syphilogy. Chicago: Year Book Medical; 1933.

2. Spergel JM. Epidemiology of atopic dermatitis and atopic march in children. Immunol Allergy Clin North Am 2010;30(3):269–80.

3. Sampson HA, Scanlon SM. Natural history of food hypersensitivity in children with atopic dermatitis. J Pediatr 1989;115(1):23–7.

4. Burks AW, Mallory SB, Williams LW, et al. Atopic dermatitis: clinical relevance of food hypersensitivity reactions. J Pediatr 1988;113(3):447–51.

5. Burks W. Skin manifestations of food allergy. Pediatrics 2003;111(6 Pt 3):1617–24.

6. Wood RA. The natural history of food allergy. Pediatrics 2003;111(6 Pt 3):1631–7.

7. Fleischer DM, Conover-Walker MK, Christie L, et al. The natural progression of peanut allergy: Resolution and the possibility of recurrence. J Allergy Clin Immunol 2003;112(1):183–9.

8. Fleischer DM, Conover-Walker MK, Matsui EC, et al. The natural history of tree nut allergy. J Allergy Clin Immunol 2005;116(5):1087–93.

9. Hill DJ, Hosking CS, de Benedictis FM, et al. Confirmation of the association between high levels of immunoglobulin E food sensitization and eczema in infancy: an international study. Clin Exp Allergy 2008;38(1):161–8.

10. Rona RJ, Keil T, Summers C, et al. The prevalence of food allergy: a meta-analysis. J Allergy Clin Immunol 2007;120(3):638–46.

11. Eigenmann PA, Sicherer SH, Borkowski TA, et al. Prevalence of IgE-mediated food allergy among children with atopic dermatitis. Pediatrics 1998;101(3):E8.

12. Guillet G, Guillet MH. Natural history of sensitizations in atopic dermatitis. A 3-year follow-up in 250 children: food allergy and high risk of respiratory symptoms. Arch Dermatol 1992;128(2):187–92.

13. Bath-Hextall F, Delamere FM, Williams HC. Dietary exclusions for improving established atopic eczema in adults and children: systematic review. Allergy 2009;64(2):258–64.

14. Barnes KC. An update on the genetics of atopic dermatitis: scratching the surface in 2009. J Allergy Clin Immunol 2010;125(1):16–29 e1–11; quiz 30–1.

15. Hamid Q, Boguniewicz M, Leung DY. Differential in situ cytokine gene expression in acute versus chronic atopic dermatitis. J Clin Invest 1994;94(2):870–6.

16. Hamid Q, Naseer T, Minshall EM, et al. In vivo expression of IL-12 and IL-13 in atopic dermatitis. J Allergy Clin Immunol 1996;98(1):225–31.

17. Bieber T. Atopic dermatitis. N Engl J Med 2008;358(14):1483–94.

18. Niggemann B, Reibel S, Wahn U. The atopy patch test (APT) – a useful tool for the diagnosis of food allergy in children with atopic dermatitis. Allergy 2000;55(3):281–5.

19. Mehl A, Rolinck-Werninghaus C, Staden U, et al. The atopy patch test in the diagnostic workup of suspected food-related symptoms in children. J Allergy Clin Immunol 2006;118(4):923–9.

20. Leung DY, Boguniewicz M, Howell MD, et al. New insights into atopic dermatitis. J Clin Invest 2004; 113(5):651–7.

21. Fox AT, Sasieni P, du Toit G, et al. Household peanut consumption as a risk factor for the development of peanut allergy. J Allergy Clin Immunol 2009;123(2): 417–23.

22. Rodriguez E, Baurecht H, Herberich E, et al. Meta-analysis of filaggrin polymorphisms in eczema and asthma: robust risk factors in atopic disease. J Allergy Clin Immunol 2009;123(6):1361–70 e7.

23. Marenholz I, Kerscher T, Bauerfeind A, et al. An interaction between filaggrin mutations and early food sensitization improves the prediction of childhood asthma. J Allergy Clin Immunol 2009; 123(4):911–6.

24. Torgerson TR, Linane A, Moes N, et al. Severe food allergy as a variant of IPEX syndrome caused by a deletion in a noncoding region of the FOXP3 gene. Gastroenterology 2007;132(5):1705–17.

25. Kusunoki T, Okafuji I, Yoshioka T, et al. SPINK5 polymorphism is associated with disease severity and food allergy in children with atopic dermatitis. J Allergy Clin Immunol 2005;115(3):636–8.

26. Zitnik SE, Ruschendorf F, Muller S, et al. IL13 variants are associated with total serum IgE and early sensitization to food allergens in children with atopic dermatitis. Pediatr Allergy Immunol 2009;20(6): 551–5.

27. Greer FR, Sicherer SH, Burks AW. Effects of early nutritional interventions on the development of atopic disease in infants and children: the role of maternal dietary restriction, breastfeeding, timing of introduction of complementary foods, and hydrolyzed formulas. Pediatrics 2008;121(1):183–91.

28. Lack G, Fox D, Northstone K, et al. Factors associated with the development of peanut allergy in childhood. N Engl J Med 2003;348(11):977–85.

29. Atherton DJ, Sewell M, Soothill JF, et al. A double-blind controlled crossover trial of an antigen-avoidance diet in atopic eczema. Lancet 1978;1(8061):401–3.

30. Juto P, Engberg S, Winberg J. Treatment of infantile atopic dermatitis with a strict elimination diet. Clin Allergy 1978;8(5):493–500.

31. Lever R, MacDonald C, Waugh P, et al. Randomised controlled trial of advice on an egg exclusion diet in young children with atopic eczema and sensitivity to eggs. Pediatr Allergy Immunol 1998;9(1):13–9.

32. Mankad VS, Williams LW, Lee LA, et al. Safety of open food challenges in the office setting. Ann Allergy Asthma Immunol 2008;100(5):469–74.

33. Burks AW, James JM, Hiegel A, et al. Atopic dermatitis and food hypersensitivity reactions. J Pediatr 1998;132(1):132–6.

34. Wilson S, Walzer M. Absorption of undigested proteins in human beings, IV: absorption of unaltered egg protein in infants. Am J Dis Child 1935;50:49–54.

35. Sampson HA, Jolie PL. Increased plasma histamine concentrations after food challenges in children with atopic dermatitis. N Engl J Med 1984;311(6):372–6.

36. Suomalainen H, Soppi E, Isolauri E. Evidence for eosinophil activation in cow's milk allergy. Pediatr Allergy Immunol 1994;5(1):27–31.

37. Magnarin M, Knowles A, Ventura A, et al. A role for eosinophils in the pathogenesis of skin lesions in patients with food-sensitive atopic dermatitis. J Allergy Clin Immunol 1995;96(2):200–8.

38. Sampson HA, Broadbent KR, Bernhisel-Broadbent J. Spontaneous release of histamine from basophils and histamine-releasing factor in patients with atopic dermatitis and food hypersensitivity. N Engl J Med 1989;321(4):228–32.

39. Abernathy-Carver KJ, Sampson HA, Picker LJ, et al. Milk-induced eczema is associated with the expansion of T cells expressing cutaneous lymphocyte antigen. J Clin Invest 1995;95(2):913–8.

40. Gdalevich M, Mimouni D, David M, et al. Breast-feeding and the onset of atopic dermatitis in childhood: a systematic review and meta-analysis of prospective studies. J Am Acad Dermatol 2001;45(4):520–7.

41. Hattevig G, Kjellman B, Sigurs N, et al. Effect of maternal avoidance of eggs, cow's milk and fish during lactation upon allergic manifestations in infants. Clin Exp Allergy 1989;19(1):27–32.

42. Sigurs N, Hattevig G, Kjellman B. Maternal avoidance of eggs, cow's milk, and fish during lactation: effect on allergic manifestations, skin-prick tests, and specific IgE antibodies in children at age 4 years. Pediatrics 1992;89(4 Pt 2):735–9.

43. Zeiger RS, Heller S. The development and prediction of atopy in high-risk children: follow-up at age seven years in a prospective randomized study of combined maternal and infant food allergen avoidance. J Allergy Clin Immunol 1995;95(6):1179–90.

44. Zeiger RS, Heller S, Mellon MH, et al. Effect of combined maternal and infant food-allergen avoidance on development of atopy in early infancy: a randomized study. J Allergy Clin Immunol 1989;84(1):72–89.

45. von Berg A, Filipiak-Pittroff B, Kramer U, et al. Preventive effect of hydrolyzed infant formulas persists until age 6 years: long-term results from the German Infant Nutritional Intervention Study (GINI). J Allergy Clin Immunol 2008;121(6):1442–7.

46. Alexander DD, Cabana MD. Partially hydrolyzed 100% whey protein infant formula and reduced risk of atopic dermatitis: a meta-analysis. J Pediatr Gastroenterol Nutr 2010;50(4):422–30.

47. Zutavern A, Brockow I, Schaaf B, et al. Timing of solid food introduction in relation to eczema, asthma, allergic rhinitis, and food and inhalant sensitization at the age of 6 years: results from the prospective birth cohort study LISA. Pediatrics 2008;121(1):e44–52.

48. Sicherer SH, Burks AW. Maternal and infant diets for prevention of allergic diseases: understanding menu changes in 2008. J Allergy Clin Immunol 2008;122(1): 29–33.

49. Sicherer SH, Wood RA, Stablein D, et al. Immunologic features of infants with milk or egg allergy enrolled in an observational study (Consortium of Food Allergy

Research) of food allergy. J Allergy Clin Immunol 2010;125(5):1077–1083 e8.

50. Lack G. Epidemiologic risks for food allergy. J Allergy Clin Immunol 2008;121(6):1331–6.

51. Caubet JC, Eigenmann PA. Allergic triggers in atopic dermatitis. Immunol Allergy Clin North Am 2010;30(3):289–307.

52. Schafer T, Heinrich J, Wjst M, et al. Association between severity of atopic eczema and degree of sensitization to aeroallergens in schoolchildren. J Allergy Clin Immunol 1999;104(6):1280–4.

53. Fleischer DM, Bock SA, Spears GC, et al. Oral Food Challenges in Children with a Diagnosis of Food Allergy. J Pediatr 2010 (epub).

54. Sampson HA, McCaskill CC. Food hypersensitivity and atopic dermatitis: evaluation of 113 patients. J Pediatr 1985;107(5):669–75.

55. Bock SA, Atkins FM. Patterns of food hypersensitivity during sixteen years of double-blind, placebo-controlled food challenges. J Pediatr 1990;117(4):561–7.

56. Fuglsang G, Madsen G, Halken S, et al. Adverse reactions to food additives in children with atopic symptoms. Allergy 1994;49(1):31–7.

57. Schwartz H. Food allergy: Adverse reactions to foods and food additives. In: Asthmaandfood additives. 2nd ed. Blackwell Science; 1997. In.

58. Lieberman JA, Sicherer SH. Diagnosis of Food Allergy: Epicutaneous Skin Tests, In Vitro Tests, and Oral Food Challenge. Curr Allergy Asthma Rep 2010;11(1):58–64.

59. Perry TT, Matsui EC, Kay Conover-Walker M, et al. The relationship of allergen-specific IgE levels and oral food challenge outcome. J Allergy Clin Immunol 2004; 114(1):144–9.

60. Perry TT, Matsui EC, Conover-Walker MK, et al. Risk of oral food challenges. J Allergy Clin Immunol 2004; 114(5):1164–8.

61. David TJ. Hazards of challenge tests in atopic dermatitis. Allergy 1989;44(Suppl. 9):101–7.

62. Mills EN, Mackie AR, Burney P, et al. The prevalence, cost and basis of food allergy across Europe. Allergy 2007;62(7):717–22.

63. Sicherer SH, Noone SA, Munoz-Furlong A. The impact of childhood food allergy on quality of life. Ann Allergy Asthma Immunol 2001;87(6):461–4.

64. Bock SA. The natural history of food sensitivity. J Allergy Clin Immunol 1982;69(2):173–7.

65. Savage JH, Matsui EC, Skripak JM, et al. The natural history of egg allergy. J Allergy Clin Immunol 2007;120(6):1413–7.

66. Skolnick HS, Conover-Walker MK, Koerner CB, et al. The natural history of peanut allergy. J Allergy Clin Immunol 2001;107(2):367–74.

CHAPTER 6

Food-induced Urticaria and Angioedema

Julia Rodriguez and Jesús F. Crespo

KEY CONCEPTS

- Urticaria/angioedema is the most common clinical manifestation of IgE-mediated food allergy, either alone or associated with other symptoms.

- IgE-mediated, food-induced urticaria/angioedema usually occurs following ingestion of a food allergen(s), but can also occur following topical contact, inhalation or with food ingestion followed by exercise; in some cases after a specific food or after any food.

- The most important effector cell in IgE-mediated urticaria/angioedema is the mast cell in dermis and mucosal tissues.

- Patients with food-induced IgE-mediated urticaria can have a more severe reaction in the future.

- Once the diagnosis of clinical allergy to foods is established, the only effective intervention therapy is strict avoidance of the offending food. Cross-reactive foods should be evaluated before advising the patient that they can be safely consumed.

Introduction

Adverse reactions to food can be identified as underlying causes in various urticarial diseases. IgE-dependent allergic reactions to food are known to play a role in acute urticaria, in some cases of exercise-induced urticaria and in contact urticaria. Food allergy can be defined as an adverse immune response that occurs reproducibly on exposure to a given food and is distinct from other adverse responses to food, such as food intolerance, pharmacologic reactions and toxin-mediated reactions. Allergic reactions after the ingestion of foods could result in diverse manifestations as the result of complex interactions among the causal food protein, gut, immune system and target organs. Although food initially contacts the gastrointestinal mucosa, allergic manifestations frequently occur outside the gastrointestinal tract, with symptoms or diseases affecting a variety of target sites alone or in combination. Studies that used double-blind placebo-controlled oral food challenges (DBPCFCs) have also demonstrated the variety of organ systems affected during food allergic reactions. In several recent series of oral food challenges the skin was commonly affected. There are several distinct manifestations of skin reactions caused by food allergy. Most of these disorders are mediated by food-specific IgE antibody that is bound to high-affinity IgE receptors on mast cells. A typical skin reaction after food ingestion is acute urticaria and angioedema, which represents a clinical example of a systemic symptom/disorder attributed to food hypersensitivity. In addition, urticaria and angioedema are the most common manifestations of anaphylaxis, associated with other symptoms such as respiratory compromise, reduced blood pressure or associated symptoms and/or persistent gastrointestinal symptoms. Urticaria can also appear on ingestion of a particular food or any meal followed by exercise. The clinical syndrome of food-dependent exercise-induced urticaria/anaphylaxis (FDEIA) is typified by the onset of urticaria/anaphylaxis during (or soon after) exercise that was preceded by the ingestion of the causal food allergen(s) within a specified period of time.[1,2]

CLINICAL CASE

An 18-year-old male presented to the emergency room; he had been jogging for 30 minutes when he presented with pruritus, disseminated urticaria, eyelid angioedema, conjunctival erythema, nausea, vomiting, general malaise and hypotension. He had eaten two apples 3 hours before exercise. He had not taken any medication. Results for skin prick testing for apple were positive (7 mm wheal). Specific serum IgE (CAP FEIA) for apple also elicited a positive result (1.95 kU/L). An open food challenge with two apples without subsequent exercise was negative. An exercise challenge test without prior apple consumption was negative. Given the strong evidence from the clinical history and the potential risks of anaphylaxis, no exercise challenge test following apple consumption was carried out in this patient. He was advised to allow 4 hours between apple ingestion and exercise. He has not reported any further episodes.

Acute urticaria and angioedema may be the result of a local reaction elicited by direct contact with food, and more rarely by the exposure to dust, steam, vapors and aerosolized proteins generated during cooking or boiling. These symptoms can occur at home, in restaurants or in the occupational setting.

CLINICAL CASE

A 38-year-old man reported multiple episodes since childhood with pruritus, disseminated urticaria, eyelid and lip swelling, facial erythema, difficulty swallowing, wheezing and dyspnea minutes after entering seafood restaurants and whenever shellfish was boiled at home. In many of these episodes he required treatment in the emergency room. He reported one episode of lip swelling, oropharyngeal pruritus and dyspnea minutes after ingestion of a single shrimp. He tolerated fish ingestion. Skin prick testing and serum specific IgE (CAP-FEIA) elicited positive results to shrimp (10 mm mean wheal and 25.7 kU/L, respectively). Since the last episode the patient has not entered any seafood restaurants and no shellfish has been kept at home. He has been instructed to avoid shellfish ingestion and any food that could contain shellfish, such as shellfish sauces and broth, to avoid areas where shellfish are being boiled or cooked, to always carry

epinephrine when eating out of home and to self-administer in case of inadvertent exposure/ingestion of shellfish.

CLINICAL CASE

A 29-year-old woman had worked as a cook in a seafood restaurant for the last 2 years. Two months before referral she reported ocular erythema and pruritus, facial erythema and hives, cough and dyspnea when shellfish species such as shrimp, squid, clam or mussels were being boiled and cooked. When she handled these foods, either raw or cooked, she reported hand and arm pruritus and urticaria. Minutes after the ingestion of two shrimps she reported an episode of ocular erythema, oropharyngeal pruritus and cough. Since then she has currently avoided shellfish ingestion. Skin testing (prick by prick) carried out with raw and boiled shellfish species brought in by the patient elicited positive results (mean wheal raw/boiled) to shrimp (12.5/10), squid (15/9), clam (8.5/7) and mussel (9/8.5). Specific serum IgE (CAP FEIA) was also positive to shrimp (29.1 kU/L), squid (3.29 kU/L), clam (15.3 kU/L) and mussel (17.2 kU/L). The patient was diagnosed with allergy to shellfish (crustaceae and mollusks: both cephalopods and bivalves). She was strongly advised to change her job, or at least try to avoid contact with and ingestion of shellfish and any food that could contain shellfish, such as shellfish sauces and broth, and being in areas where shellfish were being cooked, to always carry epinephrine when eating out of home, and to self-administer in case of inadvertent exposure/ingestion of shellfish.

Immunological (allergic) contact urticaria is due to immediate-type hypersensitivity; it is mediated primarily by histamine, and may be associated with systemic and potentially life-threatening symptoms. Immunological contact urticaria to food may occasionally affect those who handle food, and may be associated with development of a protein contact dermatitis.[3]

Chronic urticaria, defined as continuous wheals and/or angioedema, presenting daily or almost daily, that goes on for 6 weeks or more, is frequently perceived by patients as food-induced; however, virtually no reported food reactions in chronic urticaria patients are confirmed by double-blind placebo-controlled food challenge.[4]

Epidemiology

It is a general perception that acute urticaria and angioedema are among the most common symptoms of food-allergic reactions, although the exact prevalence of these reactions is unknown. A number of clinical studies reviewed by Bindslev-Jensen and Osterballe[5] revealed that an average of 14% of patients with confirmed food allergy has been estimated to react with urticaria upon challenge. Some insights on the prevalence of food-induced urticaria could be provided by population-based studies, including food challenge tests. A recent population-based study in 6–9-year-old urban schoolchildren living in Turkey estimated a prevalence of food-induced urticaria of 0.6%, although the prevalence of actual food allergy was 0.8%.[6] As for the frequency of food-induced urticaria and angioedema in the emergency department, a recent study analyzed food-allergic and anaphylactic events from 34 participating centers in the National Electronic Injury Surveillance System (USA) in a 2-month pilot program. There were 141 medical records, including children and adults, that reported food allergy-induced symptoms, the majority of which were skin related. Urticaria and angioedema were the most common: urticaria accounted for 38% if cases; facial edema (face, tongue, eyes, oral cavity) 48%; general edema 4%; and laryngeal edema (swelling of throat/uvula) 15%.[7]

Most cases of food-induced contact urticaria occur in the occupational setting. In fact, bakers and preparers of processed food were found to rank among those most commonly affected by occupational contact urticaria in Finland.[8] In the same way, food was recognized as the second major cause, after natural rubber latex, of occupational contact urticaria in Australian patients with occupational skin disease.[9]

Exposure to food allergens through inhalation can also cause food hypersensitivity reactions, with symptoms that typically include respiratory manifestations such as rhinoconjunctivitis and asthma, particularly in the occupational setting. In addition, a limited number of investigations have reported allergic reactions in the form of acute urticaria that have occurred following exposure to fumes or vapors from cooked foods, such as fish and legumes (see Chapter 8).[10,11]

Urticaria/angioedema are the most frequent symptoms seen in food-dependent exercise-induced anaphylaxis (FDEIA). In a survey carried out in a national hospital in Korea, this accounted for 13.2% of 138 anaphylactic reactions. Urticaria (82%) and angioedema (70%) were the most common symptoms observed and buckwheat was the most frequent causal food.[12] An epidemiological study carried out in junior high-school students reported a frequency of 0.017% FDEIA. All cases showed urticarial symptoms, which were also documented in further challenges. The most frequent causative foods were crustaceans and wheat.[13] In a 10-year follow-up study of patients with exercise-induced anaphylaxis,[14] one-third of the cohort reported food triggered attacks. Urticaria, pruritus and angioedema accounted for more than 80% of symptoms. Shellfish, tomatoes and wine were the most frequently reported culprits.

Pathogenesis

The most important effector cell in urticaria/angioedema is the mast cell in dermis and mucosal tissues. This cell expresses high-affinity IgE receptors that bind to the constant region domain of IgE, C3. Food allergens, whether ingested, through skin contact or inhaled, react with IgE bound to the patient's tissue mast cells, and trigger the reaction upon re-exposure to the antigen. This event elicits mast cell degranulation and the subsequent release of vasoactive mediators. Histamine, released by preformed granules, is the major mediator of urticaria and angioedema. It elicits vasodilation and vascular permeability, which is seen clinically as a wheal. An axon reflex, caused by the release of the neuropeptide substance P from type C cutaneous fibers, increases the extent of the reaction. Substance P also further stimulates mast cells to increase their histamine release. Other membrane-derived mediators such as prostaglandins and leukotrienes are subsequently released, contributing respectively to vasodilation and an increase in microvascular permeability, all of which allows fluid leakage into the superficial tissues. In the case of FDEIA, exercise may favor intestinal absorption of causative food allergens or have some effect on the mast cell itself, which can be detected in patients' sera during the food–exercise combined challenge and not with the eliciting food or exercise separate challenge. Aspirin is known as an aggravating factor in FDEIA patients: it has been hypothesized that it may upregulate intestinal absorption of antigen and/or increase histamine release.[15]

Skin biopsies performed in 108 patients with acute, chronic and physical urticaria showed dermal edema and dilated lymphatic and vascular capillaries. Inflammatory infiltrates, with significantly increased numbers of neutrophils and eosinophils, were observed exclusively in the involved skin of all patients. Mast cell numbers were higher in the upper and lower dermis of lesional as well as the uninvolved skin of all patients.[16] This fact, together with increased levels of food-specific IgE bound to skin mast cells, could provide an explanation for the high frequency of urticaria/angioedema upon food ingestion. Bloodborne food allergens absorbed and processed in the gastrointestinal mucosa would reach a sensitized, mast cell-populated skin ready to react upon re-exposure.

Clinical features

After ingestion of the culprit food, urticaria and/or angioedema may appear within minutes or up to 2 hours later. Urticarial lesions, preceded by or appearing together with pruritus, are easily recognized. Wheals are intensely pruritic and involve any area of the skin; they may appear in one location and fade in another within minutes or hours. Wheals vary in shape and size from millimeters to a few centimeters. They may coalesce to form giant lesions with raised borders. An individual wheal does not persist over 24 hours. Pruritus is the hallmark, it is felt all over the skin, and worsens with scratching. Pruritus in the palms and soles, usually without wheals in those locations, may precede or appear together with disseminated urticaria. This is sometimes a warning signal of further severe symptoms. Angioedema is not usually pruritic: rather, patients describe a burning or tingling sensation. It may appear anywhere on the skin or on mucous surfaces. Angioedema may be a life-threatening symptom if airway obstruction occurs as a result of laryngeal edema or tongue swelling.

The most frequent foods reported as causing urticaria on ingestion in children are egg, milk, peanuts and tree nuts. In adults, fish, shellfish, tree nuts and peanuts are reported as the most common. However, the relative frequencies of different causal foods may vary across geographical areas. In a study carried out in 1537 German adults, 20% reported food allergy symptoms. Skin reactions accounted for 8.7%. The most frequently reported foods were fruits and herbs/spices.[17] A French study carried out in the general population reported urticaria and angioedema as the most frequent food-elicited symptoms. The most frequently reported foods were rosaceae fruits, vegetables, milk, crustaceans, fruit cross-reacting with latex, egg, tree nuts and peanut.[18] In a Mediterranean adult population from Turkey, vegetables, egg and fruits were the most frequent causal foods eliciting urticaria and angioedema.[19]

Food-induced contact urticaria reactions may erupt from minutes to 1 hour after exposure. A local wheal and flare appears, usually pruritic, but tingling or burning may be reported by the patient. The reaction can be exclusively local, but may progress to a disseminated urticaria or present with systemic symptoms, defined as contact urticaria syndrome.[20] Food handlers can also present with a local IgE-mediated eczematous reaction known as protein contact dermatitis, which can coexist with contact urticaria; it can affect not only the hands but the wrists and arms as well. The causal proteins have been classified into four groups, the first three of which include numerous foods, such as fruits, vegetables, spices, plants and woods; animal proteins; grains; and enzymes. Virtually any job that involves food handling can be at risk for food-induced contact urticaria and/or protein contact dermatitis: homemakers, cooks, food handlers, mushroom growers, bakers, confectionery workers, butchers, veterinarians etc.

In food-allergic patients urticaria and angioedema may appear minutes after inhalation of cooking fumes or aerosolized food particles, as an isolated symptom, together with wheezing or progressing to systemic anaphylaxis.[10,11,21]

Clinical symptoms of FDEIA usually have an onset after around 10 minutes of exercise, and within 2 hours after food ingestion. Generalized urticaria, angioedema and erythema are the first clinical manifestations and are usually followed by respiratory and systemic symptoms, evolving into systemic anaphylaxis.

Diagnosis

As with other adverse reactions to foods, the primary tools available to diagnose food-induced urticaria/angioedema include a detailed clinical history, diet diaries as appropriate, physical examination, skin testing, serum tests for food-specific IgE antibodies, trial elimination diets, and oral food challenges.[22] In the case of food ingestion, patients often identify the offending food if symptoms begin within minutes to 2 hours after consumption, especially if they have experienced more than one episode with these characteristics. It is important to note that if symptoms are reported more than 3 hours after ingestion and last for several days, a causal relationship with food is unlikely. Patients may report symptoms appearing daily or on most days. In this case, they frequently try to associate urticaria with a particular food(s); they should be questioned if hives appear on each and every ingestion of that food; if that is not the case, the causal relationship may be excluded, unless the suspected food may or may not contain a hidden allergen/contaminant, e.g. mustard in some but not all ketchup brands, lupine in some fortified pasta, scombroid fish poisoning, anisakis in seafood, etc. To search for a consistent relationship between food and symptoms in these cases, a symptom diary including frequency, timing, duration and severity of the symptoms and foods ingested previously to the episode may be kept by the patient. In the case of symptoms after a meal composed of several foods, all should be carefully listed and the patient questioned about further tolerance of any of these foods; if that is the case, they should be excluded from the suspicion list if they contain no possible hidden allergens/contaminants, e.g. fresh fruits, meat, egg. In all cases of suspected processed foods, patients should be required to bring in the food label.

Auriculotemporal syndrome is a disease occasionally misdiagnosed as food allergy. Symptoms consist of non-pruritic flushing and/or sweating in facial areas while chewing or immediately after eating, for example the cheeks or jaw supplied by the auriculotemporal nerve, which may be damaged by local trauma, such as forceps delivery, virus or surgery. Symptoms usually appear unilaterally, although some bilateral cases have been documented.[23]

If symptoms are reported after contact of the food with skin, patients usually identify the culprit food(s). Timing of the reaction and circumstances of onset should be recorded, especially in an occupational setting in which many different foods may be handled. The relationship between possible worsening at work and improvement in periods off work should be investigated.

In the case of urticaria after a particular food ingestion or any meal followed by exercise, information should be obtained on whether this food or any food consumption is tolerated without exercise, time between ingestion, exercise and onset of symptoms, which usually occurs minutes after beginning of exercise. Systemic manifestations evolving to anaphylaxis should be recorded. The concomitant administration of drugs prior to exercise, especially aspirin and other anti-inflammatory drugs, should be asked about. FDEIA urticarial lesions should be differentiated from cholinergic urticaria, which presents with pinhead-sized wheals;

therefore, patients reporting FDEIA should be questioned about the characteristics of the skin lesions. Moreover, the trigger in cholinergic urticaria is an increase in core body temperature, sweating and stress. Hot and spicy foods may increase sweating and elicit cholinergic urticaria; therefore, a distinction should be made between this symptom in patients with this condition and genuine food allergy by means of complementary diagnostic tools: skin testing and oral challenges if necessary.

In all cases patients should be questioned about the characteristics of the lesions: site, duration of individual lesions, whether they are pruritic or painful, and if there are wheals lasting for more than 24 hours. Associated angioedema should also be questioned for. A useful procedure may be to show patients photographs of urticaria and angioedema and ask them if their hives and swelling look similar. A thorough physical examination must be performed. Dermographism should be explored by lightly scratching the skin. If positive, wheals appear within 10 minutes locally. In the case of recent urticarial lesions, lineal bruising caused by scratching may be observed lasting for more than 24 hours. Any individual wheal lasting for more than 24 hours, being painful or with ecchymosis or petechiae, is concerning and should be investigated by skin biopsy as it may be a vasculitic lesion. This procedure also should be carried out in unusual patterns of urticaria with suspicion of vasculitis (fever, malaise and arthralgia). In this case the main pathological findings would be leukocytoclasis – that is, fragmentation of neutrophils with nuclear dust in the infiltrate – red blood cell extravasation, and fibrinoid degeneration of the endothelial cells. This pattern is not found in genuine urticaria.

Skin prick testing (SPT) is the most useful procedure to detect sensitization (the presence of antibody) to the suspected ingested foods, but it is not diagnostic of clinical reactivity. However, it is an excellent tool to rule out food allergy as a cause of urticaria/angioedema with 95% accuracy. A useful variant is skin testing by the prick-by-prick procedure, which yields better results than commercial extracts, particularly with fresh fruits and vegetables, as labile allergenic proteins in these foods may be lost in extract processing. In vitro assays for specific serum IgE have similar sensitivities and specificities. The increasing size of the SPT or concentration of food-specific IgE antibody by an in vitro assay may be related to the likelihood of a clinical reaction for some foods;[24] however, these values may vary depending on different age groups, different foods and different in vivo and in vitro techniques. Importantly, panels of food allergy in vivo and in vitro tests should not be performed because many clinically irrelevant positive results may be found in cross-reactive foods.

As stated above, symptom diaries look for any temporal relationship between food consumption and urticaria, which often is ruled out in the case of symptoms occurring more than 2 hours after ingestion or lasting for several days.

Elimination diets might be the best way to help the patients discard a food causal relationship for their daily or persistent urticaria/angioedema, a situation which they may desperately try to associate with ingestion of one or more particular foods.

Oral challenges administered openly, with the food in its natural form and preparation reported by the patient, are helpful in the case of several reported foods. Challenges should also be carried out in the case of single food consumption without a clear-cut temporal relationship, and/or reported reactions not evaluated by a physician when they took place. If the food is tolerated, a causal relationship is ruled out. If the patient reports subjective symptoms in the open challenge, a double-blind placebo-controlled food challenge should be carried out. In the case of a negative result a final open challenge in an amount and preparation similar to that which caused the original reaction should be given.

The diagnosis of food contact urticaria can often be confirmed by skin prick testing using commercial extracts or prick-by-prick testing with fresh foods and the open patch test, evaluating the appearance of local wheals 15–30 minutes after application of the suspected eliciting agent. Other topical application techniques, such as the chamber prick test, the scratch test and the open test, in which 0.1 mL of the test substance is spread over a 3×3-cm area of skin, can be used. Prick testing theoretically has the lowest risk of anaphylaxis because only minute amounts of allergen are introduced into the skin. The risk of other types of topical food application techniques should be carefully weighed against the risk of anaphylaxis if the patient reports extracutaneous symptoms with the suspected food. Measurement of serum-specific IgE can also be a useful diagnostic tool, especially in these cases of severe urticaria contact syndrome.

In patients reporting occasional anaphylaxis after food ingestion and exercise, challenge tests might be indicated, especially if a particular food has not been clearly identified. An oral challenge, without subsequent exercise, should be performed. If the result is positive FDEIA is excluded. In the case of a negative result, an oral challenge followed by exercise can be carried out to confirm the causative food and the diagnosis.[25] The procedure should be performed under strict medical supervision, blood pressure and pulse rate monitoring and an intravenous line. This test elicits a negative result in 30% of patients, probably because of the different temperatures, humidity, type of exercise, amount of food administered and other conditions of the reported reaction.

Treatment

Once the diagnosis of clinical allergy to ingested foods is established, the only effective therapy is strict avoidance of the offending food and all others that might contain it as a labeled component or as a hidden allergen. After a specific food has been identified and proved causal, recognition of cross-reacting allergens in other foods is an important issue. Since a very low rate of clinical cross-allergy has been demonstrated among legumes, cereal grains, egg–chicken and milk–cooked beef, it is not appropriate to restrict entire families or groups that include these foods. Avoidance of the entire food group has been suggested to patients with allergy to nut or shellfish families.[26] In the case of fruit elimination, diets limited to those proven to induce allergic symptoms might overlook the risk of potential clinical cross-reactivity, when the patient has not consumed other related fruits after the reaction. Therefore, other foods of the same plant family or antigenically related should be specifically tested by oral challenges before advising the patient that these fruits may be safely consumed.[27]

Both patients and caregivers should be informed about the risks of inadvertent consumption, especially if the food is ubiquitous; they should be instructed to correctly read and interpret labeling, which could be misleading. For a patient allergic to a particular food the term 'may contain' should mean 'contains'. In the case of foods consumed boiled, such as legumes or crustaceans, broths used to boil these foods should be avoided. Parents/patients should be instructed on the risks of inadvertent ingestion of causal foods in schools, restaurants, markets, etc.

Patients may experience a severe reaction after a subsequent exposure to a food, even if previous reactions were only cutaneous without any associated systemic symptoms. A subsequent exposure may begin with urticaria/angioedema symptoms and progress to a systemic reaction; therefore, patients should be provided with self-injectable epinephrine and instructions on its use in case of the appearance of more severe symptoms beyond urticaria/angioedema, such as dysphonia, difficulty swallowing, nausea, vomiting, abdominal cramps, dyspnea or fainting. Epinephrine should be administered early in the treatment of an anaphylactic reaction. In addition, the patient should immediately seek appropriate medical care if he or she develops a systemic reaction to a food.

Patients diagnosed with food-induced contact urticaria should avoid foods and food products that elicit symptoms. In the case of contact urticaria with raw foods, such as fish or potato, patients may tolerate ingestion of cooked food. Cosmetics may include food extracts in their formulations, which could elicit reactions; therefore, cosmetic labels should be carefully read. Patients with contact reactivity to latex should be investigated for tolerance of latex-related foods, including skin testing, serum-specific IgE assessments and oral challenges if they have not consumed those foods with tolerance after the latex reaction. In the case of contact urticaria syndrome patients may require self-injected epinephrine and subsequent medical care.

Patients with symptoms on inhalation of food cooking fumes and/or raw fish odors should carefully avoid all risk situations at home, with cooking or food handling and in fish markets. Depending on the severity of the symptoms, they should be instructed to carry self-injectable epinephrine.

In the case of FDEIA patients should avoid exercise, even milder than that which elicited symptoms, for 4–5 hours after eating the causal foods. Patients with a history of a life-threatening reaction should always carry self-injectable epinephrine.

In summary, urticaria/angioedema are recognized as one of the most common symptoms of food-allergic reactions, although their exact prevalence is unknown. The most important effector cell in IgE-mediated urticaria/angioedema is the mast cell. Urticaria/angioedema can occur not only by food ingestion but also by contact with foods; in this case, allergic reactions can be local but may also become severe and systemic. Urticaria induced by inhalation of aerosolized food particles can take place not only with fumes but also with raw foods, at home, in food markets, in restaurants and in occupational settings. Urticaria/angioedema can also occur with food ingestion followed by exercise, and be the first sign of a severe anaphylactic reaction. Diagnosis of food-induced urticaria/angioedema must include a careful, thorough clinical history and the appropriate diagnostic tools, depending on the different clinical features reported by the patient. The hallmark of treatment is avoidance of the causal food. Cross-reactive foods should be investigated before advising the patient that they can be safely consumed.

References

1. Sicherer SH. Determinants of systemic manifestations of food allergy. J Allergy Clin Immunol 2000;106(5 Suppl):S251–7.
2. Morita E, Kunie K, Matsuo H. Food-dependent exercise-induced anaphylaxis. J Dermatol Sci 2007;47(2):109–17.
3. Killig C, Werfel T. Contact reactions to food. Curr Allergy Asthma Rep 2008;8(3):209–14.
4. Zuberbier T, Balke M, Worm M, et al. Epidemiology of urticaria: a representative cross-sectional population survey. Clin Exp Dermatol 2010 Dec; 35(8):869–73.
5. Bindslev-Jensen C, Osterballe M. Other IgE- and non IgE-mediated reactions of the skin. In: Metcalfe DD, Sampson HA, Simon RA, editors. Food Allergy. Adverse Reactions To Foods And Food Additives. 4th ed. Blackwell Publishing Ltd; 2008. pp. 124–32.
6. Orhan F, Karakas T, Cakir M, et al. Prevalence of immunoglobulin E-mediated food allergy in 6–9-year-old urban schoolchildren in the eastern Black Sea region of Turkey. Clin Exp Allergy 2009;39:1027–35.
7. Ross MP, Ferguson M, Street D, et al. Analysis of food-allergic and anaphylactic events in the National Electronic Injury Surveillance System. J Allergy Clin Immunol 2008;121:166–71.
8. Kanerva L, Toikkanen J, Jolanki R, et al. Statistical data on occupational contact urticaria. Contact Dermatitis 1996;35:229–33.
9. Williams JD, Lee AY, Matheson MC, et al. Occupational contact urticaria: Australian data. Br J Dermatol 2008; 159:125–31.
10. Crespo JF, Pascual C, Dominguez C, et al. Allergic reactions associated with airborne fish particles in IgE-mediated fish hypersensitive patients. Allergy 1995;50:257–61.
11. Martínez Alonso JC, Callejo Melgosa A, Fuentes Gonzalo MJ, et al. Angioedema induced by inhalation of vapours from cooked white bean in a child. Allergol Immunopathol (Madr) 2005;33(4): 228–30.

12. Yang MS, Lee SH, Kim TW, et al. Epidemiologic and clinical features of anaphylaxis in Korea. Ann Allergy Asthma Immunol 2008;100:31–6.

13. Aihara Y, Takahashi Y, Kotoyori T, et al. Frequency of food-dependent, exercise-induced anaphylaxis in Japanese junior-high-school students. J Allergy Clin Immunol 2001;108:1035–9.

14. Shadick NA, Liang MH, Partridge AJ, et al. The natural history of exercise-induced anaphylaxis: survey results from a 10-year follow-up study. J Allergy Clin Immunol 1999;104:123–7.

15. Matsuo H, Morimoto K, Akaki T, et al. Exercise and aspirin increase levels of circulating gliadin peptides in patients with wheat-dependent exercise-induced anaphylaxis. Clin Exp Allergy 2005;35:461–6.

16. Haas N, Toppe E, Henz BM. Microscopic morphology of different types of urticaria. Arch Dermatol 1998;134:41–6.

17. Schäfer T, Böhler E, Ruhdorfer S, et al. Epidemiology of food allergy/food intolerance in adults: associations with other manifestations of atopy. Allergy 2001;56:1172–9.

18. Kanny G, Moneret-Vautrin DA, Flabbee J, et al. Population study of food allergy in France. J Allergy Clin Immunol 2001;108:133–40.

19. Gelincik A, Büyüköztürk S, Gül H, et al. Confirmed prevalence of food allergy and non-allergic food hypersensitivity in a Mediterranean population. Clin Exp Allergy 2008;38(8):1333–41.

20. Bourrain JL. Occupational contact urticaria. Clin Rev Allergy Immunol 2006 Feb;30(1):39–46.

21. Taylor AV, Swanson MC, Jones RT, et al. Detection and quantitation of raw fish aeroallergens from an open-air fish market. J Allergy Clin Immunol 1999;166–9.

22. Guidelines for the Diagnosis and Management of Food Allergy in the United States. Report of the NIAID-Sponsored Expert Panel. J Allergy Clin Immunol 2010;126:S1–58.

23. Sicherer, SH, Sampson, HA. Auriculotemporal syndrome: a masquerader of food allergy. J Allergy Clin Immunol 1996;97:851.

24. Sampson HA. Food allergy. Accurately identifying clinical reactivity. Allergy 2005;60(Suppl 79):19–24.

25. Romano A, Di Fonso M, Giuffreda F, et al. Diagnostic work-up for food-dependent, exercise-induced anaphylaxis. Allergy 1995;50:817–24.

26. Sicherer SH. Clinical implications of cross-reactive food allergens. J Allergy Clin Immunol 2001 Dec;108(6): 881–90.

27. Rodriguez J, Crespo JF. Clinical features of cross-reactivity of food allergy caused by fruits. Curr Opin Allergy Clin Immunol 2002;2:233–8.

CHAPTER 7

Pollen–Food Syndrome

Antonella Muraro and Cristiana Alonzi

Introduction

Pollen–food syndrome is a term describing associations between inhalant pollen allergies and allergic manifestations on ingestion of particular fruits, vegetables and spices. Albeit first described as far back as 1948, this kind of allergy has attracted special attention during the last few decades because of the steadily increasing prevalence of inhalant allergies in recent years. So far, several clinical syndromes have been described, such as birch–fruit, celery–mugwort–spice and latex–fruit, which have a molecular background consistent with pollen–food syndrome. The term class II food allergy was coined to describe the relationship between sensitivity to certain foods and airborne allergens. In fact, two different forms of immunoglobulin (Ig)E-mediated food allergy can be distinguished (class I and class II), based on clinical appearance, pattern of allergens, and underlying immunological mechanisms; and in class I food allergies, the sensitization process is assumed to occur via the gastrointestinal tract. The class I type of food allergy mainly affects young children and may be the presenting sign of atopic syndrome. The most important allergens are cows' milk, egg, and beans. The second type (class II), which we discuss here, develops later in life and it is believed to be the consequence of an allergic sensitization to inhalant allergens. The basis for this food allergy is an immunological cross-reactivity due to a high amino acid sequence identity and structural homology between food and pollen allergens (i.e. even from botanically unrelated plants).[1] They are often called incomplete food allergens or non-sensitizing elicitors. It is not always possible, however, to distinguish clearly between class I and II food allergens. Extreme thermostability and resistance to pepsin digestion identify lipid transfer proteins (LTPs) as potent class I food allergens, whereas pollen LTPs reportedly behave as primary sensitizing allergens in patients with IgE to both mugwort and peach LTPs, indicating an involvement of LTPs in class II food allergies as well.

These plant proteins are often referred to as pan-allergens because they are widely distributed throughout the plant kingdom and are involved in the extensive IgE cross-reactivity between antigens from unrelated plant species.[2] Several families of plant proteins have been shown to be involved in pollen–food syndrome, including profilins, pathogenesis-related proteins (PRs) and LTPs. Cross-reactions can even occur between species that are only remotely related phylogenetically, such as birch and kiwi. In most of these cases the 'oral allergy syndrome' (OAS) is the prominent clinical symptom, but reactions may range in severity from mild local symptoms to associated systemic symptoms involving distal organs, to a fatal outcome. The severity of the reaction may depend on a variety of factors, including the type of allergen, the amount ingested, its digestion and uptake in the gastrointestinal system, and individual cofactors (e.g. concomitant viral infections, physical exertion, intake of alcohol or drugs). Thermostable allergens of higher molecular weight seem responsible for more severe reactions, e.g. LTPs.[3]

The increasing availability of allergen panels derived from various sources enables a detailed analysis of individual patients' sensitization profiles – what has been termed 'component-resolved diagnostics' (CRD). The rationale behind CRD is to establish associations between specific IgE, measured by using individual allergen components (or parts of them) and clinically relevant aspects of the allergic disease.

Epidemiology

Pollen–food syndrome is the most frequent cause of food allergies in adults and adolescents.[2]

Most allergic reactions against plant-derived foods are strongly associated with several pollen allergies. Approximately 15–20% of the populations in the developed world are allergic to pollen, and 50–93% of patients allergic to birch pollen have IgE-mediated reactions to pollen-related foods. On the basis of these data, the prevalence of fruit, nut and vegetable hypersensitivity can be estimated at significantly more than 1%. The overwhelming majority of pollen-related reactions to fruits in Europe are associated with birch and hazel nut pollen allergy. Cross-reactive allergies to certain foods, for example apple, peach, tomato or peanut, have also been found in a minority of individuals with grass pollen allergy. Allergies to several foods related to birch pollen (such as celery, carrot and spices) can occur in patients allergic to mugwort pollen but not to birch pollen, but some studies have shown that this phenomenon is rare.[4] Enrique et al.[5] reported an association between plantain pollinosis and plant food allergy, with 50% of their patients allergic to the pollen being allergic to at least one plant. The foods most frequently implicated were hazelnuts, fruits (e.g. peach, apple, melon and kiwi), peanuts, maize, chick peas, and some vegetables (e.g. lettuce and green beans). There are few reports of specific food allergies being associated with wall pellitory (Parietaria) and trees from the Oleaceae family, although these pollens are common elicitors of pollen allergies in the Mediterranean area, Liccardi et al.[6] described associations between sensitization to pistachio and Parietaria allergy. In 2002, Florido Lopez and coworkers evaluated 40 patients with Olea pollinosis

and adverse reactions to plant-derived foods (21 of them with OAS, 19 with anaphylactic reactions): all the patients were positive on the skin prick test (SPT) against one or more *Olea europaea* allergens. Sensitization to Ole e 7 (an LTP in Olea pollen) was significantly more common in anaphylactic patients, whereas sensitization to Ole e 2 (a profilin) was more frequent in the OAS group.[7] Sensitization to Amb a 4, ragweed homolog of Art v 1, the major pollen allergen of the composite plant mugwort (*Artemisia vulgaris*) has been reported to trigger reactions to the Cucurbitaceae family (watermelon, cantaloupe, honeydew melon, zucchini and cucumber) and banana. So far the cross-reactive allergens have not been characterized. However, the pan-allergen profilin or glycoallergens or LTPs seem involved in the clinical manifestations of this ragweed–melon–banana association. Although the symptoms are usually mild, patients with severe systemic reactions have been described.[1]

Clinical presentation

Oral allergy syndrome: also known as pollen–food syndrome

The most frequent symptom of food allergy, particularly in adults, is the so-called OAS. This has been demonstrated in double-blind placebo-controlled food challenge (DBPCFC) studies involving hazelnut, apple and cherry allergies.[8]

OAS is a condition characterized by IgE-mediated allergic symptoms restricted to the oral mucosa, which may involve itching and vascular edema of the lips, tongue, palate and pharynx. It is sudden in onset and may be associated with itching of the ear and a sense of tightness in the throat.[9] Symptoms usually develop within minutes and then gradually fade within an hour. Although oral itching can be elicited by any food allergen, the classic OAS is associated with sensitization to heat- and pepsin-labile plant-derived proteins in patients with a pollen-related food allergy, in which case cross-reactivity between homologous plant-derived proteins in pollens and vegetable foods is the basis of the syndrome.[10]

Most allergens involved in such cross-reactivity reactions are easily destroyed by pepsin digestion and heat, which explains why symptoms of pollen-related food allergy are generally mild and the majority of patients with OAS have no problem if they ingest the offending foods after cooking or other heat treatments. OAS can also be induced by stable allergens, so a subset of patients with this specific type of food allergy may sometimes experience generalized and even life-threatening reactions.

Anaphylaxis

Pollen–food allergy syndrome is often associated with systemic and severe reactions in addition to OAS. This is the case when nsLTP, the most important family of pollen stable allergens, is involved. Patients may experience a generalized life-threatening reaction within minutes of ingesting the food.[11]

Studies focusing particularly on celery and carrot allergies in subjects allergic to pollens have reported systemic reactions in approximately 50% of patients according to case histories, and up to 50% of patients experienced systemic reactions when challenged, even if the DBPCFC was performed using a stepwise 'spit and swallow' protocol, which was suspended at the lowest food dose reproducibly causing symptoms.[12] It has also been reported that a member of the PR-10 protein family from soybean, Gly m 4, can induce severe allergic reactions.[13] Anaphylactic reactions are not rare in mugwort–birch–celery syndrome.[4]

In conclusion, these studies demonstrate that the symptoms of pollen-related allergy to certain foods may be more severe than is commonly assumed.

Gastrointestinal disorders

The digestive tract can also be involved in pollinoses which can cause a Th2-mediated inflammatory response in the gut, and may even be responsible for eosinophilic esophagitis, a disorder characterized by a dense eosinophilic infiltrate with squamous epithelial hyperplasia in the absence of any gastric or intestinal mucosal anomalies. It has been demonstrated that colonoscopic Bet v 1 challenge can induce intestinal inflammation in patients with birch pollen allergy. Magnusson et al.[14] have concluded that in patients with birch pollinosis and a birch + plant food syndrome, a duodenal biopsy obtained during the pollination season shows a greater eosinophil and mast cell infiltration than in biopsies taken at other times of year.

Pan-allergens

As reported by Breiteneder and Ebner,[15] plant-derived proteins responsible for food allergy include few protein families (Table 7.1). Many allergens belong to the cupin (seed storage proteins) or prolamin superfamilies (2S albumins, α-amylase inhibitors, non-specific (ns)LTPs, and prolamin storage proteins of cereals). The pathogenesis-related proteins are a miscellany of 14 plant protein families involved in plant resistance to pathogens or adverse environmental conditions. Then there are the profilins, a number of unrelated families of structural and metabolic plant proteins. Several of these proteins are widely distributed throughout the plant kingdom and may consequently be involved in extensive IgE cross-reactivity between antigens from taxonomically unrelated plant species, a phenomenon described in the pan-allergen theory.[16] IgE cross-reactivity may be clinically manifest or irrelevant. The clinical signs seem to be influenced by a number of factors, including the host's immune response and exposure to the allergen, and the type of allergen involved. The proteins' structural characteristics are major cross-reactivity determinants, so pollen–food syndrome develops as a consequence of shared features at primary and tertiary protein structure level. It has been claimed that proteins with >70% sequence identity are often cross-reactive, whereas those with <50% sequence identity rarely cross-react, although there are a few exceptions. Other factors influencing the clinical correlations of pollen–food syndrome include allergen concentrations and their differential expression during ripening, and their stability on cooking. A brief description of the cross-reactive pan-allergens involved in pollen–food allergy (Table 7.2) is given below.

The prolamin superfamily

The prolamin superfamily is the most prominent of all the protein families with allergenic members, including the nsLTP family, the 2S albumin storage proteins, the cereal α-amylase/trypsin inhibitors, and the soybean hydrophobic protein. Prolamins are a group of seed storage proteins and the main storage proteins in cereals and other members of the grass family. They are stable in response to thermal processing and enzyme proteolysis as they are rich in cysteine. Since they were first described

Table 7.1 Biological classification of the main vegetable food allergens. Allergen nomenclature: Act c (kiwi), Ana o (cashew), Api g (celery), Ara h (peanut), Ber e (Brazil nut), Bra r (rapeseed), Cas a (chestnut), Cor a (hazelnut), Cuc m (melon), Jug r (walnut), Lyc e (tomato), Mal d (apple), Pers a (avocado), Pru av (cherry), Pru p (peach), Pyr c (pear), Sec c (rye), Ses i (sesame), Tri a (wheat). Adapted from Asero et al. Plant food allergies: a suggested approach to allergen-resolved diagnosis in the clinical practice by identifying easily available sensitization markers. Int Arch Allergy Immunol. 2005; 138: 1–11.

Main vegetable food allergens	Cupin superfamily	2.2 Vicilins	Ara h 1, Ses I 3, Jug r 2, Ana o 1, Cor a 11
		Legumins	Ara h 3–4, Jug r 4, Ana o 2, Cor a 9
	Prolamin superfamily	2S albumins	Ara h 2–6-7, Jug r 1, Ana o 3, Ric c 1–3, Sin a 1, Bra j 1, Ber e 1
		Ns LTP	Pru p 3, Jug r 3, Cor a 8, Mal d 3,
		α-amylase inh	Rice
		Prolamins of cereals	Tri a 19, Sec c 20
	Defense system proteins (I)	Pathogenesis-related protein	PR-2 (Hev b 2)
			PR-3 (Hev b 6.02, Pers a 1, Cas s 5)
			PR-4 (Bra r 2)
			PR-5 (Pru av 2, Mal d 2, Cap a 1, Act c 2)
			PR-9 (Tri a Bd)
			PR-10 (Mal d 1, Api g 1)
			PR-14 (LTP)
	Defense system proteins (II)	Thiol proteases	Papain-like cysteine proteases (Act c 1) Gli (Gly credo) m Bd
			Subtilisin-like serine proteases (Cuc m 1)
		Protease inhibitors	Type Kunitz (soy)
			α-amylase inhs (cereals)
	Structural and metabolic proteins	Storage proteins	Patatin (Sola t 1)
		Enzymes	Phenylcoumaran benzyl eth. reductase (Pyr c 5)
			Cyclophilin (carrot)
			Oxydases (Api g 5)
			Liases (garlic)
		Profilins	Api g 4, Mal d 4, Ara h 5

in 1999[17] they have been the object of considerable research in view of their clinical relevance.

Lipid transfer proteins

LTPs are members of the prolamin superfamily (PR-14) with low-molecular-weight proteins (9–10 kDa) and are contained in large amounts (as much as 4% of the total soluble proteins) in higher plants. LTPs are characterized by a conserved pattern of 6–8 cysteines, forming three to four disulfide bridges. They are named after their capacity to transfer lipids between membranes. More than 100 plant nsLTPs have been sequenced. Plant LTPs have a total number of amino acids varying from 91 to 95 residues and exhibit strong structural homologies.[18] Nevertheless, no sequence homology has been found between LTPs from mammalian and plant LTPs.

LTPs are important food allergens, especially in Mediterranean areas. In northern and central Europe, fruit allergies are mainly described as a cross-reactive phenomenon resulting from sensitization to homologous allergens from (birch) pollen, and patients usually have only mild symptoms restricted to the oral cavity (OAS), whereas patients in Mediterranean countries also suffer from fruit allergies unrelated to pollens and frequently have systemic reactions. The nsLTPs have been suggested as a model allergen for true food

Table 7.2 Class II food allergens. Adapted from Mothes N, Horak F, Valenta R. Transition from a botanical to a molecular classification in tree pollen allergy: implications for diagnosis and therapy. Int Arch Allergy Immunol. 2004; 135: 357–373.

Allergen	kDa	Family	Cross-reactivity	
			Source	**Molecule**
Bet v 1	17	PR-10	Fruits:	
			Apple	Mal d 1
			Cherry	Pru av 1
			Apricot	Pru ar 1
			Pear	Pyr c 1
			Vegetables:	
			Celery	Api g 1
			Carrot	Dau c 1
			Soybean	Gly m 4
			Nuts:	
			Hazelnut	Cor a 1
			Peanut	Ara h 8
			Others:	
			Parsley	Pc PR 1 and 2
			Spices	
Bet v 2	14	Profilin	Fruits:	
			Cherry	Pru av 4
			Peach	Pru p 4
			Pear	Pyr c 4
			Vegetables:	
			Celery	Api g 4
			Tomato	Lyc e 1
			Soybean	Gly m 3
			Potato	
			Others:	
			Spices	Cap a 2
			Latex	Hev b 8
LTP	9	PR-14	Fruits:	
			Apple	Mal d 3
			Apricot	Pru ar 3
			Peach	Pru p 3
			Plum	Pru d 1
			Others:	
			Corn	Zea m 14
TLP	23–31	PR-5	Fruits:	
			Apple	Mal d 2
			Cherry	Pru av 2
			Kiwi	Act c 2

allergy[19] because of their high resistance to heat treatment and proteolytic digestion. Sensitization to LTPs has also been reported in patients with no pollen allergies, which supports their role as a sensitizing food allergen. LTPs were first identified by Lleonart[20] and his group in 1992, who discovered a low-molecular-weight (~10 kDa) allergen in peach skin that later turned out to be the nsLTP recently designated Pru p 3. In the last 15 years, several studies have shown an immunologic cross-reactivity within LTPs from Rosaceae[17] and between LTPs from Rosaceae and botanically unrelated plant-derived foods.[21] The spectrum of foods in which the role of LTP as an allergen is being studied is increasing rapidly. IgE antibodies against food LTPs have been shown to express variable degrees of cross-reactivity, which has been identified between LTPs in latex and some pollens (e.g. Par j 1 and Par j 2, the major Parietaria allergens, are LTPs) as well. Peach seems to be responsible for the primary sensitization to this allergen (as no patients allergic to LTPs but not sensitized to peach have been described to date) and the cross-reactivity to LTPs of botanically unrelated plant foods seems to depend on the level of peach LTP-specific IgE (as in class I allergies).[22,23] This finding has been questioned, as in some patients with mugwort pollinosis it appears that the antigenicity common to mugwort and peach LTP was due primarily to mugwort pollen (i.e. a class II food allergy).[24]

CLINICAL CASE

A 10-year-old girl reported tingling and pruritus of the lips, mouth and oropharynx after ingestion of peach, carrot, apple, cherry and tomato. The symptoms appeared less than 5 minutes following the ingestion of these foods, were mild and subsided spontaneously in less than 15 minutes. She had never had gastrointestinal or respiratory complaints. The girl was already on an elimination diet for these fruits and vegetables, both raw and cooked. From the age of 4 years she had suffered from rhinitis and asthma with sensitization to grass pollen, Bermuda grass, birch and hazel pollen. In vitro specific IgE tests show the following results:

Tomato	8.0 kU/L
Carrot	29.9 kU/L
Apple	37.7 kU/L
Peach	47.3 kU/L
Cherry	25.5 kU/L
Birch	>100 kU/L
Hazel	>100 kU/L
Olive	89.5 kU/L
Grass	>100 kU/L

Prick-by-prick test with fresh fruits and vegetables was positive for peach, cherry and carrot, but negative for tomato as evaluated in mm wheal/erythema.

Peach	3/6	Carrot	5/10
Cherry	5/10	Apple	7/10
Tomato	Neg		
Histamine	4/20	Neg control	Neg

Discussion

The most important challenge in pollen–food syndrome is to identify those patients with a high risk for systemic reactions.

Considering that the girl had a positivity to birch (>100 kU/L), apple, cherry and peach, which belong to the Rosaceae family, it is important to investigate the presence of IgE antibodies to Bet v 1 and nsLTP to evaluate the risk for serious systemic reactions.

Bet v 1 is the major allergen component found in birch pollen, which belongs to a group of plant proteins termed pathogenesis-related protein family number 10 (PR-10), sensitive to heat and proteases. Bet v 1 is correlated with symptoms restricted to the mouth.

nsLTP (non-specific lipid transfer proteins) are very stable allergens widespread in plants. The important characteristic of nsLTP is the high resistance to heat and protease, correlated with severe clinical symptoms, such as urticaria/angioedema, asthma and anaphylaxis.

CRDs evaluation has shown:

Bet v1	>100 kU/L
Peach LTP (Pru p 3)	0.16 kU/L

Conclusion

The time course of the pollen and food allergies suggests a primary sensitization through the inhalation route to pollen with the generation of cross-reactive IgE to pollen profilin.

Considering these results, we can suppose that the patient will have only oral symptoms (oral allergy syndrome). Furthermore, the reactions are only induced by fresh fruits and the processed fruits and vegetables, such as commercial fruit juices, peach in syrup or cooked foods are tolerated.

Pathogenesis-related proteins

PRs form a heterogeneous collection of 14 plant protein families. They are not a protein superfamily but a set of unrelated protein families that function as part of the plant defense system.

Proteins homologous to Bet v 1

About 98% of patients allergic to birch pollen are sensitized to the major allergen Bet v 1, an 18-kDa PR-10, and proteins homologous to Bet v 1 have been detected in a number of plant-derived foods. Bet v 1 is a member of the PR-10 family.

Approximately 70% of individuals allergic to birch pollen suffer from pollen–food syndrome and have IgE cross-reactivity to Bet v 1 and its food homologs.[15] The taxonomic distribution of allergens related to Bet v 1 is fairly limited. Pollen allergens are found exclusively in the birch and beech families, whereas the food allergens described come from fruits in the Rosaceae families (including apple, pear, peach, cherry, plum, apricot and almond), and vegetables in the Apiaceae (including celery, carrot, fennel and parsley) and Fabaceae (peanut and soybean). The cross-reactivity of Bet v 1 with the major apple allergen Mal d 1 occurs not only at B-cell but also at T-cell level. Bet v 1 also contains the major T-cell activating region of Api g 1, confirming that Bet v 1 is responsible for initializing an allergic response to the major celery allergen. The epitopes of the hazelnut allergen Cor a 1.04 appear to be less related to the hazel pollen allergen Cor a 1 than to the Bet v 1 from birch pollen. Virtually all patients allergic to birch pollen are positive by SPTs with many of these fresh fruits and vegetables, but only a proportion of them have food allergies (generally those reporting severe allergy-related respiratory symptoms or showing the highest levels of birch pollen-specific IgE). This is particularly true of allergies to vegetables that are botanically distant from Rosaceae, such as those of the Apiaceae. Many vegetable food proteins homologous to Bet v 1 (and those from fruits of the Rosaceae in particular) are extremely labile and easily destroyed by heat, oxidation, extraction procedures and pepsin digestion. Clinically, this translates into a good tolerance of heat-processed foods and commercial fruit juices, and the symptoms of a reaction rarely amount to more than OAS. Not all Bet v 1-homologous proteins are equally heat- and/or pepsin-sensitive, however: celery (Api g 1) and soybean (Gly m 4) antigens have been reported to cause severe systemic symptoms.

Celery allergy is common in Europe, and reportedly a major cause of food-induced anaphylaxis in Switzerland.[25] Heating does not change its allergenicity. Birch and mugwort pollens are known to be cross-reactive to celery and are considered sensitizing antigens. Whereas the allergens in celery also include Api g 4 and Api g 5, the major allergen is Api g 1, which belongs to the above-mentioned PR-10. The reason why Api g 1 is stable on heating – unlike other allergens in the same group, such as Bet v 1 – remains to be thoroughly clarified.

In 2002, Kleine-Tebbe et al.[13] reported that 20 patients with birch pollinosis developed allergic symptoms, including anaphylactic shock, soon after the initial ingestion of soybean protein. Their symptoms included facial swelling (17 patients), OAS (14 patients), dyspnea (six patients), urticaria (six patients) and drowsiness (five patients), and occurred within 20 minutes of their first taste of the soy product. The majority of patients reported symptoms during the tree pollen season. The authors produced a very pure recombinant SAM22 protein (Gly m 4) to prove the hypothesis that a pollen-related allergen in soybean was responsible for the allergic reactions to the food product. They concluded that there was strong evidence to suggest that a protein from soy related to birch pollen could trigger adverse reactions to soy in patients with high IgE titers to Bet v 1. A follow-up study by Mittag et al.[26] confirmed that Gly-m-4-specific IgE testing was positive in 21 of 22 birch pollinosis patients who developed soybean allergy, and that it inhibited IgE binding to soybean protein by 60% or more in nine of 11 patients, indicating that Gly m 4 was the major allergen. Moreover, as the binding of IgE to soybean protein was inhibited by 80% or more after adding birch pollen protein in nine of the 11 patients, the authors suggested that birch pollen is the main culprit responsible for the antigenicity shared by the two allergens. According to their report, the Gly m 4 content in soybean increased during ripening and storage, and was no longer detectable in highly fermented soy foods (e.g. miso and soy sauce) or roasted soybeans, whereas it was still detectable in tofu, soy flakes, and a dietary powder containing soybean. Gly m 4 also revealed a certain degree of stability to moderate heating, i.e. its content in soybeans was reduced after 30 minutes of cooking, but it was only after 4 hours of cooking that no Gly m 4 was detectable.

Thaumatin-like proteins (TLPs)

TLPs are members of the PR-5 family. Thaumatin is highly water-soluble and stable on heating and under acidic conditions.

Mal d 2 is an important allergenic TLP in apple that is associated with IgE-mediated symptoms in individuals with apple allergy. Purified recombinant Mal d 2 displayed the ability to bind IgE from individuals with apple allergy in the same way as natural Mal d 2. The TLP of sweet cherry, Pru av 2, has also been identified as a major allergen, and a grape TLP with an amino acid sequence very similar to that of Mal d 2 and Pru av 2, and a kiwi TLP described as the allergen Act c 2, have been identified as minor allergens.

Profilins

Profilin is a monomeric, largely cross-reacting 12–15-kDa actin-binding and cytoskeleton-regulating protein contained in all eukaryotic cells.[27] Allergenic profilins are found exclusively in flowering plants and are minor pollen allergens. Several studies have shown that only 10–20% of patients with pollen allergy are sensitized to profilins, but they react to a broad range of inhalant and food allergens. Actually, profilins form a family of highly cross-reactive allergens in monocot and dicot pollens, plant foods and *Hevea latex*. An example of profilin is the birch pollen allergen Bet v 2. Patients sensitized to Bet v 2 or to grass pollen profilin often have oral symptoms on ingesting apple, pear, carrot and celery, in response to IgE cross-linking by the homologous profilins contained in these foods.[15] In the mugwort–celery–spice syndrome, patients sensitized to mugwort cross-react to the profilins in celery and spices of the Apiaceae, or Umbelliferae, family (carrots, caraway seeds, parsley, coriander, aniseed and fennel seeds).[1]

Although many pollen–food syndromes are related to profilins, it is difficult to purify natural profilins from fruit and vegetables, and only a few isolated recombinant profilins have been described. Asero et al.[28] performed skin tests in 200 pollinosis patients using purified palm profilin (Pho d 2) and observed a positive reaction in one-third, who were also positive to pollens from a wide range of plants; more than half of them also exhibited OAS, with fruit allergy symptoms and no symptoms on ingesting cooked or processed foods.

Cross-reactive carbohydrate determinants (CCDs)

The *N*-linked carbohydrate groups of glycoproteins induce IgE, leading to cross-reactivity between foods and pollens.[29]

Carbohydrates with an IgE-binding capacity have also been reported in plant proteins with no allergenicity, e.g. bromelain in pineapple, horseradish peroxidase, polyamine oxidase in corn, ascorbic acid oxidase in *Cucurbita pepo*, and phytohemagglutinin in haricot bean.[1]

Cross-reactive IgE directed against the glycosyl portion of glycoproteins seem to have a poor biological activity. Many CCDs are monovalent and do not form bridges of IgEs on the mast cells, so they are generally assumed not to induce histamine release. The identification of anti-CCD IgE will improve allergy diagnostics in vitro by discriminating specific IgE positive to foods without any apparent clinical significance in patients sensitized to pollen.

Because of the variable biological activity of cross-reactive IgE in relation to carbohydrates, the debate over their importance in allergy remains open.

CLINICAL CASE

A 10-year-old girl with a history of mild to moderate atopic dermatitis, allergic asthma and rhinitis and food allergy for kiwi was admitted to the pediatric allergy clinic for a reaction to hazelnut, with angioedema of the lips and itching in her mouth. She reported having experienced the same symptoms 2 weeks as well as 1 year before the current episode which did not require medical intervention.

She had suffered from a cows' milk allergy until 5 years of age and subsequently developed multiple sensitizations to grass pollen, birch and hazel pollen, and dust mites.

The diagnostic work-up included prick-by-prick testing, in vitro specific IgE tests and evaluation of relevant CRDs.

Prick-by-prick test results (wheal and erythema size in mm)

Cashew	3/5
Pistachio	4/20
Sesame	3/15
Hazelnut	Negative
Brazil nuts	Negative
Walnut	Negative
Peanut	Negative
Histamine	3/20
Control	Negative

Specific IgE results

Timothy grass	27.40 kUa/L
Orchard grass	34.10 kUa/L
Perennial ryegrass	41.50 kUa/L
Velvet grass	36.90 kUa/L
Birch	46.10 kUa/L
Hazel	38.00 kUa/L
Bet v 1	52.40 kUa/L

Specific IgE results	
Profilin	<0.10 kUa/L
Bet v 4	0.18 kUa/L
Sesame	1.31 kUa/L
Peanut	0.50 kUa/L
Hazelnut	39.60 kUa/L
Brazil nut	0.69 kUa/L
Cashew	2.68 kUa/L
Pistachio	4.14 kUa/L
Walnut	4.99 kUa/L
Kiwi	4.97 kUa/L
rCor a 8 LTP hazelnut	0.79 kUa/L
rCor a 1 PR-10 hazelnut	39.00 kUa/L
rAra h 8 PR10	4.54 kUa/L
rAra h 1 peanut	<0.10 kUa/L
rAra h 2 peanut	0.20 kUa/L
rAra h 3 peanut	<0.10 kUa/L

Discussion

In this case the patient was positive for birch and hazel pollen and for hazelnut, but prick-by-prick testing with fresh hazelnut was negative. Moreover, the specific IgE for Bet v 1 and rCor a 1 PR-10 hazelnut was very high, whereas rCor a 8 LTP hazelnut IgE resulted very low.

Bet v 1	52.40 kUa/L
Hazel	38.00 kUa/L
Hazelnut	39.60 kUa/L
rCor a 1 PR-10 hazelnut	39.00 kUa/L
rCor a 8 LTP hazelnut	0.79 kUa/L

The major allergen from hazel pollen, Cor a 1, a Bet v 1 homolog, was reported to have similar IgE-binding properties as the major hazelnut allergen.

Bet v 1 (the major birch pollen allergen) is a pathogenesis-related protein that is responsible for oral allergy syndrome (OAS) in patients with birch pollinosis and was strongly correlated with apple, peach, hazelnut and carrot. Patients allergic to birch and hazel pollen may have symptoms to hazelnut.

Conclusion

In patients sensitized to *Rosaceae* food allergens or having clinical symptoms to *Rosaceae* foods, it is important to investigate the presence of IgE antibodies to Bet v 1 and nsLTP to evaluate the risk for severe systemic reactions. Bet v 1 homologs, unlike nsLTPs, are often associated with local symptoms (OAS) and rarely with life threatening reactions. In spite of this, it could be misleading to predict a clinical reaction only on the basis of positivity to Bet v 1 above all, in the presence of high concentration of IgE antibodies to this recombinant allergen.

In this light an oral food challenge with hazelnut should strongly be considered.

Diagnosis

The class II food allergy is difficult to diagnose and currently available diagnostic tools are inadequate, mainly because commercially available food extract preparations are generally not suitable for performing diagnostic tests. The major allergens involved in this type of food allergy are susceptible to degradation processes and are easily destroyed during the extraction procedure. Recombinant DNA technologies have enabled a number of these allergens to be produced in a pure and stable form, and several recombinant allergens involved in class II food allergies have been tested for their suitability for use in in vivo and/or in vitro diagnostic process. The use of these molecules should lead to important advances, moving on from an extract-based diagnosis to a CRD, which may provide refined information on cross-reactivity patterns and the potential severity of symptoms. Molecular analysis of allergen sensitization patterns may help us to improve the predictive and prognostic power of allergy diagnostics based on IgE antibodies.

In northern European populations, for example, sensitization to Rosaceae fruits is characteristically directed against Bet v 1-related food allergens and the symptoms are usually mild, but in the Mediterranean area (where sensitization to Rosaceae is mainly related to nsLTPs) is often accompanied by systemic food reactions.[8] Although certain allergens are known to be strongly predictive of manifest allergic disease, others (typically cross-reactive determinants such as profilins or particular glycan structures) are considered only weakly associated with clinical reactivity. Given its use of purified natural or recombinant allergen molecules rather than crude natural extracts,[30] an intrinsic advantage of CRD lies in its higher diagnostic sensitivity, which has been demonstrated in several cases. The use of such potent reagents in routine diagnostic tests would have a positive effect on their diagnostic efficacy in clinical practice.

In vivo, SPT, oral food challenges (open and DBPCFC), and in vitro tests (food-specific IgE assay and basophil studies) are primary tools for the diagnosis of food allergy in daily practice (Fig. 7.1).

In vivo tests

Prick test

For plant-derived foods, commercial extracts for use in SPT have a limited sensitivity and give rise to

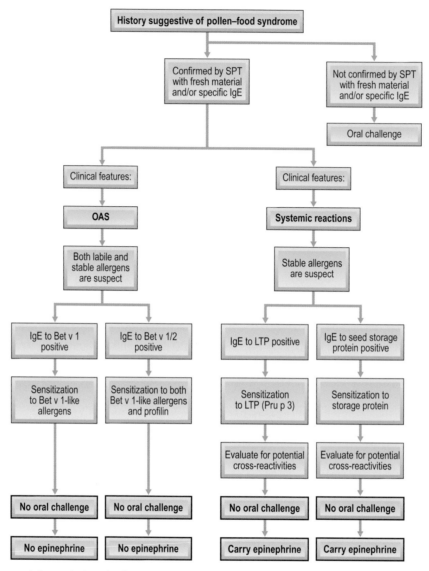

Figure 7.1 Proposed diagnostic algorithm for patients with suspected pollen–food syndrome.[10]

high false-negative rates. Most allergens involved in class II food allergy are easily degraded during the extraction process. The enzymes are released during the mechanical crushing of the food and certain allergens may be degraded even before extraction begins. The degradation may also continue during lengthy periods of storage, thereby progressively changing the composition of the initial food extract. The final amount of an allergen in an extract depends on the raw material used and the method adopted to extract the proteins. For instance, an optimal content of LTP is achieved when they are extracted from fruit peel or skin. On the other hand, using this approach will mean that allergens belonging to the PR-10 family and profilins will be under-represented in the final extract, because they are located mainly in the flesh of fruits. The same problem applies to the pH conditions during the extraction process. Whereas optimal amounts of PR-14 family proteins are obtained under slightly acidic conditions, members of the PR-10 protein family are ideally extracted at a pH of 8.6. In addition, different plant strains may contain different quantities of allergens, as shown in the case of apples.[31] The standardization of food extracts by total protein content, single allergen content or allergenic activity is therefore unfeasible in many cases. Several attempts have successfully been made to improve this situation. Unfortunately, these approaches demand complex extraction procedures so they are not suitable for use in the routine preparation of food extracts.

Skin testing with native foods using the prick-prick technique clearly produces better results. In this test, the lancet is plunged several times into the peel and/or flesh of the food immediately before pricking the patient's skin. This is currently the most reliable in vivo test as far as labile allergens are concerned (e.g. fruit and vegetables). Prick-prick tests are also useful when there are discrepancies between a suggestive case history and a negative SPT result obtained with a commercial extract, or when a specific food extract is unavailable. The main drawbacks of the prick-prick test are the low specificity, resulting in high false positive rates, and the impossibility of standardizing the source of the allergen. Among other reasons, the test's limited specificity is also an expression of IgE cross-reactivity with pollen or other related foods, and the only way to ascertain the clinical relevance of positive SPT findings is by means of controlled oral challenges. As the concentration of labile allergens in commercial extracts of plant-derived foods falls considerably whereas the stable allergens persist, it has been suggested that this observation be exploited for the differential diagnosis between patients sensitized to stable (e.g. LTP, seed storage proteins etc.) versus labile (e. g. Bet v 1-like, profilin) allergens.[10]

When recombinant Api g 1, the major allergen of celery, was used in skin tests, the results indicated that this protein enabled an accurate in vivo diagnosis of celery allergy in areas where birch trees are common.[32] Very recently, taking cherry as a model food, a panel of three recombinant allergens (Pru av 1, Pru av 3, and Pru av 4) was tested for their ability to diagnose cherry allergy by SPT by comparison with DBPCFC. The commercially available cherry extract prompted a positive skin prick response in 20% of cases, whereas the panel of recombinant proteins reached a sensitivity of 96%.

Food challenges

Besides all the difficulties of obtaining a reliable serological diagnosis of class II food allergy, oral provocation tests may also produce questionable results. In this respect, the diagnosis of OAS is particularly difficult to handle, as the food should not be swallowed immediately but kept in the mouth for a certain time. The oral challenge is a diagnostic test that usually provides strong evidence of a food allergy, and enables clinicians to recommend suitable dietary restrictions.

Oral food challenges may be performed in open or single-blind fashion, or as a DBPCFC, which is usually considered the gold standard for diagnosing food allergies. Owing to the 'instability' of most class II food allergens and their rapid degradation by endogenous enzymes in the food, truly allergic patients may have a negative response to the probe of the DBPCFC but react positively to an open challenge with the fresh food. Different challenge models may also differ in sensitivity and the number of placebo reactions. Additional problems concern how to find suitable ingredients to conceal the food being assessed in the meal used for the challenge, so as to minimize the patient's subjective bias. In 2000, Ballmer-Weber developed a two-step 'spit and swallow' protocol to verify allergies to celery, carrot and cherry. The patient must initially retain the allergen in increasing amounts in his mouth, spitting it out after 1 minute. The amount is doubled every 15 minutes. After an interval of 1 hour, the procedure is repeated with a placebo. If patients consistently report OAS symptoms three times in response to the allergen, but not to the placebo, they are regarded as responders. Patients who complain of no symptoms during this spitting phase go on to step 2 of the DBPCFC, in which they ingest the allergen in increasing amounts at 15-minute intervals. Between the two steps of the challenge there must be an interval of at least 24 hours. This protocol not only considers the specific clinical features of OAS but is also safer for the patients. The need for standardized challenge models and suitable recipes for challenge and placebo preparations nevertheless remains.

In vitro tests

Allergen-specific IgE antibodies are the main components of food allergy reactions. They are easy to measure in blood samples from individuals suspected of having a food allergy using commercially available assays, and assessing specific IgE is a frequently used important element in the clinical investigation and diagnosis of food allergy. In vitro allergen-specific IgE tests (including the radio-allergosorbent test (RAST) and the enzyme aller-gosorbent test (EAST)) are used to test serum for IgE-mediated food allergies.

Commercial ImmunoCAP extracts have a low diagnostic sensitivity in pollen–food syndrome. Several studies based on the CRD concept using pure allergen molecules have been published.

Using recombinant Pru av 1 and Pru av 4, EAST revealed 97% positive results in 101 patients allergic to cherry, as opposed to only 17% identified by CAP/RAST.[33]

Sera from 43 patients with DBPCFC-proven allergy to hazelnuts were investigated with either hazelnut extract or recombinant major allergen Cor a 1.0401.[34] EAST with recombinant Cor a 1.0401 yielded a sensitivity of 95%, as opposed to 70% obtained with the commercially available CAP/RAST system, which is based on a total food extract.

Ballmer-Weber et al.[35] examined the IgE antibody response in carrot allergy in 40 patients carefully selected according to their clinical history, specific IgE and a positive DBPCFC result. Two isoforms of Dau c 1 (Dau c 1.0104 and Dau c 1.0201), the profilin Dau c 4 and a reagent for CCDs were used to assess sensitization, and the birch pollen allergens Bet v 1 and Bet v 2 were used for comparison. The results confirmed that Dau c 1 is a major allergen in carrot allergy. Although sensitization to the Dau c 1.0104 isoform was more prevalent among the individuals studied, the Dau c 1.0201 isoform showed the best correlation to the clinical situation.

Gly m 4 and Ara h 8 have recently been identified as Bet-v-1-related molecules in soybean and peanut, respectively, and they have been produced in recombinant form.[26] In addition to extending the panel of soybean and peanut allergens, Gly m 4 in particular has prompted a marked improvement in diagnostic sensitivity when used as an ImmunoCAP reagent. Whereas only 10 of 22 individuals (45%) with pollen-related allergy to soybean tested positive with the soybean extract-based test, all but one (96%) showed IgE binding to rGly m 4 coupled with streptavidin-coated ImmunoCAP tests.

Asero et al.[22] suggested that peach LTP (Pru p 3) could be important as a general marker of allergies to plant-derived food. Studying 40 patients with LTP reactivity, they found a correlation between specific IgE levels to Pru p 3 and the extent of clinical reactivity to an increasing number of plant-derived foods. Bolhaar et al.[36] described cases of severe reactions to Sharon fruit and identified homologs of Bet v 1 and Bet v 2 as the main IgE-binding molecules in Sharon fruit extract. The results of mediator release experiments conducted with Bet v 1 and Bet v 2 led indirectly to the conclusion that Bet v 1-related structures, but not profilins, were biologically active allergens in Sharon fruit and responsible for the clinical reactivity to this food.[36]

Basophil activation test

Skin and serological assays indicate sensitization but are not clinically relevant to IgE reactivity. Information on the biological function of observed IgE reactivity can be obtained by means of the basophil activation test (BAT), which has been used in a number of clinical studies on plant food allergy and CRDs. There are reports of BAT flow cytometry being of diagnostic value in allergies to airborne allergens (pollen and house dust mites), hymenoptera venoms, drugs (muscle relaxant allergy and β-lactams), food and latex. For pollen-associated food allergy the method has been evaluated in only a few studies. Erdmann and collaborators[37] focused on a panel of Bet v 1 homologs from apple, carrot and celery (respectively Mal d 1, Dau c 1.01 and Api g 1.01), also considering Bet v 1 and Bet v 2 for comparative purposes. A functional BAT with pure allergen molecules was compared with Immuno-CAP™ measurements using whole allergen extracts, revealing clinical sensitivities and specificities of 60–75% and 64–86%, respectively, for the IgE assay and 65–75% and 68–100%, respectively, for the BAT assay. The patients were not selected on the basis of challenge tests, and unlike in the Ballmer-Weber[35] study, no control group (patients with birch pollen allergy without food allergy) was included in the evaluation of the test's diagnostic performance. The authors concluded that, although a better characterization of the study participants would have been useful, the use of CRD and the inclusion of biological assays such as BAT might help to identify the clinically most relevant allergens for in vitro tests. Bet v 1 and Bet v 2 have also been included in a CRD study dealing with grass pollen allergy. Recording detailed case histories and determining IgE reactivity to various pollen extracts and recombinant birch pollen allergens helped to identify different subsets of individuals allergic to grass pollens, with or without food allergies, and with or without co-sensitization to birch pollen allergens.

Recombinant food allergens have improved our knowledge of the chemical and immunological features of these proteins and given us a better idea of the immunological mechanisms underlying class II food allergies, but this is not enough. Data on the use of recombinant allergens strongly support the conviction that they are molecules suitable for replacing food extracts in the future. But positive serological test and SPT results do not necessarily reflect a clinically relevant food allergy. The finding of allergen-specific IgE does not always correlate with symptoms when a given food is ingested. So, in the end, although recombinant food allergens improve the reliability and accuracy of the diagnostic material to use in SPT and serological assays, the gold standard for confirming clinical symptoms against certain foods remains the oral food challenge.

Management

There is no agreement among clinicians on how to manage pollen–food syndrome. One survey among allergists found that 53% recommended complete avoidance of the offending foods, 38% reported giving recommendations tailored to each patient, and 9% did not advocate food restrictions; 4% of the clinicians recommended avoiding potentially cross-reactive foods.[38] Several studies have assessed cross-reactivity, particularly in the Rosaceae family of fruits: from 46% to 63% of patients with confirmed pollen–food syndrome to one fruit revealed a clinical reactivity to other Rosaceae fruits.[39] Based on these studies and others, Rodriguez et al.[39] recommended that, if a reported reaction is confirmed, tolerance to other Rosaceae fruits (particularly apricot, apple and plum) should be assessed unless patients have already eaten them without developing any symptoms at any time after their initial reaction.

Patients with pollen–food syndrome generally tolerate cooked forms of the fruit or vegetable to which they are allergic, and allergists often recommend that they cook reactive fruits and vegetables before ingesting them.[40,41] Thermal processing of PR-10-like food proteins induces a denaturation of the proteins and a disruption of their conformation that translates into a loss of IgE-binding capacity, thereby making these foods clinically tolerable. Bohle et al.[41] found that food allergens soon lost their capacity to bind IgE and cause mediator release after cooking, but these same cooked food allergens retained their ability to stimulate Bet-v-1-specific T cells.[40,41] T-cell epitopes are short, linear peptides that tend to survive gastrointestinal digestion and thermal processing.[40] This may be important for several reasons. One is that patients with atopic dermatitis and pollen–food syndrome who eat cooked fruits and vegetables may experience an exacerbation of their atopic dermatitis due to the activation of Bet v 1-specific T cells that can migrate to the skin and induce effector responses.[40] Second, the ingestion of cooked fruit and vegetables may cause perennial pollen-specific T- and B-cell activation, leading to perennially increased allergen-specific IgE levels in patients allergic to pollen even outside the pollen season.[41] Pollen allergy is often treated with subcutaneous immunotherapy. Because the clinical symptoms of pollen–food syndrome relate to a cross-reactivity between food allergens and pollen IgE, it has been hypothesized that immunotherapy for pollen allergy may treat pollen–food syndrome too. Several studies have addressed this issue with regard to birch pollen and pollen–food syndrome, with varying results. Asero[42] conducted one of the most successful studies, in which 84% of patients who were sensitive to birch pollen and had pollen–food syndrome in relation to apple reported a significant reduction or the disappearance of their oral symptoms in response to apples after being treated with birch pollen subcutaneous immunotherapy. In addition, 88% of these patients showed a marked reduction in their reactivity to SPTs with apple.[42] In another study, 87% of birch-allergic patients with pollen–food syndrome who were treated with subcutaneous immunotherapy could eat significantly more apple or hazelnut without developing allergic signs or symptoms, though the amount of apple or hazelnut they tolerated was still small.[43] In contrast to the above studies, Moller[44] found no significant improvement in food allergy symptoms during a course of subcutaneous or oral birch pollen immunotherapy in a group of children with birch pollen allergy and pollen–food syndrome compared with a control group, although the treatment group's pollen-related rhinoconjunctivitis improved substantially. In another study on birch subcutaneous immunotherapy and apple allergy, two of 12 patients developed pollen–food syndrome and five of 12 developed IgE to Bet v 2 at some point during the therapy,[45] whereas there was no evidence of pollen–food syndrome or Bet v 2 IgE in controls not submitting to birch immunotherapy. The authors concluded that the treatment could induce allergies to additional components in the pollen immunotherapy preparations that might cause new symptoms (e.g. pollen–food syndrome).[45]

Other investigators examined the effects of sublingual immunotherapy with birch pollen on pollen–food syndrome to apple to ascertain whether administering birch pollen directly at the site of food allergy symptoms might enhance the treatment's efficacy against pollen–food allergy. No improvement in oral symptoms to apple ingestion was seen in nine patients whose scores for nasal reaction to birch pollen improved after sublingual immunotherapy.[46] The debate therefore continues on the therapeutic benefits of pollen immunotherapy in pollen–food syndrome.

Conclusions

The pollen–food syndrome is increasingly common and should always be considered in patients with pollinosis. The clinical manifestations range from mild symptoms, limited to the oropharynx, to more severe reactions resulting in anaphylaxis. The management of the food pollen-related symptoms depends on the type of offending allergen. When labile allergens are the triggers of the reaction the cooked food can be tolerated and exclusion of raw fruits and vegetables only is required. However, this is also questioned, as some cooked labile food allergens can retain their ability to activate pollen-specific T cells at the gastrointestinal tract, inducing exacerbations of chronic symptoms. In addition, when nsLTPs are involved, instructions to peel the fruit and vegetables as well as managing severe reactions should also be provided.

The role of immunotherapy is still controversial in spite of some promising results with subcutaneous immunotherapy in birch sensitive patients with reactions to apple or hazelnut. The use of component-resolved diagnostics (CRD) in characterizing the specific IgE profile of the patient has proved to be a promising approach that in the future might allow the treatment of this syndrome to be customized.

Acknowledgements

The authors would like to thank Dr Francesca Lazzarotto and Dr Francesca Barbon for their contribution to the case studies evaluation and Ms Catherine Crowley for editorial assistance.

References

1. Egger M, Mutschlechner S, Wopfner N, et al. Pollen–food syndromes associated with weed pollinosis: an update from the molecular point of view. Allergy 2006;61:461–76.
2. Ma S, Sicherer SH, Nowak-Wegrzyn A. A survey on the management of pollen–food allergy syndrome in allergy practices. J Allergy Clin Immunol 2003;112:784–8.
3. Wuthrich B, Stager J, Johansson SG. Celery allergy associated with birch and mugwort pollinosis. Allergy 1990;45:566–71.
4. Lüttkopf D, Ballmer-Weber BK, Wüthrich B, et al. Celery allergens in patients with positive double-blind placebo-controlled food challenge. J Allergy Clin Immunol 2000;106:390–9.
5. Enrique E, Cisteró-Bahíma A, Bartolomé B, et al. Platanus acerifolia and food allergy. Allergy 2002;57:357–6.
6. Liccardi G, Russo M, Mistrello G, et al. Sensitization to pistachio is common in Parietaria allergy. Allergy 1999; 54:643–6.
7. Florido Lopez JF, Quiralte Enriquez J, Arias de Saavedra Alías JM, et al. An allergen from Olea europaea pollen (Ole e 7) is associated with plant-derived food anaphylaxis. Allergy 2002;57(Suppl 71):53–9.
8. Ballmer-Weber BK, Scheurer S, Fritsche P, et al. Component-resolved diagnosis with recombinant allergens in patients with cherry allergy. J Allergy Clin Immunol 2002;110:167–73.
9. Mari A, Ballmer-Weber BK, Vieths S. The oral allergy syndrome: improved diagnostic and treatment methods. Curr Opin Allergy Clin Immunol 2005;5:267–73.
10. Asero R. Plant food allergies: A suggested approach to allergen-resolved diagnosis in the clinical practice by identifying easily available sensitization markers. Int Arch Allergy Immunol 2005;138:1–11.
11. Sampson HA, Muñoz-Furlong A, Campbell RL, et al. Second symposium on the definition and management of anaphylaxis: summary report – Second National Institute of Allergy and Infectious Disease/Food Allergy and Anaphylaxis Network symposium. J Allergy Clin Immunol 2006;117:391–7.
12. Ballmer-Weber BK, Wüthrich B, Wangorsch A, et al. Carrot allergy: double-blind placebo-controlled food challenge and identification of allergens. J Allergy Clin Immunol 2001;108:310–7.
13. Kleine-Tebbe J, Vogel L, Crowell DN, et al. Severe oral allergy syndrome and anaphylactic reactions caused by a Bet v 1-related PR-10 protein in soybean, SAM22. J Allergy Clin Immunol 2002;110:797–804.
14. Magnusson J, Lin XP, Dahlman-Höglund A, et al. Seasonal intestinal inflammation in patients with

birch pollen allergy. J Allergy Clin Immunol 2003;112: 45–50.

15. Breiteneder H, Ebner C. Molecular and biochemical classification of plant derived food allergens. J Allergy Clin Immunol 2000;106:27–36.

16. van Ree R. Clinical importance of cross-reactivity in food allergy. Curr Opin Allergy Clin Immunol 2004;4:235–40.

17. Sánchez-Monge R, Lombardero M, García-Sellés FJ, et al. Lipid-transfer proteins are relevant allergens in fruit allergy. J Allergy Clin Immunol 1999;103: 514–51.

18. Désormeaux A, Blochet JE, Pézolet M, et al. Amino acid sequence of a non-specific wheat phospholipid transfer protein and its conformation as revealed by infrared and Raman spectroscopy: role of disulfide bridges and phospholipids in the stabilization of the α-helix structure. Biochim Biophys Acta 1992;1121:137–52.

19. Van Ree R. Clinical importance of nonspecific lipid transfer proteins as food allergens. Biochem Soc Trans 2002;30:910–3.

20. Lleonart R, Cistero A, Carreira J, et al. Food Allergy: Identification of the major IgE-binding component of peach. Ann Allergy 1992;69:128–30.

21. Asero R, Mistrello G, Roncarolo D, et al. Immunological cross-reactivity between lipid transfer proteins from botanically unrelated plant-derived foods: a clinical study. Allergy 2002;57: 900–6.

22. Asero R, Mistrello G, Roncarolo D, et al. Relationship between peach lipid transfer protein IgE levels and hypersensitivity to non-Rosaceae vegetable foods in patients allergic to lipid transfer protein. Ann Allergy Asthma Immunol 2004;92:268–72.

23. Pastorello EA, Ortolani C, Farioli L, et al. Allergenic cross-reactivity among peach, apricot, plum, cherry in patients with oral allergy syndrome. An in vivo and in vitro study. J Allergy Clin Immunol 1994;94: 699–707.

24. Lombardero M, Garcia-Selles FJ, Polo F, et al. Prevalence of sensitization to Artemisia allergens Art v 1, Art v 3 and Art v 60 kDa. Cross-reactivity among Art v 3 and other relevant lipid-transfer protein allergens. Clin Exp Allergy 2004;34:1415–21.

25. Rohrer CL, Pichler WJ, Helbling A. Anaphylaxis: clinical aspects, etiology and course in 118 patients. Schweiz Med Wochenschr 1998;128:53–63.

26. Mittag D, Vieths S, Vogel L, et al. Soybean allergy in patients allergic to birch pollen: clinical investigation and molecular characterization of allergens. J Allergy Clin Immunol 2004;113: 148–54.

27. Van Ree R, Voitenko V, van Leeuwen WA, et al. Profilin is a cross-reactive allergen in pollen and vegetable foods. Int Arch Allergy Immunol 1992;98: 97–104.

28. Asero R, Monsalve R, Barber D. Profilin sensitization detected in the office by skin prick test: a study of prevalence and clinical relevance of profilin as a plant food allergen. Clin Exp Allergy 2008;38: 1033–7.

29. Foetisch K, Westphal S, Lauer I, et al. Biological activity of IgE specific for cross-reactive carbohydrate determinants. J Allergy Clin Immunol 2003;111: 889–96.

30. Bohle B, Vieths S. Improving diagnostic tests for food allergy with recombinant allergens. Methods 2004;32:292–9.

31. Vieths S, Jankiewicz A, Schoning B, et al. Apple allergy: the IgE-binding potency of apple strains is related to the occurrence of the 18-kDa allergen. Allergy 1994;49:262–71.

32. Hoffmann-Sommergruber K, Demoly P, Crameri R, et al. IgE reactivity to Api g 1, a major celery allergen, in a Central European population is based on primary sensitization by Bet v 1. J Allergy Clin Immunol 1999;104:478–84.

33. Vieths S, Scheurer S, Reindl J, et al. Optimized allergen extracts and recombinant allergens in diagnostic applications. Allergy 2001;56(Suppl 67): 78–82.

34. Luttkopf D, Muller U, Skov PS, et al. Comparison of four variants of a major allergen in hazelnut (Corylus avellana) Cor a 1.04 with the major hazel pollen allergen Cor a 1.01. Mol Immunol 2002;38: 515–25.

35. Ballmer-Weber BK, Wangorsch A, Bohle B, et al. Component-resolved in vitro diagnosis in carrot allergy: does the use of recombinant carrot allergens improve the reliability of the diagnostic procedure? Clin Exp Allergy 2005;35:970–8.

36. Bolhaar S, van Ree R, Ma Y, et al. Severe allergy to Sharon fruit caused by birch pollen. Int Arch Allergy Immunol 2005;136:45–52.

37. Erdmann SM, Sachs B, Schmidt A, et al. In vitro analysis of birch-pollen associated food allergy by use of recombinant allergens in the basophil activation test. Int Arch Allergy Immunol 2005;136:230–8.

38. Ma S, Sicherer S, Nowak-Wegrzyn A. A survey on the management of pollen–food allergy syndrome in allergy practices. J Allergy Clin Immunol 2003;112:784–8.

39. Rodriguez J, Crespo JF, Lopez-Rubio A. Clinical crossreactivity among foods of the Rosaceae family. J Allergy Clin Immunol 2000;106:183–9.

40. Bohle B. The impact of pollen-related food allergens on pollen allergy. Allergy 2007;62:3–10.

41. Bohle B, Zwolfer B, Heratizadeh A. Cooking birch pollen-related food: divergent consequences for IgE- and T cell-mediated reactivity in vitro and in vivo. J Allergy Clin Immunol 2006;118:242–9.

42. Asero R. Effects of birch pollen-specific immunotherapy on apple allergy in birch pollen-hypersensitive patients. Clin Exp Allergy 1998;28:1368–73.

43. Buchner X, Pichler WJ, Dahinden CA, et al. Effect of tree pollen specific, subcutaneous immunotherapy on the oral allergy syndrome to apple and hazelnut. Allergy 2004;59:1272–6.

44. Moller C. Effect of pollen immunotherapy on food hypersensitivity in children with birch pollinosis. Ann Allergy 1989;62:343–5.

45. Modrzynski M, Zawisza E. Possible induction of oral allergy syndrome during specific immunotherapy in patients sensitive to tree pollen. Med Sci Monit 2005;11:CR351–5.

46. Kinaciyan T, Jahn-Schmid B, Radakovics A, et al. Successful sublingual immunotherapy with birch pollen has limited effects on concomitant food allergy to apple and the immune response to the Bet v 1 homolog Mal d 1. J Allergy Clin Immunol 2007;119:937–43.

CHAPTER 8

The Respiratory Tract and Food Allergy

John M. James

Introduction

CLINICAL CASE

A 15-month-old boy presents to your clinic with a history of atopic dermatitis and allergy to cows' milk. Previous reactions following the ingestion of cows' milk have provoked exacerbations of eczema and urticaria. Following a recent accidental ingestion of cows' milk, when the infant was given a sibling's cup of cows' milk instead of soy milk, he experienced immediate generalized urticaria, emesis, coughing and significant wheezing requiring management in a local emergency department. Medical therapies included one dose of intramuscular epinephrine, oral antihistamines every 4 hours (i.e. three doses), nebulized albuterol and two doses of systemic corticosteroids 12 hours apart. The infant was observed in the hospital for 24 hours and then discharged home in good condition.

This clinical case provides a good introduction to respiratory manifestations of food allergy. Skin and gastrointestinal tract symptoms are commonly observed with allergic reactions to foods, but respiratory tract symptoms may also be involved, as illustrated above.[1-3] Specific respiratory symptoms that can be observed include nasal congestion, rhinorrhea, sneezing, pruritus of the nose and throat, coughing, wheezing and asthma. Anaphylactic reactions can also occur. Exposure is typically through ingestion, but in some cases inhalation of food allergens may also precipitate these reactions.[4] In fact, an increasing number of medical publications have highlighted allergic reactions to food allergens that have occurred following inhalation. Food allergy in early childhood does appear to be a good marker for later respiratory allergy, including asthma. In addition, studies have demonstrated that food-induced allergic reactions can provoke recurrent asthmatic responses, as well as persistent asthma. Food allergy can also increase asthma morbidity in adults and children,[5] therefore, evaluation for food allergy should be considered in patients with difficult to control or otherwise unexplained acute severe asthma exacerbations and in patients with asthma and other manifestations of food allergy (e.g. anaphylaxis, moderate to severe atopic dermatitis). As highlighted in the clinical case above, anaphylactic reactions to foods in children almost always include respiratory tract symptoms, and these often determine the severity and outcome of the reaction. This highlights the importance of documenting respiratory tract symptoms as part of a food allergic reaction (Clinical Pearl 1)

CLINICAL PEARL #1

FOOD ALLERGY/RESPIRATORY TRACT/ANAPHYLAXIS

General Caveats

- Exposure through ingestion of food allergen(s) provokes most reactions
- Inhalation of food allergen(s) can lead to respiratory symptoms
- Consider food allergy evaluation in patients with chronic asthma and unexplained, acute asthma exacerbations
- Anaphylaxis almost always involves the respiratory tract
- Respiratory manifestations of food-induced anaphylaxis often determine severity and outcome of reaction

Epidemiology

Overview

Adverse reactions to foods can commonly provoke clinical signs and symptoms involving the skin, the gastrointestinal tract, the respiratory tract, and in some cases the cardiovascular system. These reactions consist of any abnormal clinical responses following the ingestion of a food or food additive, and can be further divided into two major categories.[1] The vast majority can be categorized as adverse physiologic reactions or food intolerances, which are not mediated by specific immunologic mechanisms (e.g. an exaggerated physiological reaction following the ingestion of lactose in cows' milk causing abdominal distension, gas and diarrhea). In contrast, food allergy is an immunologic-mediated food reaction unrelated to any physiologic effect of the food or additive. The two broad groups of immune reactions are IgE mediated and non-IgE mediated. The IgE-mediated reactions are usually divided into immediate-onset and immediate plus late-phase reactions, which involve an immediate onset of symptoms followed by prolonged or ongoing symptoms. Typical examples of immediate-onset IgE-mediated reactions include allergic reactions following the ingestion of peanuts, tree nuts, shellfish or sesame seeds resulting in laryngeal edema, coughing and/or wheezing. Non-IgE-mediated reactions are typically delayed in onset (i.e. 4–48 hours) and most frequently involve the gastrointestinal tract (e.g. celiac disease or gluten-sensitive enteropathy). It is imperative to understand the specific terminology and basic classification of adverse food reactions to properly interpret the scientific studies implicating food allergy in respiratory tract symptoms and anaphylaxis.

Prevalence

Over the past 20 years there has been an increase in the prevalence of food allergy and its clinical expression.[1,6] The exact prevalence of respiratory tract symptoms induced by food allergy, however, has been difficult to establish. For many years there has been a public perception that food allergy-induced asthma is common, but this has not been substantiated when careful objective investigations, including food challenges, have been undertaken to confirm patient histories.[7,8] When the specific focus has been on the role of food allergy and respiratory tract manifestations, the incidence has been estimated to be between 2% and 8% in children and adults with asthma.[5,9,10] Using a cross-sectional epidemiologic study design in 1141 randomly selected young adults ranging in age from 20 to 45 years, Australian investigators evaluated the prevalence of IgE-mediated food allergy and the relationships with other atopic disease.[11] Those with probable IgE-mediated peanut allergy were more likely to have current asthma, wheeze and a history of eczema, and those with probable IgE-mediated shrimp allergy were also more likely to have current asthma and nasal allergies. No relationships were observed between those subjects with probable IgE-mediated cows' milk, wheat and egg allergy and allergic diseases because of small numbers of subjects with these food allergies. They concluded that further research, with larger numbers of subjects demonstrating IgE-mediated food allergy, would be required to confirm these results.

To examine the strength of the association and temporal relationships between food allergy and asthma, investigators followed 271 children over 6 years of age and 296 children less than 6 years from a family-based food allergy cohort in Chicago.[12] Food allergy status was determined based on the type and timing of clinical symptoms after ingestion of a specific food and results of specific IgE to foods using skin prick testing and allergen-specific IgE. Symptomatic food allergy was associated with asthma in both older (odds ratio (OR) = 4.9, 95% confidence interval (CI): 2.5–9.5) and younger children (OR = 5.3, 95% CI: 1.7–16.2). The association was stronger among children with multiple or severe food allergies, especially in older children. Children with food allergy developed asthma earlier and at a higher prevalence than children without food allergy. No associations were seen between asymptomatic food sensitization and asthma. Independent of markers of atopy (e.g. aeroallergen sensitization and family history of asthma), there was a significant association between food allergy and asthma.

To determine the prevalence, clinical features, specific allergens and risk factors of food allergy, a population study including 33 110 persons completing a questionnaire was conducted in France.[13] The overall prevalence of food allergy was estimated to be 3.24%, with rhinitis and asthma documented in 6.5% and 5.7% of respiratory reactions, respectively. In addition, the clinical expression of food allergy was dependent on the existence of sensitization to pollens and was typically expressed in the form of rhinitis, asthma and angioedema. Another survey found that 17% of 669 adult respondents in Australia reported food-induced respiratory symptoms.[14] Whereas the patients with asthma did not report food-related illness more frequently than those without asthma, those reporting respiratory symptoms following food ingestion were more likely to be atopic.

CLINICAL CASE

A family presents to your clinic with a 10-month-old girl who has a clinical history and course very compatible with allergy to egg protein. Following the ingestion of scrambled eggs on two prior occasions, the infant has had emesis and urticaria without anaphylactic manifestations. The infant is otherwise healthy and does not have atopic dermatitis or other atopic conditions. Both parents have a history of allergic rhinitis. The parents specifically ask about the likelihood of their infant developing allergic respiratory diseases such as asthma and allergic rhinitis later in childhood. This clinical case illustrates a very important point that children with a family history of atopy and sensitization to food proteins in early infancy may have a higher risk of developing subsequent respiratory allergic disease.[15] Investigators from the Isle of Wight reported that egg allergy in infancy predicts respiratory allergic disease by 4 years of age.[16] In a cohort of 1218 consecutive births followed until 4 years of age, 29 (2.4%) developed egg allergy by 4 years of age. Increased respiratory allergy (e.g. rhinitis, asthma) was associated with egg allergy (OR: 5.0, 95% CI: 1.1–22.3; p < 0.05) with a positive predictive value of 55%. Furthermore, the addition of the diagnosis of eczema to egg allergy increased the positive predictive value to 80%. Rhodes et al.[17] conducted a prospective cohort study of subjects at risk of asthma and atopy in England. Of 100 babies of atopic parents who were recruited at birth, 73 were followed up at 5 years, 67 at 11 and 63 at 22 years of age. Skin sensitivity to hen's egg, cows' milk or both in the first 5 years of life was predictive of asthma (OR: 10.7; 95% CI: 2.1–55.1; p = 0.001, sensitivity 57%; specificity 89%).

One specific focus area of the National Cooperative Inner City Asthma Study examined the degree of food allergen sensitization to six common foods (egg, milk, soy, peanut, wheat and fish) in 504 inner-city patients 4–9 years of age (median 6 years) with asthma.[18] Children sensitized to foods had higher rates of asthma hospitalization (p <0.01) and required more steroid medications (p = 0.25). In addition, sensitization to foods was correlated with sensitization to more indoor and outdoor aeroallergens (p < 0.001). The association of increased asthma morbidity with at least one food sensitization and findings that patients with sensitization to multiple foods had significantly more asthma morbidity than those with single-food sensitization suggests that food allergen sensitivity may be a marker for increased asthma severity.

An investigation by Sicherer and colleagues[19] summarized data from a voluntary registry of 5149 individuals (median age 5 years) with peanut and/or tree nut allergy. The primary objective was to characterize clinical features including respiratory reactions in the registrants. Respiratory reactions, including wheezing, throat tightness and nasal congestion, were reported in 42% and 56% of respondents as part of their initial reactions to peanuts and tree nuts, respectively. One half of the reactions involved more than one system and more than 75% required some form of medical treatment. Interestingly, registrants with asthma were significantly more likely than those without asthma to have severe reactions (33% versus 21%; p < 0.0001). Moreover, another investigation by the same group estimated the prevalence of seafood allergy in the United States using a nationwide, cross-sectional random telephone survey and standardized questionnaire. A total of 5529 households completed the survey, representing a census of 14 948 individuals. Fish or shellfish allergy was reported in 5.9% of households. Recurrent reactions were common. Shortness of breath and throat tightness was reported by more than 50% of those surveyed and 16% were treated with epinephrine[20] (Clinical Pearl 2).

CLINICAL PEARL #2

ROLE OF FOOD ALLERGY IN RESPIRATORY MANIFESTATIONS
Epidemiology
- Incidence estimated at approximately 2–8% of patients with asthma
- Pollen sensitization may be an associated risk factor
- Family history of atopy and sensitization to food allergens in early infancy increase the risk of future allergic respiratory disease (e.g. asthma, allergic rhinitis)
- Allergic sensitization to some foods may be a marker for increased asthma severity

Pathogenesis

Mechanisms

Our understanding of how food allergy causes a significant disruption of normal oral tolerance continues to evolve. Recently, it has become evident that the gut, which is the classic site of sensitization to foods, is only responsible for primary sensitization in a subset of patients. These patients are generally younger and exhibit their first symptoms shortly after initial exposures to the relevant food. In contrast, a newly recognized route of sensitization for food-allergic patients is by initial exposure to allergens through inhalation, mostly pollens, with secondary clinical reactions following ingestion of specific cross-reactive foods. In these patients, many years may elapse before the first respiratory symptoms appear. Investigations from Europe suggest that lipid transfer proteins (LTP) may induce significant allergic sensitization through the respiratory tract due to inhalation, and this may precede the onset of relevant food allergy.[21,22] For example, inhalation of LTP from specific fruits (e.g. peaches and apples) may lead to allergic sensitization and ultimately allergic reactions following the oral ingestion of these foods.

Allergens

Specific foods are more often implicated in food allergic reactions involving respiratory symptoms and have subsequently been confirmed in well-controlled, blinded food challenges.[7,23,24] These foods include chicken egg, cows' milk, peanut, fish, shellfish and tree nuts (Clinical Pearl 3). For example, one group of young children who were allergic to cows' milk was followed from 1 year of age until 5 years.[25] These patients did develop early respiratory symptoms, including nasal symptoms and cough, without skin or gastrointestinal symptoms, and 69% did ultimately develop allergic sensitivities to common indoor aeroallergens. In addition, anaphylactic reactions to foods, including significant respiratory symptoms, and rarely fatal anaphylactic reactions have been reported.[26–29] Some food allergens seem to be more prone to present with respiratory tract symptoms, such as peanuts and tree nuts,[19] fish and shellfish[20] or sesame.[30] Finally, there have been many food allergens implicated as the cause of respiratory tract allergy symptoms following inhalation as opposed

> **CLINICAL PEARL #3**
>
> ### COMMON FOOD ALLERGENS HAVE BEEN IMPLICATED IN RESPIRATORY DISEASE
>
> - Chicken egg, cows' milk, peanut, fish, shellfish and tree nuts have been the main foods responsible for food allergen-induced respiratory reactions
> - Peanuts, tree nuts, sesame seed and shellfish have most often been responsible for near-fatal and fatal anaphylactic reactions following food ingestion

to ingestion.[4] Common examples include fish, shellfish and eggs.[31]

Baker's asthma is among one of the most common occupational diseases and results from inhalation of relevant wheat allergens. Thus far, however, little is known about those allergens. Only a few of the suspected causative wheat allergens have been characterized on the molecular level. The aim of a recent investigation in Germany was to identify and characterize unknown wheat allergens related to baker's asthma to improve the reliability of diagnostic procedures.[32] Of the asthmatic bakers studied, 33% showed sensitization to native total gliadin. Gliadins represent a newly discovered family of inhaled allergens in baker's asthma and these water-insoluble proteins might represent causative allergens. The presence of asthma induced by inhaled flour is not strictly related to occupational exposure and may also occur in subjects not displaying asthma among symptoms induced by wheat ingestion.[33]

A high percentage of patients with asthma perceive that food additives contribute to worsening of their respiratory symptoms.[34] Several different food additives, including monosodium glutamate, sulfites and aspartame, have been implicated in adverse respiratory reactions,[35] but well-controlled investigations in this area have reported a prevalence rate of < 5%.[9,23] Food additives as a trigger for asthma have been a controversial area, with few data to support a cause and effect,[36] and studies have shown the prevalence to be much less than 1% of the total population. There are more than 2500 food additives, but only a few are known to be triggers of asthma. Sulfites and monosodium glutamate (MSG) are the most often implicated and the most studied. Sulfites are used as a preservative and found in many foods, including dried fruits, wine, sauerkraut, white grape juice, dried potatoes and fresh shrimp. Overall, the prevalence of sulfite-induced asthma responses appears to be < 3.9%.

Monosodium glutamate (MSG) is the flavor enhancer that has been held responsible for the 'Chinese restaurant syndrome', which is clinically manifested by headache, numbness, chest discomfort, weakness, flushing and abdominal discomfort after eating Chinese food. Focusing on conflicting evidence that some people with asthma are more likely to have adverse effects from monosodium glutamate than the general population, Woods and co-workers[37] were unable to demonstrate MSG-induced immediate or late asthmatic reactions in 12 adult asthmatics reporting food additive-induced symptoms. In addition, no significant changes in bronchial hyperresponsiveness or soluble inflammatory markers (e.g. eosinophil cationic protein, tryptase) were observed during these challenges. In an investigation utilizing double-blind placebo-controlled oral MSG challenges in subjects who had histories of adverse reactions to MSG,[38] no specific upper or lower respiratory complaints were observed, but 22 (36.1%) of the 61 subjects had confirmed adverse reactions to MSG including headache, muscle tightness, numbness, general weakness and flushing.

Route of exposure and subsequent respiratory symptoms

Oral ingestion of food allergens

Oral ingestion is the primary route of exposure to foods that can cause or exacerbate respiratory symptoms (e.g. cough, laryngeal edema and asthma). The vast majority of published reports, highlighted in this chapter, focus on respiratory tract symptoms following the ingestion of food allergens.

Inhalation of food allergens

CLINICAL CASE

A 33-year-old man was evaluated at his family physician's office for a recent adverse food reaction. He was at a shopping mall and stopped to have lunch in a designated food court area. There were several different types of food being served, including pizza, Chinese food, fried shrimp and sushi, and there was a strong aroma of all of these foods in the court. He had a past history of anaphylactic reactions following the ingestion of shrimp. While he was eating a salad without any seafood, he noticed itching in his mouth and throat, a swelling sensation in his throat and repetitive coughing. If this patient did not ingest any shrimp, could this still represent an allergic reaction to shrimp?

This clinical case is an example of how some food-allergic individuals may react when exposed to airborne allergens in a restaurant when fish or shellfish are cooked in a confined area.[31,39] Seafood allergens aerosolized during food preparation are a source of potential respiratory and contact allergens.[40] A number of reports highlight allergic reactions associated with airborne fish particles,[41,42] including one using air sampling and an immunochemical analytic technique to detect fish allergen in the air of an open-air fish market.[43] Avoidance of a food allergen should include the prevention of exposure to aerosolized particles in relevant environments. Finally, an internet-based survey of 51 anaphylactic reactions to foods showed that whereas most reactions (40–78%) occurred after ingestion, eight (16%) reactions occurred following exclusive skin contact and three (6%) after inhalation.[44]

Children with IgE-mediated food allergy can develop asthma following inhalational exposure to aerosolized food allergens during the cooking process.[45] Twelve food-allergic children developed asthma following the inhalation of relevant food allergens. Foods implicated included fish, chickpea, milk, egg and buckwheat. Five of nine bronchial challenges were positive with objective clinical features of asthma, and two children developed late-phase symptoms with a decrease in lung function. Positive reactions were seen with fish, chickpea and buckwheat; there were no reactions to the seven placebo challenges. These data demonstrate that inhaled food allergens can produce both early- and late-phase asthmatic responses. Finally, Sicherer and colleagues[46] have reported that patients with allergy to peanuts and tree nuts might experience adverse respiratory reactions when they are exposed on airline flights serving peanut and tree nut snacks. Such exposures can include accidental ingestion, inhalation or skin contact during the flight. Of the allergic reactions reported, some were severe, requiring medications including epinephrine.

Differential diagnosis of food-induced respiratory syndromes (Table 8.1)

Many questions remain when evaluating respiratory manifestations that may be a clinical manifestation of food allergy. Unlike cutaneous symptoms (e.g. urticaria, angioedema), respiratory manifestations may be immediate, delayed or chronic, mostly

Table 8.1 Differential Diagnosis of Food-Induced Respiratory Syndromes

1. Eczema within the first 2 years of life and risk of developing asthma and allergic rhinitis
2. Food allergy in infancy and risk for wheezing and hyperactive airways in childhood
3. Acute asthma induced by food allergy
4. Respiratory symptoms contributing to the severity of acute allergic reactions to foods
5. Patients with recurrent or chronic asthma
6. Food allergy and predisposition to bronchial hyperreactivity (BHR)
7. Recurrent or chronic rhinitis induced by food allergy
8. Recurrent or chronic otitis media induced by food allergy
9. Dyspnea associated with anemia in infants

due to the pattern of inflammatory manifestations of the respiratory tract. This section will review potential manifestations of food allergy in the respiratory tract.

Recurrent or chronic rhinitis induced by food allergy

In a large group of children undergoing double-blind placebo-controlled food challenges[47] acute rhinitis accounted for 70% of the overall respiratory symptoms observed. These symptoms typically occur in association with other clinical manifestations (e.g. cutaneous and/or gastrointestinal symptoms) during allergic reactions to foods; they rarely occur in isolation.[23,47] Chronic or recurrent rhinitis, mostly in preschool children, is sometimes associated with allergic reactions, mostly to milk. Although some patients claim of a significant decrease in symptoms after starting an avoidance diet, a clear association has not been reproduced by double-blind studies.

Recurrent or chronic otitis media induced by food allergy

Serous otitis media has multiple etiologies, viral upper respiratory tract infections being the most common. Allergic inflammation in the nasal mucosa may cause eustachian tube dysfunction and contribute to subsequent otitis media with effusion. Studies investigating a food-allergic mechanism in recurrent serous otitis media are inconclusive.[48,49]

Dyspnea associated with anemia in infants

In 1960, Heiner[50] reported a syndrome in infants consisting of recurrent episodes of pneumonia associated with pulmonary infiltrates, hemosiderosis, gastrointestinal blood loss, iron-deficiency anemia and failure to thrive. This syndrome is most often associated with a non-IgE-mediated hypersensitivity to cows' milk proteins. Although increased peripheral blood eosinophils and multiple serum precipitins to cows' milk are commonly observed, the specific immunologic mechanisms responsible for this disorder are not known.[51] The diagnosis is suggested by infiltrates on chest X-ray, anemia, hemosiderosis evidenced by bronchoalveolar lavage and the presence of the precipitating antibodies to milk (in most cases). This food-induced syndrome is only very rarely observed even in referral clinics for childhood food allergy.

Eczema within the first 2 years of life and risk of developing asthma and allergic rhinitis

The presence of persistent eczema in infancy has been identified as an important risk factor for the development of allergic rhinitis and asthma. In one study,[52] children with atopic eczema had a significantly greater risk of asthma (OR = 3.52, 95% CI = 1.88–6.59 and allergic rhinitis OR = 2.91, 95%CI = 1.48–5.71). This risk was not observed in the control patients.

Although a family history of atopy, including the presence of atopic dermatitis and food allergy, appears to contribute to the development of asthma, it is unclear when the airways become involved with the atopic process and whether airway function relates to the atopic characteristics of the infant. In one study of 114 infants (median age 10.7 months; range 2.6–19.1), atopic status was determined by the presence of specific IgE to foods or aeroallergens and total IgE levels.[53] Exhaled nitric oxide (eNO), forced expiratory flow at 75% exhaled volume (FEF75) and airway reactivity to inhaled methacholine were measured in these infants. Compared to non-atopic controls, infants sensitized to egg or milk had lower flow rates (FEF75: 336 vs 285 mL/s, p < 0.003) and lower lnPC(30) (mg/mL) provocative concentrations to decrease FEF(75) by 30% (−0.6 vs −1.2, p < 0.02) but no difference in eNO levels. This suggests that atopic characteristics of the infant might be important determinants for the development of asthma.

Food allergy in infancy and risk for wheezing and hyperactive airways in childhood

Children allergic to common food allergens in infancy may be at increased risk of wheezing and bronchial hyperreactivity later in childhood. A case–control study was conducted with 69 children aged 7.2–13.3 years with allergy to egg (n = 60) and/or fish (n = 29) in the first 3 years of life.[54] A control group consisted of 154 children (70 sensitized to inhaled allergens) with no history of food allergy in the first 3 years of life. Asthma symptoms were reported more frequently in the study group than in controls. Children in the study group showed a significantly increased frequency of positive responses to methacholine challenge than the control group. Multivariate logistic regression analysis showed that bronchial hyperresponsiveness, as well as reported current asthma symptoms, was associated with early wheezing and early sensitization to inhaled allergens but not with atopic dermatitis in infancy or persistence of egg or fish allergy. Therefore, children allergic to egg or fish in infancy may be at increased risk for wheezing illness and hyperactive airways in the school years.

Acute asthma induced by food allergy

CLINICAL CASE

A very frustrated young couple decides to seek the opinion of an allergy specialist regarding their 3-year old daughter. She has a long-standing history of eczema and has recently been diagnosed with asthma. Her parents believe that some of her acute exacerbations of asthma may have been provoked by the accidental ingestion of cows' milk protein. Their primary care physician informed them that this is not very likely because asthma exacerbations in this age group are typically caused by viral upper respiratory infections. They are seeking an expert opinion about the role of food allergy in acute asthma.

The wide use of standardized food challenges has provided a better view of the type and frequency of respiratory reactions in food allergy. Hill and colleagues[55] challenged 100 milk-allergic patients with a mean age of 16.2 months and elicited cough and/or wheeze in 20, rhinitis in 12 and stridor in two. Cough and wheezing were more frequent in the

patients who initially presented with chronic eczema and recurrent bronchitis, and with urticaria and eczema. Lower respiratory symptoms were only observed in two of 53 patients (4%). In another study of 410 children with a history of asthma, 279 (68%) had a history of food-induced asthma.[56] There were positive food challenges in 168 (60%) of the 279 patients. This investigation documented that 67 (24%) of the 279 children with a history of food-induced asthma had a positive blinded food challenge that included wheezing. The most common foods responsible for these reactions included peanut (19), cows' milk (18), egg (13) and tree nuts (10). Interestingly, only five (2%) of these patients had wheezing as their only objective adverse symptom. In addition, 10 of the group of 188 children without a history of asthma had wheezing elicited by the food challenge, showing a tendency for a bronchial response in the absence of a concomitant asthma.

A total of 320 subjects presenting primarily with atopic dermatitis undergoing blinded food challenges were monitored for respiratory reactions.[47] The subjects, aged between 6 months and 30 years, were highly atopic and had multiple allergic sensitivities to foods, and over half had a prior diagnosis of asthma. In the 205 (64%) patients with food allergy confirmed by blinded challenges, almost two-thirds experienced respiratory reactions during their positive food challenges (e.g. nasal 70%, laryngeal 48%, pulmonary 27%). Overall, 34 (17%) of 205 subjects with positive food challenges developed wheezing as part of their reaction. Furthermore, 88 of these patients were monitored with pulmonary function testing during positive and negative food challenges. Thirteen (15%) developed lower respiratory symptoms, including wheezing in 10, but only six had a > 20% decrease in FEV_1. Wheezing as the sole manifestation of a food-induced respiratory reaction was rare.

In a series of 163 children in which 385 DBPCFC were performed,[57] 250 challenges (65%) were positive to peanuts (31%), hens' egg (23%) and cows' milk (9%). Cutaneous symptoms were observed in most positive challenges (59%), but respiratory reactions were also frequent (24%). Among the respiratory reactions, oral symptoms (5%), rhinitis and conjunctivitis (6%) and asthma (10%) were observed. Again, isolated asthma was rare, i.e. 2.8% of the challenges. Furthermore, investigations from Italy suggest that asthma and/or rhinitis as part of the initial presentation of allergy to cows' milk may be an independent predictor of persistence of this food allergy and a failure to develop oral tolerance.[58]

Food allergy and predisposition to bronchial hyperreactivity (BHR)

Observations have been made that asthma symptoms have improved in patients with atopic dermatitis and food allergy who are following a food avoidance diet, despite the absence of respiratory symptoms during specific food challenges. This prompted a series of investigations on bronchial hyperreactivity (BHR) in food-allergic patients without acute respiratory symptoms following food ingestion. In one investigation, 26 children with asthma and food allergy were evaluated using methacholine inhalation challenges for changes in their BHR before and after blinded food challenges.[59] Of the 22 positive blinded food challenges, 12 (55%) involved chest symptoms (cough, laryngeal reactions and/or wheezing). Another 10 (45%) positive food challenges included laryngeal, gastrointestinal and/or skin symptoms without any chest symptoms. Significant increases in BHR were documented several hours after positive food challenges in seven of the 12 (58%) patients who experienced chest symptoms during these challenges. During the actual food challenges decreases in FEV_1 were not observed in these seven patients, suggesting that significant changes in BHR can occur without significant pulmonary function changes in a preceding food challenge. These data confirmed that food-induced allergic reactions may increase airway reactivity in a subset of patients with moderate to severe asthma, and may do so without inducing acute asthma symptoms.

A more recent investigation hypothesized that children allergic to common food allergens in infancy are at increased risk of wheezing illness and bronchial hyperresponsiveness during the school years.[60] A case–control study of 69 children aged 7.2 to 13.3 years allergic to egg (n = 60) and/or fish (n = 29) in early life (first 3 years) was conducted. The children received follow-up for 1 year and were evaluated by parental questionnaire, skin prick testing, spirometry and metacholine bronchial challenge. A control group consisted of 154 children (70 sensitized to inhaled allergens) from a general population sample with no history of food allergy during their first 3 years. Food-allergic patients showed a significantly increased frequency of positive response to metacholine bronchial challenge compared to the control group as a whole. Children allergic to egg or fish in infancy are at increased risk for wheezing illness and hyperactive airways at school age; asthma and bronchial hyperresponsiveness seem to be mostly determined by wheezing and sensitization to inhaled allergens in early life, regardless of atopic dermatitis in infancy or retention of food allergy.

In contrast, another study of 11 adult asthmatics with a history of food-induced wheezing and positive skin tests to the suspected food concluded that food allergy is an unlikely cause of increased BHR.[61] An equal number of patients had increased BHR, as determined by methacholine inhalation challenges, 24 hours after blinded food challenges to either food allergen or placebo. However, the small number of patients evaluated and the lack of environmental controls prior to the repeat methacholine challenges limit their conclusions.

Two more recent studies indicate that patients with food allergy in the absence of asthma might develop increased BHR. In 35 non-asthmatic patients with food allergy, 10 of 19 (53%) were found to have BHR by methacholine inhalation challenges.[62] Similarly, Kivity et al.[63] investigated patients with food allergy with or without asthma and/or allergic rhinitis by spirometry, methacholine challenges and sputum-induced cell analysis. BHR by methacholine challenge was observed in all patients with asthma, and in 40% of patients with food allergy alone. They also found mainly eosinophils in the sputum of patients with asthma, and neutrophils in the patients with food allergy but no asthma. This observation has been confirmed by other investigators, who also observed an increased proportion of neutrophils and increased levels of IL-8 in non-asthmatic food-allergic patients.[64]

An animal study came to a similar conclusion, as mice sensitized by intraperitoneal injection of ovalbumin in the presence of alum and orally challenged to ovalbumin had significant airway inflammation for up to 12 days following a single intranasal challenge to ovalbumin.[65] Interestingly, an unrelated antigen, house dust mite, did induce a similar inflammatory response. Taken together, these observations suggest that food sensitization with non-respiratory manifestations of food allergy may also enhance inflammation in other mucosal tissues. Hence, non-asthmatic patients diagnosed with food allergy should be carefully evaluated for bronchial inflammation in order not to delay appropriate anti-inflammatory treatment if necessary.

Respiratory symptoms contributing to the severity of acute allergic reactions to foods

CLINICAL CASE

A 17-year-old male college student experienced a severe anaphylactic reaction while eating in the cafeteria in his dormitory. He had a past history of peanut allergy, as well as moderate persistent asthma requiring combination therapy with an inhaled corticosteroid and a long-acting bronchodilator. He ingested chili which contained peanut butter as a flavoring agent and developed immediate, generalized urticaria, emesis, and an exacerbation of his asthma with significant respiratory distress. He was transported to a local emergency room for medical management, including two doses of intramuscular epinephrine, and was ultimately admitted for a 2-day hospital stay.

This case example makes the point that although the specific cause of anaphylaxis is frequently undetermined, food allergens can be responsible for these severe reactions in a significant number of cases.[29,66] Until two decades ago, fatal food-induced anaphylaxis had mainly consisted of anecdotal reports of isolated cases. In 1988, Yuninger et al.[27] reported a series of seven cases identified over a 16-month period. Five patients reacted to tree nuts or peanuts. Four years later, Sampson et al.[26] reported 13 fatal and near-fatal anaphylactic reactions in children and adolescents. Again, most patients reacted to tree nuts or peanuts, and all had a history of asthma. Moreover, respiratory symptoms were prominent in all patients, and most probably contributed to the outcome of the reaction. More recently, Bock et al.[67] analyzed the circumstances of 32 deaths after food-induced anaphylaxis reported to a national registry. Allergies to peanuts and tree nuts were responsible for most. In addition, all but one patient with adequate information were known to have asthma. These reports highlight an increased risk for severe food-induced anaphylaxis in patients with asthma, in particular those requiring maintenance medications. Follow-up visits in these patients should emphasize the importance of good asthma control, and should assure the availability and proper instruction of the use of self-injectable epinephrine.

To determine whether self-reported food allergy is significantly associated with potentially fatal childhood asthma, medical records from 72 patients admitted to a pediatric intensive care unit (PICU) for asthmatic exacerbation were reviewed and compared in a case–control study.[68] Two control groups included randomly selected groups of 108 patients admitted to a regular nursing floor for asthma and 108 ambulatory patients with asthma. Factors evaluated included self-reported food allergy, gender, age, residence in a poor area, race/ethnicity, inhaled steroid exposure, tobacco exposure, length of hospital stay, psychological comorbidity and season of admission. At least one food allergy was documented for 13% (38/288) of the patients. Egg, peanut, fish/shellfish, milk and tree nut accounted for 78.6% of all food allergies. Children admitted to the PICU were significantly more likely to report food allergy (p = 0.004) and 3.3 times more likely to report at least one food allergy than children admitted to a regular nursing floor. Furthermore, the study subjects were significantly more likely to report food allergy (p < 0.001) and 7.4 times more likely to report at least one food allergy than children seen in the ambulatory setting. Self-reported food allergy is an independent risk factor for potentially fatal childhood asthma. Asthmatic children or adolescents with food allergy are a target population for more aggressive asthma management. Finally, a 5-year retrospective review from Australia summarized reports of children presenting with anaphylaxis to a local emergency department.[69] There were 123 cases of anaphylaxis in 117 patients; one fatality was reported. Foods were by far the most common trigger (86%), with peanuts and tree nuts leading the list. Respiratory symptoms were the principal presenting symptom (97%).

Patients with recurrent or chronic asthma: routine testing for food allergy

Foods are often suspected in the quest for allergic triggers of recurrent or chronic asthma. A clear link between ingestion of a specific food and worsening of asthma is only rarely reported. In one investigation,[9] 300 consecutive patients with asthma (age range 7 months to 80 years) were evaluated in a pulmonary clinic; 25 (12%) had a history of food allergy suggested by clinical symptoms, and/or positive tests of food-specific IgE antibodies. Food-induced wheezing was documented in six (2%) of the cases; all were children aged 4–17 years. In another investigation, 140 children, aged 2–9 years, with asthma were screened by clinical history and testing for food-specific IgE antibodies.[70] Of these children, 32 were able to undergo blinded food challenges; 13 (9.2%) had food-induced respiratory symptoms and eight (5.7%) had specific asthmatic reactions documented during food challenges. Only one patient had asthma as the sole symptom during a positive food challenge. Interestingly, the patients with food allergy and asthma were generally younger and had a past medical history of atopic dermatitis.

In a similar investigation, Oehling and co-workers[71] reported that food-induced bronchospasm was present in 8.5% of 284 asthmatic children evaluated. The majority of the allergic sensitization occurred in the first year of life and was caused by a single food, especially egg. In addition, Businco and colleagues[72] evaluated 42 children (age range 10–76 months) with atopic dermatitis and milk allergy. Eleven (27%) of these patients developed asthmatic symptoms during a positive food challenge. Finally, an investigation from Turkey confirmed that food allergy can elicit asthma in children less than 6 years of age; the incidence was 4%. The most common food allergens implicated were egg and cows' milk.[73]

In order to evaluate food allergy as a risk factor for severe asthma, Roberts and colleagues[74] investigated 19 children with exacerbations of asthma needing ICU ventilation. Compared to controls, these patients had an increased risk of food allergy (OR 8.58; 95% CI 1.85–39.71), multiple allergic diagnoses (OR 4.42; CI 1.17–16.71) and frequent asthma admissions (OR 14.2; CI 1.77–113.59). The authors concluded that food allergy and frequent asthma admissions appear to be significant independent risk factors for life-threatening asthmatic events. As noted earlier, the association of increased asthma morbidity with at least one food sensitization and the increasing morbidity with sensitization to increasing numbers of foods indicates that food allergen sensitivity may be a marker for increased asthma severity[18] (Clinical Pearl 4).

Diagnosis/management

Medical history

The importance of a comprehensive medical history in patients suspected of having food allergy or anaphylaxis will be reviewed in detail in Chapters 4 and 12. This history should include questions about the timing of the reaction in relation to food ingestion,

---

CLINICAL PEARL #4

KEY POINTS RELATED TO FOOD ALLERGY AND THE RESPIRATORY TRACT

- Food-induced respiratory tract symptoms are typically accompanied by either cutaneous or gastrointestinal symptoms; they rarely occur as isolated symptoms
- Allergic sensitization or clinical reactions to foods in infancy predict the later development of respiratory allergies and asthma
- Food-induced asthma is more common in young pediatric patients than in older children and adults
- Children with atopic dermatitis, especially those with food allergy confirmed during blinded food challenges, are at increased risk for food-induced asthma
- Food-induced allergic reactions may increase airway reactivity in some patients with moderate to severe asthma and may do so without inducing acute asthma symptoms
- Asthmatic reactions induced by food allergy are considered risk factors for fatal and near-fatal anaphylactic reactions

---

the minimum quantity of food required to cause symptoms, specific upper and lower respiratory signs and symptoms, the reproducibility of the symptoms, and a current or past clinical history of allergy to specific food allergens (e.g. egg).[1,31,75] A family history of allergy and/or asthma can be a useful historical point. When there is a history of an unexplained sudden asthma exacerbation, details about preceding food ingestion should be elicited. A history of a severe or anaphylactic reaction following the ingestion of a food may be sufficient to indicate a causal relationship. Finally, the specific treatment received and its response should be documented.

Physical examination

In evaluating patients with respiratory complaints that may be induced by food allergy, the physical examination can be useful. Findings here are helpful in assessing overall nutritional status, growth parameters and any signs of allergic disease, especially atopic dermatitis. Moreover, this examination will help rule out other conditions that may mimic food allergy.

Testing for food allergy

When used in conjunction with standard criterion of interpretation, skin testing (e.g. percutaneous) can give reliable clinical information in a short period of time (i.e. 15–20 minutes), and should provide useful information in the overall evaluation of a patient with suspected food allergy-induced respiratory tract reactions. This specific issue, as well as other diagnostic testing for food allergy, is very thoroughly addressed in Chapter 13. The routine use of skin testing to foods in patients presenting with asthma is not appropriate. Of children evaluated in a tertiary care hospital emergency room, 97 patients with asthma or bronchiolitis were skin tested to common foods and aeroallergens. These results were compared to similar testing in 60 control patients without any respiratory disease.[76] Most specific IgE antibody responses in wheezing children were to aeroallergens and the prevalence of specific IgE antibodies to food allergens was low. Laboratory assessment of food allergy may include the measurement of food-specific IgE in the serum. When highly sensitive assays are used, the sensitivity and specificity are similar to those of skin tests.[77–79] In contrast, basophil histamine release assays, which are mainly limited to research settings, have not been shown conclusively to be a reproducible, diagnostic test for food allergy.[80]

Food challenges

When there is clinical suspicion of a food-induced respiratory tract reaction and the test for specific IgE antibody to the food is positive, an elimination diet may be implemented to see if there is a resolution of clinical symptoms. Confirming this association, however, can be very difficult. Food challenges can be very useful and reliable in the diagnostic evaluation of a patient with food-induced respiratory symptoms. Chapter 14 provides an excellent overview of oral food challenge procedures (Clinical Pearl 5).

Treatment

Once a food allergy has been confirmed as a cause for respiratory tract symptoms, strict avoidance of the offending food is necessary.[1,23,80] A properly managed elimination diet can lead to resolution of clinical symptoms such as chronic asthma. Appropriate nutritional counseling is important to ensure that an elimination diet is well balanced, to provide appropriate substitutes for foods that are eliminated from the diet, and to avoid any anticipated nutritional deficiencies, such as calcium deficiency.[36]

CLINICAL PEARL #5

KEY POINTS RELATED TO THE EVALUATION OF FOOD ALLERGY AND RESPIRATORY SYMPTOMS

- The medical history supplemented with appropriate laboratory testing and well-designed food challenges can provide useful information in the workup of patients with respiratory symptoms that may be induced by food allergy; a diagnosis based solely on history or skin testing/allergen-specific IgE levels is not acceptable.
- If no specific foods are implicated in the history and if skin tests to foods are negative, further workup for IgE-mediated allergy is not generally indicated.
- With positive skin tests and/or respiratory symptoms associated with specific foods, an elimination diet may be instituted for 7–14 days; if symptoms persist, food is not likely to be the problem, except in some cases of atopic dermatitis or chronic asthma.
- Symptoms recurring after a regular diet is resumed should be evaluated with a properly designed food challenge.

Growth parameters should be closely monitored, especially in infants and children on elimination diets. An overview of the management of food allergy and the development of an appropriate anaphylaxis treatment plan, including the use of injectable epinephrine for anaphylactic symptoms, is addressed in Chapter 15.

Summary and conclusions

Previous investigations have clearly established the pathogenic role of food allergy in respiratory tract symptoms. These symptoms are typically accompanied by skin and gastrointestinal manifestations and rarely occur in isolation. Specific foods have been implicated in these reactions, and a small well-identified subset of foods has been associated with anaphylactic reactions. Allergic sensitization to foods in infancy may predict the later development of respiratory allergies and asthma. Asthmatic reactions to food additives can occur but are uncommon. Food-induced asthma is more common in younger, pediatric patients, especially those with atopic dermatitis, than in older children and adults. Asthma may be triggered by the inhalation of relevant food allergens at all ages. Asthma, induced by food allergens, is considered a significant risk factor for fatal and near-fatal anaphylactic reactions.

Studies have demonstrated that foods can elicit airway hyperreactivity and asthmatic responses; therefore, evaluation for food allergy should be considered in patients with difficult to control asthma or otherwise unexplained acute severe asthma exacerbations; asthma triggered following ingestion or inhalation of particular foods; and in asthmatic patients with other manifestations of food allergy (e.g. anaphylaxis, moderate to severe atopic dermatitis). Practice parameters for the diagnosis and treatment of asthma have highlighted the potential role of food allergy in asthma in some patients.[81,82]

References

1. Sicherer SH, Sampson HA. Food Allergy. J Allergy Clin Immunology 2006;117:S470–5.
2. Lack G. Clinical practice. Food allergy. N Engl J Med 2008;359:1252–60.
3. Bahna SL. Clinical expressions of food allergy. Ann Allergy Asthma Immunol 2003;90(Suppl 3):41–4.
4. James JM, Crespo JF. Allergic reactions to foods by inhalation. Curr Allergy Asthma Rep 2007;7:167–74.
5. Ozol D, Mete E. Asthma and Food Allergy. Curr Opin Pulm Med 2008;14:9–12.
6. Nowak-Wegrzyn A, Sampson HA. Adverse reactions to foods. Med Clin N Am 2006;90:97–127.
7. Bock SA. Prospective appraisal of complaints of adverse reactions to foods in children during the first 3 years of life. Pediatr 1987;79:683–8.
8. Niestijl Jansen JJ, Kardinaal AFM, Huijbers G, et al. Prevalence of food allergy and intolerance in the adult Dutch population. J Allergy Clin Immunol 1994;93:446–56.
9. Onorato J, Merland N, Terral C, et al. Placebo-controlled double-blind food challenges in asthma. J Allergy Clin Immunol 1986;78:1139–46.
10. Nekam KL. Nutritional triggers in asthma. Acta Microbiol Immunol Hung 1998;45:113–7.
11. Woods RK, Thien F, Raven J, et al. Prevalence of food allergies in young adults and their relationship to asthma, nasal allergies and eczema. Ann Allergy Asthma Immunol 2002;88:183–9.
12. Schroeder A, Kumar R, Pongracic JA, et al. Food allergy is associated with an increased risk of asthma. Clin Exp Allergy 2009;39:261–70.
13. Kanny G, Moneret-Vautrin D-A, Flabbee J, et al. Population study of food allergy in France. J Allergy Clin Immunol 2001;108:133–40.
14. Woods RK, Abramson M, Raven JM, et al. Reported food intolerance and respiratory symptoms in young adults. Eur Respir J 1998;11:151–5.
15. Peroni DG, Chatzimichail A, Boner AL. Food allergy: what can be done to prevent progression to asthma? Ann Allergy Asthma Immunol 2002;89:44–51.
16. Tariq SM, Matthews SM, Hakim EA, et al. Egg allergy in infancy predicts respiratory allergic disease by 4 years of age. Pediatr Allergy Immunol 2000;11:162–7.
17. Rhodes HL, Sporik R, Thomas P, et al. Early life risk factors for adult asthma: a birth cohort study of subjects at risk, J Allergy Clin Immunol 2001;108:720–5.
18. Wang J, Visness CM, Sampson HA. Food allergen sensitization in inner-city children with asthma. J Allergy Clin Immunol 2005;115:1076–80.
19. Sicherer SH, Furlong TJ, Munoz-Furlong A, et al. A voluntary registry for peanut and tree nut allergy: Characteristics of the first 5149 registrants. J Allergy Clin Immunol 2001;108:128–32.
20. Sicherer SH, Munoz-Furlong A, Sampson HA. Prevalence of seafood allergy in the United States determined by a random telephone survey. J Allergy Clin Immunol 2004;114:159–65.
21. Borghesan F, Mistrello G, Roncarolo D, et al. Respiratory allergy to lipid transfer proteins. Int Arch Allergy Immunol 2008;147:161–5.
22. Fernandez-Rivas C, Gonzalez-Mancebo E, de Durana DA. Allergies to fruits and vegetables. Pediatr Allergy Immunol 2008;19:675–81.
23. Bock SA, Atkins FM. Patterns of food hypersensitivity during sixteen years of double-blind placebo-controlled oral food challenges. J Pediatr 1990;117:561–7.
24. Burks AW, James JM, Hiegel A, et al. Atopic dermatitis and food hypersensitivity reactions. J Pediatr 1998;132:132–6.
25. Huang SW. Follow-up of children with rhinitis and cough associated with milk allergy. Pediatr Allergy Immunol 2007;18:81–5.
26. Sampson HA, Mendelson L, Rosen JP. Fatal and near-fatal food anaphylaxis reactions in children. N Engl J Med 1992;327:380–4.
27. Yunginger JY, Sweeney KG, Sturner WQ, et al. Fatal food-induced anaphylaxis, J Am Med Assoc 1988;260:1450–2.
28. James JM. Anaphylactic reactions to foods. Immunol Allergy Clin N Am 2001;21:653–67.
29. Wang J, Sampson HA. Food anaphylaxis. Clin Exp Allergy 2007;37:651–60.
30. Gangur V, Kelly C, Navuluri L. Sesame allergy: a growing food allergy of global proportions? Ann Allergy Asthma Immunol 2005;95:4–11.
31. Sicherer SH. Is food allergy causing your patient's asthma symptoms? J Respir Dis 2000;21:127–36.
32. Bittner C, Grassau B, Frenzel K, et al. Identification of wheat gliadins as an allergen family related to baker's asthma. J Allergy Clin Immunol 2008;121:744–9.
33. Salvatori N, Reccardini F, Convento M, et al. Asthma induced by inhalation of flour in adults with food allergy to wheat. Clin Exp Allergy 2008;38:1349–56.
34. Abramson M, Kutin J, Rosier M, et al. Morbidity, medication and trigger factors in a community sample of adults with asthma. Med J Aust 1995;162:78–81.
35. Weber RW. Food additives and allergy. Ann Allergy 1993;70:183–90.
36. Bird JA, Burks AW. Food allergy and asthma. Prim Care Respir J 2009;18:258–65.

37. Woods RK, Weiner JM, Thien F, et al. The effects of monosodium glutamate in adults with asthma who perceive themselves to be monosodium glutamate-intolerant. J Allergy Clin Immunol 1998;101:762–71.

38. Yang WH, Drouin MA, Herbert M, et al. The monosodium glutamate symptom complex: Assessment in a double-blind, placebo-controlled, randomized study. J Allergy Clin Immunol 1997;99:757–62.

39. Ramirez DA, Bahna SL. Food hypersensitivity by inhalation. Clinical Molecular Allergy 2009;7:4.

40. Goetz DW, Whisman BA. Occupational asthma in a seafood restaurant worker: cross-reactivity of shrimp and scallops. Ann Allergy Asthma Immunol 2000;85:461–6.

41. Crespo JF, Pascual C, Dominguez C, et al. Allergic reactions associated with airborne fish particles in IgE-mediated fish hypersensitive patients. Allergy 1995;50:257–61.

42. Pascual CY, Reche M, Flandor A, et al. Fish allergy in childhood. Pediatr Allergy Immunol 2008;19;573–9.

43. Taylor AV, Swanson MC, Jones RT, et al. Detection and quantification of raw fish aeroallergens from an open-air fish market. J Allergy Clin Immunol 2000;105:166–9.

44. Eigenmann PA, Zamora SA. An internet-based survey on the circumstances of food-induced reactions following the diagnosis of IgE-mediated food allergy. Allergy 2002;57:449–53.

45. Roberts G, Golder N, Lack G. Bronchial challenges with aerosolized food in asthmatic food-allergic children. Allergy 2002;57:713–7.

46. Sicherer SH, Furlong TJ, DeSimone J, et al. Self-reported allergic reactions to peanut on commercial airliners. J Allergy Clin Immunol 1999;104:186–9.

47. James JM, Bernhisel-Broadbent J, Sampson HA. Respiratory reactions provoked by double-blind food challenges in children. Am J Respir Crit Care Med 1994;149:59–64.

48. Bernstein JM. The role of IgE-mediated hypersensitivity in the development of otitis media with effusion: A review. Otolaryngol Head Neck Surg 1993;109:611–20.

49. Nsouli TM, Nsouli SM, Linde RE, et al. Role of food allergy in serous otitis media. Ann Allergy 1994;73:215–9.

50. Heiner DC, Sears JW. Chronic respiratory disease associated with multiple circulation precipitins to cow's milk. Am J Dis Child 1960;100:500–2.

51. Heiner DC, Sears JW, Kniker WT. Multiple precipitins to cow's milk in chronic respiratory disease: A syndrome including poor growth, gastrointestinal symptoms, evidence of allergy, iron deficiency anemia and pulmonary hemosiderosis. Am J Dis Child 1962;103:634–54.

52. Lowe AJ, Hosking CS, Bennett CM, et al. Skin prick test can identify eczematous infants at risk of asthma and allergic rhinitis. Clin Exp Allergy 2007;37:1624–31.

53. Tepper RS, Llapur CJ, Jones MH, et al. Expired nitric oxide and airway reactivity in infants at risk for asthma. J Allergy Clin Immunol 2008;122:760–5.

54. Priftis KN, Mermiri D, Papadopoulou A, et al. Asthma symptoms and bronchial reactivity in school children sensitized to food allergens in infancy. J Asthma 2008;45:590–5.

55. Hill DJ, Firer MA, Shelton MJ, et al. Manifestations of milk allergy in infancy: clinical and immunological findings. J Pediatr 1986;109:270–6.

56. Bock SA. Respiratory reactions induced by food challenges in children with pulmonary disease. Pediatr Allergy Immunol 1992;3:188–94.

57. Rance F, Dutau G. Asthma and food allergy: report of 163 cases. Arch Pediatr 2002;9:402–7.

58. Fiocchi A, Terracciano L, Bouygue GR, et al. Incremental prognostic factors associated with cow's milk allergy outcomes in infant and child referrals: the Milan Cow's Milk Allergy Cohort study. Ann Allergy Asthma Immunol 2008;101:166–73.

59. James JM, Eigenmann PA, Eggleston PA, et al. Airway reactivity changes in asthmatic patients undergoing blinded food challenges, Am J Respir Crit Care Med 1996;153:597–603.

60. Prifits KN, Mermiri D, Papadopoulou A, et al. Asthma symptoms and reactivity in school children sensitized to food allergens in infancy. J Asthma 2008;45:590–5.

61. Zwetchkenbawn JF, Skufca R, Nelson HS. An examination of food hypersensitivity as a cause of increased bronchial responsiveness to inhaled methacholine. J Allergy Clin Immunol 1991;88:360–4.

62. Thaminy A, Lamblin C, Perez T, et al. Increased frequency of asymptomatic bronchial hyperresponsiveness in nonasthmatic patients with food allergy. Eur Respir J 2000;16:1091–4.

63. Kivity S, Fireman E, Sage K. Bronchial hyperactivity, sputum analysis and skin prick test to inhalant allergens in patients with symptomatic food hypersensitivity. Isr Med Assoc J 2005;7:781–4.

64. Wallaert B, Gosset P, Lamblin C, et al. Airway neutrophil inflammation in nonasthmatic patients with food allergy. Allergy 2002;57:405–10.

65. Brandt EB, Scribner TA, Akel HS, et al. Experimental gastrointestinal allergy enhances pulmonary responses to specific and unrelated allergens. J Allergy Clin Immunol 2006;118:420–7.

66. Webb LM, Lieberman P. Anaphylaxis: a review of 601 cases. J Allergy Clin Immunol 2006;97:39–43.

67. Bock SA, Munoz-Furlong A, Sampson HA. Fatalities due to anaphylactic reactions to foods. J Allergy Clin Immunol 2001;107:191–3.

68. Vogel NM, Katz HT, Lopez R, et al. Food allergy is associated with potentially fatal childhood asthma. J Asthma 2008;45:862–6.

69. de Silva IL, Hehr SS, Tey D, et al. Paediatric anaphylaxis: a 5 year retrospective review. Allergy 2008;63:1071–6.

70. Novembre E, de Martino M, Vierucci A. Foods and respiratory allergy. J Allergy Clin Immunol 1988;81:1059–65.

71. Oehling A, Baena Cagnani CE. Food allergy and child asthma. Allergol Immunopathol 1980;8:7–14.

72. Businco L, Falconieri P, Giampietro P, et al. Food allergy and asthma. Pediatr Pulmonary Suppl 1995;11: 59–60.

73. Yazicioglu M, Baspinar I, Ones U, et al. Egg and milk allergy in asthmatic children: assessment by immulite allergy panel, skin prick tests and double-blind placebo-controlled food challenges. Allergol et Immunopathol 1999;27:287–93.

74. Roberts G, Patel N, Levi-Schaffer F, et al. Food allergy as a risk factor for life-threatening asthma in childhood: a case-controlled study. J Allergy Clin Immunol 2003;112:168–74.

75. Sicherer SH, Teuber S. Current approach to the diagnosis and management of adverse reactions to foods. J Allergy Clin Immunol 2004;114:1146–50.

76. Price GW, Hogan AD, Farris AH, et al. Sensitization (IgE antibody) to food allergens in wheezing infants and children. J Allergy Clin Immunol 1995;96: 266–70.

77. Sampson HA, Ho DG. Relationship between food-specific IgE concentrations and the risk of positive food challenges in children and adolescents. J Allergy Clin Immunol 1997;100:444–51.

78. Sampson HA. Utility of food specific IgE concentrations in predicting symptomatic food allergy. J Allergy Clin Immunol 2001;107:891–6.

79. Wraith DG, Merret J, Roth A, et al. Recognition of food-allergic patients and their allergens by the RAST technique and clinical investigation, Clin Allergy 1979;9:25–36.

80. James JM, Sampson HA. An overview of food hypersensitivity, Ped Allergy Immunol 1992;3:67–78.

81. Chapman JA, Bernstein IL, Lee RE, et al. Food allergy: a practice parameter. Ann Allergy Asthma Immuonol 2006;96:S1–S68.

82. Spector SL, Nicklas RA, editors. Practice parameters for the diagnosis and treatment of asthma. J Allergy Clin Immunol (supplement) 1996;96:707–869.

CHAPTER 9

Food-induced Anaphylaxis and Food Associated Exercise-induced Anaphylaxis

Motohiro Ebisawa

KEY CONCEPTS

- The most common food triggers for anaphylaxis are peanut, tree nuts, cows' milk, hens' egg, fish and shellfish. However, in some regions wheat, buckwheat, lipid transfer protein-related fruits and bird's nest can also provoke food-induced anaphylaxis.

- The incidence of food-dependent exercise-induced anaphylaxis has increasingly been reported during the past three decades. Wheat, crustaceans and vegetables are the most common food triggers for the disease in recent reports.

- Comorbidities (e.g. asthma) and risk factors (NSAIDs, exercise etc.) may affect symptom severity and

- treatment response in patients with food-induced anaphylaxis or food-dependent exercise-induced anaphylaxis.

- Adrenaline is the first line of therapy and its administration is strongly recommended in all cases as soon as the first symptoms of anaphylaxis are recognized.

- Long-term management, including avoidance of causative foods and an emergency management prescription including self-injectable adrenaline, is essential in patients with food-induced anaphylaxis.

Introduction

Historical background

Fatal allergic reactions were reported more than 1000 years ago, but it was only 100 years ago that the term of 'anaphylaxis' was fully established. In 1902, Portier and Richet[1] first described the sudden death of several dogs involved in immunization trials against the venom of the sea anemone. As this phenomenon represented the opposite of the intended 'prophylaxis' of immunization, they created the term 'anaphylaxis', meaning a phenomenon without or against the protection. In 1969, 10 cases of anaphylaxis following the ingestion of various foods, including different legumes, fish and milk, were reported. Furthermore, the natural course of near-fatal and fatal food-induced anaphylactic reactions has been further reported by US researchers in the last 30 years.[1]

The first case of food-dependent exercise-induced anaphylaxis (FEIAn or FDEIA) was reported by Mauliz et al. in 1979.[2] This patient was a runner who often developed anaphylactic reactions after having meals with shellfish prior to his routine running activity. Since this initial case report, the incidence of FDEIA appears to be increasing over the past few decades.

Definition of anaphylaxis

Based on the World Health Organization (WHO) definition, anaphylaxis is 'a severe, life-threatening generalized or systemic hypersensitivity reaction'.

However, this definition can be problematic, given that the term 'life-threatening' may be interpreted differently by different healthcare providers. A recent meeting in the US sponsored by the National Institute of Allergy and Infectious Disease (NIAID) and the Food Allergy and Anaphylaxis Network (FAAN) has established a consensus definition to satisfy epidemiological, research and clinical needs.[3] According to this definition, anaphylaxis is considered likely if any one of the following three criteria is present within minutes to hours after the onset of the reaction (Table 9.1).

Symptoms of anaphylaxis can include cutaneous, respiratory, cardiovascular and gastrointestinal (GI) signs and symptoms either isolated or in combination. A grading system evaluating the severity of food-induced anaphylaxis might be helpful and is shown in Table 9.2.[4]

The clinical syndrome of FDEIA is characterized by the rapid onset of anaphylaxis during (or soon

Table 9.1 Definition of anaphylaxis (Sampson HA, Muñoz-Furlong A, Campbell RL, et al. Second symposium on the definition and management of anaphylaxis: summary report. J Allergy Clin Immunol 2006; 117: 391–7.)

1. Acute onset of illness with cutaneous and/or mucosal involvement AND at least one of the following:
   a. Respiratory compromise (e.g. dyspnea, bronchospasm, stridor, hypoxia)
   b. Cardiovascular compromise (e.g. hypotension, collapse)
2. Two or more of the following occur rapidly after exposure to a likely allergen (minutes to several hours):
   a. Involvement of skin or mucosa (e.g. generalized hives, itch, flushing, swelling)
   b. Respiratory compromise
   c. Cardiovascular compromise
   d. Or persistent gastrointestinal symptoms (e.g. crampy abdominal pain, vomiting)
3. Hypotension after exposure to known allergen for that patient (minutes to several hours): age-specific low blood pressure* or > 30% decline from baseline (or less than 90 mmHg for adults).

*Hypotension for children is defined as systolic blood pressure <70 mmHg from 1 month to 1 year, <(70 mmHg+[2×age]) from 1 to 10 years, and <90 mmHg from 11 to 17 years.

Table 9.2 Grading of food-induced anaphylaxis according to severity of clinical symptoms (Sampson HA. Anaphylaxis and emergency treatment. Pediatrics. 2003; 111: 1601–8.)

Grade	Skin	GI Tract	Respiratory tract	Cardiovascular	Neurological
1	Localized pruritus, flushing, urticaria, angioedema	Oral pruritus, oral 'tingling', mild lip swelling	–	–	–
2	Generalized pruritus, flushing, urticaria, angioedema	Any of the above, nausea and/or emesis × 1	Nasal congestion, and/or sneezing	–	Change in activity level
3	Any of the above	Any of the above plus repetitive vomiting	Rhinorrhea, marked congestion, sensation of throat pruritus or tightness	Tachycardia (increase >15 bpm)	Change in activity level plus anxiety
4	Any of the above	Any of the above plus diarrhea	Any of the above, hoarseness, 'barky' cough, difficulty swallowing, dyspnea, wheezing, cyanosis	Any of the above, dysrhythmia and/or mild hypotension	'Light headedness', feeling of 'pending doom'
5	Any of the above	Any of the above, loss of bowel control	Any of the above, respiratory arrest	Severe bradycardia, and/or hypotension or cardiac arrest	Loss of consciousness

after) exercise which was preceded by the ingestion of the causal food(s). Both the food allergen and exercise are independently tolerated.[5]

Epidemiology

Food-induced anaphylaxis

The true prevalence of food-induced anaphylaxis is not well established, since it was only recently that International Classification of Diseases Code (ICD) for food-induced anaphylaxis was defined. Therefore, it is still difficult to obtain reliable information regarding its prevalence, incidence or mortality rates. Furthermore, it is suspected that adults with less severe cases of food-induced anaphylaxis, tend to avoid causative foods without consulting physicians.

Accordingly, limited information on food-induced anaphylaxis is currently available. This chapter will review recent reports on food-induced anaphylaxis, and data will be summarized in four categories described below. Most data on food-induced anaphylaxis were obtained from hospital ED (emergency department) based-studies or questionnaires in selected populations.

Reports on children

Reports from various areas of the world on foods involved in anaphylaxis in children are summarized in Table 9.3. In reports from the USA, the most frequent food to cause anaphylaxis are peanuts, followed by tree nuts, cows' milk and cows' milk protein-based products, as well as shellfish. Data from the USA were mostly collected in hospital emergency departments (ED) or referral outpatient clinics. Two reports from Australia, with ED-based analysis, were using the corresponding ICD codes for anaphylaxis. Similarly to the USA, the most common causative foods were peanuts, cows' milk, cashew nuts and eggs. More reports were from Asia,

Table 9.3 Causes of food-induced anaphylaxis in children

Study	Country	Publication year	Most frequent causative foods			Cases (n)	Ref.
			1st	**2nd**	**3rd**		
Järvinen KM et al.	USA	2008	Peanuts	Cows' milk	Nuts	95	J Allergy Clin Immunol 122: 133–138
Rudders SA et al.	USA	2010	Peanuts	Cows' milk	Nuts	846	J Allergy Clin Immunol 126: 385–388
Russell S et al.	USA	2010	Peanuts	Shellfish	Cows' milk	124	Pediatr Emerg Care 26: 71–76
Braganza SC et al.	Australia	2006	Dairy	Egg	Peanuts	57	Arch Dis Child 91: 159–163
de Silva IL et al.	Australia	2008	Peanuts	Cashew nut	Cows' milk	104	Allergy 63: 1071–1076
Goh DL et al.	Singapore	1999	Bird's nest	Crustacean seafood	Egg and milk	124	Allergy 54: 84–86
Piromrat K et al.	Thailand	2008	Prawn				Asian Pac J Allergy Immunol 26: 121–128
Imai T	Japan*	2004	Hen's egg	Cows' milk	Wheat	408	Arerugi 52: 1006–1013

*Infant only.

Table 9.4 Causes of food-induced anaphylaxis in adults

Study	Country	Publication year	Most frequent causative foods			Cases (n)	Ref.
			1st	**2nd**	**3rd**		
Greenhawt MJ et al.	USA	2009	Cows' milk	Nuts	Shellfish	104	J Allergy Clin Immunol 124: 323–327
Asero R et al.	Italy	2009	Peach	Shrimp	Nuts	58	Int Arch Allergy Immunol 150: 271–277
Moneret-Vautrin DA et al.	France	1995	Hen's egg	Fish or crustaceans	milk or fruit-latex group	794	Ann Gastroenterol Hepatol 31: 256–263
Brown AF et al.	Australia	2001	Fish and Seafood	Nuts	Mango or Lemon drink	22	J Allergy Clin Immunol 108: 861–866
Imai T	Japan	2004	Fish	Buckwheat	Meat	130	Arerugi 52: 1006–1013

including Singapore and Japan (the latter one with hospital ED-based data). Unlike the USA and Australia, the common causative foods in children were hens' eggs, cows' milk and wheat products. Interestingly, bird's nest and crustaceans were reported as the top two foods responsible for food-induced anaphylaxis in Singapore. These data clearly show geographically and environmentally related causes for food-induced anaphylaxis in children.

Reports in adults

Reports on food-induced anaphylaxis in adulthood are less frequent than those for children. As shown in Table 9.4, reports from the USA involved college students, with common food triggers being cows' milk, tree nuts, shellfish and peanuts. In Italy, hospital ED-based reports revealed that peach was the most common food to induce anaphylaxis, followed by shrimp, tree nuts and legumes other than peanut. In France, hen's egg, fish, crustaceans and cows' milk were reported to be common foods to induce anaphylaxis. In Australia, fish and seafood were reported to be the most common causative foods, followed by tree nuts and mango- or lemon-containing drinks. In Japan, fish and buckwheat were reported to be the top two causative foods in hospital ED-based surveys. These data were mostly obtained from multicenter or single-hospital ED-based studies, suggesting a potential population bias.

Reports including all age groups

Table 9.5 summarizes four reports on the incidence of food-induced anaphylaxis including both children and adults from various different regions of the world. In the USA, similarly to the previously cited reports, tree nuts, crustaceans and peanut were the top three causative foods. In Korea, wheat, buckwheat and seafood are top of the list. Buckwheat seems to be a common food trigger to induce anaphylaxis in both Korea and Japan, where noodles made of buckwheat are commonly eaten. Buckwheat-like wheat can be not only a food allergen but also an aeroallergen, especially for workers in buckwheat noodle factories. As buckwheat is now becoming a common food in countries such as the USA and France, one might suspect a progression of buckwheat allergy throughout the world. In Japan, cows' milk, hen's egg, and wheat products were reported to be the three major food suspects; the study included more children than adults

Reports on fatal cases of anaphylaxis

Although detailed data on fatal anaphylaxis are limited, several recent publications from the USA, UK, Australia and Japan report on fatal food-induced anaphylaxis (Fig. 9.1). A careful search for fatal cases of food-induced anaphylaxis in the UK revealed 48 deaths between 1999 and 2006. A

Table 9.5 Causes of food-induced anaphylaxis from childhood to adulthood

Study	Country	Publication year	Age	Most frequent causative foods			Cases (n)	Ref.
				1st	**2nd**	**3rd**		
Ross MP et al.	USA	2008	2–66 y	Seafood	nuts		23	J Allergy Clin Immunol 121: 166–171
Yang MS et al.	Korea	2008	5–76 y	Wheat flour	Buckwheat	Seafood	29	Ann Allergy Asthma Immunol 100: 31–36
Imamura T et al.	Japan	2008	0–93 y	Milk	Eggs	Wheat	319	Pediatr Allergy Immunol 19: 270–274
Cianferoni A et al.	Italy	2001	?	Seafood			113	Ann Allergy Asthma Immunol 87: 27–32

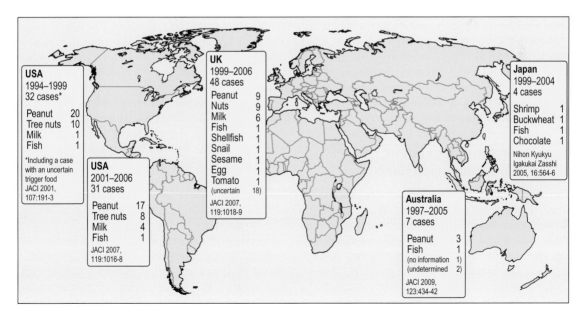

Figure 9.1 Worldwide cases of fatal food-induced anaphylaxis.

voluntary registry initiated by the American Academy of Allergy, Asthma and Immunology (AAAAI) and the Food Allergy and Anaphylaxis Network (FAAN) collected 32 cases of fatal food-induced anaphylaxis between 1994 and 1999 and a further 31 cases between 2001 and 2006. There were 112 anaphylaxis fatalities in Australia between 1997 and 2005, of which seven (6.3%) were attributed to food. Through the national mortality reporting system in Japan, each year several cases of food-induced anaphylaxis fatalities have been reported in the last 15 years. Compared to the number of anaphylaxis deaths in the UK or the USA, food-induced anaphylaxis reports are relatively less frequent in Australia and Japan. In the USA, the UK and Australia, peanut was reported to be the most frequent food to cause fatal anaphylaxis. Other than peanut or tree nuts, any kind of food, such as shellfish, fish and cows' milk, can be a potential trigger for fatal food-induced anaphylaxis. It needs to be pointed out that in the reports cited above, most of the individuals did not have epinephrine available at the time of their fatal reaction. With regard to comorbid conditions, asthma was reported to be the most important risk factor for death.

Summarized from these data on food-induced anaphylaxis from childhood to adulthood, the most common foods involved are peanut, tree nuts, cows' milk, hen's egg, fish, and crustacean shellfish. However, in some regions, wheat, buckwheat, lipid transfer protein (LTP)-related fruits such as peach or Kiwi fruit, and bird's nest were commonly identified triggers. Also, the incidence may vary according to age, regional diet, food preparation, amount of exposure, and timing of first exposure.

Reports on food-dependent exercise-induced anaphylaxis

The incidence of FDEIA seems to be increasing since the first report by Mauliz et al. in 1979.[2] Reports from all over the world are summarized in Table 9.6. Wheat, crustaceans and vegetables are reported as the most common triggers. Aihara[6] reported the prevalence of (FEIAn or FDEIA) in junior high-school students in Japan to be 0.017% (13/76229). He also reported on 84 cases from various countries which occurred between 1979 and 2004.[7] As shown in Figure 9.2, FDEIA was most frequently seen in teenagers and young adults, and the most common causative foods were wheat, vegetables and tree nuts (Table 9.7).

Pathogenesis

Causative food allergens absorbed in the gut may lead to anaphylaxis through a mechanism that involves cross-linking of IgE and aggregation of FcεRI on mast cells and basophils (described in more detail in Chapter 1). In humans, food-induced anaphylaxis is mostly IgE driven. Intracellular events, including activation of tyrosine kinases and calcium influx in mastocytes and basophils, result in the rapid release of preformed mediators such as histamine, tryptase and chymase. Activation of phospholipase A2, COXs, and lipooxygenases leads to the production of arachidonic acid metabolites, including prostaglandins and leukotrienes, and synthesis of platelet-activating factor. Various cytokines and chemokines are further synthesized and released, which may play a role in the late-phase reaction. Increased permeability of the endothelial barrier through endothelial Gq/G11-mediated signaling has been identified as a critically important process leading to symptoms of anaphylaxis in several organs.[8]

Relatively few protein families account for the vast majority of allergic reactions. A study by Jenkins et al.[9] comparing food allergens of animal origin and their human homologs (by analyzing protein families, sequence analysis and evolutionary features) disclosed that sequence identities to human homologs > 62% typically excluded the protein from being allergenic in humans. It has been shown that major food allergens share a number of common features: they are water-soluble glycoproteins, 10–70 kDa in size, and relatively stable to heat, acid and proteases.

Host conditions, including diseases, medications, infections and exercise, have also been associated with the pathogenesis of food-induced anaphylaxis, as discussed later in this chapter.

Overall, the pathogenesis of FDEIA is not well understood. One possible explanation for FDEIA would be increased gut permeability during exercise, resulting in larger amounts of potentially allergenic proteins reaching the host's gut-associated immune system. Gut permeability has been shown to be increased in food-allergic and food-intolerant children.[5]

Table 9.6 Summary of worldwide multiple food-dependent exercise-induced anaphylaxis case reports

Study	Country	Publication year	Age	Foods triggering FEIAn			Cases (n)	Ref.
				1st	2nd	3rd		
Kano H et al.	Japan	2000	9–43 y	Wheat	Shrimp	Shellfish or fish	18	Arerugi 49: 472–478
Harada S et al.	Japan	2000	>20 y	Wheat	Shrimp		167	Arerugi 49: 1066–1073
Harada S et al.	Japan	2000	<20 y	Shrimp	Wheat		167	Arerugi 49: 1066–1073
Aihara Y et al.	Japan	2001	12–15 y	Shrimps and crab	Wheat	Grapes, vegetables, buckwheat	13	J Allergy Clin Immunol 108: 1035–1039
Yang MS et al.	Korea	2008	5–76 y	Wheat	Apple or shrimp		18	Ann Allergy Asthma Immunol 100: 31–36
Teo SL et al.	Singapore	2009	9–20 y	Shellfish			5	Ann Acad Med Singapore 209: 905–909
Mathelier-Fusade P et al.	France	2002	?	Wheat	Corn, barley, shrimp, apple, paprika, mustard		7	Ann Dermatol Venereol 129: 694–697
Romano A et al.	Italy	2001	?	Tomatoes	Wheat	Peanuts	54	Int Arch Allergy Immunol 125: 264–272
Shadick NA et al.	USA	1999	13–77 y	Shellfish	Alcohol	Tomatoes	279 (EIA patients)	J Allergy Clin Immunol 104: 123–127

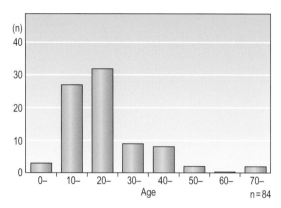

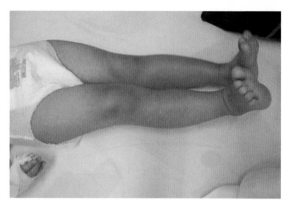

Figure 9.2 Age distribution of food-dependent exercise-induced anaphylaxis reported from 1979 to 2004. Aihara Y. [Food-dependent exercise-induced anaphylaxis]. Arerugi. 2007 May; 56(5): 451–6.

Figure 9.3 Food-induced anaphylaxis (after wheat challenge). 4-year-old boy with a skin rash, wheezing and dyspnea.

Table 9.7 Causative foods of FEIAn reported from 1979 to 2004. Aihara Y. [Food-dependent exercise-induced anaphylaxis]. Arerugi. 2007 May; 56(5): 451–6.

Food	Case (n)	(%)
Wheat	29	(38.2)
Vegetable	24	(31.6)
Nut	16	(21.1)
Fruit	7	(9.2)
Plant oil	4	(5.3)
Shellfish	3	(3.9)
Others	6	(7.9)
Total	76	

Clinical features

Food-induced anaphylaxis

The symptoms of anaphylaxis are generally related to the skin, the respiratory or GI tracts and the cardiovascular system.[10] Figure 9.3 shows a patient with typical skin symptoms. The patient is a 4-year-old boy who experienced anaphylaxis after receiving the initial dose of wheat challenge during an in-hospital test. In addition to skin symptoms, he developed wheezing and oxygen saturation <90%. He received intramuscular epinephrine twice, and recovered from his anaphylactic reaction. Skin symptoms, which occur in most patients, may include itching, flushing, urticaria and angioedema. However, it is important to realize that anaphylaxis can occur without skin manifestations. Respiratory symptoms, which frequently occur in anaphylaxis, include nasal symptoms, laryngeal edema, choking, wheezing, coughing and dyspnea. Gastrointestinal symptoms include abdominal pain and cramping, nausea, vomiting and diarrhea. Cardiovascular symptoms, such as hypotension and shock, are less common as early manifestations of food-induced anaphylaxis. The time course of the reaction and the perception of symptoms and signs differ among individuals.[1]

Biphasic allergic reactions, defined as a second reaction occurring 1–72 hours after recovery from the initial reactions, were reported in 11% of children treated for anaphylaxis in a pediatric ED. Biphasic reactions were reported in 25% of cases of fatal and near-fatal food-induced reactions and 23% of drug/biological-induced reactions, but in only 6% of anaphylaxis due to other causes. They are uncommon after insect stings. It is important to note that biphasic reactions rarely occur without initial hypotension or airway obstruction.[11]

Food-dependent exercise-induced anaphylaxis

CLINICAL CASE

Figure 9.4 illustrates a case of FDEIA . The patient is a 14-year-old student in junior high school who ate seafood

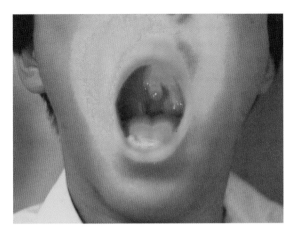

Figure 9.4 A case of food-dependent, exercise-induced anaphylaxis. A 14-year-old junior high-school student developed anaphylaxis after eating seafood for lunch, followed by playing football with his friends.

for lunch and played football with his friends immediately afterwards. During the game his skin began to itch he developed a strange feeling in his mouth. He also developed severe eyelid edema, laryngeal edema and a blister on the uvula. He had difficulty in breathing and lost consciousness during transfer to the ED owing to a drop in his blood pressure to 80 mmHg systolic. He received appropriate treatment in the ED, including several injections of intramuscular epinephrine, and was carefully monitored, including an overnight stay for further careful observation. A case series of Japanese schoolchildren reported the following symptoms among those with food-dependent exercise-induced anaphylaxis: pruritus (92%), urticaria (86%), angioedema (72%), flushing (70%), shortness of breath (51%), dysphagia (34%), chest tightness (33%), fainting (32%), profuse sweating (32%), headache (28%), gastrointestinal symptoms (colic, nausea and diarrhea) (28%), and upper airway symptoms (choking, hoarse, throat constriction)(25%).[11] Although FDEIA may lead to life-threatening anaphylaxis with airway obstruction and/or hypotensive shock, reports of fatalities are rare and restricted to adults. However, fatalities may be underestimated due to the rarity of the disease and the difficulty of making a diagnosis.

Unusual variants

Late-onset food-induced anaphylaxis

Onset of an anaphylactic reaction usually occurs within 30 minutes after exposure to the relevant allergen. Isolated late anaphylactic reactions without early-phase reactions are rarely reported in patients with food-induced anaphylaxis. Two specific conditions might be highlighted.

- Natto (soybeans fermented by the bacteria *Bacillus natto*) anaphylaxis. Inomata et al.[12] reported the first case of IgE-mediated skin, respiratory and abdominal symptoms occurring 10–12 hours after consuming natto.
- Meat anaphylaxis. Commins et al.[13] described a cohort of 24 patients with IgE antibodies to α-gal who experienced delayed symptoms of anaphylaxis, angioedema or urticaria after eating mammalian meat. The patients described a similar history of anaphylaxis or urticaria 3–6 hours after the ingestion of meat and reported fewer episodes or complete recovery when following an avoidance diet. Skin prick tests to mammalian meat produced wheals of usually <4 mm, whereas intradermal or fresh-food skin prick tests elicited larger and more consistent wheal responses. In vitro testing revealed positive specific IgE antibodies to beef, pork, lamb, cows' milk, cat and dog, but not to turkey, chicken or fish.

Associated condition worsening food-induced anaphylaxis or food-dependent exercise-induced anaphylaxis

Associated conditions and risk factors may affect symptom severity and treatment response in patients with food-induced anaphylaxis or FDEIA[8] (Table 9.8). Bronchial asthma is the most important risk factor for a more severe outcome. Persistent asthma, especially if not well controlled, is an important risk factor for fatal anaphylaxis, in particular in adolescents and young adults. Cardiovascular disease is also an important risk factor, especially in elderly patients. Common viral or bacterial infections are also known to affect symptom severity, especially in cases of gastrointestinal infections. Various medications, such as β-blockers, angiotensin-converting enzyme inhibitors, α-adrenergic blockers, and non-steroidal anti-inflammatory drugs (NSAIDs), may also affect symptom severity and treatment response in patients with food-induced anaphylaxis. Non-steroidal anti-inflammatory drugs have also been shown to enhance the symptoms of FDEIA. Alcohol intake, fatigue, stress and exercise are known to worsen symptoms and the severity of food-induced anaphylaxis or FDEIA.[8]

Table 9.8 Comorbid conditions and risk factors for food-induced anaphylaxis and food-dependent exercise-induced anaphylaxis

Factors		FIA	DEIA	Ref.
Disease	Asthma*	o		J Allergy Clin Immunol. 2009; 124: 625
	Cardiovascular disease	o		Clin Exp Immunol. 2008; 153: 7
				Curr Opin Allergy Clin Immunol. 2007; 7: 337
	Infection	o	o	J Allergy Clin Immunol. 2010; 125: S161
	Other disorder**	o		J Allergy Clin Immunol. 2010; 125: S161
Medication	β-Adrenergic antagonists	o		Curr Allergy Asthma Rep. 2008; 8:·37
	Angiotensin-converting enzyme (ACE) inhibitors	o		Curr Allergy Asthma Rep. 2008; 8: 37
	α-Adrenergic blockers	o		Curr Allergy Asthma Rep. 2008; 8: 37
	Antidepressants	o		Curr Allergy Asthma Rep. 2008; 8: 37
	NSAIDs, aspirin	o	o	J Dermatol Sci. 2007; 47: 109
				Br J Dermatol. 2001; 145: 336
Other	Alcohol intake	o	o	Addict Biol. 2004; 9: 195
	Fatigue	o	o	J Allergy Clin Immunol. 2010; 125: S161
	Stress	o	o	J Allergy Clin Immunol. 2010; 125: S161
	Type of exercise	o	o	J Allergy Clin Immunol. 2010; 125: S161
	Atmospheric and seasonal conditions		o	J Allergy Clin Immunol. 2010; 125: S161

* In particular if poorly controlled.

** 1) Mastocytosis and clonal mast cell disorder, 2) chronic lung disease, 3) anatomical airway obstruction , 4) depression and other psychiatric disease.

Diagnosis

Food-induced anaphylaxis

The diagnosis of food-induced anaphylaxis is based on clinical findings and a detailed description of the acute episode, in association with known or suspected food exposure.[1] As mentioned in the Introduction, new diagnostic criteria for anaphylaxis were published recently with the intention to help clinicians both to recognize the spectrum of signs and symptoms that comprise anaphylaxis and to establish a more systematic diagnostic and management approach.[3] As shown in Table 9.1, the presence of any one of three clinical criteria indicates that anaphylaxis is highly likely. As already mentioned (Table 9.2), a grading system evaluating the severity of food-induced anaphylaxis might be useful.[4]

Laboratory tests are of limited value in the acute phase of anaphylaxis. The clinical diagnosis may be supported by the measure of serum tryptase within 6–8 hours after the beginning of the reaction. Further tests at a follow-up visit will help to identify the culprit food allergen. Skin prick and serum allergen-specific IgE testing (e.g. ImmunoCAP) may provide information about a specific food allergy sensitization, but do not provide definite information regarding the cause of or risk for anaphylaxis. Oral food challenge tests (ideally a double-blind placebo-controlled food challenge) are useful for a definite diagnosis in selected cases.

Food-dependent exercise-induced anaphylaxis

A detailed clinical history is essential, and skin prick and serum allergen-specific IgE testing may also provide information regarding sensitization to a specific food. The combination of the clinical history and the support of allergy testing may provide enough information to make an accurate diagnosis. However, some patients with FDEIA may have negative results on allergy testing. In the case of wheat-dependent exercise-induced anaphylaxis, it has been

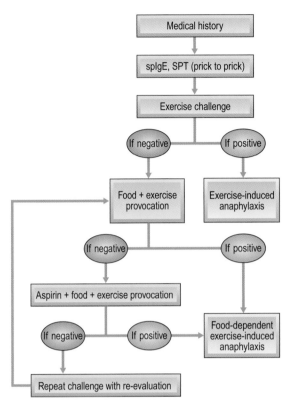

Figure 9.5 Flowchart for the diagnosis of food-dependent exercise-induced anaphylaxis. Modified from: Japanese Pediatric Guideline for Oral Food Challenge Test in Food Allergy 2009. *Allergol Int.* 2009; 58: 467–74.

identified that measurement of the concentration of specific IgE antibodies to ω-5 gliadin is more useful than measuring IgE antibodies to wheat or gluten.[14] In food challenge tests for the diagnosis of FDEIA the reproducibility of the results is not consistent. If causative foods are not identified by provocation tests, in our experience this diagnostic procedure may need to be repeated (Fig. 9.5). NSAIDs are known to enhance the symptoms of FDEIA.[15] In the *Japanese Pediatric Guideline for Oral Food Challenge Test in Food Allergy 2009*, the flowchart for the diagnosis of FDEIA includes an aspirin challenge prior to food plus exercise challenge, if the patients do not react to the suspected foods during the regular challenge procedure (Fig. 9.5).

Treatment/management

Treatment and management of food-induced anaphylaxis or FDEIA can be subdivided into acute (pharmacological management followed by careful observation) and long-term. Long-term management consists of the measures that provide the best quality of life for the patient.

Pharmacological

Most of the treatments for anaphylaxis currently used are based on consensus rather than high-quality evidence. Due in part to the difficulty in performing well-designed randomized control trials, few evidence-based studies have so far been published in this field. Furthermore, according to Cochrane Review findings, there is insufficient evidence to support the use of adrenaline, antihistamines (H$_1$ agonists) and glucocorticosteroids in the treatment of anaphylaxis. However, intramuscular epinephrine has relatively few side-effects in anaphylaxis and is acknowledged as the first line of therapy both in hospital and in the community.[4,8,10,16] An example of a protocol for the initial management of anaphylaxis in the hospital setting is shown in Figure 9.6.[16]

Epinephrine (adrenaline)

Epinephrine should be administered to all patients with an anaphylactic reaction involving any respiratory and/or cardiovascular symptoms or signs. However, acute management should be tailored to the individual. For example, if a patient has recurrent episodes of anaphylaxis commencing with severe abdominal pain, the earlier use of epinephrine would be justified if they developed severe abdominal pain after a subsequent ingestion of the same allergen. Also, an earlier use of epinephrine is justified in patients with a history of asthma, particularly in those needing regular asthma medication.

In general, the same indications apply for patients and carers as for physicians. Families finding it difficult to identify early symptoms and signs of severity should be told to administer epinephrine without waiting for severe symptoms to develop, as delayed treatment has been associated with fatalities. Unfortunately, many patients and carers do not use epinephrine, even when patients have previously experienced a life-threatening anaphylactic reaction.

The intramuscular route is preferred initially in all settings because intramuscular epinephrine

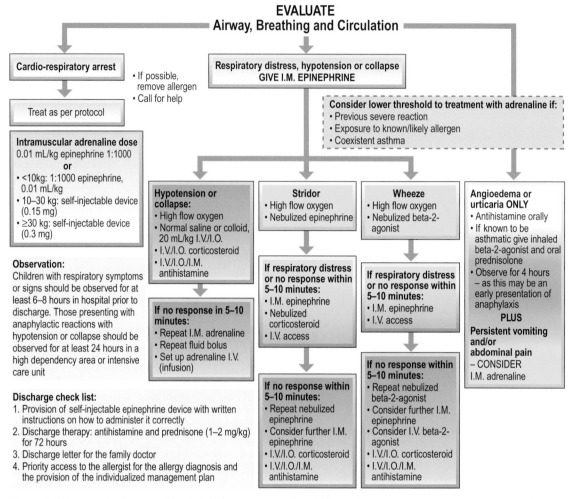

Figure 9.6 An example of a protocol for the initial management of anaphylaxis in the emergency department. Muraro A, Roberts G, Clark A, et al. The management of anaphylaxis in childhood: position paper of the European academy of allergology and clinical immunology. Allergy. 2007 Aug; 62(8): 857–71.

is rapidly bioavailable, with peak concentrations occurring within 10 minutes of administration, and has a much better safety profile and longer-lasting action than intravenous adrenaline. The recommended site for self-injectable epinephrine is the anterior lateral thigh, as there are neither major arteries nor nerves in that area.

For the intramuscular route, 1 : 1000 epinephrine (1 mg/mL) should be used at a dose of 0.01 mL/kg body weight (maximum single dose 0.3–0.5 mg). This dosage can be repeated at short intervals (every 5–10 min) until the patient's condition stabilizes. If intravenous adrenaline is used, a dose of 0.1 µg /kg/min has been recommended.[16]

Fluid support

Severe episodes of anaphylaxis often involve the cardiovascular system, resulting in tachycardia and decreased arterial blood pressure. They should be treated with both adrenaline and volume support.

Inhaled β_2-agonist

A β_2-agonist inhaled through a spacer device or by nebulizer is a useful adjuvant for treating bronchospasm associated with anaphylaxis. However, these provide treatment only for the bronchospasm, whereas anaphylaxis is a systemic disease. Delivery of β_2-agonists may be impaired by acute bronchospasm and systemic adrenaline must always be considered the first-line therapy.

Antihistamine (H₁)

Antihistamines (H₁ antagonists) should be given promptly if a patient has been exposed to an allergen or develops clinical symptoms or signs of an allergic reaction. However, there is no research-supported evidence of their efficacy in anaphylaxis.

Glucocorticosteroid

Corticosteroids should not be considered as a first-line treatment for anaphylaxis. They do not act fast enough and their efficacy in reducing the risk of late-phase reactions has not been fully proven.

Observation period

There is no consensus in the literature regarding the optimal period that a patient who has been successfully treated for anaphylaxis should be observed prior to discharge from the hospital. All patients who receive epinephrine for food-induced anaphylaxis should proceed to an emergency facility for observation and additional treatment if needed. A reasonable period for observation is 4–6 hours in most patients who have experienced anaphylaxis and have received epinephrine. An overnight hospital stay should be considered for patients with severe or prolonged symptoms.[8,10,16]

Long-term management in the community

Avoidance of causative foods

Patients or parents should be informed of the possibility of a subsequent allergic reaction after ingestion, contact with or inhalation of food allergens. Patients should be carefully instructed about hidden allergens, potential cross-reactions to other allergens, and situations that constitute a special hazard for those with food allergy, such as exposure to foods at school, daycare, the homes of friends or relatives and restaurants.[9,10,16]

Education for specific for FDEIA

The main strategy for the prevention of FDEIA is avoidance of the causative food allergen for up to 4 hours prior to exercise.[5,10]

Risk management plan

Prior to discharge patients should be given a written anaphylaxis emergency action plan that contains information about self-injection of epinephrine.[8] An example of an action plan is available at www.foodallergy.org.

Self-injectable adrenaline

All patients experiencing food-induced anaphylaxis should be provided directly with an epinephrine autoinjector, or with a prescription for it, and the advice to fill it immediately. Several different brands of device are available in many countries. Current worldwide availability of devices such as EpiPen, Anapen and Twinject is summarized in Table 9.9. A new device, Jext, will be available in European countries in 2011. Unfortunately, there is no self-injectable epinephrine device for infants under 15 kg body weight, but mild overdosing with self-injectable adrenaline in a young child device does not represent a major risk in otherwise healthy children. The physician should weigh the risk of severe anaphylaxis over the potential side effects of adrenaline.

Immunomodulation (oral immunotherapy for food-induced anaphylaxis)

Primary food-induced anaphylaxis could theoretically be modulated by allergen desensitization through immunotherapy, similarly to bee sting anaphylaxis. However, immunotherapy in food allergy desensitization remains experimental, and although several trials of oral tolerance induction are under way, this procedure is not yet recommended in routine clinical practice. Significantly increased thresholds to food-induced allergic reactions after oral immunotherapy were reported in almost all of those with milk and egg allergy and more than 90% of those with peanut allergy. It is likely that this increased threshold is dependent on ingestion of the food and reflects desensitization but not true tolerance. The efficacy of the immunotherapy, extent of desensitization versus tolerance, and the quantity/frequency of allergen consumption required to maintain this effect are currently unknown.[11]

Acknowledgement

The author wishes to thank Ms Chizuko Sugizaki and Dr Sakura Sato for their support in the writing of this chapter.

Table 9.9 Adrenaline auto-injector worldwide availability

Area	Country	EpiPen/Fastjekt	Anapen	Twinject
Europe	Austria	O	O	
	Germany	O	O	
	Hungary	O	O	
	Netherlands	O	O	
	Poland	O	O	
	Portugal	O	O	
	Sweden	O	O	
	Switzerland	O	O	
	Belgium	O		
	Czech Republic	O		
	Denmark	O		
	Finland	O		
	Italy	O		
	Luxemburg	O		
	Norway	O		
	Slovakia	O		
	Slovenia	O		
	Spain	O		
	UK	O		
	France		O	
	Greece		O	
North America	USA	O		O
	Canada	O		
South America	Argentina	O		
	Chile	O		
Africa and Middle East	Israel	O		
	South Africa	O		
Asia	Japan	O		
	Malaysia	O		
	Singapore	O		
	Thailand	O		
Oceania	Australia	O	O	
	New Zealand	O		

References

1. Metcalfe DD, Sampson HA, Simon RA. Food Allergy: Adverse Reactions to Foods and Food Additives. 4th ed. Blackwell Publishing, 2008.

2. Maulitz RM, Pratt DS, Schocket AL. Exercise-induced anaphylactic reaction to shellfish. J Allergy Clin Immunol 1979;63(6):433–4.

3. Sampson HA, Muñoz-Furlong A, Campbell RL, et al. Second symposium on the definition and management of anaphylaxis: summary report – Second National Institute of Allergy and Infectious Disease/Food Allergy and Anaphylaxis Network symposium. J Allergy Clin Immunol 2006;117(2):391–7.

4. Sampson HA. Anaphylaxis and emergency treatment. Pediatrics 2003;111(6 Pt 3):1601–8.

5. Du Toit G. Food-dependent exercise-induced anaphylaxis in childhood. Pediatr Allergy Immunol 2007;18(5):455–63.

6. Aihara Y, Takahashi Y, Kotoyori T, et al. Frequency of food-dependent, exercise-induced anaphylaxis in Japanese junior-high-school students. J Allergy Clin Immunol 2001;108(6):1035–9.

7. Aihara Y. [Food-dependent exercise-induced anaphylaxis]. Arerugi 2007;56(5):451–6.

8. Simons FE. Anaphylaxis: Recent advances in assessment and treatment. J Allergy Clin Immunol 2009; 124(4):625–36; quiz 637–8.

9. Sicherer SH, Sampson HA. Food allergy. J Allergy Clin Immunol 2010;125(2 Suppl. 2):S116–25.

10. Ebisawa M. Management of food allergy in Japan 'food allergy management guideline 2008 (revision from 2005)' and 'guidelines for the treatment of allergic diseases in schools'. Allergol Int 2009; 58(4):475–83.

11. Ben-Shoshan M, Clarke AE. Anaphylaxis: past, present and future. Allergy 2011;66(1):1–14.

12. Inomata N, Osuna H, Ikezawa Z. Late-onset anaphylaxis to Bacillus natto-fermented soybeans (natto). J Allergy Clin Immunol 2004;113(5): 998–1000.

13. Commins SP, Satinover SM, Hosen J, et al. Delayed anaphylaxis, angioedema, or urticaria after consumption of red meat in patients with IgE antibodies specific for galactose-alpha-1,3-galactose. J Allergy Clin Immunol 2009;123(2):426–33.

14. Matsuo H, Dahlström J, Tanaka A, et al. Sensitivity and specificity of recombinant omega-5 gliadin-specific IgE measurement for the diagnosis of wheat-dependent exercise-induced anaphylaxis. Allergy 2008; 63(2):233–6.

15. Shirai T, Matsui T, Uto T, et al. Nonsteroidal anti-inflammatory drugs enhance allergic reactions in a patient with wheat-induced anaphylaxis. Allergy 2003;58(10):1071.

16. Muraro A, Roberts G, Clark A, et al. The management of anaphylaxis in childhood: position paper of the European academy of allergology and clinical immunology. Allergy 2007; 62(8):857–71.

CHAPTER 10

Eosinophilic Gastroenteropathies (Eosinophilic Esophagitis, Eosinophilic Gastroenteritis and Eosinophilic Colitis)

Dan Atkins and Glenn T. Furuta

KEY CONCEPTS

- Mucosal eosinophilia is an increasingly common diagnostic finding that must be interpreted in the appropriate clinical context.

- Eosinophilic esophagitis (EoE) is a clinicopathological disease characterized by reflux-like symptoms, feeding difficulties, food impaction and dysphagia in the setting of dense esophageal eosinophilia (>15 eosinophils/hpf).

- Pathophysiological mechanisms of EoE relate to the food/environmental induction of epithelial eotaxin-3

- overexpression, which leads to chronic inflammation with a predominant mucosal eosinophilia.

- Treatment of EoE is directed at either nutritional exclusion of suspected food allergens or the application of topical steroid to the esophageal mucosa.

- Eosinophilic gastroenteritis can affect the mucosa, muscular or serosal layers of the gastrointestinal tract.

Eosinophilic gastrointestinal diseases (EGIDs)

The emergence of eosinophilic esophagitis as an increasingly encountered entity among allergists and gastroenterologists has generated a renewed interest in the role of eosinophils, not only in the esophagus where they are normally absent, but also in other areas of the gastrointestinal tract, including the stomach and small and large intestine, where they normally reside in benign numbers. Gastroenterologists encounter eosinophilic gastrointestinal diseases (EGIDs) as a result of the endoscopic evaluation of patients presenting with a variety of common gastrointestinal complaints, whereas the allergist often sees them as they present to discern whether food allergies are the cause of their discomfort. EGIDs have significantly increased the interplay between gastroenterologists and allergists,

as eosinophils are often considered the harbinger of allergic disease and an increasing body of clinical and research evidence suggests that many of these patients are indeed allergic.[1]

To date, the exact clinicopathological features that define EGIDs remain under deliberation.[2] Because eosinophils are normal inhabitants of the GI tract other than the esophagus, the definition of what constitutes normal or abnormal is contingent upon a number of different factors[3–6] (Table 10.1). When the degree of eosinophilic infiltrate is deemed excessive, the relevance of this finding must be interpreted in the clinical context of why the biopsy was obtained, as mucosal eosinophilia can be associated with a number of different diseases, including inflammatory bowel diseases, infections and allergic inflammatory responses.

When other diseases associated with mucosal eosinophilia have been excluded, the diagnosis of EGIDs is assigned. EGIDs can be subdivided

Table 10.1 Etiologies for intestinal eosinophilia

Esophagus	Small intestine and colon
Gastroesophageal reflux disease	Food hypersensitivity
Eosinophilic esophagitis	Eosinophilic gastroenteritis
Eosinophilic gastroenteritis	Inflammatory bowel disease
Crohn's disease	Celiac disease
Connective tissue disease	Infectious: *Ancylostoma duodenale*, anisakiasis, basidiobolomycosis, *Enterobius*
Hypereosinophilic syndrome	*vermicularis*, *Helicobacter pylori*, schistosomiasis, *Toxocara canis*,
Infectious: *Candida*, herpes virus	Malignancy
Drug hypersensitivity response	Churg–Strauss syndrome
	Systemic lupus erythematosus

Table 10.2 Symptoms associated with eosinophilic esophagitis

Children	Adolescent and adult
Abdominal pain	Dysphagia
Feeding difficulty	Reflux symptoms unresponsive to medical/
Reflux symptoms unresponsive to medical/surgical management	surgical management
Esophageal food or foreign body impaction	Esophageal food or foreign body impaction

according to the area of the GI tract involved. Eosinophilic esophagitis affects only the esophagus, whereas eosinophilic colitis affects only the colon and eosinophilic gastroenteritis can affect multiple parts of the GI tract. These distinctions are important, as pathophysiological mechanisms, natural history and therapeutic interventions can differ between EGIDs. This chapter will focus on clinical features, the role of allergy and therapeutic interventions for EGIDs, with a special emphasis on the most common EGID, eosinophilic esophagitis (EoE).

Eosinophilic esophagitis

Clinical features/diagnosis

Originally a clinical curiosity, increasing clinical experience and research studies have transformed eosinophilic esophagitis (EoE) into a well-characterized clinicopathological entity.[7] Multidisciplinary diagnostic and therapeutic recommendations for EoE were developed at the First International Gastrointestinal Eosinophil Research Symposium at Orlando, Florida, in October 2006 (www.naspghan.org for slide set of program). At the time of this process, EoE was characterized as a clinicopathological disease requiring symptoms and isolated esophageal eosinophilia manifested

by a minimum of 15 intraepithelial eosinophils in the most densely involved high-power microscopic field (400×). Because of its significant prevalence, gastroesophageal reflux disease (GERD) should be ruled out as a potential cause for esophageal eosinophilia with either a trial of proton pump inhibition or pH/impedance monitoring of the distal esophagus before the diagnosis of EoE is made.[8,9]

A number of different names have been associated with eosinophilic esophagitis, including eosinophilic oesophagitis, primary eosinophilic esophagitis, allergic eosinophilic esophagitis and idiopathic eosinophilic esophagitis. Although some still refer to eosinophilic esophagitis as EE, EoE has been increasingly used by gastroenterologists to avoid confusion because of the historical use of EE to refer to erosive esophagitis. As a result, EoE will be used here.

EoE in children has several different patterns of clinical presentation (Table 10.2). Infants or toddlers may present with feeding difficulties,[10–14] which may manifest as feeding refusal or problems with advancing the diet to include a broader array of new textures (see Clinical Case 1). Other children may complain of GERD-like symptoms unresponsive to acid blockade.[14–16] Symptoms can include vomiting, regurgitation, waterbrash, epigastric abdominal pain, heartburn or chest pain. Older children, teenagers and adults may develop intermittent or chronic dysphagia or present acutely with food impaction.

CLINICAL CASE 1

AT is a 3-year-old boy brought for evaluation of inadequate growth. His mother reports that he had gastroesophageal reflux as an infant that resolved at 1 year of age, but since then he has been difficult to feed. Initially, he would put food in his mouth but not swallow it. More recently, he has refused to eat most foods and prefers only soft foods and liquids. His pediatrician reports that over the last 6 months his weight has dropped from the 35th percentile to the 10th. His physical examination is unremarkable except for eczema. Initial laboratory testing is normal. Nutritional evaluation reveals that he is not meeting his caloric needs. Two months of taking lansoprazole did not alter his growth pattern or eating preferences. An upper endoscopy revealed white exudates on his esophageal mucosa, and 33 eosinophils/hpf in the esophageal epithelia with normal gastric and duodenal biopsies. Serum food-specific IgE levels and skin prick tests to foods he was eating revealed sensitization to wheat and eggs, so these foods were removed from his diet. He was evaluated and treated by a feeding specialist. Over the course of the next 6 months, his appetite and eating behaviors normalized and his weight began to follow the 30th percentile.

Toddlers with EoE may present with feeding difficulties and behaviors that at a minimum lead to family unrest at mealtimes and in some circumstances result in growth disturbances. Even after inflammation has resolved as a result of appropriate elimination diets and/or other therapies, feeding dysfunction can persist and may require the expertise of a feeding specialist.

The most common presentation of recalcitrant GERD-like symptoms was first documented through a unique collaboration between allergists and gastroenterologists over 15 years ago, when Kelly and colleagues reported 10 patients with severe GERD, six of whom remained symptomatic despite fundoplication.[17] These patients developed clinicopathological remission when placed on an elemental formula and symptoms returned upon food challenge. Orenstein's[18] detailed analysis of 30 children with esophageal eosinophilia identified vomiting, abdominal pain and dysphagia as the most common associated symptoms. Over 60% of the patients had concomitant asthma, recurrent upper respiratory illnesses and pneumonias, suggesting an association of EoE with other allergic and/or airway diseases. Liacouras et al.[15] described their findings in one of the largest pediatric series of 381 children with EoE, of whom over 300 had

GERD-like symptoms while 69 presented with dysphagia.

EoE also commonly presents with an isolated esophageal food impaction that is thought to occur secondary to either a fixed anatomical stricture or intermittent esophageal spasm[19-24] (see Clinical Case 2). Studies in both adults and children have documented that EoE is a common etiology for esophageal food impaction. For instance, Desai[19] reported that 17 of 31 adult patients presenting with an acute esophageal food impaction had > 20 eosinophils per hpf.

Recalcitrant GERD-like symptoms, dysphagia and food impaction, especially when encountered in patients with other atopic diseases, should raise the suspicion for EoE (see Clinical Case 3).

CLINICAL CASE 2

TL is a 15-year-old boy who was seen in the emergency room for food impaction. He had been on a hunting trip in the mountains when he ate turkey jerky that became lodged in his esophagus, preventing him from being able to swallow his saliva. He did not experience respiratory distress. A detailed history of his eating habits revealed that he always drank three to four glasses of water during meals to wash his food down. Typically he avoided meats because they were difficult to swallow, but he enjoyed eating jerky, particularly while hunting. Endoscopic analysis revealed that his proximal esophagus was obstructed by a food bolus that was removed. Distal to the bolus an esophageal stricture was identified and mucosal biopsies were obtained that revealed >15 eosinophils/hpf in the squamous epithelium. He was started on omeprazole 2 mg/kg/day and returned for esophageal dilation. Mucosal eosinophilia persisted and he was treated with topical fluticasone (220 μg) two puffs sprayed into the back of his throat and swallowed twice a day, without brushing his teeth or eating or drinking for 30 minutes afterward. He declined food allergy testing and was symptom free on swallowed fluticasone alone.

The long-term use of complex coping behaviors related to eating is surprisingly common in adolescents with EoE, for example avoiding densely textured foods such as meats, eating slower than others, using sauces as lubricants, and drinking large amounts of liquids during meals. In these patients an acute presentation with food impaction is unpredictable, often leading to diagnostic and therapeutic endoscopy and esophageal dilation. Proximal esophageal strictures are highly unusual and can result from caustic ingestions, surgical procedures, congenital anomalies or EoE. Not all food impactions are related to esophageal strictures: some patients may have a non-obstructive mucosa where the impaction is thought to result from transient esophageal contractions. Whether the inciting foods are the allergic trigger for these presentations is unknown.

CLINICAL CASE 3

HE is an 18-year-old boy with a 4-year history of dysphagia and heartburn. Use of over-the-counter antacid treatments did not provide adequate relief of his symptoms. Over the course of the last year his dysphagia has increased to the point that he was unable to swallow solid foods without pounding on his chest and drinking copious amounts of liquids. This led to social embarrassment, and he frequently eats alone because it takes him so long to complete a meal. He also has mild eczema and allergic rhinitis. When he takes fluticasone for his asthma and allergic rhinitis, his swallowing improves slightly. Endoscopic analysis when he is not taking any topical steroid preparations reveals 51 eosinophils/hpf and a pH/impedance monitoring study of his distal esophagus is normal. A diagnosis of EoE was made and subsequent food allergy testing revealed positive skin tests to cows' milk and soy. Upon elimination of these foods his symptoms resolved, and re-examination of his esophageal mucosa revealed complete resolution of inflammation.

This case illustrates a number of clinical clues for the diagnosis of EoE. EoE is more common in boys, with over 75% of patients being male. A long-standing history of dysphagia, especially in a patient with an atopic background, is often found. Partial clinical responses to topical steroids used for treatment of asthma and allergic rhinitis also support further evaluation because a portion of these preparations are swallowed and may inadvertently reduce esophageal inflammation. Since gastroesophageal reflux is more common than EoE, and can present with a similar clinical and histological pattern, GERD should be ruled out in all patients in whom EoE is considered. Skin testing can reveal food sensitivities that often identify the allergen(s) inciting EoE.

Epidemiology

Over 75% of patients with EoE are male. EoE occurs at any age without obvious predilection, and has been reported on all continents except Africa. Noel estimated a disease incidence of ~1 : 10 000 children per year in Ohio, USA, and Straumann estimated an increase from 2 to 27 per 100 000 adults in Olten, Switzerland.[25,26]

Pathophysiology

Basic studies provide a link between fibrotic cascades and eosinophil-derived mediators. Eosinophils contain mediators capable of both inducing fibrotic molecules such as TGF-β and stimulating tissue contraction such as major basic protein. Aceves[27] provided translational evidence supportive of a fibrotic pattern in affected children. In this study, five patients with EoE and evidence of fibrosis were compared to two with non-fibrotic EoE, seven with GERD and seven normal patients. Patients with fibrotic EoE showed increased subepithelial fibrosis, TGF-β, VCAM-1 and phospho-SMAD2/3 expression compared to GERD and normal control patients. During a 14-year follow-up in adult patients with EoE, esophageal cancer has not been reported.[28]

Patterns of genetic influence on EoE are emerging. Zink[29] reported 17 patients from seven families with dysphagia and gastrointestinal eosinophilia. Of these, 12 patients spanning two generations were shown to have EoE. Patel[30] described three brothers with intermittent dysphagia and 20–40 eosinophils per hpf in the esophageal epithelium. In a case report, Meyers[31] documented an 80-year-old man and his 52-year-old daughter who both had dysphagia and >40 esophageal eosinophils/hpf. Thus, increasing clinical experience and case descriptions suggest a familial pattern and genetic predisposition.

Blanchard[32] hypothesized that a genetic profile existed for patients with EoE. Microarray analysis of esophageal tissues from patients with EoE and GERD identified a unique EoE gene signature, with the most upregulated gene being eotaxin-3. Eotaxin-3 levels correlated with mucosal eosinophilia and a single nucleotide polymorphism suggested susceptibility to EoE. The results of this study, and that of Mishra, emphasize the potential for novel therapeutic targets such as CCR-3 receptor or IL-5 antagonist, for selected patients with EoE.[33,34] Using gene array analysis, recent studies determined the potential role of filaggrin, mast cells and thymic stromal lymphopoetin in the pathogenesis of EoE.[35–37]

The esophageal mucosa affected by EoE has undergone further molecular characterization. Straumann[38,39] determined that the esophageal eosinophils from EoE patients expressed increased IL-4 and IL-13 compared to normal controls, and Gupta[40] found that esophageal mRNA expression in 11 patients with EoE expressed more IFN-γ, eotaxin-1 and IL-5 than in normal children. Initial reports have been followed by a number of studies to determine the impact of these and other cytokines, including IL-13 and IL-15.[41–43]

Radiology

Interestingly some of the first EoE reports originated in the radiology literature (Table 10.3). Picus[44] described a 16-year-old boy with increasing

Table 10.3 Radiological signs observed in EoE

Strictures: proximal, middle and/or distal
Longitudinal narrowing
Small caliber esophagus
Esophageal polyp or diverticulum
Concentric rings
Schatzki ring

Table 10.5 Histological features of EoE

Mucosal eosinophilia and degranulation
Eosinophil microabscesses
Superficial accumulation of eosinophils
Basal zone hyperplasia
Lymphocytosis
Mast cell accumulation

Table 10.4 Endoscopic findings seen in EoE

White exudates
Esophageal strictures
Concentric rings, trachealization, feline esophagus
Vertical lines of the esophageal mucosa
Crepe paper mucosa/linear shearing of mucosa

dysphagia, proximal esophageal narrowing, esophageal eosinophilia and peripheral eosinophilia who underwent remission when treated with systemic corticosteroids. Feczko[45] described three adults with dysphagia, allergic diseases, proximal esophageal strictures and eosinophilic esophageal inflammation that required both dilation and corticosteroid treatments. Nurko[46] reported the association of Schatzki ring and EoE in a 12-year retrospective review. Of 18 children with Schatzki ring, eight were found to have clinicopathological features consistent with EoE. Thus, any esophageal narrowing, especially proximal esophageal strictures, should raise suspicion for the diagnosis of EoE (see Case 2).

Endoscopy

Although the early literature suggests that endoscopic appearances may be normal in EoE, increased recognition of the disease documents a number of mucosal findings, including concentric ring formation (trachealization); longitudinal linear furrows or vertical lines on the esophageal mucosa; patches of small, white papules on the esophageal surface; and esophageal strictures (Table 10.4). Whitish granular patterns on the mucosa were traditionally thought to be associated only with *Candida* infection, but this finding is now also recognized as evidence of eosinophilic inflammation. Sundaram[47] reported that the esophageal epithelium of 13 children with EoE had white specks representing

an underlying epithelium containing 25–100 eosinophils per hpf without fungal elements. In a later report, Straumann,[48] in an analysis of 30 adults with EoE, showed that white exudates were consistent with eosinophilic inflammation. In contrast, Ngo[49] reported a child with clinicopathological features of EoE, including white exudates and large numbers of eosinophils in the squamous epithelium, who responded to proton pump inhibition. Thus, if white material is reported on the esophageal mucosa, peptic disease, *Candida* infection and EoE should be diagnostic considerations.

Histology

It is unusual that the number of a specific cell type is critical to the diagnosis of an inflammatory disease (Table 10.5). To date, the diagnosis of EoE rests on the finding of a dense eosinophilic inflammation of the esophageal epithelium in the proper clinical setting.[3] The ideal density has been the subject of much discussion and consists of a threshold ranging from 15 to 24 eosinophils per hpf. Variables affecting this number include size of the high-power field, characterization of the eosinophils observed, and the number of high-power fields considered.[50,51]

Another finding supporting a diagnosis of EoE is eosinophil activation as evidenced by degranulation. Mueller[52,53] reported that specific staining for eosinophil granule-derived major basic protein (MBP) significantly enhanced eosinophil visualization in adults with EoE. Desai[19] showed that extracellular MBP deposition significantly distinguished adults with EoE from those with GERD. Protheroe[54] demonstrated the impact of a novel scoring system that used antibody staining for eosinophil peroxidase (EPX) in the analysis of the epithelia in EoE. In this study, EPX scoring was able to separate patients with EoE from those with GERD and normal controls to a significant degree. Similar findings were reported in another recent study.[55] Despite these studies, it is important to note that eosinophil degranulation can occur during biopsy procurement and processing. Lymphocytic inflammation occurs more significantly in EoE patients than in those with GERD. In addition, mast cell infiltration and activation is more common in EoE than in patients with GERD.

To date, the only documented long-term complication associated with EoE is isolated or long segment esophageal narrowing. Adult and pediatric reports have identified evidence of tissue remodeling in the form of proximal and distal esophageal strictures. Typically, symptoms in these patients date back to childhood, suggesting that the development of lesions requires decades of persistent or intermittent inflammation.

Role of allergy

Allergic manifestations

Several lines of indirect and direct evidence support a likely role for allergic inflammation in EoE. Eosinophils are commonly observed in the mucosal surfaces in asthma, allergic rhinitis and eczema. An increasing number of studies associate EoE with comorbid IgE-mediated allergic disease such as food allergy, eczema, allergic rhinitis and asthma, including two that demonstrate the potential role of aeroallergens in EoE. In line with the findings of genome-wide association studies (GWAS), a family history of EoE in affected children is not uncommon.

The direct application of foods to the esophageal mucosa, along with an increasing amount of clinical experience and research, supports a causative role for food allergy in EoE. Food allergies coexist in up to 73% of children with EoE. Food allergens including milk, egg, wheat, soy, peanuts, beans, rye and beef are most often identified during skin testing, but a number of other foods may play a role as well. In addition, allergic sensitization to more than one food occurs frequently. When examining compiled case series of 786 EoE patients in whom larger panels of food skin tests were applied, the mean number of identified food allergens varied from 2.7 ± 3.3 to 6 ± 4.2. In adults, patterns may differ both in range of sensitization and patterns of suspected foods, perhaps reflecting cross-reactivity among foods and inhaled pollen allergens, a common finding in patients with EoE. Case reports have correlated pollen skin test results and seasonal changes in symptoms and numbers of mucosal esophageal eosinophils. Thus, pollen sensitization could potentially promote esophageal mucosal eosinophilia either through direct exposure to pollen swallowed after inhalation during the pollen season or by the ingestion of plant-derived foods that contain cross-reacting allergens. For example, a ragweed-allergic EoE patient could potentially experience an increase in symptoms in the fall during the ragweed pollen season, or after ingesting bananas or melons that contain allergens cross-reacting with those found in ragweed pollen.

Immune mechanisms underlying food allergic reactions are categorized as IgE-mediated, non-IgE-mediated or combined. IgE-mediated food allergies occur when a genetically predisposed host is exposed to a food leading to the generation of allergen-specific IgE. This IgE binds to and occupies high-affinity IgE receptors on mast cell and basophil cell surface membranes, resulting in sensitization. Upon re-exposure to this food, cell surface allergen-specific IgE molecules cross-link, thereby bridging their high-affinity receptors with subsequent release of preformed and newly synthesized mediators, some of which are eosinophil chemoattractants. Translational studies support the presence of increased IgE-bearing mast cells in the epithelia of patients with EoE, but in addition to IgE-mediated responses, non-IgE-mediated immune mechanisms are also considered to be involved in the pathophysiology of EoE. Careful histories for symptoms suggestive of IgE-mediated reactions should be taken, as EoE patients may have comorbid IgE-mediated reactions to foods; discussions focusing on avoidance of these foods and treatment of anaphylactic reactions resulting from accidental exposure are warranted.

Typically, non-IgE-mediated reactions coordinated by Th2 lymphocytes are slower in onset, evolve over hours to days, and can result in mucosal eosinophil accumulation. This delay in symptom onset complicates accurate identification of offending foods in non-IgE-mediated food allergy. EoE symptoms are often consistent with those seen in non-IgE-mediated reactions in that they are localized to the gastrointestinal tract and can be delayed rather than immediate in onset.

Because EoE is considered a combined disorder involving both IgE- and non-IgE-mediated immune mechanisms, suggested methods to document sensitization to foods after obtaining a thorough history include skin prick testing, measurement of serum food allergen-specific IgE antibodies and atopy patch testing. Skin prick testing is essentially a bioassay performed by introducing minute amounts of allergen into the epidermis and monitoring for a localized cutaneous allergic reaction. If mast cells in the patient's skin have IgE on their surface specific for the allergen being tested, binding to these IgE antibodies by the allergen triggers mast cell degranulation, accompanied by histamine release and mediator generation resulting in the rapid formation of a cutaneous wheal surrounded by an erythematous flare. In the absence of IgE specific for the allergen, no reaction occurs. Glycerinated commercial food extracts are widely available for skin testing to many common food allergens. In addition, fresh food extracts, prepared by crushing the food in an aliquot of saline, are occasionally used.[56] Alternatively, the 'prick-to-prick' technique, which involves pricking a food such as a fruit or vegetable with the skin test device, followed immediately by pricking the patient's skin, can be used.[57] Fresh extract testing can be useful when testing for sensitivity to fruits or vegetables containing labile allergens susceptible to degradation during the extraction process used in the preparation of commercial extracts, or when a commercial extract of the suspected food is unavailable. The potential for irritant reactions can be ruled out when necessary by skin testing others not sensitive to the food using the same extract. After pricking the skin of the back or arm with a disposable bifurcated skin test device that introduces a small amount of allergen, any resultant wheal and erythema observed at the site after approximately 15 minutes is recorded. A histamine skin test is applied as a positive control with a saline skin test serving as the negative control. A skin test is considered positive if a wheal 3 mm larger than the negative control is observed. Skin testing to all or at least the majority of foods in the patient's diet is encouraged when evaluating patients with EoE to ensure that all foods to which the patient could potentially react have been identified. In addition, skin testing to environmental allergens is beneficial because of the potential for aeroallergens to affect esophageal inflammation, either through direct exposure or through cross-reactivity with certain plant-derived foods in the diet. Benefits of skin testing include the relatively low cost, immediate results, and the relatively high negative predictive accuracy. However, commercial food extracts and fresh food extracts are not standardized. In addition, the positive predictive accuracy of skin testing is considered to be relatively low, meaning that some patients with a positive skin test are sensitized but not allergic, and would not react clinically upon exposure to the food. Alternatively, given that exposure to the esophageal mucosa occurs as the food is swallowed, without further digestion or processing, topical reactions observed in skin testing might theoretically be more predictive of reactions in EoE than in classic food allergy. These considerations occasionally increase the difficulty of interpreting skin test results in patients with EoE. The positive and negative predictive accuracies of skin testing to selected foods in patients with EoE has been reported by Spergel.[58]

In addition to skin testing, the level of serum food-specific IgE can be measured to document IgE-mediated sensitivity to a particular food. These assays are useful when medications that affect skin testing cannot be discontinued or when widespread skin disease is present, precluding the use of skin testing. Measuring serum food-specific IgE levels to a particular food longitudinally may provide evidence that sensitization to a food is increasing or waning. In classic IgE-mediated food allergy clinical studies have identified serum food-specific IgE levels to selected common food allergens above which most patients would react.[59] Studies to determine corresponding IgE levels for selected foods in populations of patients with EoE have not been performed.

In an effort to identify a test that might predict non-IgE-mediated reactions, the use of the atopy patch test (APT) in the evaluation of patients with EoE has been explored.[58,59] The APT is performed by applying the intact food allergen to non-inflamed skin on the back under occlusion in a small aluminum cup. After 48 hours the patch test is removed and the resulting reaction is assessed and recorded, initially at 20 minutes and again at 24 hours after patch removal. The reactions are graded based on the degree of erythema and the presence of papules or vesicles. Although side effects are uncommon, irritant reactions and contact urticaria have been reported.[60] Other aspects that have hindered widespread use of the APT include lack of standardization of the procedure, including standardized reagents, in addition to the time and expertise required for the accurate performance of the test.[60] However, Spergel and others[58] have reported success using a combination of skin prick testing and atopy patch testing to identify foods best eliminated from the diet, as evidenced by improvement in patients placed on diets based on the results of this approach.

The most supportive evidence for a role for food allergy in EoE arises from the multiple observations and clinical studies that demonstrate clinicopathological improvement of EoE following the use of several types of elimination diets. Diets in which the six most common food allergens are excluded (dairy products, egg, wheat, soy, peanuts, fish/shellfish) lead to a clinicopathological response in 74% of patients. Elimination diets based on both skin prick testing and atopy patch testing results were effective in the majority of children with EoE. The use of elemental diets, consisting of amino acid-based formulas, led to the resolution of symptoms and mucosal eosinophilia in more than 95% of children with EoE. In spite of these successes, nutritional management in adults and older children poses challenges with compliance and the impact on their quality of life.

Because of the association of allergic diseases with EoE and that allergens probably play a role in the pathogenesis of EoE, a thorough history and assessment of comorbid allergic diseases is an important part of the care of patients. Allergy consultation is indicated not only to aid in identifying, characterizing and treating comorbid allergic disease, but also to identify food and environmental allergens that may contribute to esophageal inflammation.

Treatment/management

Although symptom reduction/resolution remains a clear therapeutic endpoint, the clinical decision making with regard to mucosal eosinophilia remains controversial.[61] In practice, clinicians are wary of performing repeated endoscopies as it is not certain that persistent eosinophilia has untoward consequences. Alternatively, others are concerned that unresolved eosinophilia will lead to esophageal strictures and therefore must be repeatedly assessed. Future research is needed to clarify this issue.

Effective and safe therapeutic approaches to the treatment of EoE include corticosteroids and nutritional management.

Nutritional management

The rationale for using nutritional management in EoE is based on the research that supports a role for food allergens in esophageal eosinophilic inflammation. In this regard, a number of studies support the use of elemental formulas and elimination of specific foods in EoE treatment. Kelly[17] reported the successful use of an amino acid-based diet in the treatment of EoE. Ten children were treated for 10 weeks: all underwent clinicopathological remission and redeveloped symptoms when the diet was extensively liberalized. Two other studies with larger patient cohorts showed that more than 92% of children were treated successfully with this approach.[62–64] Poor compliance has led to the use of feeding tubes, and some children may have behavioral issues associated with this form of treatment.

Corticosteroids

Corticosteroids are effective in resolving the clinicopathological features in most patients with EoE. Mechanisms of action for eosinophilic inflammation include induction of eosinophil apoptosis, downregulation of chemotactic factors and inhibition of proinflammatory mediator synthesis and release. A limited number of patients require systemic corticosteroids, but most can be treated with an alternative preparation delivered from a metered-dose inhaler (MDI) that allows the medication to be swallowed and thereby deliver a topical application to the esophageal mucosa. It is thought that this technique limits systemic circulation of steroids because of reduced absorption and first pass metabolism.

Liacouras[65] reported the impact of systemic corticosteroids in 20 of 21 children who experienced a significant reduction of symptoms within 7 days. Faubion[66] reported the first use of a metered-dose inhaler of fluticasone for children with EoE in the hope of limiting steroid exposure. This novel method reported the successful impact of spraying fluticasone from an MDI into the mouth without inhaling and without the use of a spacer in four children with EoE. The study used fluticasone propionate (up to 880 µg/day) or beclomethasone twice a day. Since then, a number of other studies have demonstrated a positive impact of this approach on clinicopathological features of EoE.[67,68] Konikoff performed a randomized double-blind placebo-controlled study comparing fluticasone to placebo in 36 pediatric patients.[69] Twice-daily dosing for 3 months induced remission in 50% of the fluticasone group. When MDIs are used, patients should spray the MDI in their mouth with their lips sealed around the device and not eat, drink or rinse for 30 minutes afterward, in an effort to prevent loss of the delivered dose. An alternative method of topical steroid delivery has been recently developed. Aceves[70,71] prepared a viscous mixture of budesonide with sucralose, also termed oral viscous budesonide (OVB). Both retrospective and prospective studies have shown that children undergo successful clinicopathological remission with OVB. Corticosteroids resolve acute clinicopathological features of EoE, but when discontinued, EoE recurs. Side effects reported to date include dry mouth, cataracts and esophageal candidiasis.

Others

The use of leukotriene receptor antagonists and mast cell inhibitors has been reported in small series but not shown to be effective at pharmacological doses.[72] Biologicals, including anti-IL-5 antibodies, have undergone recent study. The rationale for using these agents relates to basic studies revealing a key role for IL-5 in mucosal esophageal eosinophilia. Studies to date demonstrate a significant impact on mucosal eosinophilia and a trend toward symptom improvement.[73]

Eosinophilic gastroenteritis

Eosinophilic gastroenteritis (EOG) represents a heterogeneous group of rare disorders characterized by various intestinal symptoms and gastrointestinal eosinophilia.[74] Other reasons for intestinal eosinophilia must be excluded before a diagnosis of EOG can be made.[2] Traditional classification grouped diseases into three categories, mucosal, muscular and serosal,[75] providing a clinical and pathophysiological paradigm for patients with these diseases. Patients with mucosal disease typically have symptoms including nondescript abdominal pain, vomiting, and non-bloody, watery diarrhea. Symptoms can be quite minor compared to the associated significantly abnormal laboratory findings. In some circumstances patients may present with severe anemia and/or hypoalbuminemia, alone or in combination with mild gastrointestinal complaints. Peripheral eosinophilia is an inconsistent finding, but other causes, such as hypereosinophilic syndrome or malignancy, should be ruled out. Radiological findings include polyps,

mucosal edema and ulcers. Endoscopic evaluation can reveal all of these findings or may appear normal, but histological analysis reveals dense eosinophilia in the lamina propria (see Clinical Case 4).

CLINICAL CASE 4

LH is an 8-year-old girl with chronic diarrhea and abdominal pain. She has grown well but frequently develops cramping, diffuse abdominal pain that is relieved with the passage of mucousy stools. Symptoms were reportedly associated with egg ingestion. She had no coincident systemic symptoms such as joint pain or fevers, but she had a long-standing history of asthma and eczema. Further investigations revealed mild peripheral eosinophilia and flocculation of the small bowel on upper gastrointestinal series. At endoscopy, her upper and lower intestinal mucosa appeared normal but histopathology revealed dense eosinophilia of the lamina propria of the duodenal mucosa. Skin testing to foods in her diet was negative, but the removal of eggs from her diet led to a reduction in her symptoms.

As with EoE, children with other EGIDs may present with common symptoms and thus escape diagnosis for years. The ingestion of certain foods may trigger symptoms in some patients but not all, and the use of topical steroids or other anti-inflammatory medications may be necessary. Follow-up of patients with lower tract EGIDs is critical, as some have later been discovered to have inflammatory bowel diseases.

When eosinophilia affects the muscular layer, symptoms associated with obstruction, such as vomiting and bloating, predominate. These patients are particularly difficult to diagnose as they may have normal mucosal biopsies; deeper biopsies procured at surgery demonstrated eosinophilia of the muscularis. Thus, in a patient with peripheral eosinophilia, a history of allergic diseases, no other identifiable causes for gastrointestinal symptoms and intestinal thickening on radiological imaging, along with a response to corticosteroids or dietary elimination, a provisional diagnosis can be made.

Serosal eosinophilic gastroenteritis is extremely rare, presenting with abdominal bloating and a fluid wave on physical examination. A peritoneal tap of the ascitic fluid reveals eosinophilia.

Pathophysiological mechanisms of eosinophilic gastroenteritis are still poorly defined. A number of translational studies have provided immunohistochemical descriptions. For instance, mucosal biopsies from these patients demonstrate deposition of eosinophil granule proteins and increased expression of IL-5. Chehade[76] demonstrated increased mast cells in the small intestine of children with severe protein-losing enteropathy and eosinophilic gastroenteritis. Murine studies identified roles for eotaxin-1 and Th2 lymphocytes in the pathogenesis of eosinophilic inflammation.[77]

Standardized criteria defining the histological features of eosinophilic gastroenteritis are lacking. Two studies have documented normal values for mucosal eosinophils, but no diagnostic guidelines exist.[5,6] Corticosteroids are the primary medical treatment for eosinophilic gastroenteritis, but controlled trials have not yet been performed. Topical steroids may be beneficial in small intestinal disease. Ketotifen, cromolyn and montelukast have been reported to be helpful in isolated case reports. The utility of food elimination diets in treating patients with eosinophilic gastroenteritis is unknown but may benefit some patients, especially younger patients who have abnormal skin testing for food allergens.

Eosinophilic colitis

Eosinophilic colitis can be categorized in a variety of different ways. For instance, allergic proctitis is a self-limited inflammatory disease presenting during infancy as blood-streaked stools in an otherwise healthy infant. The colonic mucosa contains increased eosinophils in the lamina propria without evidence of chronic changes. Milk proteins (cows', soy or breast milk) are the usual offending agents, and upon their removal the blood loss stops. On the other hand, inflammatory bowel diseases, Crohn's disease and ulcerative colitis are chronic inflammatory diseases that are manifest by abdominal pain, bloody stools, diarrhea, and in some circumstances malnutrition. Mucosal inflammation is characterized by neutrophilic inflammation with crypt abscesses and chronic inflammation of the lamina propria. Eosinophils are increased in the mucosa but are not the predominant cell type. Patients require immunosuppression with corticosteroids or other agents to induce remission. Finally, eosinophilic colitis is a somewhat vague term describing a histological finding that can occur in a number of different clinical settings. As a histological finding, eosinophilic inflammation of the colonic mucosa is characterized by a predominance of eosinophils in the lamina propria without chronic features. This can be associated with food allergies, autoimmune diseases, immunodeficiencies, drug hypersensitivity reactions, infections and eosinophilic gastrointestinal diseases. Thus, this histological finding must be interpreted in the clinical context in which it was obtained.

Summary

Allergists in practice are increasingly encountering eosinophilic gastrointestinal diseases. Although much information has been obtained over the last decade regarding eosinophilic esophagitis, eosinophilic inflammation of the remainder of the GI tract has remained relatively understudied. Despite the fact that diagnostic features of EoE are now better recognized, specifics of the allergic evaluation and treatment paradigms remain to be elucidated. Longitudinal multicentered studies involving a number of subspecialists such as pediatric and adult gastroenterologists, allergists, pathologists and radiologists will be critical to providing answers that will ultimately lead to cures and improve the quality of life of patients with EGIDs.

References

1. Rothenberg ME. Eosinophilic gastrointestinal disorders (EGID). J Allergy Clin Immunol 2004 Jan;113(1):11–28, quiz.

2. Fleischer DM, Atkins D. Evaluation of the patient with suspected eosinophilic gastrointestinal disease. Immunol Allergy Clin North Am 2009 Feb;29(1):53–63.

3. Collins MH. Histopathologic features of eosinophilic esophagitis. Gastrointest Endosc Clin N Am 2008 Jan;18(1):59.

4. Collins MH. Histopathology associated with eosinophilic gastrointestinal diseases. Immunol Allergy Clin North Am 2009 Feb;29(1):109.

5. DeBrosse CW, Case JW, Putnam PE, et al. Quantity and distribution of eosinophils in the gastrointestinal tract of children. Pediatr Dev Pathol 2006 May–Jun;9(3):210–8.

6. Lowichik A, Weinberg A. A quantitative evaluation of mucosal eosinophils in the pediatric gastrointestinal tract. Mod Pathol 1996;9(2):110–14.

7. Furuta GT, Liacouras CA, Collins MH, et al. Eosinophilic esophagitis in children and adults: a systematic review and consensus recommendations for diagnosis and treatment. Gastroenterology 2007 Oct;133(4):1342–63.

8. Ngo P, Furuta GT, Antonioli DA, et al. Eosinophils in the esophagus – peptic or allergic eosinophilic esophagitis? Case series of three patients with esophageal eosinophilia. Am J Gastroenterol 2006 Jul;101(7):1666–70.

9. Rodrigo S, Abboud G, Oh D, et al. High intraepithelial eosinophil counts in esophageal squamous epithelium are not specific for eosinophilic esophagitis in adults. Am J Gastroenterol 2008 Feb;103(2):435–42.

10. Duca AP, Dantas RO, Rodrigues AA, et al. Evaluation of swallowing in children with vomiting after feeding. Dysphagia 2008 Jun;23(2):177–82.

11. Haas AM, Maune NC. Clinical presentation of feeding dysfunction in children with eosinophilic gastrointestinal disease. Immunol Allergy Clin North Am 2009 Feb;29(1):65–75.

12. Mukkada VA, Haas A, Maune NC, et al. Feeding dysfunction in children with eosinophilic gastrointestinal diseases. Pediatrics 2010 Sep;126(3): e672–7.

13. Pentiuk SP, Miller CK, Kaul A. Eosinophilic esophagitis in infants and toddlers. Dysphagia 2007 Jan;22(1):44–8.

14. Spergel JM, Brown-Whitehorn TF, Beausoleil JL, et al. 14 years of eosinophilic esophagitis: clinical features and prognosis. J Pediatr Gastroenterol Nutr 2009 Jan;48(1):30–6.

15. Liacouras CA, Spergel JM, Ruchelli E, et al. Eosinophilic esophagitis: a 10-year experience in 381 children. Clin Gastroenterol Hepatol 2005 Dec;3(12):1198–206.

16. Putnam PE. Eosinophilic esophagitis in children: clinical manifestations. Gastroenterol Clin North Am 2008 Jun;37(2):369–81.

17. Kelly KJ, Lazenby AJ, Rowe PC, et al. Eosinophilic esophagitis attributed to gastroesophageal reflux: improvement with an amino acid-based formula. Gastroenterology 1995 Nov;109(5):1503–12.

18. Orenstein SR, Shalaby TM, Di Lorenzo C, et al. The spectrum of pediatric eosinophilic esophagitis beyond infancy: a clinical series of 30 children. Am J Gastroenterol 2000 Jun;95(6):1422–30.

19. Desai TK, Stecevic V, Chang CH, et al. Association of eosinophilic inflammation with esophageal food impaction in adults. Gastrointest Endosc 2005 Jun;61(7):795–801.

20. Focht DR, Kaul A. Food impaction and eosinophilic esophagitis. J Pediatr 2005 Oct;147(4):540.

21. Luis AL, Rinon C, Encinas JL, et al. Non stenotic food impaction due to eosinophilic esophagitis: a potential surgical emergency. Eur J Pediatr Surg 2006 Dec; 16(6):399–402.

22. Nonevski IT, Downs-Kelly E, Falk GW. Eosinophilic esophagitis: an increasingly recognized cause of dysphagia, food impaction, and refractory heartburn. Cleve Clin J Med 2008 Sep;75(9):623–6, 629–33.

23. Straumann A, Bussmann C, Zuber M, et al. Eosinophilic esophagitis: analysis of food impaction and perforation in 251 adolescent and adult patients. Clin Gastroenterol Hepatol 2008 May;6(5):598–600.

24. Hurtado CW, Furuta GT, Kramer RE. Etiology of esophageal food impactions in children. J Pediatr Gastroenterol Nutr 2011 Jan;52(1):43–6.

25. Noel RJ, Putnam PE, Rothenberg ME. Eosinophilic esophagitis. N Engl J Med 2004 Aug 26;351(9):940–1.

26. Straumann A, Simon HU. Eosinophilic esophagitis: escalating epidemiology? J Allergy Clin Immunol 2005 Feb;115(2):418–9.

27. Aceves SS, Newbury RO, Dohil R, et al. Esophageal remodeling in pediatric eosinophilic esophagitis. J Allergy Clin Immunol 2007 Jan;119(1):206–12.

28. Straumann A. The natural history and complications of eosinophilic esophagitis. Gastrointest Endosc Clin N Am 2008 Jan;18(1):99–118, ix.

29. Zink DA, Amin M, Gebara S, et al. Familial dysphagia and eosinophilia. Gastrointest Endosc 2007 Feb;65(2):330–4.

30. Patel SM, Falchuk KR. Three brothers with dysphagia caused by eosinophilic esophagitis. Gastrointest Endosc 2005 Jan;61(1):165–7.

31. Meyer GW. Eosinophilic esophagitis in a father and a daughter. Gastrointest Endosc 2005 Jun;61(7):932.

32. Blanchard C, Wang N, Stringer KF, et al. Eotaxin-3 and a uniquely conserved gene-expression profile in eosinophilic esophagitis. J Clin Invest 2006 Feb 1;116(2):536–47.

33. Mishra A, Hogan SP, Brandt EB, et al. An etiological role for aeroallergens and eosinophils in experimental esophagitis. J Clin Invest 2001 Jan;107(1):83–90.

34. Mishra A, Hogan SP, Brandt EB, et al. IL-5 promotes eosinophil trafficking to the esophagus. J Immunol 2002 Mar 1;168(5):2464–9.

35. Abonia JP, Blanchard C, Butz BB, et al. Involvement of mast cells in eosinophilic esophagitis. J Allergy Clin Immunol 2010 Jul;126(1):140–9.

36. Rothenberg ME, Spergel JM, Sherrill JD, et al. Common variants at 5q22 associate with pediatric eosinophilic esophagitis. Nat Genet 2010 Apr;42(4):289–91.

37. Sherrill JD, Gao PS, Stucke EM, et al. Variants of thymic stromal lymphopoietin and its receptor associate with eosinophilic esophagitis. J Allergy Clin Immunol 2010 Jul;126(1):160–5.

38. Straumann A, Bauer M, Fischer B, et al. Idiopathic eosinophilic esophagitis is associated with a T(H)2-type allergic inflammatory response. J Allergy Clin Immunol 2001;108(6):954–61.

39. Straumann A, Kristl J, Conus S, et al. Cytokine expression in healthy and inflamed mucosa: probing the role of eosinophils in the digestive tract. Inflamm Bowel Dis 2005 Aug;11(8):720–6.

40. Gupta SK, Fitzgerald JF, Kondratyuk T, et al. Cytokine expression in normal and inflamed esophageal mucosa: a study into the pathogenesis of allergic eosinophilic esophagitis. J Pediatr Gastroenterol Nutr 2006 Jan;42(1):22–6.

41. Blanchard C, Stucke EM, Burwinkel K, et al. Coordinate interaction between IL-13 and epithelial differentiation cluster genes in eosinophilic esophagitis. J Immunol 2010 Apr 1;184(7):4033–41.

42. Zhu X, Wang M, Mavi P, et al. Interleukin-15 expression is increased in human eosinophilic esophagitis and mediates pathogenesis in mice. Gastroenterology 2010 Jul;139(1):182–93.

43. Zuo L, Fulkerson PC, Finkelman FD, et al. IL-13 induces esophageal remodeling and gene expression by an eosinophil-independent, IL-13R alpha2-inhibited pathway. J Immunol 2010 Jul 1;185(1):660–9.

44. Picus D, Frank PH. Eosinophilic esophagitis. Am J Roentgenol 1981 May;136(5):1001–3.

45. Feczko P, Halpert R, Zonca M. Radiographic abnormalities in eosinophilic esophagitis. Gastrointest Radiol 1985;10:321–4.

46. Nurko S, Teitelbaum JE, Husain K, et al. Association of Schatzki ring with eosinophilic esophagitis in children. J Pediatr Gastroenterol Nutr 2004 Apr; 38(4):436–41.

47. Sundaram S, Sunku B, Nelson SP, et al. Adherent white plaques: an endoscopic finding in eosinophilic esophagitis. J Pediatr Gastroenterol Nutr 2004 Feb;38(2):208–12.

48. Straumann A, Spichtin HP, Bucher KA, et al. Eosinophilic esophagitis: red on microscopy, white on endoscopy. Digestion 2004;70(2):109–16.

49. Ngo P, Furuta GT, Antonioli DA, et al. Eosinophils in the esophagus–peptic or allergic eosinophilic esophagitis? Case series of three patients with esophageal eosinophilia. Am J Gastroenterol 2006 Jul;101(7):1666–70.

50. Dellon ES, Aderoju A, Woosley JT, et al. Variability in diagnostic criteria for eosinophilic esophagitis: A systematic review. Am J Gastroenterol 2007 Oct; 102(10):2300–13.

51. Dellon ES, Fritchie KJ, Rubinas TC, et al. Inter- and intraobserver reliability and validation of a new method for determination of eosinophil counts in patients with esophageal eosinophilia. Dig Dis Sci 2010 Jul;55(7):1940–9.

52. Mueller S, Aigner T, Neureiter D, et al. Eosinophil infiltration and degranulation in oesophageal mucosa from adult patients with eosinophilic oesophagitis: a retrospective and comparative study on pathological biopsy. J Clin Pathol 2006 Nov;59(11):1175–80.

53. Mueller S, Neureiter D, Aigner T, et al. Comparison of histological parameters for the diagnosis of eosinophilic oesophagitis versus gastro-oesophageal reflux disease on oesophageal biopsy material. Histopathology 2008 Dec;53(6):676–84.

54. Protheroe C, Woodruff SA, de Petris G, et al. A novel histologic scoring system to evaluate mucosal biopsies from patients with eosinophilic esophagitis. Clin Gastroenterol Hepatol 2009 Jul;7(7):749–55.

55. Kephart GM, Alexander JA, Arora AS, et al. Marked deposition of eosinophil-derived neurotoxin in adult patients with eosinophilic esophagitis. Am J Gastroenterol 2010 Feb;105(2):298–307.

56. Ortolani C, Ispano M, Pastorello EA, et al. Comparison of results of skin prick tests (with fresh foods and commercial food extracts) and RAST in 100 patients with oral allergy syndrome. J Allergy Clin Immunol 1989 Mar;83(3):683–90.

57. Dreborg S, Foucard T. Allergy to apple, carrot and potato in children with birch pollen allergy. Allergy 1983 Apr;38(3):167–72.

58. Spergel JM, Brown-Whitehorn T, Beausoleil JL, et al. Predictive values for skin prick test and atopy patch test for eosinophilic esophagitis. J Allergy Clin Immunol 2007 Feb;119(2):509–11.

59. Sampson HA. Utility of food-specific IgE concentrations in predicting symptomatic food allergy. J Allergy Clin Immunol 2001 May;107(5):891–6.

60. Spergel JM, Brown-Whitehorn T. The use of patch testing in the diagnosis of food allergy. Curr Allergy Asthma Rep 2005 Jan;5(1):86–90.

61. Aceves SS, Furuta GT, Spechler SJ. Integrated approach to treatment of children and adults with eosinophilic esophagitis. Gastrointest Endosc Clin N Am 2008 Jan;18(1):195–217.

62. Markowitz JE, Spergel JM, Ruchelli E, et al. Elemental diet is an effective treatment for eosinophilic esophagitis in children and adolescents. Am J Gastroenterol 2003 Apr;98(4):777–82.

63. Spergel JM, Andrews T, Brown-Whitehorn TF, et al. Treatment of eosinophilic esophagitis with specific food elimination diet directed by a combination of skin prick and patch tests. Ann Allergy Asthma Immunol 2005 Oct;95(4):336–43.

64. Spergel JM, Shuker M. Nutritional management of eosinophilic esophagitis. Gastrointest Endosc Clin N Am 2008 Jan;18(1):179–94.

65. Liacouras C, Wenner W, Brown K, et al. Primary eosinophilic esophagitis in children: successful treatment with oral corticosteroids. J Pediatr Gastroenterol Nutr 1998;26:380–5.

66. Faubion WA Jr, Perrault J, Burgart LJ, et al. Treatment of eosinophilic esophagitis with inhaled corticosteroids. J Pediatr Gastroenterol Nutr 1998 Jul;27(1):90–3.

67. Arora AS, Perrault J, Smyrk TC. Topical corticosteroid treatment of dysphagia due to eosinophilic esophagitis in adults. Mayo Clin Proc 2003 Jul;78(7):830–5.

68. Teitelbaum J, Fox V, Twarog F, et al. Eosinophilic esophagitis in children: immunopathological analysis and response to fluticasone propionate. Gastroenterology 2002;122:1216–25.

69. Konikoff MR, Noel RJ, Blanchard C, et al. A randomized, double-blind, placebo-controlled trial of fluticasone propionate for pediatric eosinophilic esophagitis. Gastroenterology 2006 Nov;131(5): 1381–91.

70. Aceves SS, Bastian JF, Newbury RO, et al. Oral viscous budesonide: A potential new therapy for eosinophilic esophagitis in children. Am J Gastroenterol 2007 Oct; 102(10):2271–9.

71. Aceves SS, Dohil R, Newbury RO, et al. Topical viscous budesonide suspension for treatment of eosinophilic esophagitis. J Allergy Clin Immunol 2005 Sep;116(3):705–6.

72. Attwood SE, Lewis CJ, Bronder CS, et al. Eosinophilic oesophagitis: a novel treatment using Montelukast. Gut 2003 Feb;52(2):181–5.

73. Straumann A, Conus S, Grzonka P, et al. Anti-interleukin-5 antibody treatment (mepolizumab) in active eosinophilic oesophagitis: a randomised,

placebo-controlled, double-blind trial. Gut 2010 Jan; 59(1):21–30.

74. Talley NJ, Shorter RG, Phillips SF, et al. Eosinophilic gastroenteritis: a clinicopathological study of patients with disease of the mucosa, muscle layer, and subserosal tissues. Gut 1990 Jan;31(1):54–8.

75. Klein NC, Hargrove RL, Sleisenger MH, et al. Eosinophilic gastroenteritis. Medicine (Baltimore). 1970 Jul;49(4):299–319.

76. Chehade M, Magid MS, Mofidi S, et al. Allergic eosinophilic gastroenteritis with protein-losing enteropathy: intestinal pathology, clinical course, and long-term follow-up. J Pediatr Gastroenterol Nutr 2006 May;42(5):516–21.

77. Hogan S, Mishra A, Brandt E, et al. A pathological function for eotaxin and eosinophils in eosinophilic gastrointestinal inflammation. Nat Immunol 2001; 2:353–60.

CHAPTER 11

Food Protein-Induced Enterocolitis Syndrome, Food Protein-Induced Enteropathy, Proctocolitis, and Infantile Colic

Stephanie Ann Leonard and Anna Nowak-Węgrzyn

KEY CONCEPTS

- Food protein-induced enterocolitis syndrome (FPIES), proctocolitis and enteropathy are non-IgE-mediated gastrointestinal food allergy disorders which in a majority of cases resolve by age 3 years.
- FPIES is usually caused by cows' milk and soy, but may also be caused by cereal grains (rice, oats and barley), egg, fish, molluscs, poultry and vegetables.
- Food protein-induced proctocolitis is a benign transient disorder of infancy considered to be one of the major causes of rectal bleeding under age 1 year.

- Classic infantile food protein-induced enteropathy is caused by cows' milk, soy and wheat. Recent reports describe subtle enteropathy in children with multiple IgE-mediated food allergies, as well as in older children and adults with delayed food allergy to cows' milk and cereal grains.
- Infantile colic is a benign self-limiting condition which usually resolves by age 3–4 months. A subset of cases may be food protein-induced, particularly by cows' milk and/or soy.

Food protein-induced enterocolitis syndrome

Food protein-induced enterocolitis syndrome (FPIES) is a non-IgE-mediated gastrointestinal food hypersensitivity that manifests as profuse vomiting and diarrhea.[1] Although it has been established as a distinct clinical entity, features of FPIES, especially the chronic form, overlap with food protein-induced proctocolitis and enteropathy (Table 11.1).

Epidemiology

In a large birth cohort conducted in Israel 0.34% (44/13,019) of infants developed FPIES[2]. In general, gastrointestinal immune reactions to cows' milk proteins that are mediated by T lymphocytes with or without contribution from specific IgE antibody are estimated to account for up to 40% of milk protein hypersensitivity in infants and young children.[3] A family history of atopy is positive in 40–80% of patients; family history is positive for food allergy in about 20% of the cases. Approximately 30% of infants with FPIES develop atopic diseases such as eczema (23–57%), asthma or rhinitis (20%) or drug hypersensitivity later in life, similar to the general population.

Pathogenesis

It is hypothesized that local inflammation caused by ingestion of food allergens leads to increased intestinal permeability and fluid shift. However, baseline antigen absorption is normal and does not

Table 11.1 Food protein-induced enterocolitis syndrome (FPIES), proctocolitis and enteropathy

	FPIES	Proctocolitis	Enteropathy
Age at onset	1 day–1 year	1 day–6 months	Dependent on age of exposure to antigen; Cows' milk and soy up to 2 years
Food proteins implicated			
Most common	Cow's milk, soy	Cow's milk, soy	Cow's milk, soy
Less common	Rice, chicken, turkey, fish, pea	Egg, corn, chocolate	Wheat, egg
Multiple food hypersensitivities	>50% both cows' milk and soy	40% both cows' milk and soy	Rare
Feeding at the time of onset	Formula	>50% exclusive breastfeeding	Formula
Atopic background			
Family history of atopy	40–70%	25%	Unknown
Personal history of atopy	30%	22%	22%
Genetics	Unknown	Unknown	Unknown
Symptoms			
Emesis	Prominent	No	Intermittent
Diarrhea	Moderate-severe*	No	Moderate
Bloody stools	Moderate-severe*	Moderate	Rare
Edema	Acute, severe	No	Moderate
Shock	15%	No	No
Failure to thrive	Moderate	No	Moderate
Laboratory findings			
Anemia	Moderate	Mild	Moderate
Hypoalbuminemia	Acute	Rare	Moderate
Methemoglobinemia	May be present	No	No
Acidemia	May be present	No	No
Leukocytosis	May be present	No	No
Thrombocytosis	May be present	No	No
Allergy evaluation			
Food prick skin test	Negative	Negative	Negative
Serum food-allergen IgE	Negative	Negative	Negative
Total IgE	Normal	Normal	Normal
Peripheral blood eosinophilia	No	Occasional	No
Biopsy findings			
Villous injury	Patchy, variable	No	Variable, increased crypt length
Colitis	Prominent	Focal	No
Mucosal erosions	Occasional	Occasional, linear	No

*Diarrhea may be present in acute cases and can be severe if chronic

Table 11.1 Food protein-induced enterocolitis syndrome (FPIES), proctocolitis and enteropathy—cont'd

	FPIES	Proctocolitis	Enteropathy
Lymph. nodular hyperplasia	No	Common	No
Eosinophil infiltration	Prominent	Prominent	Few
Food Challenge	Vomiting in 1–3 hours; diarrhea in 2–10 hours	Rectal bleeding in 6–72 hours	Vomiting and/or diarrhea in 40–72 hours
Treatment	Protein elimination, ≥80% respond to casein hydrolyzate and symptoms clear in 3–10 days; rechallenge in 1.5–2 years	Protein elimination, symptoms clear in 3 days with casein hydrolyzate; resume/continue breastfeeding on maternal antigen-restricted diet	Protein elimination, symptoms clear in 1–3 weeks; rechallenge and biopsy in 1–2 years
Natural history	Cow's milk: 60% resolved by 2 years Soy: 25% resolved by 2 years	Resolved by 9–12 months	Most cases resolve in 2–3 years
Reintroduction of the food	Food challenge under physician supervision with secure intravenous access	At home, gradually advancing from 1 oz to full feedings over 2 weeks	Home, gradually advancing

Reprinted with permission from Food Allergy, 4th edition; chapter 16. Eds. Metcalfe DD, Sampson HA, and Simon RA. Blackwell Publishing, 2008.

predispose to FPIES.[4] Currently, the diagnosis of FPIES is based on clinical criteria; endoscopy and biopsy are not routinely performed. However, previous endoscopic evaluations and biopsies in infants with FPIES identified diffuse colitis with variable degrees of ileal involvement.[1] Intestinal inflammation in FPIES may involve activation of peripheral blood mononuclear cells (PBMCs), increased TNF-α, and decreased expression of TGF-β receptors in the intestinal mucosa[1] (Table 11.2).

Systemic humoral antibody responses are usually not detected in FPIES. The potential role of IgE antibody produced locally in the intestinal mucosa in facilitating the antigen uptake and local intestinal inflammation requires further study, but systemic IgE is usually not detected in FPIES. A decrease in serum IgG antibody and an increase in serum food-specific IgA levels has been noted; lower levels of serum milk-specific IgG_4 (p < 0.05) and a trend for higher serum IgA antibody levels were found in children with milk FPIES compared to the control group.[5]

Clinical features

FPIES manifests as profuse emesis and diarrhea in young infants and is most commonly caused by milk and soy; over 50% react to both foods (Clinical Vignette 1). However, in a recent birth cohort in Israel none of the 44 infants with cow's milk FPIES showed sensitivity to soy.[2] Symptoms usually begin

Table 11.2 Pathologic findings in FPIES

Endoscopy

Friable mucosa
Minute spontaneous hemorrhage

Biopsy

Crypt abscesses
Villous atrophy
Tissue edema
Increased lymphocytes
Increased eosinophils and mast cells

Immunohistochemical

IgM- and IgA-containing plasma cells

In vitro studies

Increased activation of peripheral blood mononuclear cells
Increased TNF-α
Decreased expression of TGF-β receptors

Reprinted with permission from Food Allergy, 4th edition; chapter 16. Eds. Metcalfe DD, Sampson HA, and Simon RA. Blackwell Publishing, 2008.

in early infancy (1–3 months, up to 1 year of age), typically within 1–4 weeks following the introduction of milk or soy protein into the diet. Later onset usually results from delayed introduction of milk, soy, or solid foods in breastfed infants. FPIES to milk and soy in infants that are exclusively breastfed is extremely rare, suggesting an important protective role of breastfeeding.[6,7,8] FPIES to solid foods such as grains, meats, fish, egg and vegetables have

MILK FPIES

A 10-month-old boy who was born full term without complications presented for evaluation. He was breastfed from birth on an unrestricted maternal diet, although he had received cows' milk formula in the neonatal nursery as supplementation as well as cows' milk formula for a couple of days at 2 months of life. Solids were introduced and tolerated starting at 5 months and included cereals, vegetables and fruits. At 8 months of age, yogurt was introduced. Approximately 2 hours after eating two spoonfuls of yogurt, he developed irritability and repetitive, non-bloody, non-bilious vomiting. In addition, he developed diarrhea later in the day. He did not have associated fever. He was taken to the emergency department, where he was found to be hypotensive and listless. Examination revealed marked pallor. An intravenous line was placed and normal saline given. Given the extreme symptoms, a 'rule out sepsis' work-up was conducted and intravenous antibiotics were started. Serum chemistry revealed dehydration. Complete blood count revealed leukocytosis with a left shift. His stools were guaiac positive.

Within 2 hours of IV fluids the patient's condition improved and his behavior returned to baseline. He was admitted to the hospital for observation and IV antibiotics. He was discharged when cultures were negative for 48 hours.

Two weeks after his admission, he ate a piece of cheese. Again, he developed excessive vomiting and diarrhea within 2–3 hours. He was brought to the emergency department, where he required intravenous fluid resuscitation, and within a few hours his baseline behavior returned. His mother was certain that the symptoms were the result of the cheese that he had eaten. Upon discharge from the ER, recommendations included the continuation of breastfeeding, milk avoidance, and evaluation by an allergist.

Allergy evaluation revealed no concomitant atopic disease such as atopic dermatitis or asthma. Family history was significant for paternal allergic rhinitis and penicillin allergy. Physical examination was unremarkable. Skin prick testing was negative to milk with a negative saline control and a positive histamine control. The diagnosis of milk protein-induced enterocolitis syndrome was made based on the clinical history. Recommendations included strict milk avoidance and follow-up evaluation in approximately 1 year.

been reported usually with onset at 4–7 months of age; onset of symptoms at older ages may occur with some foods, such as fish or molluscs.[9]

In the most severe cases, symptoms may start within the first days of life with bloody diarrhea, lethargy, abdominal distension, weight loss, dehydration, metabolic acidosis, anemia, elevated white

RICE FPIES

A 7-month-old girl presented for allergy evaluation. She was initially breastfed with no maternal dietary restriction. When she was supplemented with cows' milk-based formula she developed emesis and formula was discontinued. She remained well on exclusive breastfeeding and at 5 months solids were started. Rice cereal was tolerated for about 2 weeks without any problems. Thereafter, she developed multiple episodes of forceful emesis within 2 hours of ingesting rice cereal. During the first episode, emesis lasted for about 1.5 hours and she became pale and lethargic. Ten days later, she was again fed rice cereal and 2 hours later developed forceful, non-bloody and non-bilious emesis; she passed a loose stool with blood. She became lethargic, pale and diaphoretic, but had no wheezing or skin rash. She was rushed to the pediatrician's office where she was treated with epinephrine, dexamethasone and oxygen, and was then sent to the emergency department, where she improved with vigorous intravenous hydration. Rice allergy was suspected, but allergy skin prick test and serum rice-specific IgE were negative. The diagnosis of rice FPIES was made. Fruits and vegetables were gradually introduced to her diet at home and were tolerated well. Wheat and cows' milk were introduced to her diet at 1 year of age without any problems. She had no reactions to any other foods. She continued to avoid rice.

blood count with left shift and eosinophilia, and hypoalbuminemia. Among those with a recorded complete blood count, 65% had thrombocytosis $>500 \times 10^9/L.$[10] Intramural gas may be seen on abdominal radiographs, prompting a diagnosis of necrotizing enterocolitis, sepsis evaluation and treatment with antibiotics. Overall, 75% of infants with FPIES appear acutely ill; about 15% are hypotensive and require hospitalization.[1]

Transient methemoglobinemia was reported in about one third of young infants with severe reactions and acidemia; some required treatment with methylene blue and bicarbonate. Methemoglobinemia may be caused by an elevation of nitrites resulting from severe intestinal inflammation and reduced catalase activity. In 24% of acute FPIES episodes, young infants manifested with hypothermia $<36\,^\circ C.$

Symptomatic infants improve within 3–10 days with intravenous fluids or with casein hydrolyzate-based formula. Food reintroduction induces acute symptoms; usually, repetitive emesis starts within 1–3 hours following ingestion, and diarrhea starts within 2–10 hours (mean onset 5 hours),

Table 11.3 Clinical characteristics of cows' milk and soy FPIES

Chronic manifestations during continued ingestion of the food	Acute manifestations upon ingestion following a period of food avoidance
Onset: days to 12 months	Onset: days to 12 months
Intermittent, chronic emesis	Repetitive emesis, onset 1–3 hours following ingestion
Chronic watery diarrhea with blood and mucus	Diarrhea, onset about 5 hours following ingestion
Lethargy	Lethargy, dusky appearance
Dehydration	Dehydration
Hypotensive shock (15%)	Hypotension in 15%
Acidemia	Acidemia
Methemoglobinemia/clinical cyanosis	Methemoglobinemia
Abdominal distension, hypoactive bowel sounds, ileus*	Abdominal distension, hypoactive bowel sounds, ileus*
Anemia	Frank or occult fecal blood
Elevated white blood count with eosinophilia	Elevated PMN count
Hypoalbuminemia	Thrombocytosis >500 × 10⁹/L
Failure to thrive	Sheets of leukocytes and eosinophils in stool
Carbohydrate malabsorption (stool positive for reducing substances)	Hypothermia <36°C in 24% of infants
	Gastric juice leukocytosis (>10 cells/hpf)

*Ileus has been reported in extreme cases, typically newborns and young infants <3 months of age.
Reprinted with permission from Food Allergy, 4th edition; chapter 16. Eds. Metcalfe DD, Sampson HA, and Simon RA. Blackwell Publishing, 2008.

with blood, mucus, leukocytes, eosinophils and increased carbohydrate content in the stool.[11] However, not all patients develop diarrhea. Peripheral blood neutrophil counts are elevated in positive challenges, peaking at 6 hours. The typical features of chronic and acute cows' milk and soy FPIES are presented in Table 11.3.

FPIES may be caused by solid foods such as rice, oats, barley, chicken, turkey, molluscs, fish, egg white, green pea and peanut[1] (Clinical Vignette 2). Rice is the single most common solid food inducing FPIES.[12] Among infants with solid food FPIES, 65% were previously diagnosed with milk and/or soy FPIES and fed with casein hydrolyzate- or amino acid-based formula; 35% were breastfed.[6] Mean age at onset of solid food FPIES tends to be higher than the mean age of onset of milk and soy FPIES.[12] In our experience, solid food FPIES usually starts at 4–7 months. Infants often present with multiple reactions and extensive evaluations for alternative etiologies (infectious, toxic or metabolic) before the diagnosis of FPIES is considered. Delayed diagnosis may be due to the low index of suspicion, since grains such as rice and oats, and vegetables are believed to have low allergenic

potential and are not suspected as culprits in severe allergic reactions. In addition, a lack of definitive diagnostic tests and the unusual nature of symptoms may contribute to the delay in diagnosis. In one study, infants with rice FPIES had severe symptoms and were more likely to receive fluid resuscitation upon presentation than those with milk or soy FPIES (42% versus 15%, p = 0.02).[12] In adults, shellfish (including crustacean and molluscs) and fish hypersensitivity may provoke a similar syndrome, with severe nausea, abdominal cramps, protracted vomiting and diarrhea.[9]

Diagnosis

Diagnosis is based on the history, clinical features, exclusion of other etiologies, and food challenge (Table 11.4). The majority (>90%) of patients have negative skin prick tests and undetectable food-specific IgE. Based on the presumed pathophysiology involving T cells, atopy patch test (APT) was evaluated in 19 infants aged 5–30 months with FPIES confirmed by an oral food challenge (OFC).[13] APT predicted the outcome of an OFC in 28/33 instances; all positive OFCs had a positive APT, but

Table 11.4 Oral food challenge in FPIES

Challenge protocol
- *High-risk procedure, requires physician supervision and immediate availability of fluid resuscitation, secure intravenous access*
- Baseline peripheral neutrophil count
- Gradual (over 1 hour) administration of food protein 0.06–0.6 g/kg body weight, generally not to exceed 3–6 g of protein or 10–20 g of total food for an initial feeding
- If no reaction in 2–3 hours, administer a regular age-appropriate serving of the food followed by several hours of observation
- Majority (>50%) of positive challenges require treatment with intravenous fluids and steroids

Criteria for a positive challenge
- *Symptoms*
  - *Emesis (typically in 1–3 hours)*
  - *Diarrhea (typically in 2–10 hours)*
- *Laboratory findings*
  - Increase in peripheral neutrophil count > 3500 cells/mm^3 peaking at 6 hours
  - Fecal leukocytes
  - Fecal eosinophils
  - Gastric juice leukocytes >10 cells/hpf

Interpretation of the challenge outcome
- *Positive challenge: three of five criteria positive*
- *Equivocal: two of five criteria positive*

Reprinted with permission from Food Allergy, 4th edition; chapter 16. Eds. Metcalfe DD, Sampson HA, and Simon RA. Blackwell Publishing, 2008.

five patients with positive APT did not react to an OFC. Similar results have not been confirmed by other investigators; therefore, the role of APT in the diagnosis of FPIES requires further evaluation. Although OFC is the gold standard for diagnosing FPIES, most infants do not need to undergo confirmatory challenges for the initial diagnosis, especially if they have a classic history of severe reactions and become asymptomatic following elimination of the suspected food. However, physician-supervised OFCs are necessary to determine whether FPIES has resolved, and whether the food may be reintroduced into the diet.

Hypoalbuminemia and weight gain <10 g/day were identified as independent predictors of milk-FPIES in young infants with chronic symptoms.[14] Stool examination in infants with chronic diarrhea is non-specific and shows occult blood, intact polymorphonuclear neutrophils, eosinophils, Charcot–Leyden crystals and reducing substances.

Prior to establishment of the diagnostic criteria, endoscopy in symptomatic infants with cows' milk- and or soy FPIES showed rectal ulceration and bleeding, with friable mucosa. In infants with chronic diarrhea, rectal bleeding and/or failure to thrive, radiographs showed air–fluid levels, non-specific narrowing and thumb-printing of the rectum and sigmoid, and thickening of the plicae circulares in the duodenum and jejunum with excess luminal fluid. In the cases of ileus, in which laparotomy was performed, distension of small bowel loops and thickening of the wall of jejunum distal to Treitz's ligament with diffuse subserosal bleeding was reported. Follow-up studies performed on a restricted diet in asymptomatic patients documented resolution of radiological abnormalities.[1]

OFCs can be used to establish a diagnosis of FPIES or to evaluate the possibility that FPIES has resolved. According to one conservative approach, follow-up challenges are usually recommended every 18–24 months in patients without recent reactions.[3] Korean investigators recommended a more accelerated course, as they reported that among 27 infants with milk FPIES, 64% tolerated milk at 10 months and 92% tolerated soy at 10 months.[15] They suggested that in milk FPIES the first milk challenge should be done after age 12 months, whereas the first soy challenge could be done between 6 and 8 months.

Oral food challenge

Guidelines for the preparation and interpretation of the OFC for FPIES are presented in Table 11.4. During an OFC, the total dose of 0.06–0.6 g/kg food protein is administered in three equal portions over 45 minutes.[16] Generally, the amount served initially does not exceed 3–6 g of food protein or 10–20 g of total food weight (usually <100 mL of liquid food such as cows' milk or infant formula). The patient is observed for approximately 2–3 hours and, if asymptomatic, a second feeding, typically an age-appropriate regular serving, may be given followed by observation for several hours.[3] OFC in FPIES should be performed under physician supervision with secure intravenous access for fluid resuscitation.[16] Rapid intravenous hydration (20 mL/kg boluses) is the first-line therapy. Intravenous corticosteroids are often used for severe reactions, based on the presumed T-cell-mediated intestinal inflammation.[3] Epinephrine should be available for potential severe cardiovascular reactions with hypotension and shock. However, our unpublished experience is that prompt administration of epinephrine does not improve the symptoms of emesis and lethargy, which do, however, resolve promptly with vigorous intravenous fluid administration.

Gastric juice analysis was proposed as an additional confirmatory test in the equivocal oral challenges.[15] Gastric juice leukocytes >10 cells/high power field (hpf) were observed in 15 of 16 positive milk challenges after 3 hours, including two infants without emesis or lethargy, whereas none of the eight age-matched control infants had gastric juice leukocytes >10/hpf. This observation needs to be validated in larger groups of subjects.

Management

Management relies on avoidance of the offending food. Extensively hydrolyzed casein formula is recommended for infants that cannot be breastfed because concomitant milk and soy FPIES occur in over 60% of cases. The majority of patients with milk and or soy FPIES experience resolution of symptoms within 3–10 days of starting extensively hydrolyzed casein formula. Rarely, patients need amino acid-based formula or temporary intravenous fluids.

Because about one third of infants with cows' milk or soy FPIES develop a reaction to solid food, the introduction of yellow fruits and vegetables, instead of cereals, at 6 months has been suggested.[3,6] Infants with solid food FPIES are likely to react to other foods: 80% are reactive to more than one food protein, 65% react to milk and/or soy, and those with a history of reactions to one grain have at least a 50% chance of reacting to other grains. Empirically, infants with solid food FPIES may benefit from avoidance of grains, legumes and poultry in the first year of life.[3] In one approach the introduction of milk and soy in infants without a prior history of reactivity to these foods may be attempted at an age older than 1 year, preferably under physician supervision. Tolerance to one food from each 'high-risk category', such as soy for legumes, chicken for poultry, or oat for grains, might be considered as an indication of increased likelihood of tolerance to the remaining foods from the same category.[3]

Milk FPIES resolves in 60%–90% and soy FPIES resolves in 25% of patients by age 3 years (Clinical Vignette 3).[2,6,16] Resolution of solid food FPIES by age 3 years occurred in 67% for vegetables, 66% for oat and 40% for rice. FPIES rarely develops to foods upon initial feeding beyond 1 year of age, although onset of FPIES to fish and shellfish has been

CLINICAL VIGNETTE 3

NATURAL HISTORY OF FPIES

After 1 year of milk avoidance, our patient from Vignette 1 returned for follow-up evaluation. He had had no adverse reactions to foods since his last visit; however, he had had accidental ingestions of foods that contained milk (i.e. cookie, bread prepared with butter). An oral food challenge to milk was recommended and conducted approximately 6 months after the follow-up visit (18 months from his original evaluation).

On the day of the food challenge, an intravenous line was placed prior to feeding milk. The patient tolerated two separate feedings of milk (total of 0.6 g of protein per kg). He was observed for 3 hours following the second feeding. On discharge from the challenge, the family was advised to add milk into the diet.

reported in older children and adults. For example, wheat allergy has not been reported in infants with oat- or rice-induced FPIES, but the introduction of wheat was significantly delayed, presumably avoiding the 'window of physiologic susceptibility' for FPIES development.[3,6] Patients presenting initially or developing food-specific IgE antibodies after the diagnosis of FPIES have a more protracted course.[6,16] It may be prudent to include skin prick testing and/or measurement of serum food-specific IgE level in the initial as well as follow-up evaluations, to identify patients at risk for persistent FPIES.

Food protein-induced proctocolitis

Food protein-induced proctocolitis is a benign transient condition which typically begins in the first few months of life with blood-streaked stools in well-appearing infants; it is considered one of the major causes of colitis under age 1 year[9] (Table 11.5).

Table 11.5 Key features of food protein-induced proctocolitis

Usually presents by 6 months of life

Blood streaked, loose stools ± diarrhea in otherwise well-appearing infants

Usually occurs in breastfed (60%) or cows'/soy milk formula-fed infants (40%)

Diagnosis is based on clinical history

Food prick skin test and serum food-IgE negative

Treatment is based on food protein elimination

Resolution of symptoms in 48–72 hours following food protein elimination

Tolerance to allergen usually occurs by 1–3 years of life

Food protein-induced proctocolitis was originally described by Lake et al. in 1982 in six exclusively breastfed infants with rectal bleeding that appeared during the first month of life.[17]

Epidemiology

In contrast to other forms of gastrointestinal food hypersensitivity, proctocolitis is prevalent in breastfed infants, making up as many as 60% of cases in published reports.[17] The exact prevalence of allergic proctocolitis is unknown; the estimated prevalence ranges from 18% to 64% of infants with rectal bleeding.[18,19] Eczema is present in about 22% of the breastfed infants. A positive family history of atopy is present in up to 25% of infants with proctocolitis, which is comparable to the general population.[20]

Pathogenesis

Food protein-induced proctocolitis most commonly affects the rectosigmoid. Endoscopy reveals focal erythema with lymphoid nodular hyperplasia. Biopsy reveals prominent eosinophilic infiltrates in the rectal mucosa; the number of eosinophils varies from 6 to >20 per 40 hpf; eosinophils are frequently degranulated and localized next to the lymphoid nodules. The pathologic findings are similar to those that can be identified in other forms of eosinophilic gastrointestinal disorders; lack of additional symptoms and a mild course support the diagnosis of allergic proctocolitis in an infant with isolated rectal bleeding. There is no correlation between the degree of peripheral blood eosinophilia and the tissue eosinophilic infiltrate within the rectosigmoid. Eosinophil mediators induce mast cell degranulation, dysfunction of vagal muscarinic M2 receptors, smooth muscle constriction, and stimulation of chloride secretion from colonic epithelium. Degranulation of the eosinophils near nerves may contribute to gastric dysmotility. Additionally, experimental eosinophil accumulation in the gastrointestinal tract is associated with the development of weight loss.[21] Table 11.6 summarizes the most important pathologic features of food protein-induced proctocolitis.

Lake[20] postulated that food protein-induced proctocolitis represents a milder form of FPIES because in both conditions the strongest inflammatory response occurs usually in the rectum. Proctocolitis in formula-fed infants would represent the mildest phenotype, whereas in breastfed infants it

Table 11.6 Pathologic findings in food protein-induced proctocolitis

Endoscopy
Rectosigmoid affected most commonly
Focal erythema and inflammation
Lymphoid nodular hyperplasia
Rectal ulcerations

Mucosal biopsy
Normal architecture preserved
Eosinophilic infiltration (6 to >20 per 40× high power field)
Features of eosinophil degranulation
Occasional eosinophilic crypt abscesses

would represent the attenuated FPIES due to the protective effects of the breast milk, such as the presence of IgA antibodies, TGF-β and partially processed food proteins. This concept is supported by the lack of published reports of classic FPIES in breastfed infants. IgA or other immunologically active components of breast milk may bind with the food allergens and release them in the rectum following cleavage by microbial IgA proteases or via other mechanisms.[20]

Clinical features

Food protein-induced proctocolitis in formula-fed infants is typically caused by cows' milk and soy proteins; in breastfed infants it is usually caused by cows' milk, soy, egg and corn proteins (Clinical Vignette 4). Infants appear healthy, but parents typically note a gradual onset of bloody stools, which increase in frequency unless the triggering food is eliminated.[20] Children with proctocolitis do not have poor weight gain but may develop mild anemia[17] or hypoalbuminemia. Some have peripheral blood eosinophilia, elevated serum IgE antibody levels and a positive family history of atopy.[22-25] Infants usually present in the first 4 months of life, usually at 1–4 weeks of age, with intermittent blood-streaked normal to moderately loose stools (Table 11.5). Breastfed infants are often older at the time of initial presentation and have less severe histologic findings. The onset may be acute (<12 hours following the first feeding of the offending food) but is more often insidious, with a prolonged latent interval between the introduction of the food protein and the onset of symptoms. The affected infants typically appear well; however, increased gas (up to 30% of patients), intermittent

FOOD PROTEIN-INDUCED PROCTOCOLITIS

An 11-month-old breastfed boy presented for evaluation of food allergy. He had been breastfed since birth without any maternal dietary restrictions, and supplemented with cows' milk-based formula, on average four to five times a week. At 8 weeks of age gross blood was noted in the stool and he appeared uncomfortable. There was no rectal fissure and no signs of an infection. Allergic proctocolitis was suspected and cows' milk formula was discontinued and milk products were eliminated from his mother's diet, with some improvement but without complete resolution of the bloody stools. The pediatric gastroenterologist suspected food protein-induced proctocolitis and recommended stopping soy in the maternal diet. Apparently, the mother had started ingesting significant amounts of soy milk to substitute for cows' milk, and when she discontinued soy milk there was a significant improvement in the amount of visible blood in the stools. His stools became entirely negative for gross blood within 4 days of elimination of delicatessen meats in the mother's diet that were suspected for probably being contaminated with traces of cheese during the process of slicing. Subsequent stool checks were negative for occult blood. He continued to be breastfed with maternal dietary restrictions for cows' milk and soy protein. The patient tolerated gradual introduction of solid foods (rice cereal, yellow fruits and vegetables) starting at the age of 6 months without any problems. His personal history of atopy was negative for atopic dermatitis, wheezing or chronic rhinitis.

On presentation to the allergy office the patient was a healthy infant, weighing 11.8 kg (90th percentile) and height 80.6 cm (>95th percentile). Allergy evaluation with skin prick tests to commercial milk and soy extract and measurement of serum milk and soy IgE (UniCap, Phadia) revealed negative results.

Based on his clinical manifestations the child was diagnosed with cows'- and soy-milk-induced allergic proctocolitis. His mother was advised to gradually introduce soy and cows' milk products into her diet, prior to directly feeding these two foods to her son after his first birthday. He tolerated soy and milk in his diet without any adverse reactions, and breastfeeding was discontinued when he was 14 months old.

emesis (up to 27%), pain on defecation (22%) or abdominal pain (up to 20%) may be present. No anatomic abnormalities are found and stool cultures are negative for pathogens. Smears of the fecal mucus usually reveal increased polymorphonuclear neutrophils.

Breastfed infants react to the cows' milk proteins consumed by the mother. Elimination of cows' milk from the mother's diet usually results in gradual resolution of symptoms in the infant and permits the continuation of breastfeeding.[17,25,26] Rarely, a casein hydrolyzate formula, or in rare instances an amino acid-based formula, may be necessary for resolution of bleeding, typically within 48–72 hours.[9]

Sometimes breastfed infants continue to have bleeding despite maternal avoidance of food(s); six of 21 of these infants developed iron deficiency anemia despite iron supplementation, but they gained weight and had normal development and by their first birthday were tolerating a regular diet.[20] The persistence of rectal bleeding despite maternal dietary restrictions may be explained by inability to remove all sources of allergen from the diet, or by an allergen that has not been identified. Alternatively, the baby might react to the human breast milk protein.

Diagnosis

Diagnosis relies on a history of rectal bleeding and response to an elimination diet which typically leads to a clinical resolution of gross bleeding within 72–96 hours.[20] Tests for IgE-mediated food hypersensitivity are negative or inconsistent, and usually not useful for the diagnosis of food protein-induced proctocolitis. Excluding causes of rectal bleeding, such as infection, necrotizing enterocolitis, intussusception or anal fissure, is important.

Management

Treatment is based on dietary restriction. In breast-fed infants, Lake[20] proposed discontinuation of breast milk and feeding with a casein hydrolyzate formula until resolution of bleeding, usually within 72 hours. Soy formula may cause bleeding in a large subset of infants reacting to cows' milk because up to 40% of infants react to both foods.[20] Most infants respond well to casein hydrolyzate formulas and only few require amino acid-based formulas. Breastfeeding mothers must strictly avoid the offending food protein in their diet. Rechallenge within the first 6 months usually induces recurrence of bleeding within 72 hours. In contrast to FPIES, no peripheral blood leukocytosis is seen following the challenge.[9,17] If food skin prick tests and serum food-specific IgE antibody levels are negative, gradual food introduction typically takes place at home, increasing from 1 oz/day to full feedings over 2 weeks.[27]

Infants with proctocolitis usually become tolerant to the offending food by 1–3 years of age and the majority achieve clinical tolerance by 1 year. Up to 20% of breastfed infants have spontaneous resolution of bleeding without changes in the maternal diet.[21] The long-term prognosis is excellent, and there are no reports of inflammatory bowel disease in infants with food protein-induced proctocolitis followed for more than 10 years.[20,28]

Food protein-induced enteropathy

Food protein-induced enteropathy is a syndrome of small bowel injury with resulting malabsorption, similar to celiac disease albeit less severe.[9] The first report of malabsorption syndrome with diarrhea, emesis and impaired growth induced by cows' milk formula in infants was published in 1905. Subsequent reports, including large series of cows' milk protein-sensitive Finnish infants, defined the clinical features of this disorder[29–35] (Table 11.7).

Epidemiology

Reports of food protein-induced enteropathy peaked in the 1960s in Finland, with virtual disappearance in the past 20 years.[36] The highest incidence of classic severe enteropathy was observed in infants fed with non-humanized milk-based formulas, and the lowest incidence was observed in breastfed infants. Infants with enteropathy typically do not have a predisposing family history of food allergy. More recently, intestinal enteropathy was reported in older children with delayed-type allergic reactions to milk, as well as in children with multiple food allergies.[37–39]

Table 11.7 Key features of protein-induced enteropathy

Onset dependent upon introduction of food antigen to diet: usually by 9 months for cows' milk
Vomiting and diarrhea mimic gastroenteritis but are protracted; may lead to failure to thrive
Usually occurs in cows'/soy milk formula-fed infants
Diagnosis is based on clinical history
Food prick skin tests and serum food-IgE are usually negative
Anemia and hypoalbuminemia are common
Treatment is based on protein elimination
Resolution of symptoms in 1–3 weeks
Tolerance to food allergen usually occurs by 2–3 years of life

Pathogenesis

Activated T lymphocytes expressing HLA-DR appear to play a central role in the pathophysiology of food protein-induced enteropathy; following milk elimination, these cells diminish.[40] Histological changes are consistent with enteropathy and allergic inflammation. The histological features of soybean- or cereal-induced enteropathy are similar to those noted for milk. Immunohistochemical studies of the mucosal biopsies in untreated and challenge-positive infants demonstrate an increase in mucosal IgA, IgG and IgM, with inconsistent increase in IgE. An elimination diet following a positive challenge results in decreased densities of IgA- and IgM-containing cells.[41] Similar changes in IgA and IgM cells were observed in soy-induced enteropathy following an oral challenge with soy and reinstitution of an elimination diet. Table 11.8 summarizes the most important pathologic and immunologic features of food protein-induced enteropathy.

Table 11.8 Pathologic findings in protein-induced enteropathy

Mucosa
Thin mucosa
Crypt hypertrophy and thinning
Villous blunting and atrophy (patchy, subtotal)
Reduced crypt:villus ratio
Shortened microvilli
Thickened basement membrane (unevenly)
Prominent intraepithelial lymphocytes
Increased mucosal lipid content
Eosinophilic infiltration (inconsistent)

Lamina propria
Increased lymphocytes, plasma cells, eosinophils
Tissue and blood vessel endothelium edema
Increased histamine content
Degranulation of mast cells and eosinophils

Immunohistochemical studies
Increased mucosal IgA, IgG and IgM
Increased mucosal IgE (inconsistent)
Increased α/β suppressor/cytotoxic CD8+ T cells
Increased density of γ/δ T cells
Activated T cells (HLA-DR+)
Increased gut homing receptor $\alpha4/\beta7$ expression on T cells

In vitro studies
Increased IFN-γ and IL-4
Decreased IL-10
Decreased TGF-β

Reprinted with permission from Food Allergy, 4th edition; chapter 16. Eds. Metcalfe DD, Sampson HA, and Simon RA. Blackwell Publishing, 2008.

CLINICAL VIGNETTE 5

FOOD PROTEIN-INDUCED ENTEROPATHY

A 9-week-old girl presented with a 4-week history of diarrhea, intermittent emesis and failure to thrive. She was breastfed exclusively for 4 weeks and then switched to cows' milk-based formula. Physical examination revealed mild eczema. Laboratory testing showed peripheral blood eosinophilia, mild anemia and low serum total protein. Stools were positive for occult blood and had increased fat content, indicating malabsorption. Endoscopy and biopsy showed subtotal villous atrophy in the proximal jejunum. The child was switched to a hypoallergenic formula and her symptoms gradually resolved in 3 weeks.

Clinical features

Food protein-induced enteropathy presents with chronic diarrhea within weeks after the introduction of milk formula, usually in the first 1–2 months of life, but may start as late as 9 months (Clinical Vignette 5). Foods such as soy, wheat and egg have also been confirmed as causes of enteropathy, frequently in children with coexistent milk protein-induced enteropathy. The affected infants have vomiting and failure to thrive; some present with abdominal distension, early satiety and malabsorption. The onset of symptoms is usually gradual; however, it may also mimic acute gastroenteritis, with transient emesis and anorexia complicated by protracted diarrhea. It may be difficult to distinguish food protein-induced enteropathy from post-enteritis-induced lactose intolerance, especially since the two conditions may overlap. Acute small bowel injury caused by viral enteritis has been postulated to predispose children to subsequent food protein-induced enteropathy, or alternatively to unmask underlying food protein hypersensitivity. Diarrhea usually resolves within 1 week of cows' milk protein elimination, although some infants require prolonged intravenous nutrition.

Moderate anemia is present in 20–69% of infants with cows' milk protein-induced enteropathy. Iron deficiency is more common than anemia, probably owing to the malabsorption of iron or folate. Bloody stools are absent, but occult blood can be found in some patients. Malabsorption with hypoproteinemia and deficiency of vitamin K-dependent factors has been reported in 35–50%. Moderate steatorrhea, manifested by increased fecal fat excretion, can be found in over 80%. The absorption of the sugar D-xylose test is abnormal in up to 80%. Lactose can be found in the urine in 55% and in the stool in 52% of cases, typically in the youngest infants. Lactose absorption normalizes promptly following the elimination of milk protein.

School-aged children with delayed gastrointestinal symptoms to milk challenge but without villous atrophy or malabsorption have been reported.[37] Twenty-seven children with suspected milk-related symptoms, such as a history of milk allergy in infancy, abdominal pains or diarrhea after consumption of dairy products, were placed on strict elimination of milk protein for 2 weeks, followed by a challenge over 1 week. All children responded clinically to milk elimination, but only 15 (mean age 10 years, range 6–14) had relapse of symptoms during 1-week challenge. Compared to control children (11 with celiac disease, 12 without gastrointestinal disease), they had a history of significantly greater food allergy at <2 years of age, gastritis and esophagitis on biopsy, as well as lymphonodular hyperplasia of the duodenal bulb. Increased γ/δ T lymphocytes were noted, but of lesser magnitude than in celiac disease. These older children may represent a subset of milder enteropathy or they may have a different disease caused by milk hypersensitivity.

Subsequent reports confirmed subtle enteropathy in children with delayed gastrointestinal symptoms following food ingestion.[38,42] One study evaluated seven children with untreated food allergy (mean age 7.3 years, range 2–13), seven with treated food allergy (mean age 8.1 years, range 1–14), and five normal controls (mean age 11.4, range 4–16). Diagnosis of food allergy was based on resolution of gastrointestinal symptoms during 2 weeks of an elimination diet and reappearance of symptoms in an open food challenge within a median 4.5 days, range 1–7 days. Children reacted to milk, cereal grains or both. Five of eight children tested had specific serum food-specific IgE >0.7 kIU/L or a positive skin prick test. Biopsies demonstrated lymphonodular hyperplasia in the small intestine in 90%. The untreated children with food allergy exhibited a higher crypt proliferation rate and HLA-DR crypt staining than the controls. In most duodenal biopsies obtained from 45 children with both immediate and delayed history of multiple food allergies, there was focal lymphocytic or eosinophilic infiltration, villous blunting and reduced crypt:villus ratio.[39]

Diagnosis

Food protein-induced enteropathy is diagnosed by finding villous injury, crypt hyperplasia and inflammation on small bowel biopsy in a symptomatic patient who is ingesting the offending food allergen. Avoidance of the allergen usually leads to resolution of clinical symptoms within 1–3 weeks. Villous atrophy usually improves within 4 weeks, but complete resolution may take up to 1.5 years. Infants with severe initial manifestations may require prolonged bowel rest and parenteral nutrition for days or weeks. Diagnostic challenges and measurement of specific serologies for celiac disease may be necessary to exclude celiac disease, or to identify multiple food allergens. In clear-cut cases OFCs are not absolutely required for diagnosis. However, challenges should be performed periodically to assess the development of oral tolerance.

Increased levels of milk serum IgA in 74% and milk serum IgG precipitins were found in 65% of infants. Milk IgA levels decreased following dietary elimination of cows' milk.[32] The diagnostic utility of these tests is unknown, particularly in view of the high prevalence of positive results in many other gastrointestinal inflammatory disorders in childhood. Food-specific serum IgE antibodies are usually undetectable and skin prick tests are negative. Patch skin tests were investigated as a screen for gastrointestinal food hypersensitivity (milk, wheat), but biopsies were not obtained and the association of positive patch tests with gastrointestinal changes remains to be determined.[43]

Serum concentrations of granzymes A (GrA) and B (GrB), soluble Fas and CD30 were measured in children with milk-sensitive enteropathy confirmed by endoscopy and biopsy.[44] These markers reflect activation of cytotoxic lymphocytes that have been shown to be upregulated in the local intestinal mucosa in food-sensitive enteropathy. Serum concentrations of GrA and GrB were significantly higher in the untreated children with food allergy and in the children with celiac disease than in the control subjects. Measurable serum GrB was present in only 20% of the control subjects but in 100% of patients with milk-sensitive enteropathy. Patients with untreated milk-sensitive enteropathy and celiac disease exhibited similarly increased CD30, whereas treated patients exhibited concentrations that were not different from those in control subjects. All groups showed similar levels of soluble Fas. The numbers of duodenal CD3+ α/β- and γ/δ-TCRs correlated with the serum granzyme and CD30 levels. These preliminary results are very encouraging for the identification of biomarkers, but must be confirmed in a larger number of patients before

measurement of serum markers of intestinal cytotoxic lymphocyte activation may be routinely used to diagnose and monitor response to elimination diets.

Treatment/management

Food protein-induced enteropathy resolves clinically in the majority of children by age 1–2 years, but the proximal jejunal mucosa may be persistently abnormal at that time.[32] Mucosal healing continues during feeding with the implicated food once clinical tolerance is achieved.[45] The majority of children with less severe disease who were diagnosed at an older age became tolerant by 3 years.[46] About 10% of infants with challenge-confirmed cows' milk-induced enteropathy were ultimately diagnosed with celiac disease that persisted beyond infancy.[32] In contrast, transient wheat enteropathy with or without associated cows' milk protein-induced enteropathy has been reported in a number of studies, including transient wheat enteropathy following enteritis.[47–49] Strict criteria for the diagnosis of transient wheat-induced enteropathy were established and include evidence of small bowel villous injury, resolution with gluten avoidance, and persistent normal small bowel mucosa for 2 or more years after the reintroduction of gluten to the diet.[50] The course of food protein-induced enteropathy in older children has not been characterized.

Infantile colic

Infantile colic is a common condition of paroxysmal, prolonged, excessive and inconsolable crying in an otherwise healthy infant. Colic lacks a formal definition or a standard set of diagnostic criteria (Table 11.9). The most commonly used criteria stem from Wessel in 1954, who described infantile colic as unexplained paroxysmal bouts of irritability, fussing or crying lasting > 3 hours a day for > 3 days a week for at least 1 week in duration, or, if severe, more than 3 weeks.[52] Excessive crying in infancy causes much distress to the infant, the family and the physician, and may have long-term implications for how the family views the child and the healthcare system. That being said, infantile colic itself is a benign and self-limiting condition.

Epidemiology

Infantile colic usually begins within the first weeks of life and resolves by 3 months of age in 60% of

Table 11.9 Diagnostic criteria for infantile colic

Wessel's rule of threes
Crying for: More than 3 hours per day
More than 3 days a week
For at least 3 weeks

Characteristics of crying episodes
Paroxysmal
Inconsolable
Excessive
Typically occurs late afternoon or early evening
Infant is normal between episodes

Physical features
Clenched fists
Stiff arms
Flexed legs, or legs drawn up
Arched back
Facial grimacing
Flushing
Abdominal distension
Passing of gas

Table 11.10 Proposed causes of infantile colic

Dietary
Food hypersensitivity
Lactose intolerance
Carbohydrate malabsorption

Gastrointestinal
Intestinal hypermotility
Feeding difficulties
Gut hormones
Imbalance of gut microflora
Gastroesophageal reflux
Excessive gas
Irritable bowel

Psychosocial
Temperament
Environmental hypersensitivity
Family stress
Parent–child interaction

infants and by 4 months in 90%.[53] The occurrence rate varies widely between 3–40%, depending on the population studied and the case definition used.[54] There seems to be no predilection for gender, full-term versus preterm, birthweight, breastfed versus formula-fed, or maternal level of education, parity or ethnicity.[52,55,56] Risk factors that have been associated with colic include living in a Western society, family stress and/or dysfunction, birth order, family history, and lack of parental confidence, all of which are probable confounders that increase the likelihood that parents will seek medical attention.[52,57]

Pathogenesis

Medical conditions account for <5% of excessive crying or irritability.[58] Pediatricians also look for simple yet often overlooked physical causes of sudden-onset crying, such as hair tourniquets (a hair wrapped around a digit), anal fissures or corneal abrasions. The cause of infantile colic is most likely multifactorial, represented by three main categories: dietary, gastrointestinal or behavioral (Table 11.10).

Colic–food hypersensitivity association

Not surprisingly, many studies have focused on diet as a cause of infantile colic owing to behavioral signs suggestive of gastrointestinal distress that often occur during crying episodes. Based on existing studies, 10–15% of infantile colic cases may be due to food allergies or intolerance.[59,60] Food hypersensitivity, particularly to milk and/or soy, may play a role in colic for a subgroup of infants (Clinical Vignette 6). Studies that have explored the colic–food hypersensitivity association are summarized in Table 11.11.

It has been suggested that infantile colic may represent an early manifestation of cows' milk allergy,[61] and that infants with a personal or family history of atopy should be given a trial off cows' milk.[62] Colic has not been associated with elevated serum

CLINICAL VIGNETTE 6

COLIC AND FOOD ALLERGY

A full-term male infant developed inconsolable crying at 2 weeks of age. He was exclusively breastfed from birth without any maternal dietary restrictions. During crying episodes, he appeared very uncomfortable and his legs were drawn up. He had frequent spit ups and frequent foul-smelling stools without blood or mucus. He had signs of cradle cap and developed an itchy rash on his cheeks and abdomen at 6 weeks, which improved slightly with topical corticosteroids. His birthweight was in the 75th percentile and gradually decreased to the 50th percentile by 2 months of age. Serum-specific IgE antibodies were detected to cows' milk 5 kIU/L and egg 1 kIU/L. Maternal restriction of cows' milk, soy and egg products resulted in resolution of his colic and significant improvement of his eczema within 1 week.

Table 11.11 Summary of studies investigating hypoallergenic diets in colic

Authors	Type of study	No. of subjects	Intervention	Results
Formula-fed				
Lothe 1982[63]	Double-blind crossover	60 formula-fed	Soy formula, if needed casein hydrolysate formula (CHF)	71% improved with formula change (18% with soy, 53% with CHF); 29% of cases not related to formula
Campbell 1989[64]	Double-blind crossover	19 formula-fed	Soy formula, if needed lactoalbumin hydrolyzate formula	69% improved with formula change (11% with soy, 2% with lactoalbumin hydrolyzate formula) vs 5% (n = 1) no change (p < 0.001); 26% (n = 6) had spontaneous improvement
Forsyth 1989[65]	Double-blind multiple crossover	17 formula-fed	Three formula changes with subjects receiving alternatively CHF or cows' milk formula	Less crying and less colic on CHF with 1st formula change (p < 0.01) Less colic on CHF with 2nd formula change (p < 0.05) No difference on 3rd formula change
Lothe 1989[66]	Double-blind crossover	27 formula-fed	CHF; challenge with whey vs placebo capsule	Less crying with formula change: 0.7 h/d in CHF group vs. 5.6 h/d in control group (p < 0.001) Increased crying with challenge: 3.2 h/d in whey group vs 1 h/d in placebo group (p < 0.001)
Iacono 1991[67]	Cohort	70 formula-fed	Soy formula	50/70 (71.4%) improved on soy formula and relapsed w/in 24 h on 2 subsequent cows' milk challenges. 8/50 showed signs of soy intolerance within 3 weeks.
Lucassen 2000[62]	RDBPCT	43 formula-fed	Whey hydrolyzate formula (WHF)	Decrease in crying by 63 min/d on WHF (p = 0.05)
Breastfed				
Evans 1981[68]	Double-blind crossover	20 breastfed	Replaced cows' milk with soy milk in maternal diet	No effect of soy milk; noted increased colic on days when mothers ate chocolate or fruit

Study	Design	Population	Intervention	Results
Jakobsson 1983[69]	Double-blind crossover	66 breastfed	Maternal elimination of cow's milk, challenge with whey vs placebo capsules	35/66 (53%) showed resolution of symptoms with elimination of cows' milk in maternal diet and 23/35 (35%) showed recurrence with reintroduction of cows' milk 9/16 (56%) infants showed increased symptoms on whey challenge
Estep 2000[70]	Cohort	6 breastfed	Amino acid formula (AAF) and maternal elimination of cows' milk, then reintroduction of breast milk	All infants improved on AAF All infants tolerated reintroduction of breast milk after maternal elimination of cows' milk
Hill 2005[71]	Randomized controlled	90 breastfed	Low allergen maternal diet (no milk, soy, wheat, egg, peanut, tree nut, fish)	Absolute risk reduction on low allergen diet was 37% (p < 0.001); based on reduction of infant distress by ≥ 25% mother's assessment indicated no difference In previous study, same group found that the effect of a low allergen maternal diet was more pronounced in infants <6 wks old (p < 0.001) vs >6 wks old (p < 0.05)
Follow-up				
Lothe 1982[63]	Double-blind crossover	60 formula-fed	Soy formula, if needed CHF	Group that responded to formula change showed higher incidence of cows' milk intolerance than normal population at 6 mo follow-up (18% vs. 1.6%) and 12 mo follow-up (13% vs. 1%)
Iacono 1991[67]	Cohort	70 formula-fed	Soy formula	22/50 (44%) of group that responded to formula change showed cows' milk intolerance at a mean follow-up time of 18 mo vs one infant (5%) in the non-responder group (p < 0.02)

RDBPCT, randomized double-blind placebo-controlled trial; CHF, casein hydrolyzate formula; WHF, whey hydrolyzate formula; AAF, amino acid formula.

total or food-specific IgE levels; however, young infants have low baseline serum-specific IgE concentrations and poor skin reactivity on skin testing, making diagnostic food allergy testing difficult at an age when they exhibit colic.[59] Some studies have reported that infants with a history of colic who responded to a change of formula have a higher likelihood of cows' milk intolerance later on (Table 11.11).[63,67]

Studies investigating the possible connection between colic and atopy have been conflicting. In a prospective cohort study of 320 children, cows' milk allergy ($p < 0.0005$) and other allergies ($p < 0.05$), but not asthma or eczema, were reported to be significantly increased in children at age 3.5 years who had a history of feeding or crying problems during infancy.[72] A prospective 10-year study on 96 children, half of whom had a history of infantile colic, found an association between infantile colic and allergic disorders (allergic rhinitis–conjunctivitis, asthmatic bronchitis, pollen allergy, atopic eczema and food allergy) ($p < 0.05$), and between infantile colic and a family history of GI and atopic disease ($p < 0.05$).[73] In contrast, the Tucson Children's Respiratory Study found no association between infantile colic and markers of atopy, asthma, allergic rhinitis, wheezing or peak flow variability at any age.[56]

Clinical features and diagnosis

Commonly observed patterns in colic include the time of day when crying episodes occur and associated physical behavior (Table 11.9). Crying episodes most often occur in the late afternoon or early evening.[52,57,74] Hypertonia, exhibited as clenched fists, stiff arms, flexed legs, arching of the back and facial grimacing, along with signs of flushing, abdominal distension, regurgitation and passing of gas, is typical.[51] The diagnosis of colic is made predominantly by history, and often using a version of Wessel's criteria.

Treatment

As in studies on causal factors of infantile colic, a wide diversity of case definitions, inclusion/exclusion criteria and outcome measurements make it difficult to compare the effectiveness of different colic treatments. One systematic review of infantile colic treatments concluded that four interventions were significant: hypoallergenic diet

(number needed to treat (NNT) in order for one case of colic to improve = 6), soy formula (NNT = 2), reduced stimulation (NNT = 2) and herbal tea (NNT = 3).[75] Proposed interventions that have been studied are reviewed in Table 11.12.

Several studies concluded that hypoallergenic diets may be beneficial in infantile colic. Some studies have shown improvement of colic with the introduction of soy formula; however, because some colicky infants are sensitive to both cows' milk and soy, a hydrolyzate formula may be a better choice. No studies have compared soy formula directly with hypoallergenic formula.

Management

An otherwise healthy infant <5 months old who exhibits crying for more than 3 hours/day for more than 3 days/week may be considered colicky. Table 11.13 lists strategies for managing a colicky infant. When evaluating an infant who presents with excessive crying, basic needs such as feeding, diaper changing and sleeping should be addressed, and more serious medical conditions ruled out first. The next most important management step is parental support. Most techniques for soothing a crying infant are anecdotal, but typically minimally invasive and benign. Feeding techniques such as frequent burping, an upright position while feeding and special bottles that reduce air bubbles have been suggested. Other methods focus on altering stimulation with, for example, pacifiers, changes in ambient temperature or scenery, swings, warm baths, massages, crib vibrators, secure car seats on a clothes dryer, and various sources of white noise.

Hypoallergenic diets have shown some efficacy in reducing colic symptoms for a subgroup of colicky infants, although how to identify which infants fall into this subgroup is unclear. Even though data on whether colic may actually represent an early manifestation of allergy are few, it would be reasonable to try diet management in infants with a personal or family history of atopy. Diet management might also be a good option if gastrointestinal symptoms such as vomiting, cramping or diarrhea are present, or if colic symptoms are associated predominantly with feeds. If the infant is formula-fed, switching to a hydrolyzed formula rather than a soy formula may be more efficacious because of the frequent intolerance to both cows' milk and soy. If the infant is breastfed and the mother would like to attempt

Table 11.12 Interventions for infantile colic

Intervention	Current understanding of effectiveness
Dietary	
Hydrolyzed formula	Beneficial for some (several studies)*
Soy formula	Significant crossover between cows' milk and soy intolerance (several studies)*
Low-allergen maternal diet	Beneficial for some (several studies)*
Fiber-enriched formula	Lacks evidence (1 RCT)[76]
Oral lactase or lactase-treated feeds	Inconclusive (2 RCT show no benefit, 2 RCT show benefit)[77,78,79,80]
Pharmaceutical	
Antireflux medication	Lacks evidence (2 RCT)[81,82]
Simethicone	Lacks evidence (3 RCT); no adverse effects[83,84,85]
Anticholinergic	Beneficial (4 RCT); case reports of serious side effects; contraindicated[86,87,88,89]
Cimetropium bromide	Beneficial (1 RCT); side effect increased sleepiness; needs additional safety studies[90]
Alternative therapies	
Probiotics	Beneficial (2 RCT showed benefit, 1 RCT showed no benefit with different strains for a shorter period); needs additional studies[91,92,93]
Sucrose/Glucose	Beneficial (3 RCT); effects short-lived[94,95,96]
Herbal tea/extract	Beneficial (3 RCT); needs standardization and safety studies[97,98,99]
Spinal manipulation	Inconclusive (1 RCT showed benefit, 1 RDBPCT showed no benefit); not recommended[100,101]
Behavioral	
Decreased stimulation	Beneficial (1 RCT)[102]
Intensive parental training	Beneficial (2 RCT)[103,104]
Increased carrying of infants	Lacks evidence (1 RCT); still suggested for reduction of infant and parental stress[105]

RCT, randomized controlled trial.
*RDBPCT, randomized double-blind placebo-controlled trial; CHF, casein hydrolyzate formula; WHF, whey hydrolyzate formula; AAF, amino acid formula.

Table 11.13 Management of infantile colic

Non-invasive
Rule out more serious medical conditions
Parental support and coping techniques
Soothing techniques
Eliminating tobacco smoke exposure (associated with increased motilin/hypermotility)
Proposed interventions
May be trialed
Hypoallergenic diet
• Formula-fed: hydrolyzed formula
• Breastfed: maternal elimination diet
Sucrose
Probiotics
Safety needs to be assessed
Herbal tea
Anticholinergic drugs

a hypoallergenic diet, maternal elimination of cows' milk may be tried first, followed by soy if no results are seen; as a last resort, other allergenic foods such as wheat, peanut, tree nuts, fish and shellfish may be eliminated. The effect of altering the maternal diet on the duration of breastfeeding should be addressed, and breastfeeding should be encouraged for its many other benefits. For this same reason, discontinuing breastfeeding and switching a colicky infant to a hypoallergenic formula may not be advisable when additional research is needed and colic is considered a benign condition.

It is recommended that alterations in diet be undertaken as trials. If there is no improvement in colic symptoms on a hypoallergenic diet, then a regular diet can be resumed. A hypoallergenic diet may be considered beneficial if symptoms improve or resolve when suspect foods are removed and recur when they are reintroduced.[60] Because colic is self-limited and resolves in most infants by 4 months of age, and because many children outgrow early food intolerances, rechallenges with suspect foods may be attempted every 3–4 months with physician recommendation.[60]

Summary

We have reviewed the common childhood non-IgE mediated gastrointestinal conditions induced by food proteins. The prognosis is favorable, with the majority of cases resolving in the first few years of life. Diagnosis is complicated by the lack of non-invasive confirmatory tests and tests that identify the offending food proteins. Definitive diagnosis usually requires an oral food challenge. Management relies on the avoidance of the offending food and periodic reintroductions.

References

1. Nowak-Wegrzyn A, Muraro A. Food protein-induced enterocolitis syndrome. Curr Opin Allergy Clin Immunol 2009;9:371–7.
2. Katz Y, Goldberg MR, Rajuan N, et al. The prevalence and natural course of food protein-induced enterocolitis syndrome to cow's milk: A large-scale, prospective population-based study. J Allergy Clin Immunol 2011;127:647–53 e3.
3. Sicherer SH. Food protein-induced enterocolitis syndrome: case presentations and management lessons. J Allergy Clin Immunol 2005;115: 149–56.
4. Powell GK, McDonald PJ, Van Sickle GJ, et al. Absorption of food protein antigen in infants with food protein-induced enterocolitis. Dig Dis Sci 1989;34:781–8.
5. Shek LPC, Soderstrom L, Ahlstedt S, et al. Determination of food specific IgE levels over time can predict the development of tolerance in cows' milk and hen's egg allergy. J Allergy Clin Immunol 2004;114:387–91.
6. Nowak-Wegrzyn A, Sampson HA, Wood RA, et al. Food protein-induced enterocolitis syndrome caused by solid food proteins. Pediatrics 2003; 111:829–35.
7. Monti G, Castagno E, Liguori SA, et al. Food protein-induced enterocolitis syndrome by cow's milk proteins passed through breast milk. J Allergy Clin Immunol 2011;127:679–80.
8. Nomura I, Morita H, Hosokawa S, et al. Four distinct subtypes of non-IgE-mediated gastrointestinal food allergies in neonates and infants, distinguished by their initial symptoms. J Allergy Clin Immunol 2011;127:685–8 e8.
9. Sampson HA, Anderson JA. Summary and recommendations: Classification of gastrointestinal manifestations due to immunologic reactions to foods in infants and young children. J Pediatr Gastroenterol Nutr 2000;30(Suppl):S87–94.
10. Mehr S, Kakakios A, Frith K, et al. Food proteininduced enterocolitis syndrome: 16-year experience. Pediatrics 2009;123:e459–64.
11. Powell GK. Milk- and soy-induced enterocolitis of infancy. Clinical features and standardization of challenge. J Pediatr 1978;93:553–60.
12. Mehr S, Kakakios A, Kemp A. Rice: a common and severe cause of food protein-induced enterocolitis syndrome. Arch Dis Child 2009;123:e459–64.
13. Fogg MI, Brown-Whitehorn TA, Pawlowski NA, et al. Atopy patch test for the diagnosis of food proteininduced enterocolitis syndrome. Pediatr Allergy Immunol 2006;17:351–5.
14. Hwang JB, Lee SH, Kang YN, et al. Indexes of suspicion of typical cows' milk protein-induced enterocolitis. J Korean Med Sci 2007;22:993–7.
15. Hwang J-B, Song J-Y, Kang YN, et al. The significance of gastric juice analysis for a positive challenge by a standard oral challenge test in typical cows' milk protein-induced enterocolitis. J Korean Med Sci 2008;23:251–5.
16. Sicherer SH, Eigenmann PA, Sampson HA. Clinical features of food protein-induced enterocolitis syndrome. J Pediatr 1998;133:214–9.
17. Lake AM, Whitington PF, Hamilton SR. Dietary protein-induced colitis in breast-fed infants. J Pediatr 1982;101:906–10.
18. Xanthakos SA, Schwimmer JB, Melin-Aldana H, et al. Prevalence and outcome of allergic colitis in healthy infants with rectal bleeding: a prospective cohort study. J Pediatr Gastroenterol Nutr 2005;41:16–22.
19. Arvola T, Ruuska T, Keränen J, et al. Rectal bleeding in infancy: clinical, allergological, and microbiological examination. Pediatrics 2006;117:e760–8.
20. Lake AM. Food-induced eosinophilic proctocolitis. J Pediatr Gastroenterol Nutr 2000;30(Suppl):S58–60.
21. Maloney J, Nowak-Wegrzyn A. Educational clinical case series for pediatric allergy and immunology: allergic proctocolitis, food protein-induced enterocolitis syndrome and allergic eosinophilic gastroenteritis with protein-losing gastroenteropathy as manifestations of non-IgE-mediated cows' milk allergy. Pediatr Allergy Immunol 2007;18:360–7.
22. Goldman H, Proujansky R. Allergic proctitis and gastroenteritis in children. Clinical and mucosal biopsy features in 53 cases. Am J Surg Pathol 1986;10:75–86.
23. Jenkins HR, Pincott JR, Soothill JF, et al. Food allergy: the major cause of infantile colitis. Arch Dis Child 1984;59:326–9.
24. Odze RD, Bines J, Leichtner AM, et al. Allergic proctocolitis in infants: a prospective clinicopathologic biopsy study. Hum Pathol 1993;24:668–74.
25. Pumberger W, Pomberger G, Geissler W. Proctocolitis in breast fed infants: a contribution to differential

diagnosis of haematochezia in early childhood. Postgrad Med J 2001;77:252–4.

26. Machida HM, Catto Smith AG, Gall DG, et al. Allergic colitis in infancy: clinical and pathologic aspects. J Pediatr Gastroenterol Nutr 1994;19:22–6.

27. Lake AM. Food protein-induced colitis and gastroenteropathy in infants and children. In: SHSR MD, editor. Food allergy: Adverse reactions to foods.

28. Hill DJ, Ford RP, Shelton MJ, et al. A study of 100 infants and young children with cows' milk allergy. Clin Rev Allergy 1984;2:125–42.

29. Davidson M, Burnstine RC, Kugler MM, et al. Malabsorption defect induced by ingestion of beta lactoglobulin. J Pediatr 1965;66: 545–54.

30. Harrison M, Kilby A, Walker-Smith JA, et al. Cows' milk protein intolerance: a possible association with gastroenteritis, lactose intolerance, and IgA deficiency. Br Med J 1976;1:1501–4.

31. Kuitunen P. Duodenal-jejunal histology in malabsorption syndrome in infants. Ann Paediatr Fenn 1966;12:101–32.

32. Kuitunen P, Visakorpi JK, Savilahti E, et al. Malabsorption syndrome with cows' milk intolerance. Clinical findings and course in 54 cases. Arch Dis Child 1975;50:351–6.

33. Lamy M, Nezelof C, Jos J, et al. Biopsy of the intestinal mucosa in children. Initial results of a study of the malabsorption syndromes. Presse Med 1963;71:1267–70.

34. Liu H-Y, Tsao MU, Moore B, et al. Bovine milk-proteininduced intestinal malabsorption syndrome in infancy. Gastroenterology 1967;54:27–34.

35. Visakorpi J, Immonen P. Intolerance to cows' milk and wheat gluten in the primary. … Acta Pædiatrica 1967.

36. Savilahti E. Food-induced malabsorption syndromes. J Pediatr Gastroenterol Nutr 2000;30(Suppl):S61–6.

37. Kokkonen J, Haapalahti M, Laurila K, et al. Cows' milk protein-sensitive enteropathy at school age. J Pediatr 2001;139:797–803.

38. Veres G, Westerholm-Ormio M, Kokkonen J, et al. Cytokines and adhesion molecules in duodenal mucosa of children with delayed-type food allergy. J Pediatr Gastroenterol Nutr 2003;37:27–34.

39. Latcham F, Merino F, Lang A, et al. A consistent pattern of minor immunodeficiency and subtle enteropathy in children with multiple food allergy. J Pediatr 2003;143:39–47.

40. Kokkonen J, Holm K, Karttunen TJ, et al. Enhanced local immune response in children with prolonged gastrointestinal symptoms. Acta Paediatr 2004;93: 1601–7.

41. Savilahti E. Immunochemical study of the malabsorption syndrome with cows' milk intolerance. Gut 1973;14:491–501.

42. Paajanen L, Vaarala O, Karttunen R, et al. Increased IFN-gamma secretion from duodenal biopsy samples in delayed-type cows' milk allergy. Pediatr Allergy Immunol 2005;16:439–44.

43. Isolauri E, Turjanmaa K. Combined skin prick and patch testing enhances identification of food allergy in infants with atopic dermatitis. J Allergy Clin Immunol 1996;97:9–15.

44. Augustin M, Karttunen TJ, Kokkonen J. TIA1 and mast cell tryptase in food allergy of children: increase of intraepithelial lymphocytes expressing TIA1 associates with allergy. J Pediatr Gastroenterol Nutr 2001;32:11–8.

45. Iyngkaran N, Yadav M, Boey CG, et al. Effect of continued feeding of cows' milk on asymptomatic infants with milk protein sensitive enteropathy. Arch Dis Child 1988;63:911–5.

46. Verkasalo M, Kuitunen P, Savilahti E, et al. Changing pattern of cows' milk intolerance. An analysis of the occurrence and clinical course in the 60s and mid-70s. Acta Paediatr Scand 1981;70:289–95.

47. Bürgin-Wolff A, Gaze H, Hadziselimovic F, et al. Antigliadin and antiendomysium antibody determination for coeliac disease. Arch Dis Child 1991;66:941–7.

48. Meuli R, Pichler WJ, Gaze H, et al. Genetic difference in HLA-DR phenotypes between coeliac disease and transitory gluten intolerance. Arch Dis Child 1995;72:29–32.

49. Walker-Smith J. Transient gluten intolerance. Arch Dis Child 1970;45:523–6.

50. McNeish AS, Rolles CJ, Arthur LJ. Criteria for diagnosis of temporary gluten intolerance. Arch Dis Child 1976;51:275–8.

51. Barr RG. Colic and crying syndromes in infants. Pediatrics 1998;102:1282–6.

52. Wessel MA, Cobb JC, Jackson EB, et al. Paroxysmal fussing in infancy, sometimes called colic. Pediatrics 1954;14:421–35.

53. Parker S, Magee T. Colic. In: Parker S, Zuckerman B, Augustyn M, editors. The Zuckerman Parker Handbook of Development and Behavioral Pediatrics for Primary Care. 3rd ed. Philadelphia: Lippincott Williams & Wilkins; 2011. p. 182.

54. Lucassen P, Assendelft W, van Eijk J, et al. Systematic review of the occurrence of infantile colic in the community. Br Med J 2001;84:398.

55. Illingworth RS. Three-months' colic. Arch Dis Child 1954;29:165–74.

56. Castro-Rodriguez J, Stern D, Halonen M, et al. Relation between infantile colic and asthma/atopy: a prospective study in an unselected population. Pediatrics 2001;108:878.

57. Lehtonen L, Rautava P. Infantile colic: natural history and treatment. Curr Probl Pediatr 1996;26:79–85.

58. Freedman SB, Al-Harthy N, Thull-Freedman J. The crying infant: diagnostic testing and frequency of serious underlying disease. Pediatrics 2009;123:841–8. (p0795)

59. Sampson H. Infantile colic and food allergy: fact or fiction? J Pediatr 1989;115:583–4.

60. Sampson H, Burks W. Adverse Reactions to Foods. In: Adkinson NF, editor. Middleton's Allergy: Principles and Practice. 7th ed. Maryland Heights, MO: Mosby, Inc.; 2008.

61. Hill DJ, Hosking CS. Infantile colic and food hypersensitivity. J Pediatr Gastroenterol Nutr 2000;30(Suppl):S67–76.

62. Lucassen P, Assendelft W, Gubbels J, et al. Infantile colic: crying time reduction with a whey hydrolysate: a double-blind, randomized, placebo-controlled trial. Pediatrics 2000;106:1349.

63. Lothe L, Lindberg T, Jakobsson I. Cow's milk formula as a cause of infantile colic: a double-blind study. Pediatrics 1982;70:7–10.

64. Campbell JP. Dietary treatment of infant colic: a double-blind study. J R Coll Gen Pract 1989;39:11–4.

65. Forsyth BW. Colic and the effect of changing formulas: a double-blind, multiple-crossover study. J Pediatr 1989;115:521–6.

66. Lothe L, Lindberg T. Cow's milk whey protein elicits symptoms of infantile colic in colicky formula-fed infants: a double-blind crossover study. Pediatrics 1989;83:262–6.

67. Iacono G, Carroccio A, Montalto G, et al. Severe infantile colic and food intolerance: a long-term prospective study. J Pediatr Gastroenterol Nutr 1991;12:332–5.

68. Evans RW, Fergusson DM, Allardyce RA, et al. Maternal diet and infantile colic in breast-fed infants. Lancet 1981;1:1340–2.

69. Jakobsson I, Lindberg T. Cow's milk proteins cause infantile colic in breast-fed infants: a double-blind crossover study. Pediatrics 1983;71:268–71.

70. Estep D, Kulczycki A. Colic in breast-milk-fed infants: treatment by temporary substitution of Neocate infant formula. Acta Paediatrica 2000;89:795–802.

71. Hill D, Roy N, Heine R, et al. Effect of a low-allergen maternal diet on colic among breastfed infants: a randomized, controlled trial. Pediatrics 2005;116:e709.

72. Forsyth BW, Canny PF. Perceptions of vulnerability 3 1/2 years after problems of feeding and crying behavior in early infancy. Pediatrics 1991;88:757–63.

73. Savino F, Castagno E, Bretto R, et al. A prospective 10-year study on children who had severe infantile colic. Acta Paediatr Suppl 2005;94:129–32.

74. Lehtonen L, Korvenranta H. Infantile colic. Seasonal incidence and crying profiles. Arch Pediatr Adolesc Med 1995;149:533–6.

75. Garrison M, Christakis D. A systematic review of treatments for infant colic. Pediatrics 2000;106:184.

76. Treem WR, Hyams JS, Blankschen E, et al. Evaluation of the effect of a fiber-enriched formula on infant colic. J Pediatr 1991;119:695–701.

77. Kanabar D, Randhawa M, Clayton P. Improvement of symptoms in infant colic following reduction of lactose load with lactase. J Hum Nutr Diet 2001;14:359–63.

78. Kearney P, Malone A, Hayes T, et al. A trial of lactase in the management of infant colic. J Hum Nutr Diet 1998;11:281–5.

79. Ståhlberg MR, Savilahti E. Infantile colic and feeding. Arch Dis Child 1986;61:1232–3.

80. Miller JJ, McVeagh P, Fleet GH, et al. Effect of yeast lactase enzyme on "colic" in infants fed human milk. J Pediatr 1990;117:261–3.

81. Moore DJ, Tao BS, Lines DR, et al. Double-blind placebo-controlled trial of omeprazole in irritable infants with gastroesophageal reflux. J Pediatr 2003;143:219–23.

82. Jordan B, Heine RG, Meehan M, et al. Effect of antireflux medication, placebo and infant mental health intervention on persistent crying: a randomized clinical trial. J Paediatr Child Health 2006;42:49–58.

83. Danielsson B, Hwang CP. Treatment of infantile colic with surface active substance (simethicone). Acta Paediatr Scand 1985;74:446–50.

84. Sethi KS, Sethi JK. Simethicone in the management of infant colic. Practitioner 1988;232:508.

85. Metcalf TJ, Irons TG, Sher LD, et al. Simethicone in the treatment of infant colic: a randomized, placebo-controlled, multicenter trial. Pediatrics 1994;94:29–34.

86. Illingworth RS. Evening Colic in Infants: A Double-Blind Trial of Dicyclomine Hydrocholoride. The Lancet 1959;274:1119–20.

87. Grunseit F. Evaluation of the efficacy of dicyclomine hydrochloride ('Merbentyl') syrup in the treatment of infant colic. Curr Med Res Opin 1977;5:258–61.

88. Weissbluth M, Christoffel KK, Davis AT. Treatment of infantile colic with dicyclomine hydrochloride. J Pediatr 1984;104:951–5.

89. Hwang CP, Danielsson B. Dicyclomine hydrochloride in infantile colic. Br Med J (Clin Res Ed) 1985;291:1014.

90. Savino F, Brondello C, Cresi F, et al. Cimetropium bromide in the treatment of crisis in infantile colic. J Pediatr Gastroenterol Nutr 2002;34:417–9.

91. Savino F, Pelle E, Palumeri E, et al. Lactobacillus reuteri (American Type Culture Collection Strain 55730) versus simethicone in the treatment of infantile colic: a prospective randomized study. Pediatrics 2007;119:e124–30.

92. Savino F, Cordisco L, Tarasco V, et al. Lactobacillus reuteri DSM 17938 in infantile colic: a randomized, double-blind, placebo-controlled trial. Pediatrics 2010;126:e526–33.

93. Mentula S, Tuure T, Koskenala R, et al. Microbial composition and fecal fermentation end products from colicky infants-a probiotic supplementation pilot. Microb Ecol Heal Dis 2008;20:37–47.

94. Markestad T. Use of sucrose as a treatment for infant colic. Arch Dis Child 1997;76:356–7; discussion 7–8.

95. Barr RG, Young SN, Wright JH, et al. Differential calming responses to sucrose taste in crying infants with and without colic. Pediatrics 1999;103:e68.

96. Akcam M, Yilmaz A. Oral hypertonic glucose solution in the treatment of infantile colic. Pediatr Int 2006;48:125–7.

97. Weizman Z, Alkrinawi S, Goldfarb D, et al. Efficacy of herbal tea preparation in infantile colic. J Pediatr 1993;122:650–2.

98. Alexandrovich I, Rakovitskaya O, Kolmo E, et al. The effect of fennel (Foeniculum Vulgare) seed oil emulsion in infantile colic: a randomized, placebo-

controlled study. Altern Ther Health Med 2003;9: 58–61.

99. Savino F, Cresi F, Castagno E, et al. A randomized double-blind placebo-controlled trial of a standardized extract of Matricariae recutita, Foeniculum vulgare and Melissa officinalis (ColiMil) in the treatment of breastfed colicky infants. Phytother Res 2005;19:335–40.

100. Wiberg JM, Nordsteen J, Nilsson N. The short-term effect of spinal manipulation in the treatment of infantile colic: a randomized controlled clinical trial with a blinded observer. J Manipulative Physiol Ther 1999;22:517–22.

101. Olafsdottir E, Forshei S, Fluge G, et al. Randomised controlled trial of infantile colic treated with chiropractic spinal manipulation. Arch Dis Child 2001;84:138–41.

102. McKenzie S. Troublesome crying in infants: effect of advice to reduce stimulation. Arch Dis Child 1991;66:1416–20.

103. Parkin PC, Schwartz CJ, Manuel BA. Randomized controlled trial of three interventions in the management of persistent crying of infancy. Pediatrics 1993;92:197–201.

104. Dihigo SK. New strategies for the treatment of colic: modifying the parent/infant interaction. J Pediatr Health Care 1998;12:256–62.

105. Barr RG, McMullan SJ, Spiess H, et al. Carrying as colic "therapy": a randomized controlled trial. Pediatrics 1991;87:623–30.

CHAPTER 12

Approach to the Clinical Diagnosis of Food Allergy

Jonathan O'B. Hourihane

Introduction

Clinical history-taking remains the cornerstone of diagnosis of food allergy, as it does for all other medical conditions. Distinguishing different phenotypes of food allergy can be a simple task, for example a parental report of the onset of urticaria and angioedema 2 minutes after eating peanut butter, or it can be very difficult, for example distinguishing eosinophilic esophagitis from gastroesophageal reflux disease (GERD). The experienced clinician can use existing knowledge of allergy syndromes to distinguish a particular child's current allergic status, the likelihood of resolution of the index food allergy, which may require proof by formal challenge, and can give some guidance about the breadth and duration of the required exclusion diet.

The discriminating use of in vivo and in vitro diagnostic tests relies on an understanding of the relevance of a particular history and their usefulness in any particular population. Their sensitivity and specificity are related to the pre-test probability of a disease being present in the population being tested. As an example, the significance of a positive skin prick test (SPT) to hazelnut of 3 mm differs between a 12-month-old child who has suffered anaphylaxis after eating hazelnut spread and a 12-year-old child who is having allergy tests for rhinitis but has probably eaten hazelnut several times before.[1]

The skill of history-taking related to specific food allergy syndromes or scenarios means that tests, when performed, can be interpreted in a more discriminating and definitive manner. It is therefore worthwhile examining how a physician's assessment of children presenting with suspected food allergy and his/her subsequent management of the condition(s) vary as a function of the interaction between the discrete or related foods and the child as he or she grows from being exclusively dependent on breast milk or infant formula, via weaning onto a narrow range of foods, and eventually onto a fully diverse and unrestricted 'adult' diet.

First consultation

This is a critical moment for families, and attention must be given to both the medical details and the family's response to what happened to their child that prompted their attendance. It might have been anaphylaxis, which they did not recognize, or it might have been urticaria that they have attributed to a previously tolerated food, but which was in fact not related to allergies at all. Most families will have received advice from family members or will have searched the internet before their appointment with an allergist. Some of this information may be correct, but experience shows that dietary eliminations/exclusions may be too broad; the child may be undernourished, or might be living on an age-inappropriate diet due to concerns about trying new foods.

CLINICAL CASE

Other conditions can mimic food allergy

An 11-month-old girl developed urticaria and swollen lips 2 hours after eating boiled egg. This resolved without treatment. She had previously tolerated one teaspoon of less-cooked scrambled egg. At 1 year of age she developed a cough and temperature, with a maculopapular rash (Fig. 12.1). On waking the next day she had urticaria on her legs (Fig. 12.2). No new foods had been introduced, and she had not been given any form of egg again.

Skin prick testing and serum-specific IgE at 13 months were both negative for egg. A diagnosis of virus-induced urticaria was made and she was discharged from follow-up.

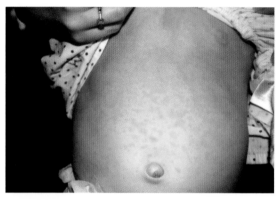

Figure 12.1 A maculopapular rash seen on day 1 of a viral illness. This is unlikely to be allergic in nature.

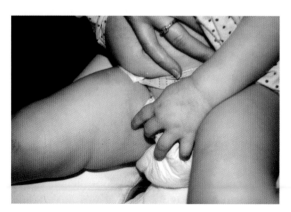

Figure 12.2 Urticaria seen in the setting of a viral illness is more likely to be due to the viremia than to a new allergy to a food previously tolerated.

Several features of this story suggest a non-allergic basis of her symptoms. This girl's initial cutaneous reaction was slightly delayed at 2 hours after contact with well-cooked egg, and she had previously eaten a less well-cooked (therefore more allergenic) form of egg without complication. The onset of a typical exanthem in the setting of fever, followed by urticaria, made it straightforward to diagnose virus-induced urticaria. The tests for egg allergy may not even have been necessary.

Mast cell membrane-bound IgE is not the only mechanism of degranulation of mast cells. Complement activation can also cause mast cell degranulation, and mast cells can respond to C5A stimulation, neurogenic stimulation and hormonal influences. Although hormonal influences are relatively irrelevant in small infants, they have high relevance in adolescent girls and may be related both to menstruation-related urticarial syndromes and also to exercise-induced anaphylaxis, with or without a food trigger.

As infants may be committed to the allergic march (see Chapters 3 and 18) for their entire childhood or longer, the pediatric allergist must ensure that he understands and addresses families' concerns; that he can remove unnecessary dietary and social restrictions; and that families remain engaged with the medical allergy service until the allergy issues are resolved or appropriate self-management strategies are in place for adolescents and young adults. For example, negative skin pricks (high negative predictive value; see Chapter 13) can be very useful in encouraging parents to relax unjustified restrictions on their child's diet.

Even at first consultation it is important for families to realize that an allergological evaluation is as much about which foods a child can be allowed to eat as about which they must rigorously avoid. A fundamental part of the clinical management of food allergy is to ensure that all foods that should be excluded are excluded, and that foods that do not need to be excluded are included, even at the time of diagnosis. An example of prudent exclusion is to advise parents that children with cows' milk allergy should not be exposed to goats' milk. The child must avoid the index food – in this case cows' milk – as reactivity is likely to be still present at first consultation, and must also avoid the associated food – goats' milk – which is highly cross-reactive with cows' milk, occasionally causing anaphylaxis in children whose presenting allergic reactions to cows' milk have only been mild.[2,3] If a child has already been exposed to goats' milk

Table 12.1 Even at first consultation, some prudent inclusions and exclusions can be advised by an experienced allergist

Index food allergen, to be avoided	Food that should be prudently excluded, unless known to have been consumed safely	Food that can be prudently included, if not previously consumed safely
Cows' milk	Goats' milk	
Unadulterated egg	Raw egg (mayonnaise, fresh ice cream)	Baked egg (cakes, muffins) Peanut*
Peanut	Tree nuts†	Other legumes, incl. soya Coconut, nutmeg‡
Cod	Other white fish	Tuna∫
Sesame	Peanut	

*Only if negative SPT with peanut.
†Consider open challenge if positive.
‡These foods are not nuts or legumes (peanut is a legume).
∫Canned tuna is tolerated by most children allergic to white fish.

without incident, then it is reasonable to allow prudent consumption of goats' milk products, although goats' milk is neither a perfect nor nutritionally complete substitute for cows' milk.

An example of early prudent inclusion is allowing continued consumption of baked egg products in children who have previously eaten them safely but have reacted to less well-cooked egg. Elimination of all egg products can be common in this scenario, but in fact safe consumption of baked egg products appears to modify the in vitro immunological profile of such children, making it more similar to those of children proven tolerant to egg than to children who remain allergic to less well-cooked egg.[4] On a practical note, the avoidance of less well-cooked egg is much easier than avoiding baked egg products, so this small liberation of an avoidance diet can have a big, early impact on family life, even while maintaining avoidance of the implicated form of egg (Table 12.1).

What immune mechanism is causing the problem in this child?

IgE is found in all body compartments, so IgE-mediated reactions often manifest in more than one body system. It is still uncertain how a locally initiated IgE-mediated reaction to a very small oral dose of food allergen becomes amplified into a multisystem reaction or even anaphylaxis.

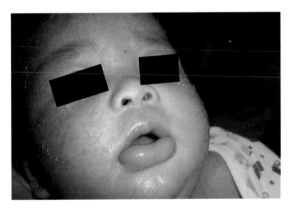

Figure 12.3 This 4-month-old boy had suffered eczema since his third day of life. He failed to thrive on breast milk, but was not brought to medical attention by his parents, who are nurses. He was offered his first infant formula at 4 months. Ten minutes later he had facial erythema, angioedema and wheeze, and was referred to hospital. Milk elimination and topical skin care were initiated as an inpatient and he is now eczema free at 7 months, on an amino acid formula and a milk-, egg- and wheat-free diet.

Similarly, it must be recognized that delayed cell-mediated responses can coexist with immediate IgE-mediated responses. So there are overlap syndromes including children who suffer both IgE-mediated, early symptoms relating to milk ingestion, and also delayed, cell-mediated reactions to milk in the forms of exacerbations of eczema or atopic dermatitis (Fig. 12.3 and Chapter 5).

Similarly, there are many infants whose parents report that dairy products and egg make their eczema worse but who have never suffered from urticaria or angioedema. Occasionally these infants and young children can tolerate small amounts of dairy, e.g. half a pot of infant yoghurt per day, but not more than this amount on a regular basis. This scenario suggests a delayed-onset reaction that is cell mediated and very unlikely to evolve into anaphylaxis. The prognosis for this type of milk allergy is generally more favorable than for IgE-mediated immediate reactions.

There are common diseases that can mimic food allergy, such as gastroesophageal reflux disease (GERD), which can cause difficulty with feeding and vomiting but is not usually associated with urticaria or angioedema. Eosinophilic esophagitis (Chapter 10) has an overlap with GERD and the diagnosis of eosinophilic esophagitis cannot be confidently made until a child has failed a trial of proton pump inhibitor.[5]

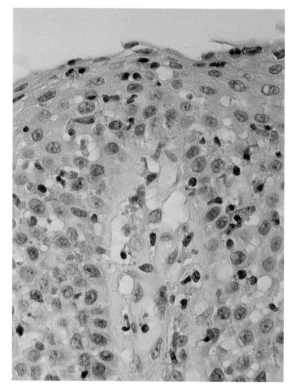

Figure 12.4 Biopsy from the mid-esophagus showing abundant eosinophils (> 15/hpf).

CLINICAL CASE

A 10-year-old boy relocated from another country where he had been under the care of an allergist since the age of 3 years, when he had apparently suffered a life-threatening reaction to banana. He had been on amino acid formula in early infancy for severe eczema and GERD. Formal food challenges had liberated restrictions related to asymptomatic peanut and tree nut sensitization. At his first interview after relocation he reported lifelong abdominal and retrosternal pain and excessive burping after eating eggs, most fruits and vegetables. SPT was positive for egg and kiwi, but negative for soya, carrot, corn, sweet potato and wheat. Because of the combination of lifelong history of feeding difficulties, and of atypical reactivity to foods that are both commonly and uncommonly seen as allergens, it was suspected he might have eosinophilic esophagitis. In a reductive way his symptomatology seemed more explicable as an intrinsic inflammatory problem in his GI tract than atypical allergic reactivity to multiple foods. Endoscopy confirmed the diagnosis (Fig. 12.4). A 6-week trial of proton pump inhibition failed to improve his symptoms, but formal exclusion of implicated foods, supported by dietetic review, remains successful.

Which foods are common allergens in this age group?

There is much practical merit in breaking down the description of clinical diagnosis into age-related groups, because there is a chronology to the associations between food and different clinical manifestations of food allergy.

Suspected allergic reactions under 6 months of age

The atopic march or marathon is well established and often starts with food allergy and eczema in the first 6 months of life (see Chapters 3 and 18). Urticaria and angioedema are unusual initial presentations of cows' milk allergy in breastfed infants who usually have enteropathic and dermatological manifestations. However, the introduction of cows' milk formula is often associated with urticarial reactions in symptomatic cows' milk-allergic infants. The reasons for this are unknown, but may be related to the presence in breast milk of immunomodulatory factors, or because the dose of allergenic cows' milk proteins is naturally higher in directly administered cows' milk-based infant formulae than in human breast milk.

Exclusion diets during pregnancy or breastfeeding are no longer recommended as protection/

prophylaxis against developing allergic disorders,[6,7] but they can be very successful in reducing or even eliminating cutaneous and other reactions in allergic children who have demonstrated clinical reactivity during breastfeeding.

Diagnosis and therapy can proceed simultaneously

A trial of maternal dietary elimination can also be part of the clinical diagnostic process as it can identify whether one food, more than one food, or any food at all, is actually implicated in the condition being presented in a breastfed infant. Professional supervision by an allergy-experienced dietitian is essential. Persistence of symptoms on a properly supervised elimination diet adhered to by the mother means that those foods are not the cause of the skin or GI symptoms and the foods can be reintroduced carefully, one at a time. It has been reported occasionally that severe reactions can be elicited during the reintroduction of excluded foods, but this is not common in breastfed infants.

The diagnostic and therapeutic dilemma then remains whether to empirically exclude a second set of foods on the same trial basis, or to abandon dietary exclusions completely. Experience shows that as the first-rank foods excluded (milk, egg, wheat, soya) are responsible for the vast majority of food-related enteropathic and skin symptoms in breastfed infants, a second trial of other empiric exclusions may not be successful, unless a particular food consumed by the mother can be implicated.

As time passes the relative nutritional importance of breastfeeding diminishes for children in developed countries, and the introduction of supplemental feeding with extensively hydrolyzed or amino acid-based infant formulas may reduce child and maternal distress considerably. This allows parents to see that their baby can grow and sleep peacefully after feeding, and can reassure them sufficiently to introduce other foods at home.

In early infancy – under 3–4 months – other food allergy syndromes can be confused with cows' milk allergy or other malabsorptive conditions. Cows' milk protein enterocolitis and proctitis can present simply with bright red blood in the diaper. These easily identified children are not unwell and respond very quickly to substitution of cows' milk with extensively hydrolyzed or amino acid formulas. IgE-based tests are usually negative and endoscopy is not required in the simplest of cases. Other infants may develop food protein enterocolitis syndrome, which is a much more complicated disease to diagnose and treat than IgE-mediated food allergy (see Chapter 11). These children can present insidiously with intractable enteropathy/diarrhea and failure to thrive, or catastrophically in a collapsed state such as cardiogenic shock, due to massive GI fluid loss. The latter responds well to high-volume fluid resuscitation. In such presentations it may not be appreciated that there may be a connection with food, as the collapse may be several hours after ingestion of the food. Rice, soya, cows' milk and wheat are the most commonly implicated foods in this condition.[8]

Suspected allergic reactions to foods 6–18 months

Weaning foods are usually introduced one at a time, even in non-allergic children, so linking suspected exposure to a witnessed reaction is not difficult. Common weaning foods are usually vegetables, fruits, and cereals such as wheat and oats. Wheat is a common allergen, and is an ingredient that must be labeled according to EU law. Wheat allergy, however, is much less common than milk or egg allergy, so it is worth investigating the implicated meal for hidden dairy products, as many weaning foods have milk powder in them. Furthermore, the interpretation of positive tests for IgE-mediated wheat allergy is more difficult than for milk, egg and peanut (see Chapter 13). Like egg and milk, wheat commonly causes delayed cutaneous reactions, such as a flare of eczema. For reasons that are based on both sound immunological principles (wheat is known to cause both immediate, IgE-mediated and delayed, cell-mediated symptoms) and on experience (IgE-based tests can be unhelpful even in immediate reactions to wheat), a supervised early food challenge in hospital is often more worthwhile for wheat (and soya for the same reasons) than for milk and egg.

Eczema is a very common disorder in infants, and parents can report that some foods cause deterioration in eczema both in the perioral area and at more remote sites. There is a strong association between eczema of more than moderate severity and food allergy.[9,10] However, many suspected foods are acidic fruits, and it appears that the flare of local and distant eczema is due to a directly irritant effect of the acidic juice on the damaged skin barrier. Skin prick testing might be needed, as

Table 12.2 Acidic foods can cause a flare of facial eczema that is often suspected to be allergic in origin

Kiwi*
Strawberry, raspberry etc*
Tomatoes*†
Citrus fruits (orange, lemon, lime)
Vegetable/yeast spreads (Marmite, Vegemite) (common in
   UK, Australia only)

*Can also cause IgE-mediated reactions, so SPT can be undertaken.
†Usually raw tomato only, with cooked tomato tolerated.

some first- and second-rank food allergens (kiwi and tomato in particular, but also strawberry) can also act in this way, so it can be prudent to do skin prick testing to demonstrate to families that the reaction is not likely to be IgE-mediated and is therefore likely to be benign and to resolve over time, when the skin barrier, especially on the face, has become better established (Table 12.2).

The introduction of other foods after weaning has started can implicate them in allergic reactions. Known allergenic foods such as lentils, hazelnuts and peanuts (in spreadable butter form rather than as whole or crushed nuts) can be introduced in this age group, but the diagnosis of allergy to these foods is usually made easily, as these foods are predominantly associated with stereotypical IgE-mediated reactions. Egg can again be implicated, in the form of boiled egg, pancakes, or raw or nearly raw in mayonnaise or ice cream, even if cooked egg has already been introduced without complication.

International and intercultural considerations

Individual foods can 'behave' differently at weaning in different geographical locations, possibly related to whether sensitization has happened de novo with the native food or secondarily via pollen allergens that are highly cross-reactive with food allergens. Hazelnut allergy is the archetype of this[11] (see also Chapter 7).

Weaning practices vary internationally too: lentils are a common weaning food for children in southern Europe but not in northern Europe. The exception to this observation is in families who are vegetarian for personal, cultural or religious reasons. Indians and Pakistanis living in northern Europe

are commonly vegetarian, and allergenic legumes including lentils and chick peas are staple weaning foods for infants, and are part of the family diet for older children and adults alike. Scandinavian families may introduce fish earlier than more southerly populations, and fish allergy was first well described in Scandinavian infants. Children of West African and Far Eastern families may consume boiled peanuts, considered to be less allergenic than roasted peanuts. Israeli Jewish children have peanut introduced to their diet much earlier than Jewish children in Britain, which has been suggested as part of the reason for a much lower prevalence of peanut allergy in the former group, though other differences in allergic conditions between the groups cannot be accounted for by the timing of introduction of peanut.[12]

New food allergies after infancy

Regular longitudinal review of existing allergies also needs to consider whether allergies established and diagnosed in infancy are persisting or have resolved (see Chapter 14 regarding the selection of children for challenge, and when and how to perform challenges). After infancy, children may encounter 'their' known allergenic foods sporadically or accidentally. Contrary to popular belief, these accidental exposures do not automatically lead to a worsening of the allergic reaction. It is more likely that variation in reaction severity is due to cofactors such as relative dose, asthma status, and the coexistence of viral infection or stressors such as exercise.[13] Such exposure may, however, give a clue to the issue of resolution or persistence of food allergies after infancy.

The onset of new allergies after infancy is a reflection of a broadening dietary repertoire (for example, peanut-allergic infants often develop allergy to tree nuts). The occurrence of accidental exposure to known allergens reflects a child's independence from (usually maternal) supervision. Although there is accumulating evidence regarding minimal eliciting doses for allergic reactions in allergic individuals,[14] there are no strong clinical or experimental data regarding the circumstances surrounding de novo sensitization in humans. Most data are derived from animal models of allergic disease,[15,16] so it is hard to be dogmatic about the advice to give to parents, beyond that outlined in Table 12.1 for infants. Regular review will allow assessment of dietary introductions that have passed without incident and those that have elicited allergic reactions.

Approximately 20% of egg-allergic children demonstrate IgE sensitization to peanut.[17] At this high rate, case finding (rather than screening) of peanut-sensitized children in an egg-allergic population with a peanut SPT or specific IgE test is worthwhile. The emergence of specific diagnostic tests for individual allergens may assist in distinguishing sensitization from likely allergy,[18,19] but at present a food challenge remains the only definitive test. This means that a lot of egg-allergic children spend a long time avoiding foods containing (or only possibly containing) peanut, to which they are sensitized but not allergic.

Other commonly allergenic foods are excluded from infant diets for reasons unrelated to their allergenicity. Peanuts and tree nuts are often consumed by infants in spread form, but peanut and nut fragments have a long and notorious history of accidental inhalation. Fish is often excluded from the diet in early life due to the fear of fish bone impaction. Shellfish (e.g. lobster) may be considered too expensive to be given to a child, who might not eat it, but, other shellfish, both molluscs and crustaceans, are available in easily deliverable form, with no financial or structural limitations on their use. However, it is not feasible to test all food-allergic children for even the major food allergens before they first consume them. Pragmatic advice must be given. As an example, unless a family is receiving advice from a dietitian to avoid it, soya is very difficult to avoid in prepared foods, such as industrially produced bread and tinned foods. It is therefore likely that it is already being tolerated by most food-allergic children. Cross-reactivity of soya with cows' milk varies from <10% to 50% of cases of cows' milk allergy in infants. Peanut and soya rarely cross-react, and peanut-allergic children should not be advised to avoid soya unless reactivity to soya is already suspected clinically. In contrast, other legumes may be problematic for soya-allergic children but are rarely so for peanut-allergic children. Egg-allergic children may not tolerate other avian eggs such as duck or goose, but these are not staple or even remotely common foods. Parents often ask about them in desperation at the apparently hopelessly narrow repertoire of foods that they can safely offer their child.

In practice, children adapt well to the limits on their dietary variety, but it must be acknowledged that there is a large impact on their overall health status-related quality of life. Growing children socialize and act more independently of their parents, but food-allergic children must become aware of the reasonable limits on their independence that comes with a diagnosis of food allergy. Such children can develop extreme anxiety when they encounter unfamiliar foods, or can experience social isolation when excluded from activities such as school outings and birthday parties.[20] Birthday parties and other social outings bring with them the risks associated with eating food prepared by people other than allergy-aware or hyper-aware parents. Reasonable planning and communication between the host parents and the food-allergic guest child can eliminate or minimize disruption to the social event (for further discussion see Chapter 15).

From a medical diagnostic perspective, new reactions in settings away from the family home can represent a greater difficulty than reactions at home in infancy. Ethnic cooking such as Chinese and Thai is a known potential source of nut and seed allergens. In restaurants and take away/carry-out stores staff awareness of food allergies may be hindered by difficulties relating to language barriers and level of education, the availability of allergy-specific food safety training and general food allergen hazard control practices.[21] Families may need to practice the advice 'If in doubt, do not eat out'.

Diagnosis of new allergies in adolescents

Older children may develop food sensitization through inhaling allergens, such as the oral allergy syndrome with birch, pollen and labile allergens in apples and hazelnuts. These are usually easy to manage on the basis of the clinical scenario relating to oral allergy syndrome, with general benign reactions related to known foods in which cross-reactivity between the food and the inhalant allergy is either known or suspected (see Chapter 7).

It should be a major focus of dialog with adolescents and young adults that risk-taking with foods is a real danger and that they are at much higher risk of death from food allergy now than when they were younger. Coexisting rejection of parental supervision/advice/support/control and a desire to both conform with a peer group and establish intimate personal relationships heighten food allergy-related risk.[22,23] Food-allergic adolescents may need to be interviewed without their parents, as they may have questions about personal relationships and other aspects of their life with and without allergies. Non-latex barrier contraception may be an issue for subjects with kiwi–latex syndrome.

Diagnosis of new allergies in adults

This area is definitely the poor relation of pediatric allergy, with few solid, challenge-proven epidemiological data to guide a diagnostic interview.[24] Diet is the most important acquired determinant of adult health, and adults are free to choose what to eat in a way that children are not: children's parents make food choices for them. However, adults with food allergy may have even more difficulty than children in accessing expert care for their allergies. Some may have food allergies that have persisted since infancy, such as peanut, or since mid-childhood, such as tree nut, fish or shellfish, or they may have developed oral allergy syndrome in adolescence.

When electively restricted diets have been excluded, such as vegan diets, the assessment of a suspected food-allergic adult must focus on whether a recognized allergy syndrome is present or not. Other conditions that are more common in adults than children may mimic allergic disorders: these include irritable bowel syndrome, wheat and milk intolerance, and again the eosinophilic disorders. Allergy to non-steroidal medication and the impact of medication use on the outcome of allergic reactions are more relevant in adults than children. Antihypertensive medications such as ACE inhibitors and β-blockers must be identified and alternatives considered in adults who have genuine IgE-mediated allergies.

Conclusion

An astute clinician can glean a lot of information from even the first encounter with a child or adult who may have experienced an allergic reaction to food. What has changed in the last decade, and what is likely to be utterly transformed in the next decade, is the amount of evidence-based information a family can be given at the same first interview. Clinicians and families embark on a health journey together. The length of this journey and the variety of possible final endpoints will continue to motivate clinical allergists for many years to come.

References

1. Roberts G, Lack G. Food allergy–getting more out of your skin prick tests. Clin Exp Allergy 2000;30(11):1495–8.
2. Pessler F, Nejat M. Anaphylactic reaction to goat's milk in a cows' milk-allergic infant. Pediatr Allergy Immunol 2004;15(2):183–5.
3. Ah-Leung S, Bernard H, Bidat E, et al. Allergy to goat and sheep milk without allergy to cows' milk. Allergy 2006;61(11):1358–65.
4. Lemon-Mulé H, Sampson HA, Sicherer SH, et al. Immunologic changes in children with egg allergy ingesting extensively heated egg. J Allergy Clin Immunol 2008;122(5):977–83.
5. Rothenberg ME. Biology and treatment of eosinophilic esophagitis. Gastroenterology 2009;137(4):1238–49.
6. Greer FR, Sicherer SH, Burks AW. Effects of early nutritional interventions on the development of atopic disease in infants and children: the role of maternal dietary restriction, breastfeeding, timing of introduction of complementary foods, and hydrolyzed formulas. American Academy of Pediatrics Committee on Nutrition; American Academy of Pediatrics Section on Allergy and Immunology. Pediatrics 2008;121(1):183–91.
7. Department of Health. Revised government advice on consumption of peanut during pregnancy, breastfeeding, and early life and development of peanut allergy. Revised August 2009. www.dh.gov.uk/en/Healthcare/Children/Maternity/Maternalandinfantnutrition/DH_104490
8. Nowak-Wegrzyn A, Muraro A. Food protein-induced enterocolitis syndrome. Curr Opin Allergy Clin Immunol 2009;9(4):371–7.
9. Hill DJ, Hosking CS. Food allergy and atopic dermatitis in infancy: an epidemiologic study. Pediatr Allergy Immunol 2004;15(5):421–7.
10. Hill DJ, Hosking C, de Benedictis FM, et al. Confirmation of the association between high levels of immunoglobulin E food sensitization and eczema in infancy: an international study. Clin Exp Allergy 2008;38(1):161–8.
11. Hansen KS, Ballmer-Weber BK, Sastre J, et al. Component-resolved in vitro diagnosis of hazelnut allergy in Europe. J Allergy Clin Immunol 2009;123(5):1134–41.
12. Du Toit G, Katz Y, Sasieni P, et al. Early consumption of peanuts in infancy is associated with a low prevalence of peanut allergy. J Allergy Clin Immunol 2008;122(5):984–91.
13. Hourihane JO'B, Knulst AC. Thresholds of allergenic proteins in foods. Toxicol Appl Pharmacol 2005;207(2 Suppl):152–6.
14. Taylor SL, Crevel RW, Sheffield D, et al. Threshold dose for peanut: risk characterization based upon published results from challenges of peanut-allergic individuals. Food Chem Toxicol 2009;47(6):1198–204.
15. Strid J, Hourihane J, Kimber I, et al. Epicutaneous exposure to peanut protein prevents oral tolerance and

enhances allergic sensitisation. Clin Exp Allergy 2005; 35(6):757–66.

16. Lack G. Epidemiologic risks for food allergy. J Allergy Clin Immunol 2008;121(6):1331–6.

17. Sicherer SH, Wood RA, Stablein D, et al. Immunologic features of infants with milk or egg allergy enrolled in an observational study (Consortium of Food Allergy Research) of food allergy. J Allergy Clin Immunol 2010;125(5):1077–83.

18. Asarnoj A, Moverare R, Ostblom E, et al. IgE to peanut allergen components: relation to peanut symptoms and pollen sensitization in 8-year-olds. Allergy 2010;65:1189–95.

19. Nicolaou N, Poorafshar M, Murray C, et al. Allergy or tolerance in children sensitized to peanut: Prevalence and differentiation using component-resolved diagnostics. J All Clin Immunol 2010;125:191–7.

20. King RM, Knibb RC, Hourihane JO'B. Impact of peanut allergy on quality of life, stress and anxiety in the family. Allergy 2009;64(3):461–8.

21. Leitch IS, Walker MJ, Davey R. Food allergy: gambling your life on a take-away meal. Int J Environ Health Res 2005;15(2):79–87.

22. Sampson MA, Muñoz-Furlong A, Sicherer SH. Risk-taking and coping strategies of adolescents and young adults with food allergy. J Allergy Clin Immunol 2006;117(6):1440–5.

23. Marklund B, Ahlstedt S, Nordström G. Health-related quality of life among adolescents with allergy-like conditions – with emphasis on food hypersensitivity. Health Qual Life Outcomes 2004;19(2):65.

24. Rona RJ, Keil T, Summers C, et al. The prevalence of food allergy: a meta-analysis. J Allergy Clin Immunol 2007;120(3):638–46.

In Vivo and In Vitro Diagnostic Methods in the Evaluation of Food Allergy

S. Allan Bock

KEY CONCEPTS

- Skin prick or puncture tests to foods are very useful when properly performed and interpreted.

- Negative prick/puncture skin tests have a high negative predictive accuracy for many foods (>95% for the common foods).

- Positive prick/puncture skin tests have a high positive predictive accuracy for egg, milk and peanut in young children, and the size of the skin test is relatively predictive.

- Food-specific serum IgE antibodies for a few foods can be used to predict the probability of a positive challenge. 'Cut-off' levels for egg, milk, peanut and fish mix have been established. There are also levels for tree nuts that are helpful but not as accurate; however, they are useful for deciding whether an individual should have a food challenge (Fleischer has suggested a level

below 2 kU/L as the level for deciding to do a challenge depending on the history).

- Measuring the annual fall in the specific IgE level for a few foods can help determine the likelihood of resolution of the food allergy.

- Food challenges may be guided by the results of skin testing and food-specific serum antibody level determination, but these measurements have not replaced oral food challenges. It remains to be determined whether or not component-resolved diagnostics can replace food challenges, or at least predict that the probability of the food being tolerated or triggering symptoms is very high.

- Patients should be followed annually as they get older to determine the chance that food allergy has been outgrown. This is an ongoing process.

This chapter focuses on skin testing and in vitro laboratory testing for food allergy. Chapter 14 discusses the ultimate gold standard, which is the oral food challenge. It is this that has helped determine the utility of the measurements discussed below. The goal of this chapter is to give the reader choices of methods depending on the setting, the training of the practitioner and the child's circumstances. Of all the areas of medicine stressed in Chapter 12, the history is the most important component of the evaluation. Ultimately and ideally, the facts gathered will be used to try to reproduce the history to confirm or refute the incriminated food as the culprit.

Skin testing

Skin testing is a technique that has been employed for decades and has been used with apparent confidence for testing aeroallergens. However, 30 years ago there were questions about the usefulness of allergy skin testing for food allergy. Part of this confusion stemmed from the fact that patients were often told that they had positive skin tests to foods that they knew they could eat without experiencing adverse clinical symptoms. This confusion did not seem to be as troublesome when patients with a positive skin test to cat found they could sleep with the cat without symptoms. Why the difference? It

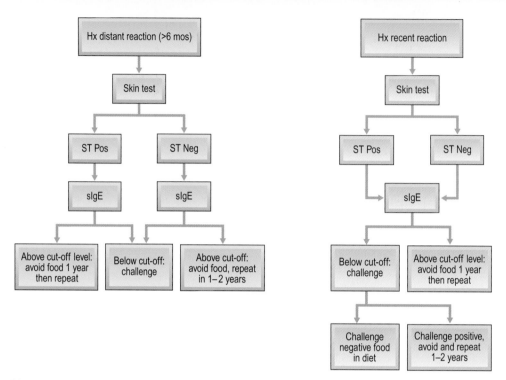

Figure 13.1 Algorithm for older subjects, >5 years of age – take a detailed history, be certain to determine most recent reaction with symptoms and severity. Levels most helpful for egg, milk, peanut and tree nuts.

may be that because you can see what you eat, food allergy testing resulted in more confusion. This is a strong argument for using an approach that only tests for foods under suspicion, rather than panels of foods (i.e. the same argument is true for measurement of serum antibody levels) as discussed below.

With regard to the specific testing method used, it is generally agreed that the 'prick/puncture' skin test gives the most accurate and helpful information regarding food allergy. However, there is not universal agreement about the technique to be used. Glycerinated extracts are available for many foods in 1 : 10 or 1 : 20 weight/volume dilutions. These are applied to the skin accompanied by positive (histamine) and negative (diluent-saline or other solution used to mix allergen extracts) controls. The skin is then pricked or punctured with one of several devices available. There are also a number of devices that are preloaded with the extract which are then applied to the skin. Skin tests are usually read 15–20 minutes after they are applied. Food allergen extract responses are considered positive when they elicit a wheal of 3 mm larger than the negative control; smaller responses are considered to be negative.

When skin tests are negative for several foods that have been well studied, they have a very high negative predictive accuracy (approximately 95% for children over 3–4 years of age) and in children older than 2 years the negative test essentially eliminates the food as a culprit in triggering immediate hypersensitive symptoms. These foods include egg, milk, wheat, peanut, most tree nuts and soy. Data for other foods are not quite as certain, but in general a negative skin test makes an immediate allergic reaction to food unlikely. However, it must be emphasized that no test can ever confidently contradict an unequivocal history, and care must be exercised in this regard (Figs 13.1 and 13.2).

CLINICAL CASE

A 2-year-old girl is seen by an allergist for possible egg allergy. The father reports that at about age 14 months she was given some scrambled egg and developed a few hives on her face. There might have been a few hives on her abdomen. There were no gastrointestinal or respiratory symptoms, but the father recalls that she stopped eating the egg after a few bites. Prior to the reaction she had consumed egg-containing baked goods without problems. Since the urticarial reaction she has had no egg and very little, if any, egg-containing food. The

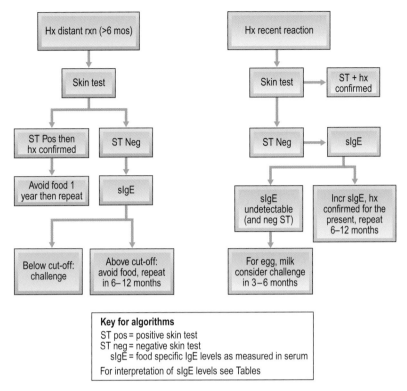

Figure 13.2 Algorithm from birth to age 3 for egg and milk – take a detailed history!

allergist performs an egg skin test with appropriate controls and finds that it is negative. Because of the history, egg-specific serum antibody levels are ordered and are found to be undetectable. The allergist schedules a food challenge, and after the equivalent of about one slice of hard-boiled egg the child breaks out in hives on her face and within a few minutes they spread to her trunk and extremities.

This scenario raises a number of important points. The first is that the history is confirmed by the food challenge. The second is that the skin test and the serum antibody level did not demonstrate sensitization that was confirmed by the challenge. The third is that if the egg-specific serum antibody level had been ordered and found to be undetectable, and if the parents had been told to feed this child egg at home, then there would have been a call to the doctor and perhaps an urgent visit to the emergency department. Even though the probability of this scenario might be less than 10%, the most conservative approach is always the best way to avoid unexpected outcomes.

The converse is not true. The positive predictive accuracy of a positive skin test is often less than 50% for most foods, depending on the population under study. Even for peanut allergy in unselected populations (i.e. not stratified by history taken by a knowledgeable allergist) the response rate to food

challenges is often less than 50%. A crucial understanding for healthcare providers and especially for patients is that a positive skin test *only detects the presence of IgE antibody* alone: it does not make a diagnosis of clinical allergy (this is also true for serum antibody levels, see below). In fact, a positive skin test or detectable antibody is common in large unselected populations and confirms sensitization that may be asymptomatic.[1-4] However, when there is a history of a severe allergic reaction or anaphylaxis to an isolated food ingestion and the skin test is positive, then the positive test may be viewed as diagnostic without the need for further allergy testing. There have been rare reports of adverse reactions to skin prick tests, but interestingly these have almost all been to aeroallergen extracts.[5] For allergists concerned about adverse reactions to skin testing, it is easy to dilute commercially available skin test extracts and use the dilutions for titrated skin testing. There is even some preliminary evidence that dilution titration skin tests might be used to enhance the predictive accuracy of food challenges.[6]

In children less than 3 years of age the negative predictive accuracy is not as high as in older children, and is probably in the range of 80–85%. However, in this age group the positive predictive accuracy of skin testing is very useful for egg, milk and peanut. In children less than 2 years of age, Hill's group[7,8] has reported that for these foods (and only these three foods) a wheal of >8 mm is diagnostic of clinical reactivity in 100% of subjects who were challenged. By contrast, Wainstein et al.[9] reported that skin prick test wheals >8 mm had a somewhat lower specificity, and cautioned that tests may need to be interpreted in the context of specific patient populations. A reasonable and practical method by which to proceed is to take a careful history, including seeking food aversions in young children, and to pay close attention to positive skin tests while being careful not to dismiss negative tests in this age group, especially those that contradict the history. After a complete history has been obtained (Chapter 19), the skin tests to be applied should be selected based on these details. As part of this selection it is useful to categorize children by age and history and then apply the known evidence base to the selection and results of skin testing.

Kagan[10] evaluated 47 children with a positive skin test to peanut extract (i.e. wheal diameter > 3mm) but no known history of reaction or accidental ingestion. In this group, 23 (49%) of the challenges were positive, inducing various symptoms. It is crucial to note, therefore, that half of the challenges were negative, and if the skin test alone was used to prescribe dietary restriction of peanut, then all of these children would be unnecessarily deprived of peanut consumption. There are numerous important issues accompanying peanut exclusion diets that alter quality of life at school, at home and in the community. Among these are the prescription and carrying of self-injectable epinephrine. Therefore, this study emphasizes the importance of not relying solely on this skin test or in vitro food-specific serum antibody levels.

Another common issue is whether the presence of one food allergy indicates the existence of others, especially in young children whose diets have not yet included some common food allergens. Dieguez[11] used skin prick tests to examine children with diagnosed milk allergy to see if any of them were sensitized to egg. They found that a number of them were, and so recommended that this group be carefully followed for the development of egg allergy. This observation then requires evaluation for symptomatic egg allergy as well as the possible resolution of milk allergy. Therefore, as

they get older children exhibiting this constellation of positive skin tests will require ongoing (longitudinal) skin testing, food-specific serum antibody level measurements and food challenges. Furthermore, allergists often skin test milk- or egg-allergic children for peanut and tree nuts, and if positive these foods will also require ongoing evaluation.

These observations reinforce the recommendation for choosing food extracts for skin testing based on the history rather than a panel of food skin tests or serum antibody levels. In very atopic children (e.g. children with atopic dermatitis) the more tests performed the more likely there are to be numerous positive results requiring systematic evaluation. Although it may be appropriate to do skin tests for foods not yet ingested in young children, healthcare providers should seek to use the best evidence base available to be judicious about these choices (Fleischer et al., unpublished observations).

Although allergen extracts have improved over the years, some are more reliable than others. Allergen extracts for the major foods – egg, milk, peanut, tree nuts and some grains – can be manufactured so that they give predictable and reproducible results in skin testing procedures. It remains incumbent upon clinicians to be certain that each lot of extract contains active allergens. As there are several manufacturers, verifying each new lot of extract that is placed into use becomes important. It is possible to purchase a bottle of allergen extract that does not contain enough material to be detected by antibody, leading to a potential for erroneous interpretation.

This reliability is especially an issue when using extracts of fresh fruits and vegetables. These are hard to produce so that they contain relevant allergens and they may lack the relevant proteins responsible for allergic reactions.[12–14] A preferable approach is to use fresh foods. This technique has been referred to as the 'prick-to-prick' technique or 'puddle' test. For the former, the food of interest is pricked and then the skin of the subject is pricked. An attempt is made to ensure that there is material from the raw food on the skin testing device. The puddle test is performed by putting a drop of the fresh food on the skin and then pricking through it with an appropriate device. A variant of this approach is to squeeze liquid from the fresh food into a small vessel and then use a syringe to put a drop of this material on the skin. The test device is then passed through the drop into the skin using the usual prick/puncture method. It is often useful to undertake these two procedures in duplicate. It is also useful to have a negative control subject so that irritant reactions can be distinguished from true immunologic responses.

There are a number of other variables to be considered when performing skin prick tests. Skin testing of surfaces that have been treated with topical steroids for atopic dermatitis may induce smaller wheals than tests performed on untreated skin; negative skin tests with commercially prepared extracts that do not support convincing histories of food reactions should often be repeated with fresh foods prior to concluding that food allergen-specific IgE antibody is absent:[15] this may include skin testing with whole milk and whole egg (and a challenge performed prior to returning the food to the diet); and there is some evidence that long-term high-dose systemic corticosteroid therapy may reduce allergen wheal size. For nuts for which there are no commercially available extracts (macadamia and pine nut are two examples), a mortar and pestle may be used to grind them to a powder, and they can then be mixed with diluent and applied to the skin. Spices are another example of important food allergens that need to be prepared for use when the need arises. Use of these non-standardized preparations is most helpful when the tests are positive, especially if they confirm the history. A negative test with a suspicious history requires a food challenge before the food is returned to the diet.

Despite these caveats, properly performed skin tests remain a very sensitive and important tool for evaluation of food allergy. They are very useful, results are immediately available, quality control is in the hands of the individual performing the test, and they are more sensitive than in vitro assays. All of these considerations make them very practical and cost-effective.

A note should be added about intradermal skin tests for foods. They have never been shown to be useful when skin prick tests are negative for the vast majority of foods. Recently, some early data have suggested that individuals reacting to a carbohydrate determinant rather than a food protein will have a positive intradermal skin test to the putative culprit.[16,17] Research in this area is ongoing, but for the vast majority of food proteins the intradermal skin test adds no useful information and has been said to potentially cause more adverse reactions than prick testing.

VARIABLES TO CONSIDER WHEN PERFORMING SKIN TESTS

- Skin tests should be interpreted with caution when performed on skin that has been treated with topical steroids. The wheals might be smaller than expected.
- Skin tests with commercial extracts that do not support the clinical history may need to be repeated with fresh foods. This may be true for milk and egg as well, and some authors recommend the use of whole milk and raw or cooked egg in skin testing procedures.
- Some foods such as spices and even some nuts will need to be prepared from the whole food by the allergist, as there are no commercially available extracts.
- A negative test with a suspicious history requires a food challenge before the food is returned to the diet (see Clinical Case above).

In vitro testing

Many of the comments about skin testing also apply to in vitro testing. The selection of tests should be guided by the history, and learning to interpret the tests in light of the history is crucial. In vitro tests are referred to using several different terms, but precision in terminology will help both practitioners and patients use and understand the results. The term commonly used is 'RAST' testing. RAST is short for radioallergosorbent test, which was one of the first in vitro tests used for diagnostic purposes. The term 'radio' stands for radioactive, in other words, this was originally a test using radioactive tracer technology. This is no longer the case: the current tests are immunoassays and should be referred to as such. The tests now use liquid or solid-phase reagents. The test currently favored by specialists is the Phadia Immunocap assay because it has been subjected to research studies that correlate the results with double-blind placebo-controlled food challenges. The test measures the amount of circulating allergen-specific IgE to individual foods and is reported in kilounits of allergen-specific IgE antibody per liter. (Laboratories also report the results in 'class levels', but these results have not been shown to be useful in clinical practice and should be ignored in favor of the kilounit levels that have been correlated with food challenges.)

Because blinded food challenges are the gold standard for making a diagnosis of food allergy (see Chapter 14), it is possible to increase the precision of this immunoassay for diagnostic purposes by performing food challenges concurrently with immunoassay measurements. With the use of a combination of skin tests and serum immunoassays, it is possible to reduce the number of food challenges that are needed. However, it is important to note that these predictive values are only for a limited number of foods, specifically egg, milk, peanut, fish, and to some degree tree nuts.

Generally skin testing appears to be the most sensitive test for the reasons discussed above, but there is one study[9] that supports the notion that skin prick tests and immunoassays have similar sensitivities and specificities. There are circumstances in which in vitro measurements may be preferred. These include patients with extensive dermographia; patients with extensive skin disease (atopic dermatitis or generalized urticaria); patients who for varying reasons cannot discontinue the use of antihistamines; and the lack of availability of skin testing in areas without allergy specialists.

The first demonstration of the utility of serum antibody levels for managing food allergy came from two important studies by Sampson,[18,19] one retrospective and one prospective. Using the CAP-RAST Fluorescent Enzyme Immunoassay (the predecessor to the current test) he demonstrated that quantification of food-specific IgE provided helpful predictive accuracies for egg, milk, peanut and fish compared to skin prick testing. These studies were meticulously performed using double-blind food challenges, skin testing and food-specific serum antibody levels. These were the first studies to establish cut-off levels that established 95% predictive values, and these levels have then been used to obviate the need for many food challenges. It is important for clinicians to note that these measurements are 95% cut-off levels and individuals with higher levels may be clinically non-reactive when culprit foods are eaten. The converse is that individuals with serum antibody levels less than the 95% cut-off values may still have reactions and should be cautioned against considering it safe to ingest suspected foods. Subsequent studies have attempted to establish lower levels of predictive accuracy, but there is no level below which it is certain that a reaction will not occur. Recent studies suggest that monitoring the allergen food-specific IgE values may be useful in predicting when individuals have 'outgrown' their specific food allergy and therefore food challenges are appropriate and likely to be negative.[20] In young children it has been shown that the 'cut-off' levels are lower for milk and egg, but there are important exceptions in all of these studies that relate to the population under consideration and the prevalence of the condition (Table 13.1).[21-23] The food-specific IgE determinations may be used prospectively in order to determine when food challenges might be appropriate in children who have been maintained on restricted diets.

Shek et al.[24] have reported that the rate of fall of the food-specific serum antibody level may be a good predictor of when challenges are appropriate for hen's egg and cows' milk. Recent studies have also supported the contention that lower levels of food-specific antibodies are associated with earlier resolution of food allergy, suggesting that some children have a different phenotype (and perhaps genotype) of their food allergy than children with

PREFERENCE FOR IN VITRO TESTS VS SKIN TESTS

- Patients with extensive dermographia
- Patients with extensive atopic dermatitis or generalized urticaria
- Patients who cannot discontinue antihistamines
- Areas where there are no allergists to perform skin testing

Table 13.1 Predictive value of food-specific IgE

Allergen	Decision point (kU$_A$/L)	Rechallenge value
Egg	≥ 7.0	≤ 1.5
≤ 2 yrs old	≥ 2.0	
Milk	≥ 15.0	≤ 7.0
≤ 2 yrs old	≥ 5.0	
Peanut	≥ 14.0	≤ 5.0
Fish	≥ 20.0	
Tree nuts	≥ 15.0	< 2.0

Notes:
1. Patients with food-specific IgE values less than the listed diagnostic values may experience an allergic reaction following challenge. Unless history strongly suggests tolerance, a physician-supervised food challenge should be performed to determine whether the child can ingest the food safely.
2. These are values that have been derived from a number of studies; these offer a practical approach to use of levels to determine whether or not challenges should be done. There have been other studies proposing other levels.

Table 13.2 Suggested interpretation of food-specific serum immunoassay levels using one specific technique. Created with the generous assistance of Staffan Ahlstedt PhD

Level undetectable: <.35 kU/L by ImmunoCAP for any individual suspected food:

Food allergy has a lower probability but must be considered in context of the history.
If there is a strong/suspicious history, refer to an allergist. Also consider other causes of symptoms. (Be careful not to tell patients that the test is negative – antibody is undetectable, the test is not negative. Be extremely careful about allowing food reintroduction at home when the history suggests a reaction has occurred.)

Level to one or more allergens: 0.35–5 kU/L by ImmunoCAP:

Possible reaction to food culprits.
Each allergen with a detectable level must be considered individually to be a trigger of symptoms.
If the history and the serum antibody level support each other, then avoid the food, educate the patient, parents, family members and caregivers, and prescribe self-injectable epinephrine if indicated.
Then schedule regular review of course, accidental exposures, and periodically repeat the serum antibody levels (perhaps annually).
At some interval after the last reaction (a year or more, depending on the age of the patient) consider referral for food challenge under observation.

Level to one or more allergens: 5–15 kU/L by ImmunoCAP:

Significant probability of reaction.
Avoid each food, educate the patient, parents, family members and caregivers, and prescribe self-injectable epinephrine if indicated.
Repeat the ImmunoCAP level every 1–2 years to see if it has fallen low enough to justify referral for possible challenge.

Level to one or more allergens: >15 kU/L:

For the major food allergens egg, milk, peanut, and possibly tree nuts there is very high probability of reaction.
Avoid the food, educate the patient, parents, family members and caregivers, and prescribe self-injectable epinephrine if indicated.
Repeat the ImmunoCAP every 1–2 years to see if it has fallen low enough to justify referral for possible challenge.
When in doubt leave it out and arrange for a food challenge under observation in a safe place.
Remind patients/parents to practice using the self-injectable epinephrine so they can respond quickly and effectively in a crisis!

higher levels.[25–28] These observations make it imperative that the clinician ordering and interpreting the test have sophistication in this area to determine when challenges are indicated, safe, and likely to be negative, in order to shorten the duration of elimination diets. Table 13.2 presents one approach to interpretation. There are certainly others, and individual circumstances must always be taken into consideration. However, the most important caveat is that it is never acceptable to send individuals home to reintroduce a food into the diet when the history contradicts the skin tests and/or the food-specific serum antibody level. Proper precautions and warnings are always necessary before the reintroduction of suspected food culprits away from medical facilities.

The studies cited above apply primarily to allergies to milk, egg, peanut, to some extent fish (but individual fish have not been examined in detail), and less so to soy and wheat, for which Sampson did not identify useful predictive values. More recently, several investigators have determined that cut-off levels for tree nuts, if interpreted judiciously, are useful in accomplishing the goal of appropriate dietary restriction and determination of the timing of food challenges to nuts.[29–32] Although these studies are not as meticulous as the Sampson retrospective study that involved a food challenge for every level measured, they do provide practical clinical data to use in the management of individual patients. Fleischer's studies propose that for levels of tree nut allergens <2 kU/L challenges could be reasonable, whereas levels >5 predict that reactions are likely enough that challenges should be postponed. The natural history of peanut allergy study suggests that 20% of a particular population will outgrow peanut allergy, whereas in a similar population of children with tree nut allergy the resolution of the problem was about 5%.[33,34] These observations help in determining and predicting how the immunoassay results should be used. Knight et al.[35] have published a study indicating that a combination of skin test size and food-specific serum antibody level to egg white may help clinicians determine the appropriate time for food challenge.

Other in vitro testing methods that have been and are under investigation but have not yet been shown to be clinically useful include the basophil histamine release assay and the intestinal mast cell histamine release assay. The basophil histamine release assay is not actually a new test, having been used in research applications for decades.[36,37] In the past, lymphocyte stimulation tests were reported to be useful for the identification of subjects with food allergy. These results have not been reproduced and clinical utility of this approach has not been demonstrated. However, cellular populations and responses are being investigated using other hypotheses. Turcanu et al.[38] found that in peanut-allergic individuals T- and B-cell response to peanut allergens were correlated. A high frequency of T-regulatory lymphocytes (Tregs) to milk allergy were reported by Shreffler et al.[39] to correlate with less severe milk-allergic reactions.

There are a number of new and potentially exciting approaches to in vitro testing for both food and aeroallergen clinical reactivity. The goal is to improve the diagnostic accuracy, especially the sensitivity, specificity and positive and negative predicative accuracies, of the tests in order to reduce the need for food challenges, and importantly to predict when food allergy has resolved.

Component-resolved diagnostic tests are being developed and preliminary studies have been reported. The idea is to measure antibody responses to individual allergen epitopes to establish individual sensitization profiles and specific 'phenotypes' of food-allergic individuals. The approach uses epitopes (pieces of the allergenic proteins) analyzed by microarray technology to predict whether the subject will or will not react to ingested food. Which of these epitopes are the most important and the levels with clinical significance are currently being determined by research studies. The goal is to characterize patient heterogeneity and predict clinically significant food allergy (symptomatic sensitization) as opposed to allergen sensitization without symptoms (asymptomatic sensitization). Thus far, several important epitopes have been identified for celery root,[40] peanut[41] and hazelnut,[42] and research is being directed toward others. Another exciting result of molecular investigations into antibodies to food has shown that persistence of food allergy is more likely if the individual reacts to linear or

sequential epitopes rather than conformational epitopes. Linear epitopes are the primary amino acid sequence and are not affected by usual cooking processes, whereas the conformational epitopes are the folded structure of the proteins and may be affected by heating. These findings are now being investigated by microarray techniques as tests to use to identify individuals whose food allergy has resolved, but they are not currently available to clinicians.[43-53]

CLINICAL CASE

A 4-year-old boy has had egg allergy since about age 1. The original symptoms were hives and vomiting when he was first fed scrambled egg. About 3 months before the current visit he had an egg challenge under observation with hard-boiled egg. At that time his skin test to egg was 4 mm mean wheal diameter and his egg-specific serum antibody level was 2.2 kU/L. At about 2 g he complained of abdominal pain and about 15 minutes later he began to break out in hives, which became generalized. The mother asked about a challenge with egg baked into something, as he had recently had a few bites of a muffin with egg in it and did not have any symptoms. A subsequent challenge was arranged with well-cooked pancakes, where the mother made a dozen pancakes containing two eggs. The child tolerated three pancakes before declaring that he was full. Over a period of observation of 2 hours no symptoms were observed. Thus during this period he tolerated about half an egg well cooked into the pancakes. The mother was instructed to begin feeding him approximately half an egg cooked into various baked goods, and if this was tolerated over a couple of weeks then to begin slowly and gradually increasing the amount of egg. Early studies have suggested that this approach might hasten resolution of the egg allergy (this has also been observed for milk) in a group of egg-allergic children who may be reacting to conformation epitopes rather than linear or sequential epitopes. (It is also probably true that these children tend to have lower egg- (or milk-) specific IgE antibody levels, but confirmation of this hypothesis requires further data.)

Numerous facilities and practitioners have been using in vitro IgG assays to diagnose food allergy and 'food intolerance' (the latter term having no specific definition in this context). Some of these tests have 'footnotes' stating specifically that they are not to be used for diagnosis of IgE-mediated food allergy. Exactly what they are identifying other than the individual's ability to produce IgG antibodies to food protein, which is a normal immune response, is completely unclear. The absence of any positive results of IgG to food proteins should raise an immediate concern of immunodeficiency or an improperly performed test. Serum food-specific IgG levels might be elevated in disorders affecting protein absorption in the intestine, such as celiac disease and perhaps inflammatory bowel disease. At present these test should not be used in clinical practice, and the individuals who claim test validity should validate their results with properly controlled challenge studies. Often these are not covered by insurance and the cost to patients may be considerable.. The European Academy of Allergy and Clinical Immunology issued a strong statement to this effect in 2008,[54] and the statement has been supported by the AAAAI.[55] IgG$_4$ (a subclass of IgG) is likely to give some information about tolerance to a food rather than a reaction, and may also indicate that regulatory cells and mediators have been activated.[56,57] It is possible that the ratio of IgE to IgG$_4$ (IgE:IgG$_4$) may have clinical utility, but this hypothesis awaits controlled study for confirmation.

References

1. Liu A, Jaramillo R, Sicherer SH, et al. National prevalence and risk factors for food allergy and relationship to asthma: Results from the National Health and Nutrition Examination Survey 2005–2006. J Allergy Clin Immunol 2010;126:298–806.

2. Arbes SJ, Gergen PJ, Elliott L, et al. Prevalence of positive skin test responses to 10 common allergens in the US population: Results from the Third National Health and Nutrition Examination Survey. J Allergy Clin Immunol 2005;116:377–83.

3. Sampson HA. Food allergy. Part 1: Immunopathogenesis and clinical disorders. J Allergy Clin Immunol 1999;103:717–29.

4. Sampson HA. Food allergy. Part 2: Diagnosis and Management J Allergy Clin Immunol 1999;103:981–89.

5. Liccardi G, D'Amato D, Canonica GW, et al. Systemic reactions from skin testing: literature review. J Investig Allergol Clin Immunol 2006;16:75–8.

6. Tripodi S, Di Rienzo Businco A, Alessandri C, et al. Predicting the outcome of oral food challenges with hen's egg through skin test end-pint titration. Clin Exptl Allergy 2009;39:1225–33.

7. Sporik R, Hill DJ, Hosking CS. Specificity of allergen skin testing in predicting positive open food challenges to milk, egg and peanut in children. Clin Exp Allergy 2000;30:1540–6.

8. Hill DJ, Hosking CS, Reyes-Benito MLV. Reducing the need for food allergen challenges in young children – comparison of in vitro with in vivo tests. Clin Exp Allergy 2001;31:1031–5.

9. Wainstein BK, Yee A, Jelley D, et al. Combining skin prick, immediate skin application and specific IgE testing in the diagnosis of peanut allergy in children. Pediatr Allergy Immunol 2007;18:231–9

10. Kagan, R, Hayami D, Lawrence J, et al. The predictive value of a positive skin prick test to peanut in atopic, peanut-naïve children. Ann Allergy Asthma Immunol 2003;90:640–45.

11. Dieguez MC, Cerecedo I, Muriel A, et al. Skin prick test predictive value on the outcome of a first known egg exposure in milk-allergic children. Pediatr Allergy Immunol 2008;19:319–24.

12. Ortolani C, Ispano M, Pastorello EA, et al. Comparison of results of skin prick tests (with fresh foods and commercial food extracts) and RAST in 100 patients with oral allergy syndrome. J Allergy Clin Immunol 1989;83:683–90.

13. Pastorello E, Ortolani C, Farioli L, et al. Allergenic cross-reactivity among peach, apricot, plum, and cherry in patients with oral allergy syndrome: an in vivo and in vitro study. J Allergy Clin Immunol 1994;94:699–707.

14. Rance F, Juchet A, Bremont F, et al. Correlations between skin prick tests using commercial extracts and fresh foods, specific IgE, and food challenges. Allergy 1997;52:1031–5.

15. Rosen J, Selcow J, Mendelson L, et al. Skin testing with natural foods in patients suspected of having food allergies … is it necessary? J Allergy Clin Immunol 1994;93:1068–70.

16. Chung CH, Mirakhur B, Chan E, et al. Cetuximab induced anaphylaxis and IgE specific for galactose alpha 1,3 galactose. N Engl J Med 2008;358:1109–17.

17. Commins SP, Santinover SM, Hosen J, et al. Delayed anaphylaxis, angioedema or urticaria after consumption of red meat in patients with IgE antibodies specific for galactose-a-1, 3- galactose. J Allergy Clin Immunol 2009;123:426–33.

18. Sampson HA, Ho DG. Relationship between food-specific IgE concentrations and the risk of positive food challenges in children and adolescents. J Allergy Clin Immunol 1997;100:444–51.

19. Sampson HA. Utility of food-specific IgE concentrations in predicting symptomatic food allergy. J Allergy Clin Immunol 2001;107:891–6.

20. Sicherer SH, Sampson HA. Cow's milk protein-specific IgE concentrations in two age groups of milk-allergic children and in children achieving clinical tolerance. Clin Exptl Allergy 1999;29:507–12.

21. van der Gugten A, den Otter M, Meijer Y, et al. Usefulness of specific IgE levels in predicting cow's milk allergy. J Allergy Clin Immunol 2008;121:631–3.

22. Garcia-Ara C, Boyano-Martinez T, Diaz-Pena JM, et al. Specific IgE levels in the diagnosis of immediate hypersensitivity to cows' milk protein in the infant. J Allergy Clin Immunol 2001;107:185–90.

23. Boyano-Martinez T, Garcia-Ara C, Diaz-Pena JM, et al. Validity of specific IgE antibodies in children with egg allergy. Clin Exptl Allergy 2001;31:1464–9.

24. Shek LPC, Soderstrom L, Ahlstedt S, et al. Determination of food specific IgE levels over time can predict the development of tolerance in cow's milk and hens' egg allergy. J Allergy Clin Immunol 2004;114:387–91.

25. Perry TT, Matsui EC, Conover-Walker MK, et al. The relationship of allergen specific IgE levels and oral food challenge outcome. J Allergy Clin Immunol 2004;113:144–9.

26. Skirpak J, Matsui EC, Mudd K, et al. The natural history of IgE-mediated cow's milk allergy. J Allergy Clin Immunol 2007;120:1172–7.

27. Savage JH, Matsui E, Skripak JM, et al. The natural history of egg allergy. J Allergy Clin Immunol 2007;120:1413–7.

28. Rottem M, Shostak D, Foldi S. The predictive value of specific immunoglobulin E on the outcome of milk allergy. Israel Med Assn J 2008;10;862–4.

29. Clark AT, Ewan PW. Interpretation of tests for nut allergy in one thousand patients in relation to allergy or tolerance. Clin Exp Allergy 2003;33:1041–5.

30. Fleischer DM, Conover-Walker MK, Matsui EC, et al. The natural history of tree nut allergy. J Allergy Clin Immunol 2005;116:1087–93.

31. Fleischer DM. The natural history of peanut and tree nut allergy. Current Allergy Asthma Reports 2007;7:175–81.

32. Maloney JM, Rudengren M, Ahlstedt S, et al. The use of serum-specific IgE measurements for the diagnosis of peanut, tree nut, and seed allergy. J Allergy Clin Immunol 2008;122:145–51.

33. Fleischer DM, Conover-Walker MK, Christie L, et al. The natural progression of peanut allergy resolution and the possibility of recurrence. J Allergy Clin Immunol 2003;112:183–9.

34. Fleischer DM, Conover-Walker MK, Christie L, et al. Peanut allergy: recurrence and its management. J Allergy Clin Immunol 2004;114:1195–210.

35. Knight AK, Shreffler WG, Sampson HA, et al. Skin prick test to egg white provides additional diagnositic utility to serum egg white-specific IgE antibody concentration in children. J Allergy Clin Immunol 2006;117:842–7.

36. May CD. High spontaneous release of histamine in-vitro from leukocytes of persons hypersensitive to food. J Allergy Clin Immunol 1976;58:432–7.

37. Sampson HA, Broadbent K, Berhnisel-Broadbent J. Spontaneous release of histamine from basophils and histamine-releasing factor in patients with atopic dermatitis and food hypersensitivity. New Engl J Med 1989;321:228–32.

38. Turcanu V, Winterbotham M, Kelleher P, et al. Peanut-specific B and T cell responses are correlated in peanut allergic but not in non-allergic individuals. Clin Exptl Allergy 2008;38:1132–9.

39. Shreffler WG, Wanich M, Maloney M, et al. Association of allergen-specific regulatory T cells with the onset of clinical tolerance to milk protein. J Allergy Clin Immunol 2009;123:43–52.

40. Bauermseister K, Ballmer-Weber BK, Bublin M, et al. Assessment of component resolved in vitro diagnosis of celeriac allergy. J Allergy Clin Immunol 2009;124:166–81

41. Nicolaou N, Poorafshar M, Clare M, et al. Allergy or tolerance in children sensitized to peanut: prevalence and differentiation using component-resolved diagnostics. J Allergy Clin Immunol 2010;125:191–7.

42. Hansen KS, Ballmer-Weber BK, Sastre J, et al. Component-resolved in vitro diagnosis of hazelnut allergy in Europe. J Allergy Clin Immunol 2009;123:1134–41.

43. Chatchatee P, Jarvinen K-M, Bardina L, et al. Identification of IgE-and IgG binding epitopes on α_{s1}-casein: differences in patients with persistent and transient cow's milk allergy. J Allergy Clin Immunol 2001;107:379–83.

44. Chatchatee P, Jarvinen KM, Bardina L, et al. Identification of IgE and IgG binding epitopes on beta- and kappa-casein in cow's milk allergic patients. Clin Exptl Allergy 2001;31:1256–62.

45. Vila L, Beyer K, Jarvinen K-M, et al. Role of conformational and linear epitopes in the achievement of tolerance in cow's milk allergy. Clin Exptl Allergy 2001;31:1599–606.

46. Jarvinen KM, Beyer K, Vila L, et al. B-cell epitopes as a screening instrument for persistent cow's milk allergy. J Allergy Clin Immunol 2002;110:293–7.

47. Beyer K, Ellman-Grunther L, Jarvinen K-M, et al. Measurement of peptide-specific IgE as an additional tool in identifying patients with clinical reactivity to peanuts. J Allergy Clin Immunol 2003;112:202–7.

48. Cocco RR, Jarvinen K-M, Sampson HA, et al. Mutational analysis of major, sequential IgE-binding epitopes in α_{s1}-casein, a major cow's milk allergen. J Allergy Clin Immunol 2003;112:433–7.

49. Shreffler WG, Beyer K, Chu T-HT, et al. Microarray immunoassay: association of clinical history, in vitro IgE function, and heterogeneity of allergenic peanut epitopes. J Allergy Clin Immunol 2004:113:446–82.

50. Shreffler WG, Lencer DA, Bardina L, et al. IgE and IgG4 epitope mapping by microarray immunoassay reveals the diversity of immune response to the peanut allergen, Ara h 2. J Allergy Clin Immunol 2005;116:893–9.

51. Cocco RR, Marvinen KM, Han N, et al. Mutational analysis of immunoglobulin E-binding epitopes of beta-casein and beta-lactoglobulin showed a heterogeneous pattern of critical amino acids between individual patients and pooled sera. Clin Exptl Allergy 2007;35:831–8.

52. Jarvinen K-M, Beyer K, Vila L, et al. Specificity of IgE antibodies to sequential epitopes of hen's egg ovomucoid as a marker for persistence of egg allergy. Allergy 2007;62:758–65.

53. Cerecedo I, Zamora J, Shreffler WG, et al. Mapping of the IgE and IgG4 sequential epitopes of milk allergens with a peptide microarray-based immunoassay. J Allergy Clin Immunol 2008;122:589–94.

54. Stapel SO, Asero R, Ballmer-Weber BK, et al. Testing for IgG4 against foods is not recommended as a diagnostic tool. EAACI task force report. Allergy 2008;63:793–6.

55. Bock SA. AAAAI support of the EAACI Position Paper on IgG4. J Allergy Clin Immunology 2010;125:1410.

56. Tomicic S, Norrman G, Flath-Magnusson K, et al. High levels of IgG4 antibodies to foods during infancy re associate with tolerance to corresponding foods later in life. Pediatr Allergy Immunol 2009;20:35–41.

57. Ruiter B, Knol EF, van Neerven RJJ, et al. Maintenance of tolerance to cow's milk in atopic individuals is characterized by high levels of specific immunoglobulin G4. Clin Exptl Allergy 2007;27:1103–10.

CHAPTER 14

Oral Food Challenge Procedures

Gideon Lack, George Du Toit and Mary Feeney

KEY CONCEPTS

- Oral food challenges (particularly double-blind placebo-controlled food challenge) represent the accepted gold standard investigation for objective diagnosis of both immediate and delayed-onset food allergy.
- Oral food challenges are clinically indicated to demonstrate allergy or tolerance to achieve safe dietary expansion or appropriate allergen avoidance.

- A particular challenge design is selected according to clinical history, age of patient and associated factors at the time of the index reaction.
- Using standardized procedures, safe and objective challenge outcomes can be achieved.

The World Allergy Organization (WAO) defines any adverse reaction to food as food hypersensitivity, which can be further divided into immune-mediated reactions (food allergy) and non-immune mediated reactions (food intolerance). Food-allergic reactions may be broadly divided into immunoglobulin E (IgE)-mediated (immediate-onset) reactions and non-IgE-mediated (delayed-onset) reactions (Table 14.1).

A diagnosis of food hypersensitivity is achieved using a combination of diagnostic modalities such as clinical history, physical examination and allergy testing. When only an equivocal diagnosis is possible, use is made of oral food challenge tests. The oral food challenge (especially double-blind placebo-controlled food challenge – DBPCFC) represents the gold standard investigation for the diagnosis of both immediate and delayed food-induced allergic reactions.[1,2]

Rationale

Oral food challenges are diagnostic tests which aim to achieve safe dietary expansion or appropriate allergen avoidance; to achieve this, the oral food challenge hopes to demonstrate an unequivocal outcome of either 'tolerance' or 'allergy'. The outcomes may include symptoms and signs that indicate IgE-mediated or non-IgE-mediated reactions.

Indications for an oral food challenge

The indications for undertaking an oral food challenge are varied but fall broadly into two categories, those where a state of either allergy or tolerance to a food is anticipated but uncertain. The rationale for these is described in Table 14.2.

Table 14.1 Classification of food hypersensitive reactions

IgE-mediated, immediate-onset symptoms and signs	
Gastrointestinal	Gastrointestinal anaphylaxis: symptoms include vomiting, pain and/or diarrhea
Cutaneous	Urticaria, angioedema, pruritus, morbilliform rashes and flushing
Respiratory	Acute rhinoconjunctivitis, wheezing, coughing and stridor
Generalized	Anaphylaxis
Mixed IgE- and cell-mediated, immediate–delayed onset symptoms and signs	
Gastrointestinal	Eosinophilic esophagitis
Cutaneous	Atopic eczema
Cell-mediated, immediate–delayed onset symptoms and signs	
Gastrointestinal	Food protein-induced enterocolitis, food protein-induced proctocolitis and food protein-induced enteropathy syndrome – which may present with a clinical picture of 'sepsis'
Respiratory	Food-induced pulmonary hemosiderosis (Heiner syndrome) (rare) – pulmonary hemosiderosis or bleeding in the lower respiratory tract.
Mechanism uncertain, immediate–delayed onset symptoms and signs	
GI dysmotility	Gastroesophageal reflux* Constipation* Infantile colic*

*Associations remain controversial.

Table 14.2 Indications for performing a food challenge

Indication	**Rationale**
Demonstrate tolerance	1. Allergy suspected to have been outgrown, e.g. the child who was previously egg allergic but now returns ever-decreasing allergy test results. 2. When the food has been tolerated in some presentations but not others e.g. baked egg in cakes tolerated but scrambled egg causes a reaction. 3. When allergy tests suggest tolerance, but food never eaten and patient and/or parent too cautious to introduce at home. 4. Cross-reactivity suspected, e.g. the child with a low positive IgE result to wheat but high positive grass pollen sensitization. 5. When the diet is restricted due to a suspicion that one or more foods is resulting in delayed allergic symptoms, e.g. eczema, gastroesophageal reflux. 6. To establish a tolerance threshold to allergen proteins (currently restricted to the research setting). 7. When multiple dietary restrictions are maintained but symptoms are subjective.
Demonstrate allergy	1. Suspected food allergic reaction but cause uncertain despite SPT and Sp-IgE testing, e.g. composite meal eaten. 2. Suspected food allergic reaction but equivocal or inconsistent symptoms following consumption of a particular food.
Monitor therapy for food allergy	To monitor response to immunomodulatory treatment in the research setting.

It has been proposed that the clinician should aim to achieve a 50% positive to negative outcome ratio when performing oral food challenges (OFCs) in adults and children with established allergies.[3] This outcome indicates that the patients who are selected for challenges are those with the highest risk to benefit ratio of having a negative challenge. OFCs are not without risk and may induce severe, occasionally life-threatening reactions or more commonly less severe symptoms such as an exacerbation of atopic dermatitis. They are also labour and resource intensive. For these reasons, to minimize the need for oral food challenges, use is made of established diagnostic modalities, of which the clinical history is the most helpful. There are, however, scenarios where the history is of limited use, such as when a food has never been eaten. The clinical history is also dependent on the disease in question and the suspected allergenic trigger. For example, hives and angioedema that develop soon after peanut ingestion make for a very likely diagnosis of peanut allergy,[4] but abdominal pain that develops 4 hours after eating wheat makes for a less certain diagnosis of IgE-mediated wheat allergy.

If the history results in an equivocal diagnosis use is then made of validated allergy tests (such as the skin prick test and/or specific IgE determination) to help attain a post-test probability of allergy or tolerance. To facilitate this process (at least for immediate-onset allergies), where possible, positive and negative predictive values (PPV, NPV) have been determined; such values are available for the diagnosis (with 90% or 95% certainty) of egg, cows' milk, peanut and fish allergy (Table 14.3).[5–7] Values could not be established for other common food

Table 14.3 Positive predictive values for food-specific IgE and skin prick tests*

≥ 95% Specific IgE levels (KU/L) positive predictive Values	
Egg	7
Infants ≤ 2 yrs	2
Milk	15
Infants ≤ 2 yrs	5
Peanut	15
Tree nuts	15
Fish	20
≥ 95% skin prick tests (wheal diameter in mm) positive predictive values	
Milk	8
Infants ≤ 2 yrs	6
Egg	7
Infants ≤ 2 yrs	5
Peanut	8
Infants ≤ 2 yrs	4

*Negative allergy tests (specific IgE levels (<0.3 kU/L) and/or skin prick tests) may still be associated with clinical reactions. Allergy tests should therefore never be interpreted in the absence of a thorough allergy history.[38]

allergens such as soy and wheat. The use of allergy test predictive values significantly reduces the need for diagnostic dietary investigations if immediate-onset allergies are under investigation, but are not of use for the diagnosis of delayed-onset food induced hypersensitivity. Predictive diagnostic values are significantly influenced by numerous variables, such as the age of the patient and atopic phenotype, e.g. the presence of eczema. The values are therefore most accurate if validated for the specific population served. Another way to overcome this problem is the use of likelihood ratios (LRs). The LR for a test result is the likelihood that a positive test would be expected in a patient with the food allergy compared to the likelihood that the same result would be expected in a patient without food allergy. LRs have been established for selected foods in different centers.[9] The advantage of this approach is that LR values are independent of the prevalence of the condition tested. LRs can therefore be used to calculate the likelihood of a disease both within a tertiary care center and in the primary care setting. Before a patient's test result can be interpreted using the LR, their pre-test probability must be estimated. This is the chance that they are food allergic based only on their clinical presentation and risk factors prior to any test result. The post-test probability of food allergy for a subject can be derived from a statistically derived nomogram (Fig. 14.1). This takes into account the subject's pre-test probability and the LR corresponding to the test result. The use of these values combined with the medical history leads to an accurate diagnosis of food allergy in 70% of patients.[8]

Despite the use of the above testing methodologies, oral food challenges are often required in order to obtain a certain diagnosis of allergy or tolerance.

Oral food challenges: design and methodology

The design and methodology by which oral food challenges can be performed varies enormously and is influenced by the indication for which the challenge is being performed.[2,10,11] It is, however, important to remember that in essence a supervised food challenge entails no more than safely exposing the patient to doses of a food allergen and, if initially tolerated, the patient continuing to eat the food over sequential days. Challenges can be performed

SPT (mm)	0–2	3–7	>8
LR (mm)	0.2	1.8	∞

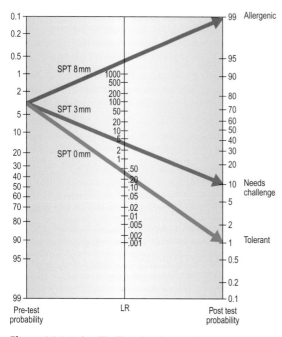

Figure 14.1 Using likelihood ratios to diagnose egg allergy. Consider a 3-year-old child who has never eaten eggs and is not atopic. Pre-test probability is estimated at 2.5% (prevalence in childhood). The LR is chosen according to SPT result. A SPT of 8 mm has a high LR and the post-test probability for egg allergy is >99%: this child is therefore considered allergic. An SPT of 3 mm has a medium LR and the child has a post-test probability of 10% allergy to egg. Diagnosis is in doubt and a DBPCFC is required. An SPT of 0 mm yields a post-test probability of <1%: this child is therefore deemed to be tolerant. With permission from Lack G. Clinical practice. Food allergy. N Engl J Med. 2008; 359(12): 1252–60.

diagnostically in the context of both suspected immediate IgE-mediated symptoms and delayed non-IgE-mediated symptoms. These challenges are broadly similar in both scenarios but with a few important differences (considerations specific to food challenges for non-IgE mediated symptoms are detailed in the section 'Oral Food Challenges for the assessment of non-IgE-mediated food (delayed) hypersensitivity'). A particular challenge design is selected according to clinical history, age of the patient and associated factors at the time of the index reaction. The variables and associated considerations that refine the choice of a particular design are described in Table 14.4.

Open vs blinded challenges

An open challenge mimics 'real-life' exposure to the food, albeit in a supervised setting. The patient is fed an age-appropriate (Table 14.5, Table 14.6) quantity of the challenge food in an open – i.e. unmasked and unblinded – manner. Depending on the risk profile, this can be performed in a single meal or in increments (incremental oral food challenge). Open oral food challenges are associated with a high degree of bias as both the patient and the observer (clinician) know what is contained in the challenge. However, the advantages of open challenges are that they are simple to carry out and reproduce 'real-life' exposure to a food in terms of the form, quantity and method of exposure. An open oral food challenge carries a high negative predictive value, i.e. when negative it is highly likely that the patient is truly tolerant of that food.[12] It is also useful if an unequivocal positive outcome (where both subjective and objective symptoms and signs are noted) is achieved. Open challenges that result in 'atypical' or 'subjective' symptoms only are less helpful, and always need to be followed by a blinded challenge; one study reports that oral food challenges produced 27% more positive challenges than DBPCFC in a group of children aged 1–15 years.[13] Subjective symptoms are reported less frequently in infants and young children ≤ 3 years, and open oral food challenges are recommended in this group; they can also be useful for preliminary screening for food allergy.[14]

Blinded challenges can be single- or double-blinded. Ideally, a food should be blinded for taste, smell, texture and appearance (consistency, color and shape). The placebo and the active (allergen-containing) food should be indistinguishable from each other, i.e. either the active food must be altered to resemble the placebo in all aspects, or vice versa.

A single-blind challenge involves masking the challenge food so that only the patient, and for younger children their family and/or carer, is unaware of what they are eating. A placebo food may also be included in the design. The staff performing the challenge are not blinded. Single blinding reduces – but does not eliminate – bias in terms of subjective symptoms reported by the patient, but does not control for any influence of observer bias by parents or staff.

A DBPCFC is achieved when the blinding process is extended to include the patient, family/carers and staff. Although DBPCFCs are considered the

Table 14.4 Variables associated with oral food challenges

Challenge-related variables	
Design • Open (single dose or incremental) • Blinded (single or double)	Design selected according to the indication and purpose for which the challenge is being performed (see section 'Open vs Blinded Challenges')
Form of challenge food	The challenge food should closely replicate the usual edible form of the food or form of the food implicated in allergic reaction. Food processing, and the food matrix can significantly influence allergenicity of the food, e.g. baked vs raw egg. For oral food challenges performed to diagnose the pollen–food syndrome, fresh fruit and vegetables should be used as the responsible proteins are commonly heat labile
Choice of food matrix	Strictly avoid use of allergenic ingredients for individual patient Minimize number of ingredients used Provide adequate allergen protein in a manageable portion size (see Table 14.6) For placebo foods sensory qualities should closely replicate those of active challenge food
Doses • Number of doses • Initial dose • Top dose • Time intervals between doses • Total duration of challenge	• If a negative outcome is anticipated and there are no safety concerns, a single dose is appropriate. If not, incremental doses increase safety due to gradual increases in exposure to food allergen • Low doses used for threshold studies in research setting or for patients at high risk of a severe reaction, higher initial doses are more practical in the clinical setting • Equivalent to an 'age-appropriate' portion, preferably a large portion, of the food (see Table 14.6) • At least 15 minutes for immediate symptoms or 24–48 hours for delayed symptoms. Adjust intervals depending on patient history • Between 2 hours (immediate symptoms) and 1–4 weeks (delayed symptoms)
Location • Day admission • Admission to hospital ward • Home	This choice depends on the risk associated and capacity to identify and treat anaphylactic reactions. Logistical dietetic factors are also important, e.g. DBPCFCs will be difficult to achieve in the home environment Low-risk challenge, cooperative patient High-risk challenge e.g. FPIES Low-risk challenge, delayed symptoms
Interpretation of challenge outcome	Challenge outcomes may be immediately apparent, i.e. within an hour of ingestion when due to IgE-mediated immune mechanisms. Delayed food-induced hypersensitivity reactions may arise over hours or even days (see Table 14.10)
Patient-related variables	
Indication for food challenge	There are many indications for performing an oral food challenge; these are listed in Table 14.2
Clinical history at last known reaction Immediate or delayed symptoms Severity of symptoms Association with other conditions, e.g. asthma	One or more of these factors have been shown to affect the severity of allergic reactions
Age	The age of the patient will affect the type of food, food volumes and number of feeds. Younger children may require less stringent blinding of foods than older children and adults

Table 14.5 Foods commonly used to disguise allergens for food challenges (other food allergens depending)

Cows' milk	Amino acid formula, extensively hydrolyzed formula, soy formula
Soy milk	Amino acid formula, extensively hydrolyzed formula, cows' milk
Egg	Blended in yogurt, ingredient in cakes or biscuits, mashed potato
Peanut	Strongly flavored biscuits or cakes, chocolate pudding, fruit smoothie
Wheat	Substitute gluten-free, wheat-free products, e.g. pasta, biscuits, oatcakes
Sesame	Hummus, chocolate pudding, soy dessert, lentil soup, beefburger
Shellfish	Beefburger, strongly flavored sauces
Meat	Alternative meat-based burger
Colorings or preservatives	Fruit juice, vegetable juice
Fruit or vegetables	Mix with alternative strong tasting fruit/vegetable

gold standard diagnostic modality[5] they require additional facilities and a skilled medical, nursing and dietetic team. In particular, dietitians are needed to develop, prepare and store blinded recipes, and need to be able to reproduce a dose if necessary. During the blinding procedure neither the patient nor the observers know which is the active food and which is the placebo (these are prepared by a third party, usually a skilled dietitian). The order of doses (active or placebo) is random and not revealed until after the challenge is completed; in the event of a negative outcome, 'unblinding' only occurs after all doses are consumed and the observation window is past, but in the event of a positive reaction unblinding occurs sooner. In the event of equivocal symptoms during the DBPCFC, the last dose should be repeated (only the dietitian who prepared the foods will be aware if this dose is active or placebo). This rigorous procedure prevents reporting bias by both parties. In order to openly prove tolerance to the patient, all negative DBPCFCs should be followed by an open feeding of age-appropriate portion of the food in its natural or 'real life' form.[20]

Owing to the practical difficulties associated with the DBPCFC, use thereof is generally limited to specific diagnostic scenarios such as clinical research, diagnosing chronic symptoms or subjective complaints, e.g. migraine, chronic fatigue syndrome.[5,21] In the clinical setting a DBPCFC is used only where there are atypical or unverifiable subjective symptoms or high levels of anxiety on the part of the patient (and/or parent).

Although efforts have been made to standardize OFCs there remains a lack of agreement in terms of the type and quantity of the food allergen to be administered, the timings between doses, observation periods and blinded recipes used.[2,11,15–17]

Form of challenge food

The common food allergens have variable sources and characteristics. Although the proportions of carbohydrate, protein and fat vary, most allergens are found in foods with a high protein content. The majority of food-induced allergic reactions arise as a result of reactions to the food proteins.[18]

The challenge food should closely resemble the usual edible form of that food and ideally mimic the food implicated in the history, as this most closely replicates the 'real-life' setting. This is particularly important for open challenges, and for the open dose given after a DBPCFC, to confirm tolerance. Careful consideration of the clinical history is essential when choosing the form of a challenge food, as processing may influence the allergenicity of a food. The effects of food processing may be allergen specific. For example, the allergenicity of egg and milk is reduced by heat processing, whereas that of peanut is increased by roasting.[19,20]

Other forms of challenge food, e.g. dried foods such as powdered egg or peanut flour, are commonly used for DBPCFC for convenience of storage, greater ease of blinding, or because of requirements for a high concentration of an allergen in a small volume, e.g. 4 g peanut protein can be provided in 8 g of peanut flour (50% peanut protein) compared to 16 g of peanut butter (25% peanut protein). This helps reduce the portion sizes required to deliver an adequate amount of allergen during the challenge. Large amounts of foods may cause symptoms such as nausea or vomiting, which could be falsely interpreted as an allergic reaction to either the challenge food or the placebo used.

It is essential to consider issues of food safety when deciding who will provide the challenge food, e.g. hospital catering service or parent. Where a catering service provides the food, the staff setting up the challenge must ensure that they have

Table 14.6 Challenge doses for common food allergens

EAACCI-proposed initial doses		Total cumulative dose for open food challenges	
Allergen	**Initial Dose**	**Dosing increments**	**Age appropriate portion sizes***
Peanut	0.1 mg	0.1 g, 0.25 g, 0.5 g, 1 g, 2 g, 4 g, 8 g, 20 g	1–2 tablespoons (15–30 g) peanut butter
Milk	0.1 mL	0.5 mL, 1 mL, 2 mL, 5 mL, 10 mL, 20 mL, 40 mL, 100 mL, 180–240 mL	180–240 mL (6–8 oz) milk or infant formula ½–1 cup yogurt ½–1 cup cottage cheese 15–30g (½–1 oz) hard cheese
Egg	1 mg	1 g, 2 g, 5 g, 10 g, 20 g, 60 g	1 hard-boiled or scrambled egg (60 g) 1 slice of French toast (1 egg per slice of bread)
Cod	5 mg	1 g, 2 g, 5 g, 10 g, 15 g, 30 g, 60 g	60–90g (2–3 oz) cooked fish
Wheat	100 mg	1 g, 2 g, 5 g, 10 g, 25 g, 80 g 1 g, 3 g, 6 g, 20 g	½–1 cup cooked pasta 15–30g (½–1 oz) wheat-based cereal ½–1 slice bread ½–1 muffin or bread roll
Soy	1 mg	0.5 mL, 1 mL, 2 mL, 5 mL, 10 mL, 20 mL, 40 mL, 100 mL	½–1 cup soy beverage ½–1 cup tofu
Shrimp	5 mg	0.5 g, 1 g, 4 g, 15 g, 60 g	60–90g (2–3 oz) shellfish
Hazelnut	0.1 g	0.25 g, 0.5 g, 2 g, 4 g, 15 g, 30 g	30–40 g crushed tree nuts or 25–30 pieces

*For older teenagers and adults larger portion sizes should be used. Adapted from Work Group report: oral food allergy challenge testing.[2]

up-to-date food safety standards and procedures in place to minimize the risk of cross-contamination. Where food is to be brought from home the patient must be informed of how to source uncontaminated and safe food products – e.g. if raw eggs are to be used these should be confirmed salmonella-free, – as well as how to best process the foods to optimize the food matrix for the challenge (see below).

Choice of food vehicle

Masking of a challenge food in a vehicle i.e. with other ingredients is sometimes required in open challenges to make the food more palatable to the patient. In DBPCFC, the use of a vehicle is always required to disguise the allergen and to ensure that the placebo food closely replicates the sensory

qualities of the active challenge food, including taste, smell, texture and appearance (consistency, color, shape).

In both instances the vehicle should avoid using allergenic ingredients. Minimizing the number of ingredients used will help avoid unknown side effects of other ingredients. A food matrix effect has been described in some preparations of challenge foods which arises as a result of the interaction between fat, carbohydrate and proteins; this may affect the allergenic characteristics of the food as well as allergen absorption and processing through the GI tract:[21,22] e.g. a higher fat recipe resulted in delayed reactions at higher doses during a peanut challenge. These characteristics need to be considered when developing these recipes.

Capsules have been used as a convenient way to disguise active and placebo foods, but safety can be significantly compromised. There is a greater chance of a severe reaction as the first immune presentation and recognition of the allergen will be in the gut at time of digestion of the full capsule dose, after having bypassed the normal physiological route of allergen detection, i.e. the oropharynx.

Challenge foods for DBPCFC

The challenge foods used for DBPCFC need to contain enough of the allergen to elicit allergic reactions and it is important that no perceivable differences between the placebo and the active food. Developing validated recipes is difficult and time-consuming and the processes for doing so have not been standardized. Until recently, available validated recipes contained amounts of allergens that were too low for many food challenge procedures. To fully validate challenge foods for clinical use, statistical modeling that incorporates advanced sensory discrimination testing, such as paired comparison, directional difference or triangle testing, is required.[23] These tests are used to determine whether a specified or unspecified difference exists between active and placebo foods.

In the case of validating foods for DBPCFC, active and placebo food samples are coded and tasted under controlled conditions in a specified order. Assessors may be asked to describe observed differences, such as taste, and estimate how large they are between samples (paired comparison or directional difference tests); or, in the case of triangle testing, they simply indicate whether they can identify which is the 'odd' sample, e.g. the one that contains peanut when presented with three samples (two active and one placebo, or one active and two placebo). Comparing the number of correct responses obtained with standardized tables helps to determine whether a perceivable difference between samples has been shown to exist. Ideally, use should be made of a large number of panelists in order to minimize bias and to optimize statistical power.[23]

Most studies to date have used adult tasting panels for sensory testing. Untrained or age-specific assessors i.e. groups more similar to those who would actually be receiving the challenge foods, could be used, and would likely show less stringent blinding to be adequate, particularly in young children; that is to say larger amounts of allergen could be blinded in a volume the child could manage. However, the power of sensory testing is generally poor and hundreds of assessors would be required to achieve adequate powering.[24]

By optimizing the conditions of sensory testing i.e. using trained tasting panels, fewer assessors are required. Recipes validated for blinding of cow's milk, egg, peanut, hazelnut and cashew suitable for children greater than 4 years old and adults (some also suitable for younger children) have been published.[23] These recipes mask a total amount of allergenic ingredient equivalent to one food serving disguised in 250 ml liquid or 125 g solid food. Validated recipes for soy and wheat are available which have managed to disguise smaller amounts of these allergens.[27]

Utility of active challenge foods also needs to be proven with respect to the ability of the food to induce an allergic reaction and the likely dose responses at which this is likely to occur in allergic individuals. It is not surprising, therefore, that few validated DBPCFC recipes exist.

Familiar foods are recommended as the starting point when developing DBPCFC recipes, as they tend to be more acceptable; however, it is important to remember that adults and children who have been on exclusion diets for many years may be reluctant to eat the challenge foods. Having been advised, sometimes for many years, to avoid a food; particularly one which has caused previous allergic reactions, they may have become averse to eating it. Alternatively, the type of food they are being asked to eat may be unfamiliar to them e.g. children who have been following egg-free diets from infancy often do not consider cakes to be 'treats' in the way that other children do as they are not familiar with them. In these situations, 'creative dietetics' may be required to disguise the food so that it does not look or taste like the food they have been avoiding e.g. disguising eggs in French toast or nuts in a flapjack. See table 14.5 for foods commonly used to disguise food allergens for challenges. A choice of more than one challenge food may also be necessary to deal with fussy eating which is relatively common among children with food allergies.

Allergenic ingredients are commonly substituted in active and placebo recipes with 'free from' alternatives which may behave quite differently from typical ingredients, affecting not only the taste of the food but other qualities such as texture and color, or even cooking time. It is therefore necessary to have a dietitian who is both creative and has a good knowledge of the use of these alternative ingredients when preparing these recipes.

Placebos

The use of placebos in allergy testing is usually restricted to older patients (adolescents and adults), research settings or after open challenges have resulted in atypical or non-specific symptoms. Their inclusion helps to increase the validity of the challenge outcome by minimizing false positive results.[27] The disadvantages of placebo use include the additional doses required for the challenge. A greater number of doses take longer to consume and may frustrate younger children; in addition, the greater total volumes required to be eaten may fill the young child before the challenge is completed. There is also a chance that the patient may be allergic to the placebo used (if different ingredients from those in the active challenge food are used).

For patients who had initially presented with objective allergic signs it may be that a single placebo dose (often given first) is sufficiently robust in providing a valid outcome; this is due to the low frequency of placebo reactions in such patients. For those with more subjective symptoms, it is recommended that placebo-controlled oral food challenges be delivered on two separate occasions. This may involve two sessions on the same day (one with active food, the other with placebo, separated by at least 2 hours) or indeed over 2 days (one day being for the administration of placebo and the other for the active food. The open dose only follows the second day's feeds).[25] Combining the two sessions by interspersing placebo doses with active doses is more practical where a prolonged challenge procedure is not feasible, e.g. using three active and three placebo or three active and two placebo doses.[2,16]

Where reported symptoms are delayed in onset, active and placebo doses should be administered on separate days, in a random order, separated by days or sometimes weeks.

Both objective and subjective placebo events have been reported; these are usually immediate, i.e. within 20 minutes.[27] Where placebo doses are given interspersed with active doses, it cannot always be certain when a reaction takes place after the administration of a placebo dose (unless it also occurs after an additional placebo dose), whether this is due to the placebo dose or whether it is a delayed reaction to one of the preceding active doses. It is therefore important to always confirm an allergy to the placebo by repeating an oral food challenge to the same placebo but in the absence of the challenge food. Reported rates of placebo reactions are 7% in threshold studies.[29,30] There are studies which report no placebo-induced reactions; this may be due to short observation periods following the administration of placebo and the active food. An interval of at least 15 minutes between doses should therefore be observed. Frequency of placebo events must not be excluded from statistical analysis, as this risks overestimating the frequency of patients having actual allergies.[5,15]

Doses

The key considerations when choosing doses for oral food challenges are the choice of initial or starting dose, incremental doses and the top dose. These should be individualized to the person(s) undergoing the challenge, thereby maximizing the reliability of the outcome and minimizing the risk of a severe reaction.

The European Academy of Allergy and Clinical Immunology (EAACI)'s proposed initial doses for common food allergens[5] (Table 14.6) are useful for threshold studies (which investigate the lowest dose of an allergen capable of eliciting an allergic reaction) or where the patient is considered at risk of a severe reaction, as very low starting doses are used. However, for most patients higher initial doses may be used which are more practical to measure and avoid food challenges being unnecessarily long (see Table 14.6). An appropriate initial dose is one smaller than the patient is known to react to.[29]

Many studies describing food challenge procedures state that tolerance is demonstrated if a total cumulative challenge dose of 8–10 g dry weight, or 60–100 mL or g 'wet weight' in children,[15] or 15 g dry weight in adults is tolerated.[2] However, these are reported with limited details of the conversion factor from dried to wet foods, and the exact nature (e.g. food matrix) of the food. Some more recent studies quantify amounts of challenge materials as an amount of allergen protein.[2,26] Additionally, as all negative DBPCFCs should be followed by an open food challenge using an age-appropriate portion of the food, the total cumulative dose in these challenges is typically twice that of open challenges. In younger children it may only be possible to achieve a lower top dose, e.g. an adolescent challenged to peanut may manage a top dose of 5 g peanut protein (equivalent to a generous spreading of peanut butter on bread), whereas a child younger than 5 years may only manage a top dose of 2 g (equivalent to a rounded teaspoon of peanut butter). The use of excess incremental feeds may upset the child or induce non-specific gastrointestinal symptoms, e.g. vomiting, which may then prove difficult to exclude as an allergic feature.

Although there is some knowledge about objective and subjective symptoms at low doses, less is known about the role of high doses in inducing symptoms. There is much debate as to the lowest starting doses for food challenges, but no data to tell us where an oral food challenge should stop. For example, a child may pass an oral food challenge giving 4 g allergen protein and be said to be tolerant, but could react at a threshold of 6 g. This phenomenon is best described as 'dose-dependent tolerance.' One audit of food challenge procedures showed that 10% of children only reacted at the top 4 g peanut protein dose (total cumulative dose 7.9 g peanut protein)[30] and a second study using DBPCFCs demonstrates that 4% of children reacted only after the open challenge dose;[31] this raises the possibility that there may be additional children who could pass a challenge ending with a 4 g or even 5 g top dose, but would react if higher doses were given. It is important, therefore, that challenges are finished with a generous 'age-appropriate portion' dose, i.e. the total cumulative challenge dose will then be higher than the patient would typically be expected to manage in daily life.

Further research is required to define an upper NOAEL (no observed adverse effect level) or top challenge dose to which no one reacts. Only tolerant patients will progress to this dose in a challenge, allergic patients will have reacted at a lower dose. This is particularly relevant in oral tolerance induction studies (specific oral tolerance induction), as research indicates that some participants in these studies react at doses that would not be tested in the typical clinical setting, e.g. a study investigating oral tolerance induction to milk in a group of milk-allergic children describes that during the maintenance phase of the study a number of patients reacted to 16 g milk protein (equivalent to 440 mL milk), which is higher than doses typically used in oral food challenges.[32]

Number of doses and interval between doses

The number of doses, and intervals between doses, should match the anticipated safety and outcome of the challenge. For example, a single-dose open challenge can be used when a negative outcome is anticipated and no safety concerns exist. Examples would include baseline challenges at the point of entry into research studies in participants with negative allergy tests and no history of reactivity to that food. An additional example would be when tests are negative but the participant and/or family are reluctant to introduce the food in an unsupervised setting. Use of a single-dose feed serves to minimize the time and resources required for the challenge.

Incremental challenges allow for more gradual exposures to the food, hence increasing safety. There is a lack of consensus as to how these doses should be increased, with some studies recommending doubling doses.[2,15,16] Other studies advise using a logarithmic mean, i.e. 1, 3, 10, 30, 100 until the top dose is reached. The choice of increment will depend on the anticipated risk. Many studies demonstrate that positive challenge symptoms (both objective and subjective) typically occur at the lower doses; this may also be true for symptom severity, i.e. more severe symptoms occurring at lower doses.[33] This justifies smaller increases in doses in the early stages of an incremental challenge. The downside of oral food challenges that make use of excessive dose protocols is that young children easily become fatigued (remembering that placebos may need to be included in the regimens). There may also be time implications, e.g. the use of four active doses and three placebo doses, with at least 15-minute observation intervals and an hour's observation post challenge, will result in a challenge duration of 195 minutes (if feeds are all eaten on time). If cannulation is required beforehand, additional time will be required for the procedure (and the use of local anesthetic creams).

Advised time intervals between doses also vary, e.g. 10–60 minutes or 15–30 minutes. The most appropriate choice depends on safety and feasibility. The use of an interval that is too short may compromise safety by not allowing enough time for an allergic reaction to present. A short interval may also complicate the interpretation of a reaction which occurs after a placebo dose, i.e. is it the placebo or the preceding dose of the food allergen that caused the reaction? We make use of an interval of 'at least 15 minutes', which reduces the above complications and minimizes the overall duration of the oral food challenge.

Site of application of first dose

There is not always absolute concordance between allergic symptoms that occur upon skin contact and symptoms upon ingestion. For this reason it is unwise to first apply the food to skin, particularly eczematous skin, prior to commencing the oral challenge. Most challenges do, however, commence with application of the food to the mucosa of the lips (which represent the start of the gastrointestinal tract and which are densely populated with allergen recognition cells).

Logistics

The oral food challenge should be considered a formal invasive medical investigation. For this reason, signed informed consent – and, when appropriate, patient assent – is mandatory prior to the commencement of an oral food challenge. Patients and their families should be reminded beforehand about the need to stop taking those medications that are contraindicated at time of challenge. Patients should always be thoroughly examined prior to the commencement of the challenge to assess for general well-being and, in particular, the presence of pre-existing rashes and/or wheezing. Failure to do so may result in difficulty in interpreting equivocal symptoms and signs during the challenge. As it is not uncommon for children who are closely observed for 6–12 hours to develop non-specific 'blotches', pre-existing rashes should be noted in detail. It should be checked that the patient has stopped all medication, such as antihistamines, that might mask allergic reactions when they occur (Table 14.7). Patients should omit medications that

Table 14.7 Guidelines for discontinuation of medications that might interfere with interpretation of oral food challenges With permission from Nowak-Wegrzyn A, Assa'ad AH, Bahna SL, Bock SA, Sicherer SH, Teuber SS. Work Group report: oral food challenge testing. J Allergy Clin Immunol. 2009; 123(6 Suppl): S365-83.

Medication†	Last dose before oral food challenge	Medication†	Last dose before oral food challenge
Oral antihistamines	3–10 d	Inhaled cromolyn sodium	48 h
Cetirizine	5–7 d	Nedocromil sodium	12 h
Diphenhydramine	3 d	Theophylline (liquid)	24 h
Fexofenadine	3 d	Theophylline long-acting	48 h
Hydroxyzine	7–10 d	Ipatropium bromide (inhaled/intranasal)	4–12 h depending on formulation and dosing interval
Loratadine	7 d		
Antihistamine nose spray	12 h	Oral/intranasal α-adrenergic agents	
Oral H$_2$ receptor antagonist	12 h		
Antidepressants	3 d–3 wk, drug-dependent and dose-dependent	Oral β-agonist	12 h
		Oral long-acting β_2-agonist	24 h
Oral/intramuscular/ intravenous steroids‡	3 d–2 wk	**Drugs that may be continued**	
Leukotriene antagonist	24 h	Antihistamine eye drops Inhaled/intranasal corticosteroids Topical steroids Topical immunosuppressive preparations: pimecrolimus, tacrolimus	
Short-acting bronchodilator (albuterol, metaproterenol, terbutaline, isoproterenol)	8 h 24 h		
Long-acting bronchodilator (salmeterol, formoterol)	8 h		

†Aspirin and other non-steroidal anti-inflammatory agents and angiotensin-converting enzyme inhibitors should be avoided because of their theoretical ability to enhance or induce allergic reactions and potential interference with an oral food challenge outcome interpretation.
‡This suggested guideline is based on concerns regarding the potential for suppression of the late-phase responses. In addition, the patient who received a short course of systemic corticosteroid may be going through an exacerbation that would either interfere with the oral food challenge interpretation or potentially worsen the severity of a reaction. In patients who receive chronic therapy with systemic steroids, such as for inflammatory/rheumatologic diseases, the risk–benefit ratio for stopping steroid therapy and substituting an alternative therapeutic agent vs performing an oral food challenge while the patient remains on steroid should be evaluated on an individual basis.

may interfere with the treatment of severe allergic reactions with adrenaline, e.g. β-blockers. See Table 14.7 for further details.

Safety and contraindications

Food challenges are not without risk.[34] To optimize safety, procedures should be in place to deal with allergic reactions and staff should be trained in the recognition and emergency management thereof. Age- and weight-appropriate emergency medications that may be required should be written up on medication charts prior to commencing the challenge.[35,36] A careful assessment of patients prior to performing the challenge, including assessment of lung function (in older children), is mandatory. Pre-existing airway inflammation, e.g. infection or asthma, is a major risk factor for severe anaphylaxis and should be excluded. Patients who are at increased risk of experiencing a severe reaction (Table 14.8) should ideally be cannulated prior to commencing a challenge[37], although cannulation was not performed or required in a study where peanut challenges were performed in children with positive peanut allergy tests and a management plan should be in place in the event of a severe reaction, i.e. resuscitation response teams should know that an 'increased risk' challenge is taking place and the location of the challenge; ICU staff may also need to be notified. Nonetheless, oral food challenges have an excellent safety record if patients are carefully assessed before an oral food challenge that is then performed by experienced staff in a safe environment. Indeed, fatalities due to oral food challenges are not reported. Table 14.9 details both absolute and partial contraindications to an oral food challenge.

Determination of oral food challenge outcome

Although oral food challenges usually result in an unequivocal outcome, indeterminate scenarios are not uncommon. Although numerous scoring systems have been devised for the evaluation of immediate-onset IgE-mediated allergic reactions, this is not the case for all of the non-IgE-mediated (delayed-onset) food hypersensitivities.

Scoring of immediate-onset IgE-mediated allergic reactions

Oral food challenge outcome assessments are easiest to make at the extremes of clinical presentation, i.e. the child who happily eats an age-appropriate portion of a food allergen in an open challenge is tolerant, as false negatives are extremely rare; likewise, the child who develops immediate-onset allergic symptoms and signs during a DBPCFC is allergic to that food. However, if the investigator's instinct is that the allergen is an unlikely trigger, then an allergy to the placebo, or accidental contamination of the food with a different food allergen, should be excluded.

The more difficult diagnostic scenarios arise when symptoms and signs are mild, subjective or atypical (this is especially true for open oral food challenges). Further complicating the interpretation of

Table 14.8 Increased risk challenge scenarios

Condition	Rationale
Food protein-induced enterocolitis syndrome (FPIES)	Elective cannulation should be performed as patients are at risk of dehydration due to excessive vomiting and/or diarrhea. Antiemetic medications and rehydration fluids should be written up on medication charts before commencing
History of severe anaphylaxis at the time of their index reaction or severe coexisting asthma	May recur at time of subsequent challenge
Where pre-challenge allergy tests may be strongly positive and suggestive of allergy, e.g. research settings	More is being learned about the predictive value of allergen component tests in determining the risk of severe reactions, e.g. r Ara h 2 may be such a marker for patients with peanut allergy[47]
Food-dependent exercise-induced anaphylaxis (FDEIA) and exercise-induced anaphylaxis (EIA)	Elective cannulation should be performed beforehand as this may prove difficult if performed for an exercise-induced reaction. Nonetheless, exercise challenges have an excellent safety record

Table 14.9 Contraindications to oral food challenge (absolute and partial)

Contraindication	Reasoning
Absolute contraindications	
Medical illness at time of challenge, e.g. viral infection, poorly controlled asthma, uncontrolled eczema	Uncontrolled asthma is a risk factor for severe food-induced allergic reactions. Underlying illness may alter anticipated thresholds and responses during the oral food challenge. Concurrent infections may result in confusing non-allergic rashes. Severe eczema exacerbations may result in false positive challenge outcomes
Underlying medical conditions where the treatment of anaphylaxis may be compromised	Cardiac disease, or cardiac disease requiring use of a β-Blocker. ACEI may be a cause of angioedema and this should be controlled for. NSAIDs, particularly aspirin, may affect allergen absorption
Medication use that may mask allergic symptoms at time of oral food challenge, e.g. antihistamines, β_2-agonists	Antihistamines may mask early signs of an allergic reaction. β_2-agonists may mask deterioration in lung function that would have been detected at time of the oral food challenge
Partial contraindications	
Individual is unwilling to continue eating the food in the event of a negative result	Food allergy may 'recur' in patients who returned a negative oral challenge but then continued to avoid the allergen
Poorly controlled rhinoconjunctivitis	Early signs of a food-induced allergic reaction commonly include rhinoconjunctivitis, hence the presence thereof may confuse the interpretation of challenge outcomes. In addition, symptom control may depend on the use of antihistamines, which are contraindicated prior to performing an oral food challenge

mild early-onset symptoms is the fact that these are usually treated early on, which may interrupt the progression to more severe unequivocal symptoms and signs. Although safety is the primary concern during such procedures it may be necessary to continue with the challenge when only mild symptoms and signs are present. This is particularly true for children with atopic eczema, who may over the course of an oral food challenge develop nonspecific rashes, perhaps related to hospital-specific factors, e.g. ambient temperature, bedding etc.

Despite the use of rigorous oral food challenge outcome criteria, great emphasis should always be placed on the experience of nurses and dietitians who frequently perform oral food challenges. Their clinical intuition, particularly when added to the parents' opinion, is often best at detecting early symptoms or those that are non-specific, e.g. emotional and behavioral changes. Whereas older children may report a 'feeling of impending doom', younger children and infants may become 'suddenly quiet' or 'clingy'; a more subtle variation of this is the 'TV sign', where young children who had been entranced by electronic entertainment of some sort suddenly lose interest and seek their parents' close attention.

More rigorous outcome criteria may be required for research studies; we include the criteria used on young children in the NIH-funded LEAP study (Table 14.10).[38]

After the challenge

Oral food challenge outcomes should be described as positive, negative or indeterminate – describing challenge outcomes as 'failed' or 'passed' may be emotive for children. The most common reason for an indeterminate challenge result is being unable to get the child to consume adequate quantities of food to demonstrate tolerance. This situation may be avoided in a number of ways. First, children should only be challenged when they are old enough for there to be a realistic expectation that they can eat enough of the allergen. It is often necessary to disguise the challenge food, as previously described. It is also worthwhile asking mothers to omit the child's breakfast and/or avoid giving snacks during the early part of the challenge (when doses are usually small), thus increasing their appetite at the time of the challenge.

It has been described that delayed biphasic allergic reactions can occur after the initial reactions,

Table 14.10 **Example of a scoring system for the diagnosis of immediate onset reactions (LEAP Study).** A positive food challenge should be made for children who experience one or more major criteria OR two or more minor criteria, an indeterminate result is made if only one minor criterion is present, and a negative food challenge is made in the absence of any criteria. Importantly, all symptoms should be of new onset and not due to ongoing disease. Symptoms must occur no later than 2 hours after the last dose

Major criteria
Confluent erythematous pruritic rash
Respiratory signs (at least one of the following):
Wheezing
Inability to speak
Stridor
Dysphonia
Aphonia
≥3 urticarial lesions
≥1 site of angioedema
Hypotension for age not associated with vasovagal episode
Evidence of severe abdominal pain (such as abnormal stillness or doubling over) that persists for ≥3 minutes

Minor criteria
Vomiting
Diarrhea
Persistent rubbing of nose or eyes that lasts for ≥3 minutes
Persistent rhinorrhea that lasts for ≥3 minutes
Persistent scratching that lasts for ≥3 minutes

typically around 4 hours post ingestion. Therefore, patients who react during a challenge should remain under observation for at least 4 hours, or longer if symptoms persist. Severe symptoms may require overnight hospital admission. Education in the identification and appropriate management of allergic reactions in the event of accidental exposure to the food, as well as strict dietary avoidance advice, is required. Where the challenge is completed with no symptoms, patients should remain for observation for at least 2 hours prior to the challenge being considered negative. Again, they should be given advice on the identification and appropriate management of allergic reactions, including late-phase reactions. They should also be advised to reintroduce the food to their diet, initially two to three portions per week, in an attempt to ensure ongoing tolerance.[4] This may be particularly difficult for patients who are averse to the food; a dietitian can help to advise on alternative, more acceptable, forms of the food, or even disguising it. Regardless of the initial outcome, all patients should be reviewed 24 hours post challenge by telephone to eliminate delayed or ongoing symptoms and to answer any questions that typically arise.

Oral food challenges for the assessment of non-IgE-mediated (delayed-onset) food hypersensitivity

Non-IgE-mediated (delayed-onset) reactions can be difficult to link to food ingestion owing to the delay in symptom onset (hours to days after eating the food) and the natural variability of the many conditions that may require an oral food challenge to accurately assess for an influence of a food allergen (see Table 14.2). Traditional allergy tests, such as SPT and specific IgE determination, even when combined with atopy patch testing (APT), may be of limited value; hence reliance is on elimination or oligoallergenic diets, with the diagnosis confirmed by a 'reintroductory' oral food challenge.[39,40]

Considerations associated with choice of challenge design (e.g. open or blinded), type of food, placebo and doses for oral food challenges are as described for IgE-mediated immediate-onset outcomes. The main differences lie in the duration and location of the challenge and in the interpretation of symptoms and signs. Oral food challenges are usually unnecessary where an elimination diet supervised by a dietitian has not resulted in an improvement after 4 weeks, and the patient may then slowly reintroduce that food. Where an improvement does occur an oral food challenge is recommended to rule out confounding factors and confirm the diagnosis.[39] Oral food challenges for non-IgE-mediated food hypersensitivity usually require repetitive provocation with the food over a period of 2 and sometimes up to 7 days. If there is no risk of immediate-type symptoms they may be carried out in the patient's home. It is important that enough time is allowed for symptoms to develop, e.g. late eczematous responses may take up to 48 hours to develop.

Scoring of non-IgE-mediated (delayed-onset) food hypersensitivity allergic reactions

Where possible, delayed symptoms should be interpreted and scored systematically using validated tools; these are best described for the outcome of atopic eczema, which is by far the most common non-IgE-mediated food hypersensitivity outcome investigated for.

Atopic eczema

Food hypersensitivity is a known trigger for eczema, particularly in infancy, and can result in immediate-type reactions, isolated late reactions (occurring hours or 1–2 days after ingestion) or a combination of the two.[39,41] Open challenges are helpful to establish a causative relationship between the food and eczema, especially for negative outcomes. For subjective outcomes use is made of DBPCFCs. Ideally, an oral food challenge would only be initiated when the patient's eczema is well controlled. Reducing the natural fluctuations of the eczema assists with clinical evaluation of the skin post challenge. However, in clinical practice it is the patient with severe and difficult to control eczema who typically undergoes this diagnostic testing. The procedures involved in an oral food challenge for atopic eczema are summarized in Table 14.11.

Where more than one food has been eliminated, and immediate-type reactions are not expected, a stepwise reintroduction of these foods could be carried out over a period of a few weeks. A new food group can be reintroduced and then retained in the

Table 14.11 Oral food challenge in atopic eczema

Prior to challenge	Strict elimination diet of the 'candidate' allergen/s for 4 weeks, under the supervision of a dietitian* Ensure best possible eczema control prior to initiating challenge Antihistamines withdrawn at least 3–10 days before challenge	
i) Open challenge	Repetitive provocation with the same food for at least 2 days is advised with patients observed for at least 48 hours following the challenge[31]	
ii) Blinded Challenge	Day 1**	Active challenge food: incremental delivery of total daily dose
	Day 2**	Active challenge food: cumulative delivery total daily dose
	Day 3	Observation
	Day 4	Observation
	Day 4***	Placebo: incremental delivery of total daily dose
	Day 5***	Placebo: cumulative delivery total daily dose
	Day 6	Observation
	Day 7	Observation
Post challenge	Scoring of delayed symptoms. Clinical evaluation must be uniform throughout the period, e.g. SCORAD to assess eczema severity. An increase of 10 SCORAD points or more indicates a significant deterioration of eczema; however, such changes may be less significant when initiating the challenge at times when the baseline SCORAD is moderate or higher, i.e. 40 points[31]	

*Oral food challenges are usually unnecessary where an elimination diet has not resulted in any improvements after 4 weeks, and the patient may then slowly reintroduce that food.
**Daily dose is equivalent to age-related average daily intake of that food; appropriate typical daily dose e.g. 20 oz (600 mL) cows' milk formula for an infant.
***In the case of DBPCFC, the active challenge food and placebo should be given on two or more consecutive days, in random order, with a 1-day interval between placebo and active challenge. Where an immediate-type reaction is suspected these should be given in an incremental fashion,[30] e.g. 7–8 doses.

Table 14.12 Confounding oral food challenge factors

Confounding oral food challenge factors	Controlled for by:
Exercise	If indicated, perform oral food challenges while controlling for exercise, i.e. with and without prior food ingestion
Medications, e.g. aspirin	Before the challenge avoid medications that may influence or mask the outcome of the allergic reactions
Alcohol	Avoid alcohol ingestion prior to oral food challenges
Emotional stress	Avoid periods of high emotional stress and anxiety
Hormonal cycles	Record hormonal status
Infection	Oral food challenges should only be performed when the subject is in good health

diet every 4 days, with observation for a deterioration of the skin. Whether this occurs at home or in the hospital setting, it should be carefully assessed by an experienced allergy team, as severe allergic reactions have been reported in children with atopic dermatitis upon reintroduction of a food after following an elimination diet for a longer period.[42]

Modified oral food challenges

It may be that additional factors are required to alter oral food challenge outcomes; examples include hormonal cycles, medications such as aspirin, exercise, emotional stress, and even infection (Table 14.12). Observations from specific oral tolerance induction studies confirm the concept of dose-dependent tolerance and tolerance that is influenced by one or more of the above-listed confounding factors.[43] Modified oral food challenges, and challenges tailored for the diagnosis of the food protein-induced enterocolitis syndrome (FPIES), deserve special mention.

Food protein-induced enterocolitis syndrome

The FPIES represents a cell-mediated gastrointestinal food hypersensitivity usually diagnosed in infancy. The syndrome is characterized by protracted diarrhea and/or vomiting and is frequently associated with additional symptoms such as pallor and/or lethargy.[44] Symptom onset varies from 1–2 hours after the ingestion of the causative food protein, but may occur up to 10 hours later. Presentation varies from mild (e.g. non-dehydrating

vomiting and/or diarrhea) to severe; indeed, hypovolemic shock is associated in up to 20% of cases. In patients with a history of severe reactions a starting dose of 0.06 g/kg of the challenge food is recommended.[45] As immediate-onset reactions are not anticipated, the entire portion may be administered gradually in three feedings over a period of 45 minutes. Patients should then be observed for at least 4 hours to allow for delayed presentations. Additional safety precautions are as in Table 14.8.

Food–exercise challenges

Exercise-induced anaphylaxis (EIA) is a rare condition where one or more factors associated with exercise results in anaphylaxis. Subclassifications include 'pure' EIA and food-dependent exercise-induced anaphylaxis (FDEIA). Although EIA occurs independently of food, the clinical syndrome of FDEIA is typified by the onset of anaphylaxis during (or soon after) exercise which was preceded by the ingestion of the causal food(s). In FDEIA, both the food allergen and exercise are independently tolerated. To diagnose and differentiate the above conditions, use is made of modified oral food challenges such as open food–exercise challenges (OFEC) and the double-blind placebo-controlled food–exercise challenge (DBPCFEC).[46] During modified food–exercise challenges patients are asked to eat the suspected food allergen prior to exercise. Confounding factors unique to the patient's presentation may be required to reproduce FDEIA, e.g. particular forms of exercise or extreme environments. Therefore, although logistically difficult, a more ideal food–exercise challenge is for the patient to repeat the exercise under similar environmental conditions to that which induced the index reaction.

It is important that all food challenge patients be followed up (either in clinic or by telephone) for the scoring of delayed symptoms, as it is not uncommon for delayed symptoms, e.g. eczema exacerbation, to develop even after an oral food challenge performed for the primary purposes of diagnosing an immediate-onset IgE-mediated food allergy.

Summary

Food challenges remain the gold standard investigation for the diagnosis and management of immediate and delayed food-induced allergic reactions and are essential to contemporary allergy practice.

The clinician should aim to achieve a 50% positive to negative outcome ratio when performing oral food challenges in patients with established allergies. This is achieved by careful patient selection.

Oral food challenges are used to confirm a diagnosis of allergy – or tolerance – where this is uncertain based on detailed history and allergy diagnostic tests. Tolerance may be confirmed by oral food challenges in the following situations: where an allergy is suspected to have been outgrown; when allergy tests suggest tolerance but the food has never been eaten; when a food is suspected to cause delayed allergic symptoms; or to clarify allergy in cases of cross-reactivity. Allergy may be confirmed by oral food challenges where the cause of a suspected food allergic reaction is uncertain or where equivocal or inconsistent symptoms occur following the consumption of a particular food. Other uses include the establishment of thresholds of reactivity and to monitor immunomodulatory treatments. Whereas a positive oral food challenge ensures appropriate allergen avoidance, a negative challenge results in safe dietary expansion.

Challenge designs exist that are adaptable for use in both research and clinical settings and can be individualized to the patient so as to maximize the reliability of the challenge outcome and minimize risk. Variations include open or blinded challenges, with or without the inclusion of placebo foods. Adjustments can also be made to initial and top doses and the choice of challenge food, depending on the indication for the challenge and the patient's circumstances.

After a negative challenge it is essential that patients are advised about late-phase reactions and how to treat them, as well as how to introduce the food into their diet. This may be difficult for those who are averse to the food and may require the skills of an experienced dietitian to identify suitable alternatives. Ongoing consumption of the food is important to avoid a possible risk of loss of tolerance to that food. Following a positive challenge, patients should be given advice on medical management in the event of accidental exposure, as well as dietary advice to facilitate careful avoidance of the food.

When performed by an experienced healthcare team, oral food challenges are safe and remain a valid and extremely helpful diagnostic modality essential to the everyday practice of allergy management.

Food Challenge Procedures

Prior to challenge

Assessment of suitability for food challenge

OFC is indicated to confirm allergy or tolerance to challenge food (see Table 14.2)

No reactions to challenge food in last year

Patient agrees to introduce the food if the challenge is negative

Patient is old enough to complete the challenge

Patient is well enough to undergo challenge procedure

Patient understands the procedure and gives consent (or parent/carer in case of children)

Assessment on arrival for challenge

Review history of reactions to challenge food, including severity

Carry out physical examination and review medical history to confirm fitness for challenge

Carry out baseline observations: weight, height, temperature, pulse, respirations, oxygen saturations, blood pressure, and peak expiratory flow rate

Confirm all relevant medications stopped prior to challenge as appropriate

Explain procedure and obtain consent from patient (or parent/carer in case of children)

Decide if high or low risk challenge and cannulate if required

Preparation for challenge

Carry out safety checks, e.g. check oxygen and suction in working order

Ensure emergency medications available and drawn up for high risk challenges

Weigh out challenge doses as below; add masking ingredients if required. NB: these must be ingredients previously tolerated by the patient

Take precautions to avoid cross-contamination

Challenge procedure

During the challenge: record all observations, time doses given, amount of each dose given

Carry out baseline observations: temperature, pulse, respirations, oxygen saturations, blood pressure, and peak expiratory flow rate

Smear a small amount of challenge food unto lips and oral mucosa. Do not smear onto obvious patches of peri-oral eczema or areas of the body affected by eczema as this may induce localized skin reactions. Some protocols do not include a lip dose and proceed to Dose 1.

Wait at least 15 minutes and repeat observations

Give dose 1 and wait at least 15 minutes. Repeat observations prior to next dose.

Continue as above, giving other doses until the top dose has been given and tolerated.

If there are signs of a reaction

Stop the challenge immediately

Administer treatment according to severity of the reaction

Observations should be repeated and patient monitored closely

If the symptoms do not meet the criteria (Table 14.10) for a positive challenge, pause until symptoms resolve then continue with the next challenge dose

Post challenge

Following a *positive* challenge

Patients should remain for observation for at least 4 hours after the challenge or until symptoms have resolved. For severe symptoms patients may need to be admitted overnight

Provide education in the identification and appropriate management of allergic reactions

Dietitian to advise on strict dietary avoidance of the food

24 hours post-challenge review by telephone to eliminate delayed symptoms

Following a *negative* challenge

Patients should remain for observation for at least 2 hours after the challenge has been completed

Provide education in the identification and appropriate management of allergic reactions, including late-phase reactions

Dietitian to advise on reintroduction of the food, particularly in those who are averse to it

24 hours post-challenge review by telephone to eliminate delayed symptoms

For doses see Table 14.13 and Table 14.14.

Table 14.13 Example 1. Open incremental challenge to peanut

Dose	Amount of challenge food: peanut or peanut butter (g)	Peanut protein equivalent (g)*
Lip dose	Rub half a peanut or smear fingertip amount peanut butter on lower lip	Trace
Dose 1	0.5	0.125
Dose 2	1.0	0.25
Dose 3	2.0	0.5
Dose 4	4.0	1.0
Dose 5	10.0	2.5
Dose 6	20.0	5.0

*Slight differences exist in the peanut content of peanuts vs peanut butter.

Table 14.14 Example 2. DBPCFC to peanut

Design	Dose	Amount of challenge food (g)	Peanut protein equivalent (g)
		Chocolate muffin*	
Blind	Active dose 1	1.6	0.1**
	Active dose 2	4	0.25
	Active dose 3	8	0.5
	Active dose 4	16	1.0
	Active dose 5	40	2.5
	Placebo doses may be randomly interspersed with active doses or given during a separate session later the same day or on a different day		
Open	Open dose	Peanut butter (20 g) sandwich or 25 whole peanuts	5.0

*40 g muffin containing 5 g peanut flour or 2.5 g peanut protein.
**Use initial challenge dose of 0.1 mg for high-risk challenges.[5]

References

1. Du Toit G, Santos A, Roberts G, et al. The diagnosis of IgE-mediated food allergy in childhood. Pediatr Allergy Immunol 2009;20(4):309–19.

2. Nowak-Wegrzyn A, Assa'ad AH, Bahna SL, et al. Work Group report: oral food challenge testing. J Allergy Clin Immunol 2009;123(6 Suppl):S365–83.

3. Perry TT, Matsui EC, Kay Conover-Walker M, et al. The relationship of allergen-specific IgE levels and oral food challenge outcome. J Allergy Clin Immunol 2004;114(1):144–9.

4. Du Toit G, Katz Y, Sasieni P, et al. Early consumption of peanuts in infancy is associated with a low prevalence of peanut allergy. J Allergy Clin Immunol 2008;122(5):984–91.

5. Sampson HA, Ho DG. Relationship between food-specific IgE concentrations and the risk of positive food challenges in children and adolescents. J Allergy Clin Immunol 1997;100(4):444–51.

6. Sporik R, Hill DJ, Hosking CS. Specificity of allergen skin testing in predicting positive open food challenges to milk, egg and peanut in children. Clin Exp Allergy 2000;30(11):1540–6.

7. Roberts G, Lack G. Diagnosing peanut allergy with skin prick and specific IgE testing. J Allergy Clin Immunol 2005;115(6):1291–6.

8. Lack G. Clinical practice. Food allergy. N Engl J Med 2008;359(12):1252–60.

9. Jaeschke R, Guyatt GH, Sackett DL. Users' guides to the medical literature. III. How to use an article about a diagnostic test. B. What are the results and will they help me in caring for my patients? The Evidence-Based Medicine Working Group. JAMA 1994;271(9):703–7.

10. Bindslev-Jensen C, Ballmer-Weber BK, Bengtsson U, et al. Standardization of food challenges in patients with immediate reactions to foods–position paper from the European Academy of Allergology and Clinical Immunology. Allergy 2004;59(7):690–7.

11. Rance F, Deschildre A, Villard-Truc F, et al. Oral food challenge in children: an expert review. Eur Ann Allergy Clin Immunol 2009;41(2):35–49.

12. Boyce JA, Assa'ad A, Burks W, et al. Guidelines for the diagnosis and management of food allergy in the United States: summary of the NIAID-sponsored expert panel report. J Allergy Clin Immunol 2010;126(6):1105–18.

13. Venter C, Pereira B, Voigt K, et al. Comparison of open and double-blind placebo-controlled food challenges in diagnosis of food hypersensitivity amongst children. J Hum Nutr Diet 2007;20(6):565–79.

14. Bindslev-Jensen C, Ballmer-Weber BK, Bengtsson U, et al. Standardization of food challenges in patients with immediate reactions to foods–position paper from the European Academy of Allergology and Clinical Immunology. Allergy 2004;59(7):690–7.

15. Bock SA, Sampson HA, Atkins FM, et al. Double-blind, placebo-controlled food challenge (DBPCFC) as an office procedure: a manual. J Allergy Clin Immunol 1988;82(6):986–97.

16. Bindslev-Jensen C, Ballmer-Weber BK, Bengtsson U, et al. Standardization of food challenges in patients with immediate reactions to foods–position paper from the European Academy of Allergology and Clinical Immunology. Allergy 2004;59(7):690–7.

17. Niggemann B, Beyer K. Pitfalls in double-blind, placebo-controlled oral food challenges. Allergy 2007;62(7):729–32.

18. Commins SP, Satinover SM, Hosen J, et al. Delayed anaphylaxis, angioedema, or urticaria after consumption of red meat in patients with IgE antibodies specific for galactose-alpha-1,3-galactose. J Allergy Clin Immunol 2009;123(2):426–33.

19. Maleki SJ, Chung SY, Champagne ET, et al. The effects of roasting on the allergenic properties of peanut proteins. J Allergy Clin Immunol 2000; 106(4):763–8.

20. Paschke A. Aspects of food processing and its effect on allergen structure. Mol Nutr Food Res 2009;53(8): 959–62.

21. Grimshaw KE, King RM, Nordlee JA, et al. Presentation of allergen in different food preparations affects the nature of the allergic reaction–a case series. Clin Exp Allergy 2003;33(11):1581–5.

22. Van Odijk J, Ahlstedt S, Bengtsson U, et al. Doubleblind placebo-controlled challenges for peanut allergy the efficiency of blinding procedures and the allergenic activity of peanut availability in the recipes. Allergy 2005;60(5):602–5.

23. Carpenter RP, Lyon DH, Hasdell TA. Guidelines for sensory analysis in food product development and quality control. •• 2000:36–43.

24. Vlieg-Boerstra BJ, Herpertz I, Pasker L, et al. Validation of novel recipes for double-blind, placebo-controlled food challenges in children and adults. Allergy 2011 epub.

25. Fiocchi, A, Brozek J, Schunemann, H, et al. World Allergy Organization (WAO) diagnosis and rationale for action against cow's milk allergy (DRACMA) guidelines. WAO Journal 2010:57–161.

26. Vlieg-Boerstra BJ, Bijleveld CM, van der HS, et al. Development and validation of challenge materials for double-blind, placebo-controlled food challenges in children. J Allergy Clin Immunol 2004;113(2): 341–6.

27. Vlieg-Boerstra BJ, van der HS, Bijleveld CM, et al. Placebo reactions in double-blind, placebo controlled food challenges in children. Allergy 2007;62(8):905–12.

28. Hourihane JO'B, Kilburn SA, Nordlee JA, et al. An evaluation of the sensitivity of subjects with peanut allergy to very low doses of peanut protein: a randomized, double-blind, placebo-controlled food challenge study. J Allergy Clin Immunol 1997;100(5):596–600.

29. Flinterman AE, Pasmans SG, Hoekstra MO, et al. Determination of no-observed-adverse-effect levels and eliciting doses in a representative group of peanutsensitized children. J Allergy Clin Immunol 2006;117(2):448–54.

30. Torr T, Gaughan M, Roberts G, et al. Food challenges: a review and audit. Paediatr Nurs 2002;14(9):30–4.

31. Sicherer SH, Morrow EH, Sampson HA. Dose-response in double-blind, placebo-controlled oral food challenges in children with atopic dermatitis. J Allergy Clin Immunol 2000;105(3):582–6.

32. Narisety SD, Skripak JM, Steele P, et al. Open-label maintenance after milk oral immunotherapy for IgE-mediated cow's milk allergy. J Allergy Clin Immunol 2009;124(3):610–2.

33. Perry TT, Matsui EC, Conover-Walker MK, et al. Risk of oral food challenges. J Allergy Clin Immunol 2004; 114(5):1164–8.

34. Perry TT, Matsui EC, Conover-Walker MK, et al. Risk of oral food challenges. J Allergy Clin Immunol 2004; 114(5):1164–8.

35. Sampson HA, Munoz-Furlong A, Campbell RL, et al. Second symposium on the definition and management of anaphylaxis: summary report–second National Institute of Allergy and Infectious Disease/Food Allergy and Anaphylaxis Network symposium. Ann Emerg Med 2006;47(4):373–80.

36. Simons FE. Anaphylaxis, killer allergy: long-term management in the community. J Allergy Clin Immunol 2006;117(2):367–77.

37. Wainstein BK, Studdert J, Ziegler, M, et al. Prediction of anaphylaxis during peanut food challenge: usefulness of the peanut skin prick test (SPT) and specific IgE level. Pediatr Allergy Immunol 2010;21:603–11. (p0380)

38. ITN032AD Learning Early About Peanut Allergy (The LEAP Study). http://www.clinicaltrials.gov/ct2/show/ NCT00329784. 2010.

39. Werfel T, Erdmann S, Fuchs T, et al. Approach to suspected food allergy in atopic dermatitis. Guideline of the Task Force on Food Allergy of the German Society of Allergology and Clinical Immunology (DGAKI) and the Medical Association of German Allergologists (ADA) and the German Society of Pediatric Allergology (GPA). J Dtsch Dermatol Ges 2009;7(3):265–71.

40. Breuer K, Heratizadeh A, Wulf A, et al. Late eczematous reactions to food in children with atopic dermatitis. Clin Exp Allergy 2004;34(5):817–24.

41. Breuer K, Heratizadeh A, Wulf A, et al. Late eczematous reactions to food in children with atopic dermatitis. Clin Exp Allergy 2004;34(5):817–24.

42. Flinterman AE, Knulst AC, Meijer Y, et al. Acute allergic reactions in children with AEDS after prolonged cow's milk elimination diets. Allergy 2006;61(3):370–4.

43. Varshney P, Steele PH, Vickery BP, et al. Adverse reactions during peanut oral immunotherapy home dosing. J Allergy Clin Immunol 2009;124(6):1351–2.

44. Nowak-Wegrzyn A, Muraro A. Food protein-induced enterocolitis syndrome. Curr Opin Allergy Clin Immunol 2009;9(4):371–7.

45. Sicherer SH, Eigenmann PA, Sampson HA. Clinical features of food protein-induced enterocolitis syndrome. J Pediatr 1998;133(2):214–9.

46. Du Toit G. Food-dependent exercise-induced anaphylaxis in childhood. Pediatr Allergy Immunol 2007;18(5):455–63.

47. Nicolaou N, Poorafshar M, Murray C, et al. Allergy or tolerance in children sensitized to peanut: prevalence and differentiation using component-resolved diagnostics. J Allergy Clin Immunol 2010;125(1):191–7.

CHAPTER 15

Management of Food Allergy and Development of an Anaphylaxis Treatment Plan

Jacqueline Wassenberg and Philippe Eigenmann

Introduction

This chapter will develop the various aspects of food allergy management, including the treatment of acute reactions, a personalized food allergy management plan to prevent and treat recurrences, and finally suggest preventive strategies in the community.

Epinephrine remains the drug of choice for the treatment of any anaphylactic reaction, the life-threatening complication of food allergy. After allergy work-up of the initial reaction, food elimination is the only actually available treatment in daily life.

Although these treatment options are well established, there are some limitations to applying the principles of evidence-based medicine to the management of food allergy, in particular to anaphylaxis, owing to the unpredictability of the episodes, to episodes commonly occurring in the community rather than in healthcare settings, and to the variability of signs and symptoms, pattern, severity and duration of episodes.[1] Obtaining randomized placebo-controlled data to evaluate a therapeutic intervention is difficult, because of unethical delays and the use of placebo in treating a condition that is life-threatening. Consequently, most of the actual evidence for the long-term risk reduction of acute episodes of food allergy are based on consensus and opinion (grade C) or at best on well-designed studies but not randomized controlled trials (grade B).[2]

As described in Chapter 4, a wide range of symptoms ranging from atopic eczema to severe life-threatening anaphylaxis are common clinical features of food allergy. Proper management should be adapted to the clinical expression and based on the risk assessment of future reactions. The age of the patient, the foods involved, the presence of comorbidities – such as asthma – and the social environment are important factors to take into account when establishing a management plan.

Dietary elimination, the prescription of epinephrine autoinjectors and the fear of potential life-threatening reactions have a clear impact on quality of life.[3] Regular reassessment of the management plan should also take this aspect into account in order to improve adherence to the medical advice. Quality of life of patients and their families can be evaluated and reassessed by food allergy-specific validated quality of life (QoL) questionnaires. Avery et al.[4] compared the impact of food allergy and insulin-dependent diabetes mellitus (IDDM) by using disease-specific QoL questionnaires. Children suffering from food allergy showed significantly worse QoL scores than those with IDDM.

Proper food allergy management implies a specialized and up-to-date follow-up, from the diagnosis of food allergy to implementation in the community by education of childcare providers.

Management of acute reactions

Clinical manifestations

Symptoms of IgE-mediated food allergy mostly occur within 30 minutes after exposure to the food. Cutaneous signs are most often present, especially in childhood. Pruritus, more specifically of the palms, feet and head, may be an early sign of a progressive acute reaction. However, it should be highlighted that anaphylaxis can occur in the absence of cutaneous manifestations.

Acute early manifestations often include acute rhinorrhea, itching of the eyes, lips and ears or facial edema. In children, life-threatening reactions are most often associated with bronchospasm. Upper airways symptoms related to laryngeal edema might also reveal a potentially severe progressive reaction. Hypotension and cardiovascular shock are less common in children than in adults; they can be accompanied by a sensation of light-headedness and loss of consciousness. Abdominal signs, such as severe abdominal pain, vomiting and/or diarrhea, are commonly present in children and can herald a severe anaphylactic reaction.

Expert panels[5,6] have proposed a severity score to ensure the diagnosis of anaphylaxis and the appropriate indication to inject epinephrine (Table 15.1).

Epinephrine administration

Rapid initiation of treatment is crucial, as one of the identified risk factors for death is the delay of epinephrine administration. Series of fatalities described by Pumphrey et al.[7] show that death occurs most often within 25–30 minutes after ingestion (from 10 minutes to 6 hours).

International and national guidelines recommend epinephrine as the first-line treatment in an acute episode.[8] It should always be administered in case of an anaphylactic reaction involving either the respiratory tract or in case of cardiovascular signs.

Epinephrine increases peripheral vascular resistance, blood pressure and coronary perfusion, while reducing angioedema and urticaria, by an α-adrenergic effect. Its β_1-adrenergic effect increases

Table 15.1 Grading of severity of anaphylactic reaction[5,6]

Grade	Severity	Skin	GI tract	Respiratory	Cardiovascular	Neurological
1	Mild	Sudden itching of eyes and nose, generalized pruritus, flushing, urticaria or angioedema	Oral pruritis, oral 'tingling', mild lip swelling, nausea or emesis or mild abdominal pain	Nasal congestion and/or sneezing, rhinorrhea, throat pruritus, throat tightness or mild wheezing	Tachycardia (increase >15 beats/min)	Change in activity level and anxiety
2	Moderate	Any of the above	Any of the above, and crampy abdominal pain, diarrhea or recurrent vomiting	Any of the above, and **hoarseness, barky cough, difficulty swallowing, stridor, dyspnoea or moderate wheezing**	As above	'Light-headedness', feeling of 'pending doom'
3	Severe	Any of the above	Any of the above, and loss of bowel control	Any of the above, and **cyanosis or saturation <92%**, or respiratory arrest	**Hypotension* and/or collapse, dysrhythmia, severe bradycardia and/ or cardiac arrest**	Confusion, loss of consciousness

*Hypotension defined as systolic blood pressure: 1 month to 1 year <70 mmHg; 1–10 years <[70 mmHg + (2 × age)]; 11–17 years <90 mmHg. The severity score should be based on the system most affected. Symptoms and signs in bold are indications for the mandatory use of adrenaline.

Table 15.2 Indications for the administration of epinephrine in the emergency room or in the community

Mandatory if ...	Consider adrenaline administration if ...
• Respiratory distress • Hypotension • Collapse	Skin, mild gastrointestinal symptoms and • Asthma • Previous severe reaction • Exposure to known/likely allergen

the heart rate and myocardial contraction, and its β_2-adrenergic effects induces bronchodilation and inhibits the release of inflammatory mediators.[6]

The use of epinephrine should take into account who will administer it, i.e. physicians in the emergency room, or parents or the patient himself. In case of a previous severe reaction with a rapid onset, epinephrine should be administered without delay. Earlier use is also justified in patients with asthma, identified as another major risk factor for anaphylaxis fatality (Table 15.2).[6]

Contraindications for epinephrine administration

Coronary heart diseases and cardiac arrhythmia are relative contraindications for administering epinephrine. In patients with these coexisting conditions the risks and benefits of epinephrine should be evaluated, taking into consideration that it can be life-saving in anaphylaxis. In children, apart from rare comorbidities such as hypertrophic obstructive cardiomyopathy associated with tachyarrythmia, there are no contraindications to epinephrine administration.

Routes of administration and dosage of epinephrine

Intramuscular injection should be preferred both in the community and in the emergency room. Epinephrine injected into the muscle is rapidly bioavailable, with peak concentrations reached within 10 minutes, and has a much better safety profile than intravenous administration. Subcutaneous injection results in significant vasospasm, which prevents the diffusion of epinephrine into the blood vessels.

The preferred injection site is the lateral side of the thigh (vastus lateralis muscle). Obese patients should be instructed to use the autoinjector in a place where the thickness of the subcutaneous tissue does not exceed 14.3 mm, the usual length of the needle.[9]

The therapeutic range of epinephrine is narrow, implying that under- and over-dosage should be carefully avoided. The usually accepted intramuscular dose for self-treatment in adults is 0.3 mg of epinephrine 1 : 1000 (1 mg/mL). For children, autoinjectors have a fixed dose of 0.15 mg. In an emergency setting, the appropriate pediatric dose is 0.01 mg/kg of body weight, with a maximum single dose of 0.3–0.5 mg. Injections can be repeated every 5–10 minutes until the patient reaches a stable condition. The use of intravenous epinephrine should be limited to severe situations, with administration of 0.1 µg/kg/min under close monitoring.

Other medications

H$_1$ antagonists

H$_1$ antagonists can be given if a patient develops mild clinical symptoms such as skin symptoms. However, it needs to be emphasized that H$_1$ antagonists have no proven efficacy in the treatment of anaphylaxis.[10] In addition, the administration of H$_1$ antagonists should never delay the administration of epinephrine. Oral forms of H$_1$ antagonists are most often preferred as they are non-sedating and long-lasting. The dose should be adapted to the weight of the patient. Rapid-onset H$_1$ antagonists (diphenhydramine or chlorpheniramine) are also available for intravenous injection, but these two first-generation H$_1$ antagonists have a much higher sedative side effect than the second-generation H$_1$ antagonists. Their use should be limited to situations in which oral treatment is not available.

Corticosteroids

Corticosteroids should not be considered as a first-line treatment in anaphylaxis. The onset of action is within hours of administration, and they are often used to prevent relapses. However, there is no proven efficacy in the prevention of long-lasting or biphasic reactions.[11]

Inhaled β_2-agonists

An inhaled β_2-agonist, with the use of a spacer or a nebulizer, can be helpful if bronchospasm is associated. However, inhaled β_2-agonists remain a second-line treatment in case of anaphylaxis. In addition, proper penetration to the airways can be reduced by acute bronchospasm. Uncontrolled or partially controlled asthma is a risk factor for severe anaphylaxis, implying that optimal asthma control should be a high priority in these patients.

Support medication

The severe reactions of food allergy can involve the cardiovascular system and may lead to tachycardia and decreased blood pressure. In these cases intravenous fluids should be added to epinephrine, starting with normal saline 20 mL/kg body weight, a dose which can be repeated. It has been shown that the need for volume expanders as well for more than one dose of epinephrine was a predictor for biphasic reactions. In addition, high-flow oxygen is essential in all patients with respiratory or cardiovascular symptoms.

After initial emergency treatment, patients with severe anaphylaxis should be monitored for 24 hours in an appropriate medical facility. With less severe reactions without respiratory or cardiovascular impairment, an observation time of 3–4 hours in the emergency room should be sufficient. In any case, a patient should be discharged from the emergency room only when the physician is fully convinced that the allergic reaction has resolved.

Comorbidities affecting the treatment of anaphylaxis

Different pharmacologic substances may either impair the efficacy of epinephrine or increase its potential side effects. A non-exhaustive list includes tricyclic antidepressants, cocaine (cardiac arrhythmia) and β-blockers (which inhibit the sympathetic effects of epinephrine).

An increased risk of fatal reactions has been associated with recent asthma exacerbations and/or overuse of short-acting β_2-agonists as well as to suboptimal long-term asthma management. Most deaths due to food allergies were found to be associated with bronchospasm and mucous plugging of the bronchioles.[7]

Exercise is a potential cofactor of severe food allergy; it could be related to increased blood flow, or increased non-allergen-induced mast cell degranulation. Ingestion of non-steroidal anti-inflammatory agents (NSAIDs) can also lower the threshold for mast cell degranulation and hence increase the severity of the reaction.

Ingestion of alcoholic beverages has been associated with severe food-induced allergic reactions, possibly due to an increasing absorption, or to an increased risk of accidental food ingestion.

Patients with mastocytosis, a rare disease associated with increased mast cell degranulation, may experience severe anaphylactic reactions.

Finally, moving from a supine to an upright position during anaphylaxis has been associated with cardiac arrest due to a sudden drop in blood pressure, implying that patients with severe food-induced anaphylaxis should be kept in a lying position.

Emergency room protocols for severe reactions (Fig. 15.1)[6]

Airways, breathing and circulation should be first assessed and regularly re-evaluated. Repeated injections of epinephrine are indicated until adequate clinical stabilization is achieved, e.g. every 10–15 minutes. Patients with respiratory symptoms should be monitored for at least 6–8 hours and those with cardiovascular involvement for at least 24 hours – as previously mentioned – before discharge.

Patients should be instructed to avoid potentially implicated allergens until the appropriate diagnostic allergy work-up. In addition, epinephrine autoinjectors should be adequately prescribed, and patients should be trained in their proper use.

It should be emphasized that allergy work-up needs to include education, which will be addressed in the next section.

Long-term anaphylaxis management

Identifying the causal factor

Patients with a history of a reaction suggestive of food allergy will need a full diagnostic work-up in order to prevent further reactions. Evaluation should be based on the history of the reaction, identifying the foods eaten during the preceding 2–4 hours. Work-up should include identification of hidden allergens (by reading labels) or 'new foods' (foods locally not consumed until recently, or new processing methods of known foods) (see Clinical Case 1). The presence of comorbidities and

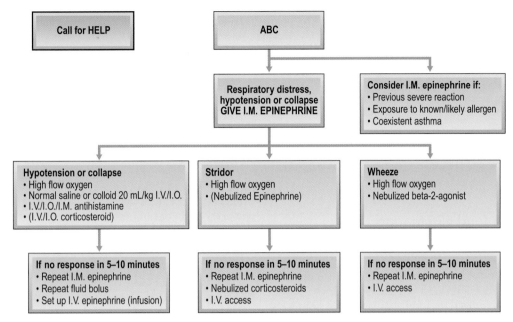

Figure 15.1 Example of the plan for initial treatment of children with anaphylaxis in the emergency room.

conditions mimicking food allergy should be considered. As outlined in Chapter 13, the allergy work-up will be conducted based on the clinical history, including specific serum IgE measurement, skin prick tests and, if needed, oral food challenges (see Chapter 14). Unnecessary food elimination diets, based on the history alone or the fear of potentially 'dangerous' foods, can cause unnecessary psychological troubles and social exclusion.[3]

CLINICAL CASE 1

A healthy but atopic 8-year-old boy with cat and grass pollen allergies presented with a sudden nasal discharge and watery eyes followed by facial edema and difficulty breathing, 30 minutes after eating a waffle in the playground. He had no history of food allergy or previous anaphylactic reactions, and was on a normal diet, including consumption of peanuts and other legumes. The factory-produced waffle contained eggs, sugar and lupin flour. The child was brought to the emergency room, where within 15 minutes he was given IV antihistamines and steroids, but no epinephrine was administered.

The allergy work-up showed skin prick tests positive to peanut but negative to soy, eggs, nuts (walnut, hazelnut, almond) and other legumes (chickpea and lentil). A prick test with native lupine flour diluted in a saline solution was strongly positive. Total IgE was 1237 UI/mL. Specific IgE antibodies were positive to lupin seeds (20.8 kU/L, norm:

<0.35 kU/L) and peanut (>100 kU/L, norm: <0.35 kU/L) (UniCAP, Phadia, Uppsala, Sweden). A diagnosis of anaphylaxis to lupin flour and a strong sensitization to peanuts was established. An oral challenge was not performed in this child with a history of a severe reaction.

The patient was instructed to strictly avoid lupin flour and seeds, as well as peanuts. Self-injectable epinephrine and oral cetirizine were prescribed in case of an accidental allergic reaction. Subsequent severe reactions due to accidental lupin ingestion occurred, thereby confirming the diagnosis. His food allergy management plan was regularly reassessed.

Discussion

An unusual food, lupin flour, triggered this severe allergic reaction. Lupin has been cultivated for more than 4000 years all over the world. It is closely related to chickpea, green pea, soy and peanuts. Lupin flour has a high protein content and offers monounsaturated fatty acids; it is a gluten-free flour. Because of its nutritional values and culinary qualities (good color, better conservation and softness), lupin is increasingly used in the preparation of industrial food (pizzas, cakes, vegetarian food, sausages).

Depending on the national regulations, lupin flour or lupin seeds – like other rare or new foods – are not always listed on food labels, unlike major allergens which must be listed. Therefore, individuals with rare food allergies are at increased risk of accidental ingestion, especially when eating manufactured products.

This child with a highly positive test to peanuts was advised to avoid this food as well.

When the patient was initially treated, no written standardized food allergy management plan was available and he and his carers were advised orally when and how to use his epinephrine autoinjector. Owing to this lack of labeling and the absence of a written food allergy management plan, the patient had subsequent severe reactions.

It might also be noted that this child did not receive epinephrine in the emergency room, which highlights the low awareness of the indication to administer epinephrine in case of anaphylaxis.

Proper food elimination

Fatal food-induced anaphylaxis has been reported even after correct use of epinephrine, therefore adequate food elimination remains the first-line advice for patients with food allergies.[9]

Correct advice for food avoidance will need to be adjusted to the age, type of food, social activities, living conditions and occupation of the patient, as well as to school and school catering settings, or to daycare centers.

Patients and their families should be informed about the symptoms as well as the severity of reactions to be expected in case of accidental ingestions, skin contact or inhalation of the allergens. They must also be instructed on how to read labels, a task which can be difficult due to the various terms for a specific allergen (for example either 'peanut' or 'arachis'), to the variety of authorized contamination thresholds between countries, and to the presence of warnings such as 'may contain …'.[12] They should also be aware of the possible presence of hidden allergens and situations of high risk for accidental ingestions, such as restaurants, or the homes of friends or relatives. Based on the UK Register of fatal reactions it has been shown by Pumphrey,[7] that one-third of fatalities due to food allergy occur at home, 25% in restaurants and the remainder in nurseries/schools/at work (15%) and at relatives' homes (12%). In the case of multiple food allergies, counseling by a dietitian knowledgeable in food allergy can provide very useful information on the minimal daily requirements for essential nutrients, food replacements, i.e. for home cooking of baked products, and proper reading of food labels. This topic will be more precisely addressed in Chapters 16 and 19. In principle, yearly follow-up visits, especially in children, are important in order to reassess the current list of allergies, accidental ingestions and their consequences in the past months, as well as to advise on minimal impact on daily activities. Such visits have been shown to reduce the rate and severity of reactions.[13,14]

Table 15.3 Special conditions increasing the risk of severe reactions

Specific foods: peanuts and tree nuts
Reactions to traces of foods
Asthma
Adolescence
Exercise
Cocaine or alcohol consumption
Medications such as β-adrenergic blockers, tricyclic antidepressants

Management of specific conditions
(Table 15.3)

As previously mentioned, there are some conditions that may increase an individual's risk of severe reactions.

A few foods, mostly peanuts and tree nuts, are responsible for the majority of severe or fatal reactions.[15] Patients reacting to traces of food are especially at risk for severe reactions and may also react to inhalation of allergens. These patients should be instructed to strictly avoid the food.

Although previous severe reactions predispose to severe or potentially fatal reactions, these might appear in patients with previously mild reactions, or at the initial episode.

Most fatalities due to food allergy are reported in children suffering from asthma, in particular patients with partially controlled or uncontrolled asthma, with a history of recent exacerbations, and recent stepping down of or non-compliance with treatment. In case of food allergy and asthma – common conditions that are frequently associated – asthma control must be regularly assessed and the risks of stepping down treatment carefully balanced against its benefits.[6]

Adolescence is a period that has been associated with severe food-induced reactions, mostly due to increased risky social behaviors, poor drug compliance and denial of food allergy. A specific follow-up especially designed for adolescents with food allergies is most helpful.

Patients should be informed of potential risk factors such as exercise, cocaine addiction, alcohol consumption or specific medications – as previously mentioned – which can increase the severity of the reactions or diminish the responsiveness to treatment.

Self-injectable epinephrine and personalized treatment plans

Despite optimal food elimination diets and long-term measures to reduce the risk of accidental ingestion, food-induced allergic reactions can recur, with symptoms even more severe than previously. Individuals, their families and their carers should be able to recognize an allergic reaction and to treat it.

The decision to prescribe an epinephrine autoinjector involves analyzing the risks of anaphylaxis, the potential benefits of rapid administration of epinephrine, the risks associated with carrying an autoinjector, and the cost to the health service or the individual family.

Who should be prescribed a self-injectable epinephrine device?

Based on current knowledge, the European Academy of Allergy and Clinical Immunology guidelines on anaphylaxis gives a list of four absolute indications to prescribe a self-injectable device (Table 15.4):[6]

- A previous cardiovascular or respiratory reaction to a food (and to other allergic triggers such as insect sting or latex)

Table 15.4 Indications for prescribing a self-injectable epinephrine device

Absolute indications	Relative indications
A previous cardiovascular or respiratory reaction to a food (and to other triggers such as insect sting or latex)	Any reactions to small amounts of a food including airborne or contact of the food allergen only via skin
Exercise-induced anaphylaxis (often related also to food)	History of previous – even mild – reactions to peanut or tree nuts
Idiopathic reactions	Remoteness of home from medical facilities
Child with food allergy and asthma	Food-allergic reaction in a teenager

- Exercise-induced anaphylaxis (often also related to foods)
- Idiopathic reactions
- A child with food allergy and asthma

as well as four relative indications:

- Any reactions to small amounts of a food, including airborne or contact only via the skin
- History of previous – even mild – reactions to peanut or tree nuts
- Remoteness of home from medical facilities
- Food-allergic reaction in a teenager.

As already mentioned, asthma is the most common risk factor for death due to food allergy, and is therefore defined as an absolute indication.

It should be emphasized that two studies evaluating the degree of severity of recurrences in tree nut- and peanut-allergic patients show that, even in mild reactions in children, the risk of anaphylaxis can reach 31% over a 6-year median period of follow-up.[15,16] This would suggest the need for all children with tree nut and peanut allergy to be prescribed self-injectable epinephrine. Unfortunately, similar data are not yet available for other foods. Deaths due to food allergy are mainly linked to tree nuts and peanut, but can also occur with milk and fruits. Known histories of reactions prior to the fatality are mainly described as mild, and the amount ingested is very variable, ranging from traces to several grams of dry food.[7]

Adolescence is another risk factor for severe reactions and has been listed as a relative indication for the prescription of self-injectable devices.

Food-induced flares of atopic dermatitis in the absence of more severe symptoms, and symptoms limited to the oral mucosa (oral allergy syndrome) are not an indication for the prescription of self-injectable epinephrine.

Which device should be prescribed?

Various devices are available in many countries. They are preset to administer a fixed dose, either 0.15 mg ('junior') or 0.3 mg of epinephrine. The 0.15 mg devices are commonly indicated for children from 15 to 25 kg body weight and the 0.3 mg devices for individuals of 25 kg and more. There is no self-injectable device for infants under 15 kg currently available. Mild overdosing should not represent a major risk for an otherwise healthy child >7.5 kg body weight (with an arbitrary maximum dose of 20 µg/kg). Providing the parents with a syringe and a vial of epinephrine is an unsafe and not easy-to-use alternative.[17] On the other hand, the 0.3 mg dose could be insufficient for overweight individuals, who should have two autoinjectors prescribed.

Devices should be stored at room temperature, remote from heat sources and direct sunlight. They have an average shelf-life of 1–2 year and should therefore be re-prescribed accordingly. However, it has been shown that epinephrine contained in recently expired devices can still be effective and used if no others are available.[18]

Risks associated with self-injectable epinephrine devices

The pharmacological effect of an appropriate dose of injected epinephrine includes side effects such as pallor, palpitations and tremor. These usually last a few minutes and remit spontaneously. Serious side effects in otherwise healthy individuals are almost always associated with overdosing. Inappropriate use of the device – such as accidental injection into a finger resulting in ischemia – can be prevented by careful education.

How many devices should a patient be prescribed?

A second dose of epinephrine should be injected within 5–10 minutes if the first one has not provided relief. It has been shown that up to 20% of people experiencing anaphylaxis had to use more than one dose of epinephrine.[19] Most of the cases were related to delayed or inappropriate administration; some children who needed more than one dose of epinephrine had poorly controlled asthma. However, few deaths have occurred after correct treatment, which brings into question the systematic prescription of two devices. The economic impact versus the potential prevention of fatalities when two devices are prescribed remains unsolved.

Schools, nurseries and separated parents often insist on being prescribed more than one device in order to make self-injectable epinephrine available at different locations. As an alternative to patients carrying their medication, anaphylaxis emergency kits could be readily stored and made accessible in schools and nurseries – after proper training for carers.[16]

In summary, the number of devices prescribed will depend on a careful evaluation of the patient's

situation; the availability of two devices potentially being recommended in case of:

- remote access to medical care
- body weight exceeding the maximum available dose
- concerns about failure to respond to the first dose
- any personal indicator suggesting an increased risk.

Other medications available in the emergency kit

It is controversial to recommend medications other than self-injectable epinephrine, such as oral steroids and antihistamines, for the patient's emergency kit, as they may delay the administration of epinephrine in the absence of evidence of their efficacy. However, a fast-acting antihistamine tablet or drops to be administered for mild symptoms is adequate for most patients, based on the recommendations of the written individualized treatment plan (see below).

Patient and family education

Management of food allergies and their most severe clinical expression, anaphylaxis, implies educating and training patients, their families and, with regard to children, their carers. At present there is still in many countries a lack of adequate support for allergic patients. Clark and Ewan,[13,14] in a large prospective study of UK children with tree nut and peanut allergies, have demonstrated that repeated and thorough education reduces the severity and frequency of reactions. Teaching should include allergen avoidance, early identification of symptoms, and appropriate emergency treatment plans. The 'community', i.e. schools and daycare, also needs careful information on the medical condition of the allergic child and adequate emergency management. Education is an ongoing process and requires regular training, adapted to the age and the psychosocial situation of the patient. It is common for patients and their carers to forget how and when to inject epinephrine, because reactions may be infrequent, they fear the needle, or because of the side effects. Regular training sessions are required to teach patients and their carers how to treat reactions in a potentially stressful situation.

A 6-year-old boy with a diagnosis of peanut allergy was on holiday with his mother's relatives. The family had taken with them H_1 antagonists but no self-injectable epinephrine device. Epinephrine had not been prescribed, as the child had had only a mild reaction after skin contact with peanuts. He then ate a cereal snack which was labeled as 'could contain traces of peanut'. Ten minutes after ingestion he developed mild angioedema, severe difficulty breathing and loss of consciousness. Intramuscular epinephrine was injected twice, with a favorable outcome.

Discussion

This child was known for a mild systemic reaction related only to peanut contact and subsequently developed a severe reaction after ingestion of a very small amount. Severe food allergy reactions may occur after previous reactions without signs of severity, in particular in peanut- or tree nut-allergic individuals. The prescription of self-injectable epinephrine should be considered in patients with nut allergies or reacting to small amounts of a food. This child therefore had two distinct indications to be prescribed epinephrine.

Food labeling should be included in the education plan of all patients and their carers. This was highlighted in our case by the fact that the child reacted after ingesting traces of peanuts.

Food labeling varies between countries, with maximal acceptable amounts of potential contamination by allergenic foods usually clearly stated. However, the regulations do not allow consumption of safe foods to highly allergic individuals. In order to avoid the risk of legal actions, the food industry increasingly labels products as 'may contain …', resulting in a reduced number of food products available without "potential risk" to food-allergic individuals.

A written individual management plan should be given to both the patient and all their carers. These have been shown to reduce the frequency and severity of further reactions. Adapted from the recommendations of the EAACI task force on the management of children's anaphylaxis,[6] a written individual treatment plan should list:

- Personal identification data (name, address, parents and doctor contact details, and, if possible, a photograph)
- Clear identification of the allergens to be avoided (including the different names used for a food, for example arachis for peanuts)
- Treatment plan written clearly in simple non-medical language with a stepwise approach:

- In case of breathing difficulty (wheezing, chest whistling, throat tightness or voice change) or collapse: give epinephrine promptly (with the identified device and dose)
- Call the emergency number (should be identified)
- Recommendation to give a second dose of epinephrine if no significant improvement after 5–10 minutes
- First symptoms of allergy (swelling, redness of the face, itching, nausea): give an antihistamine
- Monitor the patient closely for signs of breathing problems or collapse.

It is important to mention that relevant information for the food elimination diet and emergency treatment must be easily available and readable (see examples on www.foodallergy.org and www.aaaai.com and Fig. 15.2).

The epinephrine autoinjector should be readily accessible to every carer at all times.

Persons at risk for anaphylaxis in the community may also wear or carry accurate and up-to-date medical identification devices, such as bracelets or wallet cards.

Involving the community in management (Fig. 15.3)

The increasing prevalence of food allergy and anaphylaxis is a relatively recent phenomenon. Health-care professionals are not all aware that anaphylaxis occurs commonly in the community and are not all able to recognize its signs and symptoms and to treat them. Knowledge of the correct use of an epinephrine autoinjector and teaching patients how and when to use it is not always acquired.[20] Health-care professionals should be prepared to treat an acute anaphylaxis episode and also to provide patients with accurate information on potential symptoms, on the use of self-injectable epinephrine and on food elimination diets.

The lay population, including teachers, is most often not aware of the limitations on daily life for a food-allergic patient. A major effort should be made to improve risk awareness, as well as integrating individuals with food allergy into a safe community.

Management of food allergy in schools is a particular concern, as some surveys have shown that

Name : .... First Name : ....

Date of birth : ....

Address :...

Contact Person :..

| Picture |

FOODS TO BE STRICTLY AVOIDED

☐ Strict **tree nuts** avoidance
(Tree nuts, hazelnuts, almonds, cashew nuts, Brazil nuts, Macadamia nuts, pecan) including « can contain traces of... and tree nuts oil.
(coconut and nutmeg authorized)

☐ Strict **peanut/arachid** avoidance
including « can contain traces of peanut/arachid.
(peanut oil and vegetable oil authorized)

☐ Other foods avoidance
....

TREATMENT IN CASE OF ALLERGIC REACTION

Réaction	Signs	Treatment	Dose
MILD GENERALIZED	• Itching • Skin reaction • Facial or lips swelling • Oral tingling • Abdominal pain	*Anti-histamine :*	.... To be repeated if no improvement within 2 hours
SEVERE GENERALIZED	• Cough, • Difficulty to swallow, to speak, to breathe • Wheezing Asthma crisis and/or light headedness feeling • Blood pressure fall • Loss of consciousness	<u>Intramuscular injection</u>: • Epipen/Anapen or Epipen/Anapen Jr • Call Emergency number......... • *In case of loss of consciousness, place the individual in lateral security position*	To be repeated if no improvement within 5-10 minutes

<u>**Other treatments**</u> :
....

<u>**Remarks**</u> : ....

<u>**Date**</u>: ....

<u>**Physician Name and Signature**</u> : ....

Figure 15.2 Example of written food allergy treatment plan.

214

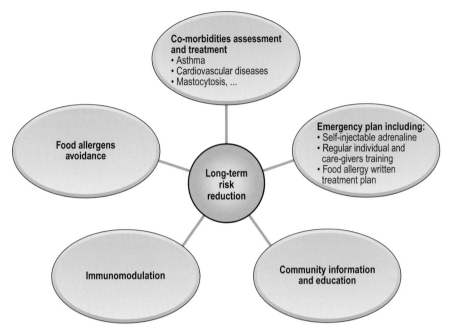

Figure 15.3 Food allergy management in the community.

16–18% of children with food allergies experience a reaction at school,[21] sometimes as a first event. School awareness of food allergy can be very diverse, depending on national and regional regulations, the presence of standardized food allergy management plans, or on previous food allergy reactions in a given school. In France, despite the availability of well-implemented and compulsory standardized food allergy management plans, it could be shown that nearly half of the children had no written food allergy management plan and only 72% carried an epinephrine autoinjector.[22] In Australia, only 40% of children known for a previous anaphylaxis reaction carried epinephrine with them and had an anaphylaxis treatment plan implemented in their school.[23]

Even if epinephrine is available at the school, it is sometimes stored far away from the child – e.g. in the school principal's office or the nurse's room. As it has been shown that many deaths are linked to late administration of epinephrine, the medication should be accessible within minutes. This implies that epinephrine should be kept near the child (for example stored by the teacher in the classroom) or directly carried by an older student.

These studies show the importance of implementing and reviewing food allergy management plans at school, as well as the need for standardized national and regional guidelines and regulations.

Teachers and other carers usually fail to recognize signs of an allergic reaction, even in countries with a higher level of awareness such as the USA. Sicherer et al.,[21] in a large study, recruited 4586 members of the US Peanut and Tree Nut Allergy Registry, 16% of whom reported reactions in school linked to delayed or inadequate treatment.

Food elimination diets might be difficult to implement in school, in particular in the catering area. The goal should be to ensure a safe environment without social exclusion. In Europe, children are most often provided with hot meals by a school cafeteria or caterer, but special meals need to be available for food-allergic children, or provided from home. In schools with on-site restaurants, too many children with food allergies are still excluded from the school restaurant by the absence of trained personnel, or because of fear of a reaction by the parents or carers.

Many reactions in school may occur in classrooms – e.g. during craft projects – and not in the cafeteria,[24] implying that foods should also be avoided in the classrooms (see Clinical Case 3).

An 8-year-old girl, known for hazelnut allergy since she was 3 years old (she initially presented with facial edema after eating hazelnut chocolate spread for the first time), was following a strict tree nut-elimination diet with yearly reassessment of her allergies. She had a personalized food allergy management plan (including a written anaphylaxis treatment plan), and training for the use of epinephrine autoinjectors was given to the family. She had also been diagnosed with allergic asthma to dust mites and furred pets, and was on daily treatment with inhaled steroids and β_2-agonists.

The food allergy management plan had been implemented at school and kept in the principal's office. However, because of the girl's young age and the fact that she was taking her meals at home, the parents decided to keep the autoinjector at home. A taste discovery week was organized at school and all children were invited to taste blindfolded different foods, including nuts. The girl did not want to participate but was reassured by her teacher, who declared that she would taste only healthy foods, such as fruits. Within 10 minutes after eating one cashew nut, the child developed facial edema and difficulty breathing, and lost consciousness. The school nurse and the teacher called her mother, who brought and injected the epinephrine. A total of three injections were necessary to stabilize her condition, followed by 24 hours' surveillance in the intensive care unit.

Discussion

This child was known for IgE-mediated tree nut allergy and allergic asthma. These two conditions, which often coexist in fatal anaphylaxis, require the compulsory prescription of a self-injectable epinephrine device and a food allergy management plan. Despite epinephrine having been prescribed, it was not available at school, suggesting insufficient patient/carer education:

- The parents kept epinephrine at home
- The school carers were not trained to recognize the forbidden foods, or to treat allergic reactions.

Probably because of the delayed epinephrine administration and the coexisting asthma, the girl's reaction was very severe and long-lasting.

This case report emphasizes the importance of educating all carers about a specific allergic child, and of community awareness of potential problems linked to food allergy. Education should be regularly repeated – we suggest a minimum of once a year – including regular training on label reading, as well as recognition of allergic symptoms and their appropriate treatment.

School or summer camps represent another activity with an increased risk necessitating well-planned organization and collaboration between parents, teachers, cooks, dietitians and healthcare professionals.

In the USA the Food Allergy and Anaphylaxis Network (FAAN), a food allergy patient organization, provides useful materials for school professionals, such as information brochures, posters and food allergy action plans. Together with the National School Board Association, the National Association of School Nurses and the National Association of School Principals, FAAN has produced a document entitled *School guidelines for managing students with food allergies* in order to provide general principles applicable to the different States' policies and education systems. A majority of American States have developed local food allergy management policies, and the US Department of Agriculture has edited a guidance document about school lunches for special needs, including severe food allergy, to ensure students have safe substitute meals available.

In Japan, *Guide-lines for the treatment of allergic diseases in schools* were published in 2008 by the Japanese Society of School Health, including *The School Life Management Certificate*, which was distributed to education boards nationwide. The availability of 'safe foods' in schools, recognition of symptoms of food allergy and their treatment will be implemented in the Japanese education system in order to improve food allergy management.

Future perspectives

There are only a few evidence-based studies for establishing guidelines on the management of food allergy, and most rely on expert opinions. Well-designed controlled trials are needed in order to increase our understanding of the mechanisms of action of the various treatments for food allergy reactions.

The self-injectable epinephrine devices have fixed doses which are not always suitable for specific conditions such as young age or overweight. Devices with doses above 0.3 and below 0.15 mg should soon be available (a device that injects 0.5 mg is newly available in some countries).

Because of their fear of needles, individuals with anaphylaxis are occasionally not adequately treated with epinephrine. Efforts must be made to educate individuals and their families about the side effects of epinephrine and indications for its use. However, no alternative methods of administration are available, and more research is needed.

National guidelines on food allergy management adapted to the local social environment should be developed and implemented.

Standardized written national or regional management plans for food allergy should be developed, and carers such as teachers and educators should be informed on an individual basis about the basics of food elimination diets and the recognition of food allergy symptoms and their treatment.[25] Politicians need to be alerted about the increasing number of anaphylactic reactions in the community in order to be able to adapt regulations and provide community funding for their implementation.

Finally, food allergy has a high emotional impact and affects the quality of life of both patients and carers. This aspect is currently insufficiently explored with regard to its professional and personal implications.

References

1. Simons FE. Anaphylaxis: evidence-based long-term risk reduction in the community. Immunol Allergy Clin North Am 2007;27:231–48.
2. Sheikh A, Shehata YA, Brown SG, et al. Adrenaline for the treatment of anaphylaxis: cochrane systematic review. Allergy 2009;64:204–12.
3. Sicherer SH, Noone SA, Munoz-Furlong A. The impact of childhood food allergy on quality of life. Ann Allergy Asthma Immunol 2001;87:461–4.
4. Avery NJ, King RM, Knight S, et al. Assessment of quality of life in children with peanut allergy. Pediatr Allergy Immunol 2003;14:378–82.
5. Sampson HA. Anaphylaxis and emergency treatment. Pediatrics 2003;111:1601–8.
6. Muraro A, Roberts G, Clark A, et al. The management of anaphylaxis in childhood: position paper of the European academy of allergology and clinical immunology. Allergy 2007;62:857–71.
7. Pumphrey R. Anaphylaxis: can we tell who is at risk of a fatal reaction? Curr Opin Allergy Clin Immunol 2004;4:285–90.
8. Kemp SF, Lockey RF, Simons FE. Epinephrine: the drug of choice for anaphylaxis. A statement of the World Allergy Organization. Allergy 2008;63:1061–70.
9. Pumphrey R. When should self-injectible epinephrine be prescribed for food allergy and when should it be used? Curr Opin Allergy Clin Immunol 2008;8:254–60.
10. Sheikh A, ten Broek V, Brown SG, et al. H1-antihistamines for the treatment of anaphylaxis with and without shock. Cochrane Database Syst Rev 2007:CD006160.
11. Mehr S, Liew WK, Tey D, et al. Clinical predictors for biphasic reactions in children presenting with anaphylaxis. Clin Exp Allergy 2009;39:1390–6.
12. Moneret-Vautrin DA, Kanny G. Update on threshold doses of food allergens: implications for patients and the food industry. Curr Opin Allergy Clin Immunol 2004;4:215–9.
13. Ewan PW, Clark AT. Efficacy of a management plan based on severity assessment in longitudinal and case-controlled studies of 747 children with nut allergy: proposal for good practice. Clin Exp Allergy 2005;35:751–6.
14. Clark AT, Ewan PW. Good prognosis, clinical features, and circumstances of peanut and tree nut reactions in children treated by a specialist allergy center. J Allergy Clin Immunol 2008;122:286–9.
15. Hourihane JO, Kilburn SA, Dean P, et al. Clinical characteristics of peanut allergy. Clin Exp Allergy 1997;27:634–9.
16. Yu JW, Kagan R, Verreault N, et al. Accidental ingestions in children with peanut allergy. J Allergy Clin Immunol 2006;118:466–72.
17. Simons FE, Chan ES, Gu X, et al. Epinephrine for the out-of-hospital (first-aid) treatment of anaphylaxis in infants: is the ampule/syringe/needle method practical? J Allergy Clin Immunol 2001;108:1040–4.
18. Simons FE, Gu X, Simons KJ. Outdated EpiPen and EpiPen Jr autoinjectors: past their prime? J Allergy Clin Immunol 2000;105:1025–30.
19. Jarvinen KM, Sicherer SH, Sampson HA, et al. Use of multiple doses of epinephrine in food-induced anaphylaxis in children. J Allergy Clin Immunol 2008;122:133–8.
20. Mehr S, Robinson M, Tang M. Doctor – how do I use my EpiPen? Pediatr Allergy Immunol 2007;18:448–52.
21. Sicherer SH, Furlong TJ, DeSimone J, et al. The US Peanut and Tree Nut Allergy Registry: characteristics of reactions in schools and day care. J Pediatr 2001;138:560–5.
22. Moneret-Vautrin DA, Kanny G, Morisset M, et al. Food anaphylaxis in schools: evaluation of the management plan and the efficiency of the emergency kit. Allergy 2001;56:1071–6.
23. Gold MS, Sainsbury R. First aid anaphylaxis management in children who were prescribed an epinephrine autoinjector device (EpiPen). J Allergy Clin Immunol 2000;106:171–6.
24. McIntyre CL, Sheetz AH, Carroll CR, et al. Administration of epinephrine for life-threatening allergic reactions in school settings. Pediatrics 2005;116:1134–40.
25. Norton L, Dunn Galvin A, Hourihane JO. Allergy rescue medication in schools: modeling a new approach. J Allergy Clin Immunol 2008;122:209–10.

CHAPTER 16

Patient Education and Empowerment

Kim Mudd and Robert Wood

Introduction

Empowerment is a process that helps people gain control over their own lives. Empowering food-allergic patients starts with education. Allergen avoidance, symptom recognition and appropriate treatment are the major educational needs to be addressed. Empowerment evolves as individuals acquire confidence in their knowledge and ability to manage their food allergy and become self-sufficient.

Avoidance

'Allergen avoidance' is a deceptively simple phrase that encompasses everything from mastering Food and Drug Administration food label laws to evaluating the effectiveness of food bans in public settings. Allergen avoidance begins with a strategy to identify foods that contain food allergens through label reading, identifying unexpected sources of food allergens and cross-contamination, and avoiding certain types of contact with food allergens.

Label reading

Avoidance starts with label reading. It is a simple concept until you consider the number of ingredient labels on foods, cosmetics, medications and pet foods in the average grocery cart. People with food allergies need to read every ingredient label, every time, and never assume that products are 'safe' because changes can be made at any time. It is also important to realize that different sizes of the same food can have different ingredients. It is no wonder that in one study of accidental exposures,[1] a quarter of the food-related reactions were directly related to the fact that no one read the label.

CLINICAL CASE 1

NS, a 4-year-old with egg allergy, was returning from the beach with his family. The family had purchased several types of 'safe' candy for the trip home. Since N had tolerated taffy candy before, the family did not read the label until N began vomiting and wheezing in the back seat. The FUN SIZE taffy is egg free. The regular-sized taffy contains albumin.

CLINICAL CASE 2

LW is a 3-year-old with a milk allergy. LW was demonstrating his newly acquired skill of chewing gum without swallowing it. His grandmother gave LW a stick of gum without reading the label. The white powder on grandma's gum contained milk. The white powder on the gum LW tolerated before was milk free. LW experienced skin, gut and respiratory symptoms.

The Food and Drug Administration (FDA) is responsible for assuring that foods sold in the United States are safe, wholesome and properly labeled. The label on packaged foods must include the principal display panel with the identity or name of the food, an ingredient list, and the contact information for the manufacturer, distributor or packer. Each part of the label is potentially useful.

The principal display is the front label that includes a picture, description or the name of the food. One should never be swayed by words such as 'non-dairy' or 'egg substitute' on the front label. These terms are not defined by the FDA, not regulated by the FDA, and do not indicate that a food is necessarily milk or egg free. The first ingredient on non-dairy coffee creamers is frequently 'milk', and egg substitutes are frequently made from egg white. Some principal display panel labels also include Kosher symbols. The basic concepts of Kosher law are no mixing of dairy and meat, no pork or pork products and no shellfish (including both crustaceans and molluscs). Manufacturers can request a review of their products by one of many Kosher reviewing agencies. The process of certifying a product as Kosher involves a review by a rabbi of the ingredients as well as the processes used to produce the food. The 'K', 'K' within a circle and 'U' within a circle are some of the most common registered trademarked symbols from Kosher certification agencies. A 'D' symbol indicates the presence of milk, and 'DE' that the equipment used also processes milk. 'Pareve' and 'Parve' indicate that the food does not contain dairy or meat. There are many different Kosher certification agencies and the level of strictness can vary. There is a case report of milk-related anaphylaxis to Pareve-labeled 'dairy-free' dessert,[2] and milk has been detected in pareve-labeled chocolates.[3] In general, milk-allergic individuals should avoid products labeled with 'D' or 'DE' and not assume that foods without these designations are milk free (Fig. 16.1).

The ingredient list on a food label lists all ingredients in descending order of predominance by weight. The Food Allergen Labeling and Consumer Protection Act (FALCPA) of 2004 requires that ingredient labels on packaged foods state in 'common or usual names' the presence of major allergens, including milk, egg, fish, crustaceans, tree nuts, wheat, peanut and soybean. (Table 16.1 and Table 16.2) Blended and hydrolyzed proteins must include all of the proteins used in the mix using common names (e.g. 'hydrolyzed soy and corn protein'). Flavors, colors and incidental additives that contain major allergens also must be declared. Highly refined oils from vegetable sources such as peanut and soy are exempt from FALCPA because the refining process removes enough of the food proteins which are the cause of allergic reactions.[4] Companies that do not comply with the FALCPA labeling requirements may be subject to both civil and criminal penalties. At a minimum, the FDA usually requires that the food product which contains the undeclared allergen be recalled by the company.

FALCPA has dramatically reduced the detective work required to find major allergens in packaged foods. Prior to the enactment of this law, ingredient lists could include words such as 'whey' (a milk protein) or 'semolina' (wheat flour) without ever including the words 'milk' or 'wheat'. FALCPA does not address the other 160+[5] allergens that have been implicated in food-allergic reactions. For instance, sesame is a common allergen frequently

Table 16.1 FDA list of tree nuts. Available at: http://www.fda.gov/Food/GuidanceComplianceRegulatoryInformation/GuidanceDocuments/FoodLabelingNutrition/ucm059116.htm

Common or usual name
Almond
Beech nut
Brazil nut
Butternut
Cashew
Chestnut (Chinese, American, European, Seguin)
Chinquapin
Coconut
Filbert/hazelnut
Ginko nut
Hickory nut
Lichee nut
Macadamia nut/bush nut
Pecan
Pine nut/piñon nut
Pili nut
Pistachio
Sheanut
Walnut (English, Persian, Black, Japanese, California), heartnut, butternut

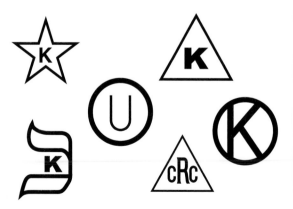

Figure 16.1 Kosher symbols.

Table 16.2 Definitions of crustaceans and molluscs

Crustacean shellfish are major food allergens and are therefore subject to the FDA's The Food Allergen Labeling and Consumer Protection Act (FALCPA)

Crustacean shellfish include all forms of crab, lobster and shrimp

Entire list of crustacean shellfish is available at: http: // www.accessdata.fda.gov/scripts/SEARCH_SEAFOOD/ index.cfm?other=complete

Molluscan shellfish are not major food allergens and are not subject to FALCPA

Molluscan shellfish include oysters, clams, mussels and scallops

found in baked goods, sushi, hummus, mole and adobo sauces. Because sesame is not on the FDA list of major allergens, the word may never appear on the ingredient list for sesame-containing ingredients, including tahini (sesame seed paste), gomashio (ground roasted sesame seed), and benne seeds (commonly used in Southern US cuisine). The FDA Food Labeling Guide is available at: http:// www.fda.gov/Food/GuidanceComplianceRegulatory Information/GuidanceDocuments/FoodLabeling Nutrition/FoodLabelingGuide/default.htm

FALCPA also does not address the issue of precautionary labeling or voluntary advisory labeling, such as 'may contain', 'manufactured on shared equipment with', or 'manufactured in the same facility with'. Advisory labeling is not regulated by the FDA, so manufacturers use different criteria to decide if and when to include various advisory statements.[6] The actual amount of allergen contained in food varies, but peanut protein has been detected in about 10% of foods bearing advisory statements regardless of the actual wording of the advisory label.[7] Milk has been found in up to a third of products such as baked goods, frozen desserts and snack foods with advisory labels, and up to 80% of dark chocolate candy.[6] The practice of including voluntary advisory labeling has become so common that for certain food categories, such as chocolate candy and cookies, up to 50% of products can contain some kind of advisory labeling.[8,9] Because of the confusion in definitions and an increase in the numbers of foods that bear advisory labeling, consumers often incorrectly assign different levels of risks to the various advisory labels or ignore them completely[7] and continue to consume foods that potentially contain significant levels of food allergens.

When both the ingredient list and the front label have failed to be helpful, the last option is to contact the manufacturer, packer or distributor. This is not generally necessary, but may be essential in trying to determine the ingredients of a generic term such as 'spices' for someone with an allergy to mustard or garlic. However, the manufacturer will frequently not share 'proprietary' or trade secret information, and in a litigious society they will not guarantee a product is 'safe'. They should be able to answer direct questions such as 'Does this product contain garlic' or 'The display label has a 'D', but milk is not listed in the ingredient list. Does this food contain milk?' Any company that cannot or will not answer this type of direct query should be avoided.

Regardless of the potential shortcoming of the current labeling system, label reading is an important piece of the avoidance strategy. Families and food-allergic individuals need to know how to read an ingredients label, to respect the advisory labeling, to use the hints offered by the Kosher designation, and when and how to contact a product manufacturer.

Cross-contamination

Cross-contamination occurs when 'safe' foods come in contact with allergens. This can occur during processing, storage, cooking or serving. Food processing cross-contamination is usually related to improper handling of products or ineffective cleaning of equipment. The food industry is very aware of potential problems and continues to make improvements in allergen control.[10] However, there is no consensus on the most effective cleaning methods and validation procedures.[11] Manufacturers are encouraged to develop an allergy control plan that reflects the most up-to-date information available on safe food handling. According to the Food Allergy and Anaphylaxis Network, An effective allergen control plan involves written policies addressing the segregation of allergenic foods or ingredients during receiving, storage, handling and processing, prevention of cross-contamination during processing, product label review and label/packaging use and control, and staff education and training (Available at: FAAN http://www.foodallergy.org/files/media/ allergen-control-plan/AllergenControlPlan.pdf). Consumers need to know to ask about a specific company's allergy control plan when they contact a manufacturer with questions about a product.

A company without an allergy control plan should be a company without customers.

Cross-contamination during the cooking and food preparation process is called allergen 'carryover' and includes things such as deep frying in oil that was previously used to cook allergenic foods. For instance, French fries can pick up contaminants of wheat, milk or egg from battered foods, or from fish or shellfish fried in the same oil. Other pieces of equipment can also be contaminated. Meats can pick up milk residue if they are cut on a slicer that was previously used for cheese. A hamburger can be contaminated with milk if the same spatula is used to flip cheese burgers and plain burgers. A steak can become contaminated with fish or shellfish if the same grill surface is used. Cross-contamination in the restaurant setting can have significant impact on the safety of food-allergic people when they eat out. In a study of restaurant personnel, more than 70% were confident in their ability to prepare a meal for a food-allergic customer despite the fact that a quarter thought it would be safe for a food-allergic patron to consume a small amount of allergen, one-third thought deep frying would destroy allergens, half thought buffets were safe if kept 'clean', and a quarter thought it was acceptable to remove allergens from a finished meal (e.g. removing nuts from a prepared salad or cheese from a 'plain' burger).[12] To address this disconnect, educational programs are being developed and disseminated. In addition, in Massachusetts legislation requires that restaurants add a menu statement about food allergies, display an educational poster on food allergy, and have restaurant workers receive training on cross-contamination issues.

Cross-contamination avoidance strategies include buying sliced meats or cheeses from delicatessens that have dedicated slicers for milk and for meat. When preparing meals at home, some families choose to maintain an allergen-free kitchen to reduce the likelihood of cross-contamination. Others use dedicated cookware and utensils to prepare food-allergy meals, or prepare the food-allergy meal first before preparing allergen-containing foods. When eating away from home, it is essential to ensure that those preparing and serving meals have proper cross-contamination prevention protocols in place. It is not feasible (or necessary) to have multiple complete kitchens and dining spaces with full utensils to accommodate people with food allergies. Food allergens can be effectively removed with household cleaners such as soap and water, sanitizing wipes and spray cleaners using usual cleaning techniques. Allergens can also be removed from hands using soap and water or wipes.[13] This means that foods can be prepared and served in a safe manner using proper cleaning and handwashing procedures. It is important to note that hand sanitizers such as antibacterial gels are not effective at removing allergens,[13] which means that hand sanitizers are not an acceptable alternative to handwashing.

The key to a successful dining experience with food allergies is planning. Many restaurants post their menus with ingredient content on their websites. Ethnic restaurants require special consideration. Asian restaurants rarely use cheese or other dairy-based ingredients, but many dishes contain sesame, nuts and/or peanuts, and a 'seasoned' wok is one that has never been scrubbed with soap and water. Vegan meals should be milk and egg free, but peanuts, tree nuts and seeds are important proteins in that style of cooking. Before dining in any establishment (or neighbor's house!) food-allergic individuals should call ahead and ask about things such as dedicated fryers, grills, utensils, kitchen preparation areas and staff training specific to food allergy. Food-allergic individuals need to avoid buffet-type serving situations, which are notorious for cross-contamination, and desserts which are a milk, egg, peanut and/or tree nut reaction waiting to happen. It is important that someone speak to the chef who actually prepares the meals, not just the server who presents the food. It is also important to be aware of high-risk situations such as high-volume times when the manager, server and chef team are less likely to be able to meet special requests. Consider using a 'chef card' such as the one available from FAAN (http://www.foodallergy.org/files/media/chef-card1/chefcardtemplate.pdf) that lists specific food ingredients to be avoided and a caution statement about food preparation which act as a visual reminder to restaurant personnel (Fig. 16.2, Table 16.3).

Avoiding contact

The greatest risk to a food-allergic individual is actually consuming an allergenic food. The amount of exposure or 'dose' of an ingested allergen may be in the microgram range, but even that small amount can cause a major reaction in a susceptible individual. Ingesting an allergen results in a far greater exposure then most topical contact or inhaled

The Food Allergy & Anaphylaxis Network | Chef Card Template

This is an interactive PDF that will allow you to type your allergens directly onto the chef card. To view the fields where you may enter information, click the "Highlight Fields" box in the upper right corner of this window.

WARNING! I am severely allergic to Peanut, Tree Nuts and Sesame

In order for me to avoid a **life-threatening reaction**, I **must avoid** all foods that contain these ingredients:

Peanut or Tree Nuts in any form	Sesame Seeds
Peanut or Nut butters	Tahini
Peanut Flour	Sesame Seed Paste
Pesto	Gomashio
Marzipan	Benne Seeds

Please ensure that my food does not contain any of these ingredients, and that any utensils and equipment used to prepare my meals, as well as prep surfaces, are thoroughly cleaned prior to use. **THANK YOU for your cooperation.**

© 2006, The Food Allergy & Anaphylaxis Network, www.foodallergy.org.

How to use your chef card:
In addition to asking a lot of questions about ingredients and preparation methods, many food-allergic teens and adults carry a "chef card" with them that outlines the foods that they must avoid. The card is presented to the chef or manager for review and serves as a reminder of the food allergy.

Print your chef card on brightly colored paper so that it will stand out in a restaurant's hectic atmosphere. Laminate your card to protect it from getting stained. Be sure to make several copies of your chef card so that if you forget to get it back, you have extra copies available.

WARNING! I am severely allergic to _____

In order for me to avoid a **life-threatening reaction**, I **must avoid** all foods that contain these ingredients:

Please ensure that my food does not contain any of these ingredients, and that any utensils and equipment used to prepare my meals, as well as prep surfaces, are thoroughly cleaned prior to use. **THANK YOU for your cooperation.**

© 2006, The Food Allergy & Anaphylaxis Network, www.foodallergy.org.

Figure 16.2 Sample chef card. Reproduced with permission from the Food Allergy and Anaphylaxis Network.

Table 16.3 High risk areas for cross-contamination

Restaurant equipment including fryers, grills and woks
Bakeries where foods are stored in racks
Food preparation areas where gloves are not changed
  between orders
Salad bars and buffets
Ice cream parlors where scoops are not washed in soap
  between orders
Delicatessen slicers
Bulk food bins

exposures. Consequently, most of the effort put into avoidance should concentrate on creating situations where food-allergic individuals do not ingest an allergenic food. There are, however, reports of allergic reactions related to contact exposure, inhalation of allergens,[14] kissing[15] and exposure to allergens during cooking.[16]

CLINICAL CASE 3

JPS is a 5-year-old with a wheat allergy. His family owns and runs an Italian restaurant. On at least two occasions JPS has had allergic reactions involving both skin and respiratory symptoms after being in the kitchen while pizza dough was prepared.

The obvious concern with a non-ingestion type of exposure is that it will be significant enough to cause a systemic reaction. To assess the relative risk, consider not only the potential dose of the exposure, but also the route of exposure. Having milk splashed directly into the eyes presents a greater risk of causing a reaction than laying an elbow in a smear of cream cheese. Inhaling wheat flour while a pizza crust is being tossed about is a much greater exposure than sitting at a table while other people eat warm buttered rolls.

Current research into non-ingestion types of exposure has focused on people with peanut allergy. Peanut is one of the most prevalent food allergies and is responsible for more severe reactions than any other food.[17,18] Peanut is also a food staple in many non-allergic diets. It is easy to see why there is concern about peanut contamination in common areas. One study looked at the amount of peanut protein present in samples collected from lunch tables, water fountains, desks and food preparation areas in six different schools. None of the eating areas, food preparation areas or desks had detectable peanut protein. In that same study, researchers tried to detect peanut protein in the air under several different conditions, including by an open peanut butter jar and as non-allergic subjects ate peanut butter and jelly sandwiches. Airborne peanut protein was not detectable.[13] When peanut-allergic children, many of whom had reported reactions to inhaled peanut, were deliberately exposed to peanut fumes, none experienced a respiratory or systemic reaction.[19] Other studies have looked at reactions in children with known peanut sensitivity who had peanut butter applied directly to their skin. None of the children experienced a systemic reaction, even those who developed a rash at the site where the peanut protein was applied.[19,20] The consensus is that the skin is a very effective barrier: 90% of highly peanut-allergic children would not experience a systemic or respiratory reaction with 'casual contact' to peanut.[19] Kissing with food allergies turns out to be more of a potential risk. Again, most of the research focuses on peanut-allergic individuals. One study showed measurable levels of peanut protein in saliva after non-peanut-allergic subjects ate peanut butter sandwiches. The amount of peanut protein varied, and brushing the teeth and chewing gum did affect the amount of detectable peanut protein, but in general, what was required was time for the peanut protein levels to fall.[15] Obviously, the type of kiss will determine the level of allergen exposure. A kiss on the cheek is a casual contact exposure that may result in a localized reaction at the site of the kiss. A kiss that involves an 'exchange of body fluids' is more likely to result in a much higher allergen dose, as well as an allergen ingestion type of reaction.

Cooking food proteins can also present a potential risk to food-allergic individuals. Food proteins can be aerosolized during the cooking process. A study that looked at children with a history of respiratory symptoms on exposure to frying, steaming or baking fish, baking chickpea, boiling milk, boiling egg and baking buckwheat found that many experienced reproducible respiratory symptoms when they were exposed to the proteins in a simulated environment.[16] Again, being in close proximity to aerosolized food as it is cooking presents a much greater exposure and risk for a reaction than being in the general vicinity.

CLINICAL CASE 4

OC is a 3-year-old with a known egg allergy. The family had always cooked and consumed egg in their home. One morning, OC's mother was frying eggs on the stovetop while holding OC on her hip. OC experienced facial swelling, hives and upper respiratory symptoms. The family has since decided not to cook eggs on the stovetop, although they continue to cook them in the oven.

The data support the focusing of avoidance efforts on allergen ingestion exposure and non-ingestion type of exposures that involve large amounts of allergens. The lack of evidence to support measurable amounts of allergens from casual exposures does not negate a common sense approach to allergen avoidance. Activities that involve allergenic foods (e.g. peanut butter bird feeders, wheat-containing modeling clay, egg-containing face paint, churning butter, using peanuts in the classroom as a counting aid) technically should not involve food ingestion, but putting food-allergic children in that situation lacks common sense. Cooking allergenic foods in food service class when a food-allergic individual is present in the classroom/workspace, or eating in a restaurant that allows patrons to throw peanut shells on the floor, also lacks sound judgment. It is small wonder that requests for food bans have become so prevalent.

Food bans take several different forms, from allergen-safe tables in the cafeteria to school-wide food-specific bans. There is evidence that 'peanut-free guidelines' are successful in reducing the amount of peanut present in lunches brought

Table 16.4 Pro/con food bans. Adapted from Young MC, Munoz-Furlong A, Sicherer SH. Management of food allergies in school: A perspective for allergists. J Allergy Clin Immunol. 2009; 124(2): 175–82.

Pro	Con
'Loaded gun' argument: reduce the chance of exposure	'No peanut detectors' to enforce food bans
Young children cannot bear responsibility of avoiding allergens	Causes an undue burden on children without a peanut allergy
Food contamination of shared equipment resulting in contact exposures	'Slippery slope' argument: if you ban peanut, why not ban other allergy foods?
Food sharing is a common behavior in children	'False sense of security' argument
School bullying difficult to control	Schools should prepare students for the 'real world'
'Community responsibility' approach to safety	Feelings of divisiveness

from home,[21] but it is not clear that such guidelines actually result in fewer allergen exposures.[22] It is clear that it is not feasible to eliminate all allergenic foods from schools, daycares, and public venues such as libraries and playgrounds. The best approach to allergen avoidance is to tailor the avoidance plan to the developmental age of the child (Table 16.4).

Young children are prone to hand-to-mouth activities, food sharing and messy eating behaviors. In this younger group, 'allergen-free' tables or classrooms are not uncommon and may provide benefit.[22] Although it is impossible to achieve an allergen-free environment, an increase in allergen awareness, combined with handwashing, cleaning of eating surfaces and high levels of supervision to prevent food sharing and to clean up spills, works well to create a safe environment. Most of these measures also have a high level of 'buy-in' from both allergic and non-allergic families. After all, everyone wants their children to have adequate supervision, clean hands and a clean table when they eat.

As children develop, the hand-to-mouth activity decreases and food-allergic children become less likely to accept shared food once they understand the potential consequences. At some point, having the entire student population wash before lunch becomes an unrealistic expectation and having a food-allergic child sit at the 'allergy table' becomes onerous. As children and their peers develop impulse control and understand the rationale for allergen avoidance, allowing food-allergic children to sit with their friends and supportive peers is much less socially isolating. Food bans and allergen-free seating are generally not necessary in upper elementary school-aged children.[22]

Food bans are also a serious issue for airline travel. Food-allergic reactions to peanut and tree nuts on airlines have been reported. One study on self-reported reactions estimated that one-third of the food-related reactions that occurred on airlines were anaphylactic.[23] Unlike exposure to peanut butter (e.g. smelling an open jar of peanut butter), where the peanut smell is due to airborne volatile organic compounds and not actual peanut protein,[22] peanut exposure on airlines is more likely to be peanut protein airborne in the dust as many packages of peanuts are opened simultaneously.[19] The major airlines have peanut policies on their websites. In general, the airlines will not guarantee that peanut-containing snacks will not be served on a flight, nor will they prevent other passengers from bringing peanut (or other allergen-containing foods) on the flight. Most airlines suggest scheduling early-morning flights when peanut snacks are less likely to be served. Some airlines will let families with food-allergic children pre-board. Families traveling with food-allergic children should wipe the tray table and arm rests with disposable wipes to address any food residue that may have been left by another passenger. Families also need to check under the seat cushions, around the floor and in the seatback pocket for stray food items that may have been missed when the plane was cleaned, especially when traveling with inquisitive children with little fingers that explore all of the nooks and crannies. In addition, food-allergic individuals need to check the policies with the specific airline, alert the reservations agent of any food allergies, arrive at the airport early, notify the gate agent of the food allergy, and avoid eating any of the snacks served by the airlines in flight. Thankfully, food-related reactions on airlines are rare,[23] but food-allergic individuals should consider traveling with multiple doses of epinephrine and antihistamines just in case.

Symptom recognition and treatment

Inevitably, even with the best avoidance plan in place, exposures to allergenic foods happen.

Table 16.5 Potential symptoms of a food allergic reaction. Adapted from Wang J, Sampson HA. Food Anaphylaxis. Clin and Exper Allergy. 2007; 37: 651–60.

Cutaneous	Urticaria, angioedema, pruritis, flushing, erythema, cyanosis or rash
Respiratory	Upper airway: rhinorrhea, congestion, sneezing, stridor, hoarseness, or 'lump in the throat'
Lower airway	Cough, wheeze, dyspnea, chest tightness, intercostal retractions
Cardiovascular	Tachycardia, arrhythmia, dizziness, syncope, hypotension, shock
Gastrointestinal	Pruritus or edema of the lips/tongue/palate/uvula, metallic taste in mouth, nausea, vomiting, abdominal cramps, reflux, nausea or diarrhea
Neurologic	Anxiety, headache, seizure, syncope, loss of consciousness, or feeling of 'impending doom'
Ocular	Pruritis, conjunctival injection, lacrimation, or periorbital edema

Table 16.6 Diagnostic criteria for anaphylaxis. Adapted from Sampson HA, Munoz-Furlong A, Campbell RL, Adkinson NF, Bock SA, Branum A, et al. Second symposium on the definition and management of anaphylaxis – Second National Institute of Allergy and Infectious Disease/Food Allergy and Anaphylaxis Network symposium. J Allergy Clin Immunol. 2006; 117(2): 391–7)

Any ONE of the following three criteria are fulfilled:
1. Acute (minutes to hours) onset of an illness with the involvement of skin, mucosal tissues, or both
   And at least ONE of the following:
   a. Respiratory compromise (dyspnea, wheeze/bronchospasm, stridor, hypoxia)
   b. Reduced BP or associated symptoms (hypotonia, syncope, incontinence)
2. TWO or more of the following that occur after exposure to a likely allergen
   a. Involvement of skin–mucosal tissue
   b. Respiratory compromise
   c. Reduced BP or associated symptoms
   d. Persistent gastrointestinal symptoms (crampy abdominal pain, nausea, vomiting)
3. ANY Reduced BP after exposure to a known allergen

Symptom recognition is the key first step to reaction management. Symptoms of a food-allergic reaction can include skin, gastrointestinal, respiratory, cardiovascular and/or neurological systems (Table 16.5). It is not uncommon to have multiple systems involved (e.g. hives and abdominal pain). Reactions can begin with minor symptoms such as a few scattered hives and increase to a multisystem anaphylactic event. Reactions can be acute and fast moving or slow to start. The majority of reactions will start within 1 hour of an exposure.[17] Although skin involvement (urticaria, angioedema, pruritis) is common, not all food-allergic reactions involve skin symptoms.

Treatment of a food-allergic reaction depends primarily on the symptoms. Minor symptoms such as an itchy mouth, scattered hives and mild pruritus may respond well to faster-acting oral antihistamines such as diphenhydramine or cetirizine. In general, liquid or chewable forms of antihistamine are preferred, for both ease of administration and speed of onset. Antihistamines do not stop or slow a reaction: they only treat the uncomfortable symptoms, such as itching and nasal congestion.

More severe reactions involving throat, lower respiratory, cardiac or neurologic systems OR combinations of systems such as hives and nausea, vomiting

and facial swelling, qualify as anaphylactic reactions.[17] Anaphylaxis is defined as 'a serious allergic reaction that is rapid in onset and may cause death'. (Table 16.6) The treatment is epinephrine[24] and must be prompt. Food-induced anaphylactic deaths do occur and frequently involve poor symptom recognition and/or a delay in epinephrine administration.[25] In one study of accidental peanut ingestions, more than half of the resulting reactions were anaphylactic and only 20% were appropriately treated with epinephrine.[18] Similar findings were reported by another group, where only 20% of systemic reactions to peanut, tree nut or milk were appropriately treated with epinephrine.[26] This may be partly explained by the fact so few patients and families know how to use an epinephrine autoinjector. Epinephrine use needs to be demonstrated with a placebo trainer and reinforced at every visit.[25]

Regardless of the severity of the symptoms and the treatment administered, food-allergic individuals need to be observed for 4–6 hours after a food-induced reaction.[27] Minor symptoms can develop into more severe reactions that warrant epinephrine. Epinephrine may treat the initial symptoms, but in about a quarter of cases additional doses are required to stop a reaction, either because of an inadequate response to the initial dose, inadequate dosing of epinephrine for body weight, delay in administration of initial dose, and/or subcutaneous administration of epinephrine.[22,26] The risk that reactions might require additional doses of epinephrine means that all reactions treated with epinephrine warrant emergency transport to a care facility for observation.[22]

Plans and paperwork

It is imperative that every food-allergic individual have a written management plan with specific instructions on symptom recognition and treatment. As it is not possible to predict the severity of a reaction based on a previous reaction,[17] it is prudent to prepare for a severe event. Food allergy action plans list potential symptoms matched with appropriate treatments, including medications, doses and monitoring plans (Fig. 16.3). Everyone who is responsible for children throughout their day must be educated on symptom recognition and plan implementation. Accidental ingestions occur in many settings, including school classrooms, school cafeterias, playgrounds, private homes, restaurants, relatives' and friends' homes. Plans need to include bus drivers, playground monitors, before and after school care providers and field trip chaperones.[18,28]

In addition to food allergy action plans, schools and daycare facilities benefit from comprehensive plans for managing food allergies. Many States and school systems have developed policies for food-allergic students. A current listing on the State guidelines is available on the Food Allergy and Anaphylaxis Network website under the advocacy tab (foodallergy.org). The existing guidelines are used as a framework to create an individualized healthcare plan (IHCP). According to the National Association of School Nurses' Position Statement, the IHCP is to specify the healthcare services required for students who have needs that 'affect or have the potential to affect safe and optimal school attendance and academic performance'. These written plans are developed collaboratively by the school nurse with input from the student, family, healthcare providers and school staff. IHCPs are used to manage the potentials risks associated with food allergy, facilitate communication and coordinate and evaluate the care specified. The plans are dynamic documents that are meant to be evaluated and revised (as appropriate) on a yearly basis. The IHCP should

include plans for allergen avoidance measures that focus on ingestion prevention and non-ingestion-type exposures that have the potential to expose food-allergic individuals to significant amounts of allergens. Since it is impossible to eliminate the potential risk of an allergen exposure, IHCPs need to specify food allergy emergency actions in classrooms, cafeterias, gymnasia, playgrounds, field trips, and extracurricular events; epinephrine administration and storage; student self-carrying of medications; emergency medical system activation; and transportation issues (Fig. 16.4).

Some situations require more than an IHCP. Section 504 of the Rehabilitation Act of 1973 is a piece of civil rights law that prohibits discrimination against individuals with disabilities in public and private programs and activities that receive financial assistance from the federal government. The Americans with Disabilities Act (ADA) prohibits discrimination against individuals with disabilities (including food allergy) and extends this protection to the full range of State and local government services, programs or activities, regardless of whether they receive federal assistance. In general, 504 Plans are used when food allergy discrimination has the potential to affect a food-allergic student's education. 504 Plans are legal documents with the backing of the US Department of Education, Office of Civil Rights.

Plans are, however, only as good as their implementation, and there are many cases of deficient plans or plans written and not followed in emergencies.[22] The school needs time to write, revise and initiate the plan, and frequently some amount of training is necessary. School nurses and teachers are not usually available in the summer, and trying to initiate a meeting and write a plan in the weeks before the school year can be challenging. The conversation about a written food allergy plan needs to be initiated well in advance of the school year. Food-allergic families need to plan to meet with school nurses and the school administration before everyone leaves for the summer holiday. A second meeting before the school year begins is helpful to ensure that training is completed, medications are in place and the plan is clear before the food-allergic child walks through the door. It is important that plans are in place before the school year starts: imagine the potential scenario if an uninformed teacher promises the class a sundae bar or pizza day as a reward for project completion and then has to refuse because of a student's food allergy.

FOOD ALLERGY ACTION PLAN

NAME:_____ DOB:____/____/_____

Child's Photograph

ALLERGY TO:_____

Asthma: ☐Yes (higher risk for a severe reaction) ☐ No.

Weight _____lbs

ANY SEVERE SYMPTOMS AFTER SUSPECTED INGESTION:

LUNG: Short of breath, wheeze, repetitive cough

HEART: Pale, blue, faint, weak pulse, dizzy, confused

THROAT: Tight, hoarse, trouble breathing/ swallowing

MOUTH: Obstructive swelling (tongue)

SKIN: Many hives over body

Or **Combination** of symptoms from different body areas:

SKIN: Hives, itchy rashes, swelling
GUT: Vomiting, crampy pain

INJECT EPINEPHRINE IMMEDIATELY

- CALL 911
-Begin Monitoring (see below)
-Additional medications:
    -Antihistamine
    -Inhaler (bronchodilator) if asthma

Inhalers/bronchodilators and antihistamines are not to be depended upon to treat a severe reaction (anaphylaxis)→ Use Epinephrine.
When in doubt, use epinephrine. Symptoms can rapidly become more severe

MILD SYMPTOMS ONLY
Mouth: Itchy mouth
Skin: A few hives around mouth/face, mild itch
Gut: mild nausea/discomfort

GIVE ANTIHISTAMINE
-Stay with child, alert health care professionals and parent
IF SYMPTOMS PROGRESS (see above), INJECT EPINEPHRINE

☐ If checked, give <u>epinephrine</u> for ANY symptoms if the allergen was likely eaten (extremely reactive).
☐ If checked, give <u>epinephrine</u> before symptoms if the allergen was definitely eaten (extremely reactive)

MEDICATIONS/DOSES
EPINEPHRINE (BRAND AND DOSE): _____

ANTIHISTAMINE (BRAND AND DOSE):_____

OTHER (e.g., inhaler-bronchodilator if asthma):_____

MONITORING: Stay with the child. Tell rescue squad epinephrine was given; request an ambulance with epinephrine. A second dose of epinephrine can be given a few minutes or more after the first if symptoms persist or recur. For a severe reaction, consider keeping child lying on back with legs raised. Treat child even if parents cannot be reached. See back/attached for auto-injection technique.

For insect sting allergy, inject epinephrine for any symptoms other than localized swelling at sting site

CONTACTS: CALL 911 (Rescue squad: (___)_____) Doctor:_____ Phone: (___)_____-_____

Parent/Guardian:_____ Phone: (____)_____

OTHER EMERGENCY CONTACT: NAME/Relationship_____ Phone: (___)_____-_____

NAME/Relationship_____ Phone: (___)_____-_____

PARENT/GUARDIAN SIGNATURE   DATE   PHYSICIAN/HEALTHCARE PROVIDER SIGNATURE   DATE

Figure 16.3 FAAN Food Allergy Action Plan. Reproduced with permission from the Food Allergy and Anaphylaxis Network.

SEVERE ALLERGIES

| Student Name: _____ DOB: _____ School: _____ |
| School Nurse: _____ Date of IHP: _____ School Year: _____ |
| Physician Name: _____ Ph. #: _____ Parent signature : _____ |

Nursing Diagnosis/Concern	Educational Goal	Plan of Action	By Whom/When
Potential for severe allergic reaction or life-threatening episode	1. Maintain optimum health and safety necessary for learning	1. Student is allergic to following: ☐ _____ ☐ _____ ☐ _____ ☐ _____ ☐ _____ Events which may trigger an allergic response: ☐ _____ ☐ _____ ☐ _____ Symptoms of student's allergic response: ☐ Respiratory distress ☐ Hives ☐ Swelling (describe) _____ ☐ Runny nose/hayfever ☐ Red, itchy, watery eyes ☐ Asthma ☐ ANAPHYLACTIC SHOCK ☐ ☐ Classroom teacher (s) will assist student to avoid exposure to allergins (food, insects, chemicals, etc) as much as possible. ☐ Student will self-monitor exposure to allergins in order to prevent allergic response-**when age/ developmentally appropriate.**	 Classroom personnel Student when age/ developmentally able

Figure 16.4 IHCP sample form. Reproduced from the New Mexico School Health Manual with permission from the New Mexico Department of Health.

Empowerment

Empowerment involves the attainment of self-sufficiency and independence. Empowerment is a process that begins when the food allergy diagnosis is made and continues through learning to read labels, making good food decisions away from home, learning to shop, cook and order in a restaurant, self-advocating, and finally leaving home for college, career and family.

The key to achieving empowerment is to understand the personality and the developmental stage of the food-allergic individual. A very verbal, outgoing young child needs a completely different approach from a shy child who is timid in new situations. An elementary school-aged child has different developmental challenges from a high-schooler. The most important thing to remember is that as they grow and develop, the plan changes and grows

with them. As they demonstrate responsibility, children earn independence.

During the early childhood stage, parents orchestrate every interaction between the food-allergic child and their environment. Children at this stage are preverbal, put everything in their mouths and are incapable of self-advocacy. What they can do is observe how the people around them cope. Families of food-allergic children are generally still dealing with the steep learning curve associated with a food-allergy diagnosis, and they are very anxious about their child's safety.[29] This anxiety is not necessarily related to the severity of previous reactions, the need to treat with epinephrine, or a food allergy-related hospital admission.[30] Parents who take a matter-of-fact approach to food allergy management that focuses on safety routines and coping strategies send the message that food allergy is manageable.[31] Although the temptation to pull up the drawbridge, build a moat, and set the alligators

229

SEVERE ALLERGIES

Student Name: _____ DOB: _____ School: _____
School Nurse: _____ Date of IHP: _____

Nursing Diagnosis/Concern	Educational Goal	Plan of Action	By Whom/When
		If symptoms of allergic response/event are noted: ☐ Student will be accompanied to the Nurse's office for appropriate assessment/intervention. ☐ Student will come to the Nurse's office for supervised administration of the following medication (s) according to written physician's orders: (Medication Authorization Policy) **Medication(s) Dose Time** All LLS procedures/policies will be followed for administration of medications. ☐ Student will have an EpiPen available during the school day in the Nurse's office. ☐ EpiPen will be administered in an emergency according to doctor's orders. Parent will be notified when supply of medication needs replacement. Student will be monitored for adverse side effects or decreased therapeutic benefit of medication such as: _____ _____ _____ .	Classroom personnel/responsible student-as needed Health office Personnel-as needed Student/School Nurse-as ordered Student/School personnel who have been designated and trained by the school nurse as ordered. Provided by office staff or health office

Figure 16.4 *Continued*

loose is overwhelming, coping with the food allergy diagnosis while staying fully engaged in social activities sets the stage for future empowerment.

During the late preschool and early school years, children are more verbal and can begin to follow rules such as 'No sharing of food'. As they develop an understanding of the potential implications of a food allergy diagnosis, children should begin to take on more responsibility for self-advocacy. It is important to give them an opportunity to practice skills such as talking to an adult outside the immediate family about their food allergies, or making food choices outside the home environment. Role playing and 'what if' situations can be helpful.[31] Involving children in the process of developing a plan for school, for birthday parties, play dates and overnights, gives them a chance to practice important management skills. Children of families who model

adaptive behavior and promote 'shared responsibility' with their food-allergic child are more likely to be ready to assume self-management.[29] 'Helicopter' parents who hover too close and anxious families who overprotect their child send the message that they lack confidence in their child. Children who perceive themselves as vulnerable are more likely to be the victims of behaviors such as being intentionally excluded or targeted as a scapegoat. Children victimized by these types of bullying often lack coping competence.[32] Children who adopt a negative attitude that focuses on limitations imposed by their food allergy are more likely to be distressed by their allergy than children who adopt a positive perspective that focuses on strengths and coping strategies.[31] Children can become overwhelmed by the process or the lack of coping demonstrated by the adults in their life. Negative attitudes towards

SEVERE ALLERGIES

Student Name: _____ DOB: _____ School: _____
School Nurse: _____ Date of IHP: _____

Nursing Diagnosis/Concern	Educational Goal	Plan of Action	By Whom/When
		If symptoms do not significantly improve in ___ minutes; Contact parent/guardian for instructions; ☐ **CALL 911 EMERGENCY RESCUE** ☐ **SERVICES** All **EMERGENCY RESCUE** personnel will be given information about student's allergies if they are called to attend student for allergic response, accident/injury or illness	
Knowledge deficit related to allergies	Student will increase responsibility in preventing and managing allergic response in school.	Student will be given information and health counseling regarding allergies and management of allergic reaction at <u>level of student's understanding.</u> Classroom teacher (s) will be provided information, support and consultation regarding management of this student's allergic condition.	School nurse-ongoing
Potential for change in medical status	Student will participate in collaboration which facilitates optimum health and safety necessary for learning.	Parent/guardian will provide school nurse with copy of current medical report or doctor's statement annually or when change in medical status occurs. The school nurse will call the student's doctor to obtain current information verbally when this is necessary to manage student's condition at school. Physician or Healthcare Provider Name: _____ Phone: _____	Parent/guardian as specified School Nurse

Figure 16.4 *Continued*

food allergy and maternal anxiety are related to greater child anxiety.[31] Children who have been programmed to be anxious by the adults in their lives have a level of anxiety surrounding their food allergy that is not in line with the severity of the allergy or the frequency of reactions.[30] Some amount of caution is necessary to maintain vigilance. Maladaptive behavior such as over-responding to perceived risk or anxiety that interferes with activity should be addressed with a healthcare professional.[31] Bullying behaviors should be addressed directly with school officials, as many schools have anti-bullying polices.

As children enter late elementary and middle school years, they need to build on their management skills with the goal of progressing towards independence. At this age, children should be responsible enough to carry autoinjectors and make appropriate food choices outside the home. Many

food-allergic children are ready to self-carry epinephrine by age 8 or 10. By age 12 or 13, children need to be well on their way to recognizing symptoms and initiating an emergency treatment plan, including self-administering epinephrine. These skills need to be in place before food-allergic children can attain the independence they desire in the teenage years, which can be challenging for both parents and teens alike. After all, being a teen or young adult is one of the risk factors of death from food-induced anaphylaxis[33] (Table 16.7).

Adolescents spend most of their time with friends, exploring their independence and taking risks. Adolescents and young adults are more concerned about fitting in with their peer group than with having a food-allergic reaction and they balance safety with quality of life issues.[34] Since teens have a poor perception of their health needs and a sense of

SEVERE ALLERGIES

Student Name: _____ DOB: _____ School: _____

School Nurse: _____ Date of IHP: _____

Nursing Diagnosis/Concern	Educational Goal	Plan of Action			By Whom/When
The Health Management Plan will be reviewed annually with parent/guardian and appropriate instructional personnel. It will be revised as needed. The school nurse in collaboration with parent/guardian will train (or arrange for training) and supervise all non-medically licensed school personnel who are delegated Responsibility for implementing any part of this health plan.	The IHP will be updated and revised annually to meet the health needs of the student.	Review Date:	RN Initials:	Parent Initials:	

Figure 16.4 *Continued*

Table 16.7 Risk factors for fatal anaphylaxis

Teen or young adult
Asthma
Peanut, tree nut or seafood allergy
Not carrying epinephrine
Delay in the use of injectable epinephrine to treat an anaphylactic reaction
Eating restaurant food
Reactions that do not involve skin symptoms
Denying symptoms
Concurrent intake of alcohol
Reliance on oral antihistamines to treat symptoms of anaphylaxis
Lack of reaction management education from healthcare providers

invulnerability,[23] they can make bad decisions. In one study of food-allergic adolescents and young adults, more than half of the adolescents reported trying a food that they knew contained a known allergen.[24] Teens and college-aged students report trying food allergens despite a history of anaphylaxis.[23]

Even when they know what the 'right' or expected behavior is, teens will still balance safety with convenience. When asked about carrying self-injectable epinephrine, two-thirds reported carrying epinephrine 'at all times'. This same group actually had epinephrine available mainly during times of travel or eating out, and not during social events such as parties and dances, sport events, or when carrying it was inconvenient because of tight clothing.[24] A study of food-allergic college-age individuals showed an alarming low number of young adults who had self-injectable epinephrine available on campus.[23]

Teens need appropriate knowledge about their food allergy and its potential implications because they will use the available information to assess the risk and make informed decisions.[34] One should never miss an opportunity to teach directly to the teen. If they do not bring it up, talk about the kissing issue. Address the fact that teens think they are invulnerable, and that they will make decisions that are socially acceptable rather than safe. Remind them that a food allergy reaction screams 'LOOK AT ME' and that the teen has the power to avoid situations that put them in the allergy spotlight. Teens value input from peers. Involving peers in the teaching and management process takes advantage of the learning style that works for teens. Obviously, sharing information on a teen's food allergy with the entire school would probably be viewed as an invasion of privacy. Having the teen teach a few friends about allergen avoidance, symptom recognition and appropriate treatment fosters independence and establishes a social safety net. There are websites maintained by groups such as the Food Allergy and Anaphylaxis Network that are specifically designed for food allergic teens (http://www. fanteen.org & www.facebook.com). These give teens an opportunity to share their experiences and learn about food allergies from their peers.

Teens also need healthy, adaptive coping skills that they can take into adulthood.[34] These skills are developed over time, with support and practice in an environment where the teens feel they can succeed. They need time and opportunity to practice coping skills and the confidence to try. Knowing that teens crave independence and that they require some kind of foundation to develop skills, consider a House Rules and Compromise approach. House rules are a list of non-negotiable rules that both teens and parents support. They include such things as 1) always carrying epinephrine autoinjector on their person when they leave home; 2) always being with at least one person who knows about the food allergy, recognizes symptoms and knows how to respond to an emergency; and 3) always checking every food (reading labels, talking to the chef or person who prepared any food) before eating anything while away from home. Every plan for every situation starts with the House Rules. The Compromise comes in the details. If the teen wants to attend an event, is the parent gong to contact the venue to check for safe foods, or is the teen? If the teen chooses not to check for safe foods, then is the teen going to bring their own, safe foods? If bringing food is not an acceptable option and eating out of a common bowl is unacceptable (breaks House Rule #3), then the teen agrees to attend the event but not eat. Even if the plan is not necessarily the plan the parent would have developed, if it meets the House Rules, it is acceptable. The House Rules approach fosters independence, allows the teen to practice planning and adaptive behaviors, and addresses the dreaded awkward social situation that a food reaction can cause.

The key to an empowered, functional young adult is to ensure that they are exposed early to appropriate modeling and balanced coping strategies. They need the opportunity to fully participate in social functions and to practice their coping skills in a supportive environment that rewards responsibility with independence.

References

1. Sheth S, Waserman S, Kagan R, et al. Role of food labels in accidental exposures in food-allergic individuals in Canada. Ann Allergy Asthma Immunol 2010;104(1):60–5.
2. Jones RT, Squillace DL, Yunginger JW. Anaphylaxis in a milk-allergic child after ingestion of milk-contaminated kosher-pareve-labeled 'dairy-free' dessert. Ann Allergy 1992;68(3):223–7.
3. Hefle SL, Lambrecht DM. Validated sandwich enzyme-linked immunosorbent assay for casein and its application to retail and milk-allergic complaint foods. J food Prt 2004;67(9):1933–8.
4. Crevel RWR, Kerkhoff MAT, Koning MMG. Allergenicity of refined vegetable oils. Food Chem Toxicol 2000; 38:385–93.
5. Hefle SL, Nordlee J, Taylor SL. Allergenic foods. Crit Rev Sci Nutr 1996;36:69–89.
6. Crotty MP, Taylor SL. Risks associated with foods having advisory milk labeling. J Allergy Clin Immun 2010;125(4):935–7.
7. Hefle SL, Furlong TJ, Niemann L, et al. Consumer attitudes and risks associated with packaged foods having advisory labeling regarding the presence of peanuts. J Allergy Clin Immun 2007;120(1):171–6.
8. Taylor SL, Hefle SL, Farnum K, et al. Survey and evaluation of pre-FALCPA labeling practices used by food manufacturers to address allergen concerns. Comp Rev Food Sci Food Safety 2007;6:36–46.
9. Pieretti M, Chung D, Pancenza R, et al. Audit of manufactured products: Use of allergen advisory labels and identification of labeling ambiguities. J Allergy Clin Immun 2009;124(2):337–41.
10. Hefle SL, Taylor SL. Food allergy and the food industry. Curr Allergy Asthma Rep 2004;4:55–9.

11. Jackson LS, Al-Taher FM, Moorman M, et al. Cleaning and other control and validation strategies to prevent allergen cross-contamination in food-processing operations. J Food Prot 2008;71(2):445–58.

12. Ahuja R, Sicherer SH. Food-allergy management from the perspective of restaurant and food establishment personnel. Ann Allergy Asthma Immunol 2007;98(4):344–8.

13. Perry TT, Conover-Walker MK, Pomes A, et al. Distribution of peanut allergen in the environment. J Allergy Clin Immunol 2004;113(5):973–6.

14. Eriksson NE, Moller C, Werner S, et al. The hazards of kissing when you are food allergic. A survey on the occurrence of kiss-induced allergic reactions among 1139 patients with self-reported food hypersensitivity. J Investig Allergy Clin Immunol 2003;13(3):149–54.

15. Maloney JM, Chapman MD, Sicherer SH. Peanut allergen exposure through saliva: assessment and interventions to reduce exposure. J Allergy Clin Immunol 2006;118(3):719–24.

16. Roberts G, Golden N, Lack G. Bronchial challenges with aerosolized food in asthmatic, food-allergic children. Allergy 2002;57:713–7.

17. Wang J, Sampson HA. Food Anaphylaxis. Clin and Exper Allergy 2007;37:651–60.

18. Yu JW, Kagan R, Verreault N, et al. Accidental ingestions in children with peanut allergy. J Allergy Clin Immunol 2006;118(2):466–72.

19. Simonte SJ, Ma S, Mofidi S, et al. Relevance of casual contact with peanut butter in children with peanut allergy. J Allergy Clin Immunol 2003;112(1):180–2.

20. Wainstein BK, Kashef S, Ziegler M, et al. Frequency and significance of immediate contact reactions to peanut in peanut-sensitive children. Clin Exp Allergy 2007;37(6):839–45.

21. Banerjee DK, Kagan RS, Turnbull E, et al. Peanut-free guidelines reduce school lunch peanut contents. Arch Dis Child 2007;92:980–2.

22. Young MC, Munoz-Furlong A, Sicherer SH. Management of food allergies in school: A perspective for allergists. J Allergy Clin Immunol 2009;124(2):175–82.

23. Greenhawt MJ, Singer AM, Baptist AP. Food allergy and food allergy attitudes among college students. J Allergy Clin Immunol 2009;124(2):323–7.

24. Sampson M, Munoz-Furlong A, Sicherer SH. Risk-taking and coping strategies of adolescents and young adults with food allergy. J Allergy Clin Immunol 2006;117(6):1440–5.

25. Kim JS, Sinacore JM, Pongracic JA. Parental use of EpiPen for children with food allergies. J Allergy Clin Immunol 2005;116(1):164–8.

26. Jarvinen KM, Sicherer SH, Sampson HA, et al. Use of multiple doses of epinephrine in food-induced anaphylaxis in children. J Allergy Clin Immun 2008;112(1):133–8.

27. Sampson HA, Munoz-Furlong A, Campbell RL, et al. Second symposium on the definition and management of anaphylaxis – Second National Institute of Allergy and Infectious Disease/Food Allergy and Anaphylaxis Network symposium. J Allergy Clin Immunol 2006;117(2):391–7.

28. McIntyre CL, Sheetz AH, Carroll CR, et al. Administration of epinephrine for life-threatening allergic reactions in school. Pediatrics 2005;116:1134–40.

29. Williams NA, Parra GR, Elkin TD. Parenting children with food allergies; Preliminary development of a measure assessing child-rearing behaviors in the context of pediatric food allergy. Ann Allergy Asthma Immunol 2009;103:140–5.

30. Cummings AJ, Knibb RC, Erlewyn-Lajeunesse M, et al. Management of nut allergy influences quality of life and anxiety in children and their mothers. Pediatr Allergy Immunol 2010;21:586–94.

31. LeBovidge JS, Strauch H, Kalish LA, et al. Assessment of psychological distress among children and adolescents with food allergy. J Allergy Clin Immunol 2009;124(6):1282–8.

32. Sapouna M, Wolke D, Vannini N, et al. Virtual learning intervention to reduce bullying victimization in primary school: A controlled trial. J Child Psychol Psychiatry 2009;51(1):104–12.

33. Munoz-Furlong A, Weiss CC. Characteristics of food-allergic patients placing them at risk for a fatal anaphylactic episode. Curr Allergy Asthma Rep 2009;9(1):57–63.

34. MacKenzie H, Roberts G, Van Laar D, et al. Teenagers' experience of living with food hypersensitivity: A qualitative study. Pediatr Allergy Immunol 2009;21:595–602.

CHAPTER 17

Future Therapies for Food Allergies

Anna Nowak-Węgrzyn and Hugh A. Sampson

At present the only treatment for food allergy is strict dietary avoidance, and so the development of therapeutic interventions for food allergy is a research priority.[1] The many promising therapies under investigation are both allergen non-specific and allergen specific.[2] Not surprisingly, these therapies focus on the foods that most frequently provoke severe IgE-mediated anaphylactic reactions (peanut, tree nuts, shellfish) and the most common food allergens, such as cows' milk and hen's egg.[3] Most promising non-specific therapies for food-induced anaphylaxis include monoclonal anti-IgE antibodies, which increase the threshold dose for peanut in peanut-allergic individuals, and Chinese herbal medications, which prevent peanut-induced anaphylaxis in an animal model and are being investigated in clinical trials. Monoclonal anti-IL-5 antibody has been tested in adults with eosinophilic esophagitis (Table 17.1). Allergen-specific therapies include oral, sublingual and epicutaneous immunotherapy (desensitization) with native food allergens (Table 17.2, Table 17.3) and mutated recombinant proteins, which have decreased IgE-binding activity, coadministered in heat-killed *E.coli* to generate maximum immune response (Table 17.4). Diets containing extensively heated milk or egg are being investigated as an alternative to oral immunotherapy.

Identifying subjects for novel food allergy therapies

Food allergy therapy is most needed for the subjects at high risk for severe anaphylaxis and those

unlikely to develop spontaneous oral tolerance. Traditional allergy tests detecting food allergen-specific IgE antibodies in serum or in the skin (skin prick test) do not reliably predict the potential severity of the allergic reaction following food ingestion or the potential for the spontaneous development of oral tolerance. Recent studies suggest that the severity of food-allergic reactions may relate to the diversity of the immune response to IgE-binding areas (IgE epitopes) on the major food allergens. A peptide microarray-based immunoassay was used to map IgE epitopes on the major peanut and milk allergens.[4–6] High epitope diversity was found in patients with a history of more severe allergic reactions. There was a positive correlation between the number of milk epitopes recognized and clinical sensitivity (r = 0.6), such that patients with the greatest epitope diversity were significantly more reactive than those with the lowest diversity (p = 0.021) (Fig. 17.1). Binding to higher numbers of IgE epitopes was associated with more severe allergic reactions during a milk challenge (Fig. 17.2). Using a competitive peptide microarray assay, milk-allergic patients demonstrated a combination of high- and low-affinity IgE binding, whereas those who had outgrown their milk allergy had primarily low-affinity IgE binding.[6] This study demonstrated that greater IgE epitope diversity and higher affinity were associated with discriminating clinical phenotypes and severity of milk allergy.

Persistent egg allergy was related to the recognition of the sequential epitopes on ovomucoid, the major egg white allergen. Subjects who generated

Table 17.1 Allergen-non-specific therapy for food allergy

Therapy	Mechanism of action	Effects	Comments
Monoclonal anti-IgE	Binds to circulating IgE and prevents IgE deposition on mast cells and blocks degranulation. Interferes with the facilitated antigen presentation by B cells and dendritic cells.	Improves symptoms of asthma and allergic rhinitis; provides protection against peanut anaphylaxis in 75% of treated patients	Subcutaneous at monthly or 2-week intervals, unknown long-term consequences of IgE elimination; food non-specific; may be used in combination with specific food allergen oral immunotherapy
Traditional Chinese medicine (TCM)	Upregulation of Th1 cytokines (IFN-γ, IL-12); downregulation of Th2 cytokines (IL-4, IL-5, IL-13); decreased allergen-IgE and T cell proliferation to peanut	Reverses allergic inflammation in the airways; protects mice from peanut anaphylaxis	Oral, generally safe and well tolerated, current studies focus on identification of the crucial active herbal components in the multiherb formulas and establishing optimal dosing in phase I and II clinical trials
Lactococcus lactis transfected with murine IL-10	Decreased serum IgE and IgG$_1$; increased IgA in the gut; increased gut and serum IL-10	Pretreatment of young mice prior to sensitization with β-lactoglobulin in the presence of cholera toxin protected against anaphylaxis on the oral food challenge	This approach was only tested in the mouse model; however, the concept of probiotic bacteria may be applied to delivery of engineered allergens in human studies
Monoclonal anti-IL-5 antibody (mepolizumab)	Reduced tenascin C (p = 0.033) and transforming growth factor β_1 (p = 0.05) expression in the esophageal epithelial layer 13 weeks after initiation of treatment	Limited improvement of symptoms was seen, although a trend was seen between 4 and 13 weeks after initiation of mepolizumab treatment	Mepolizumab was well tolerated and had an acceptable safety profile, even at the high 1500-mg dose level. Mepolizumab is currently being evaluated in children with EoE*

*EoE: eosinophilic esophagitis

IgE antibody responses against both the conformational and sequential epitopes of ovomucoid were likely to have persistent egg allergy.[7] Recognition of the specific epitopes on the cows' milk major allergen, casein, might identify children at risk for more persistent milk allergy.[8] Persistence of food allergy might also relate to high peak values of food-specific serum IgE antibodies. Two reports describing the natural history of cows' milk and egg allergy in children with multiple food allergies reported that a few children with peak cows' milk or egg white-specific IgE antibody levels ≥50 kU$_A$/L (UniCAP, Phadia) outgrew their respective allergy by teenage years.[9,10]

Allergen-non-specific therapy

Humanized monoclonal anti-IgE

Humanized monoclonal anti-IgE antibodies bind to the constant region of IgE antibody molecules and prevent the IgE from binding to high-affinity receptors, FcεRI, expressed on the surface of mast cells and basophils, and low-affinity receptors, FcεRII, expressed on B cells, dendritic cells and intestinal epithelial cells. Anti-IgE cannot interact with IgE molecules when they are bound to IgE receptors and therefore cannot induce mast cell or basophil degranulation by cross-linking IgE, thus eliminating the risk of immediate allergic reactions following the injection of anti-IgE. The decrease in free IgE molecules due to anti-IgE therapy is associated with decreased expression of high-affinity receptors for IgE (FcεRI) on mast cells and basophils and with decreased release of histamine and other inflammatory mediators.[11] In addition, anti-IgE inhibits facilitated antigen uptake by B cells and antigen-presenting cells.

A multicenter clinical trial investigated humanized monoclonal anti-IgE mouse IgG$_1$ antibody (TNX-901) in 84 adults with a history of immediate allergy to peanut.[12] Peanut allergy was confirmed by double-blind placebo-controlled oral peanut

Table 17.2 Native allergen immunotherapy for food allergy

Therapy	Mechanism of action	Effects	Comments
Conventional peanut immunotherapy	Altered T-cell responses, upregulation of suppressor cells	Increased oral peanut tolerance	Subcutaneous injections of gradually increasing doses of allergen; unacceptably high rate of serious adverse events
Birch pollen immunotherapy for oral allergy to apple	Marked reduction in skin test reactivity to raw apple; effect of immunotherapy inversely correlated with baseline skin reactivity but not with serum apple or birch IgE	Significant reduction or total resolution of oral allergy symptoms to raw Golden Delicious apple in a subset of patients receiving immunotherapy for at least 12 months	Clinical effect lasting for up to 30 months after discontinuation in >50% of patients
Oral immunotherapy (OIT)	Decreased skin test reactivity; decreased food-IgE and IL-4. Increased regulatory T cells, IL-10 and food-IgG and IgA	Oral food desensitization or increased threshold dose of food for clinical reactions up to 6 months; short-term success rate about 75%	No long-term follow-up data; many patients experience recurrence of symptoms if food not ingested on a daily basis; significant rate of moderate–severe adverse reactions; convenience of home administration of maintenance doses
Sublingual immunotherapy	Serum hazelnut-IgG$_4$ and total IL-10 increased in treated group; no change in hazelnut-IgE	Oral food desensitization or increased threshold dose on oral hazelnut challenge	Systemic side effects rate 0.2% during rush build-up phase; adverse reaction rate less than with OIT; no long-term follow-up

Table 17.3 Benefits and risks of food oral immunotherapy (OIT) for peanut and milk

	Peanut	Milk
Success*	77%	37–70%
Side effects	**Build-up**[44,46,47]	**Blinded study**[41]
	Mild oropharyngeal 69% Mild/moderate skin 62% Mild/moderate nausea or abdominal pain 44% Diarrhea/emesis 21% Mild wheezing 18%	Mild oral pruritus median 16% doses/child Gastrointestinal median 2% doses/child Epinephrine: 0.2% of total doses; 2 doses during build-up and 2 doses during home maintenance (in 4 subjects)
	Maintenance	**Open label home study**[42]
	Upper respiratory 29% Cutaneous 24% Any treatment: 0.7% of home doses Epinephrine: 2 subjects (one dose each)	1–3 months: 2.5–96.4% of doses per subject >3 months: 0–79%/subject % total doses with reactions: Oral pruritus: 17% Gastrointestinal: 3.7% Respiratory: 0.9% Cutaneous: 0.8% Multisystem: 5.5% Epinephrine: 6 reactions in 4 subjects

*Success rate is defined as the ability to ingest the significant amount of food on a regular basis for at least 6 months (desensitized state).

Table 17.4 Modified allergen immunotherapy for food allergy

Therapy	Mechanism of action	Effects	Comments
Engineered recombinant peanut immunotherapy	Binding to mast cells eliminated or markedly decreased; T-cell responses comparable to native peanut allergens	Protection against peanut anaphylaxis in mice	Improved safety profile compared with conventional immunotherapy; requires identification of IgE-binding sites
Heat-killed bacteria mixed with or containing modified peanut proteins	Upregulation of Th1 and T-regulatory cytokine responses	Protection against peanut anaphylaxis in mice, lasting up to 10 weeks after treatment	Concern for toxicity of bacterial adjuvants, excessive Th1 stimulation, and potential for autoimmunity; heat-killed *E. coli* expressing modified peanut allergens administered rectally viewed as the safest approach for future human studies
Peptide immunotherapy*	Overlapping peptides (10–20 amino-acid long) that represent the entire sequence of allergen. Binding to mast cells eliminated; T-cell responses preserved	Protection against peanut anaphylaxis in mice	Improved safety profile compared with conventional immunotherapy; does not require identification of IgE-binding epitopes
Plasmid DNA-based immunotherapy*	Induces prolonged humoral and cellular responses due to CpG motifs in the DNA backbone	Protection against peanut anaphylaxis in sensitized AKR/J mice, but induction of anaphylaxis in C3H/HeJ (H-2^K) mice; no effect on peanut-IgE antibody levels	Serious concerns regarding safety in view of strain-dependent effects in mice; concern for excessive Th1 stimulation and autoimmunity
Immunostimulatory sequences (ISS-ODN)*	Potent stimulation of Th1 via activation of antigen-presenting cells, natural killer cells and B cells; increased Th1 cytokines	Protection against peanut sensitization in mice	Not shown to reverse established peanut allergy; concern for excessive Th1 stimulation and potential for autoimmunity

*These approaches are currently no longer actively investigated.

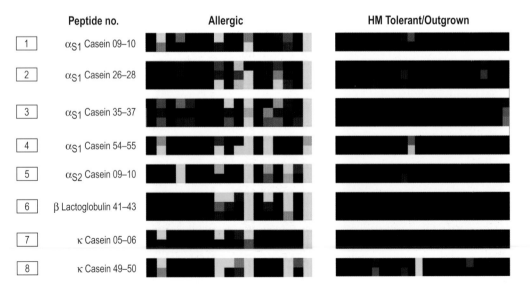

Figure 17.1 Heat map of IgE binding to candidates of informative epitopes of cows' milk peptides. (Figure courtesy of Dr. Julie Wang from the Mount Sinai School of Medicine, New York)

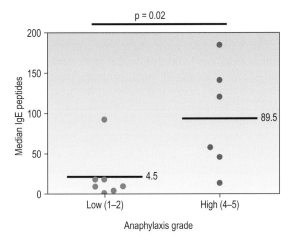

p = 0.02

89.5

4.5

Low (1–2) High (4–5)

Anaphylaxis grade

Median IgE peptides

Figure 17.2 IgE peptide-binding frequency correlated with severity of reaction during milk challenge. (Figure courtesy of Dr. Julie Wang from the Mount Sinai School of Medicine, New York)

challenges at the time of initial screening, and the threshold dose of peanut protein necessary to elicit objective symptoms was established. Subjects were randomized to either humanized monoclonal antibody TNX-901 (150, 300 or 450 mg) or placebo subcutaneously every 4 weeks for four doses. They underwent a second oral peanut challenge within 2–4 weeks following the fourth dose. The mean baseline sensitivity threshold (i.e. the amount of peanut flour that elicited objective symptoms and resulted in discontinuation of the food challenge) tended to increase in anti-IgE-treated groups, with an apparent dose response, but was statistically significant only in the highest anti-IgE dose (450 mg) group. In this group, the sensitivity threshold increased from a dose equal to approximately one half of a peanut kernel (178 mg) to a dose equal to almost nine peanut kernels (2805 mg). However, approximately 25% of subjects treated with the highest dose of TNX-901 showed no change in their sensitivity threshold. A controlled trial of a different anti-IgE humanized IgG_1 antibody (omalizumab) in children over 6 years of age with peanut anaphylaxis was initiated, but this research study was discontinued prematurely because of safety concerns related to severe anaphylactic reactions that occurred during the initial screening peanut challenge.

Combined treatment with anti-IgE and specific food allergen oral immunotherapy has also been considered because of the potential ability of anti-IgE therapy to reduce the life-threatening side effects of specific food allergen oral immunotherapy. Evaluation of this type of combination therapy has been investigated with environmental aeroallergens, but has not yet been fully assessed for food allergens. There is an ongoing study in children and adults with milk allergy.[13]

Traditional Chinese medicine (TCM)

Herbal remedies have been used in traditional Chinese medicine for centuries, albeit not for food allergies, and are reported to be effective, safe and affordable. The mechanism of action of TCM is largely unknown and it has not been evaluated in randomized clinical trials. Li and colleagues[14] have conducted the majority of work that has provided insights into the mechanism of TCM in food allergy. Food allergy herbal formula-1 (FAHF-1), a mixture of 11 herbs, was extensively tested in a mouse model of peanut allergy. Mouse models were pivotal in the initial stages of development of novel therapies for food allergy because human studies were considered unsafe owing to the risk of anaphylaxis. Mouse models of peanut allergy mimic human peanut allergy in terms of the oral route of sensitization, symptoms of anaphylaxis following ingestion, generation of peanut-specific IgE antibodies, and release of allergic mediators during the challenge test. FAHF-1 protected peanut-allergic mice against peanut-induced anaphylaxis, and reduced mast cell degranulation and histamine release. Peanut-specific serum IgE levels decreased significantly following 2 weeks of treatment, and remained lower 4 weeks after discontinuation of treatment. FAHF-1 reduced peanut-induced lymphocyte proliferation as well as the production of the pro-allergic interleukins (IL)-4, IL-5 and IL-13, but not interferon-γ (that is protective against allergy) synthesis. FAHF-1 had no observable toxic effects on the liver or kidneys.

A modified formula, FAHF-2, composed of nine herbs, completely blocked anaphylaxis to peanut challenge up to 5 months following therapy in mice.[15] This therapeutic effect was largely mediated by CD8+ T cells that produced interferon-γ.[16,17] Examination of the individual herbs revealed that each had some protective effect, but none of them offered equivalent protection from anaphylaxis compared with the complete FAHF-2 mixture. A phase I clinical safety trial in adults aged 12–45 years with peanut and tree nut allergy was recently completed. FAHF-2 was found to be safe and well tolerated.[18] A phase II efficacy trial is currently enrolling subjects aged 12–45 years with peanut, tree nut, sesame, fish or shellfish allergy. FAHF-2 is an example of allergen-non-specific treatment and is expected to exert a similar protective effect against a variety of foods. In parallel with the clinical trials, the individual active substances in each herb are being identified, their mechanism of action characterized, and their potency standardized.

Treatment with *Lactococcus lactis* expressing IL-10

Probiotic bacteria and IL-10 are presumed to play a role in the induction and maintenance of oral tolerance in the gut. *Lactococcus lactis* was transfected to secrete murine IL-10 and then given to young mice prior to oral sensitization with β-lactoglobulin (whey protein) in the presence of cholera toxin (adjuvant).[19] Symptom scores during oral challenge and serum and fecal antigen-specific antibody concentrations were measured. Antibody titers were correlated with IL-10-secreting cell numbers in the spleen and Peyers' patches. Pretreatment with *Lactococcus lactis* transfected with IL-10 diminished anaphylaxis severity and reduced β-lactoglobulin-specific serum IgE and IgG$_1$ concentrations. It also increased the production of β-lactoglobulin-specific IgA in the gut. *Lactococcus lactis* transfected with IL-10 induced IL-10 secretion in Peyers' patches in the gut and increased plasma IL-10 titers. These results suggested that a probiotic bacteria engineered to deliver IL-10 in the gut may be able to reduce food-induced anaphylaxis and provide a clinical treatment option to prevent IgE sensitization in food allergy.

Anti-IL-5 antibody (mepolizumab) in eosinophilic esophagitis

Eosinophilic esophagitis (EoE) is being increasingly diagnosed in both children and adults. EoE is a disorder of mixed pathophysiology, with both IgE- and non-IgE-mediated mechanisms involved. Although at least a subset of subjects with EoE are responsive to food elimination, available diagnostic tests do not reliably identify the triggering food allergens. Based on the pivotal role of IL-5 in the accumulation of eosinophils in the esophageal tissue, treatment with a monoclonal anti-IL-5 antibody was proposed. The results of a randomized placebo-controlled double-blinded trial of anti-IL-5

antibody (mepolizumab) in eosinophilic esophagitis were recently published.[20] Eleven adults with active EoE (>20 peak eosinophil number/high power field (hpf) and dysphagia) were randomized to receive 750 mg of mepolizumab (n = 5) or placebo (n = 6) as two intravenous infusions, 1 week apart. Those not in complete remission (<5 peak eosinophil number/hpf) after 8 weeks received two further doses 4 weeks apart, 1500 mg of mepolizumab or placebo. A marked reduction of mean esophageal eosinophilia (p = 0.03) was seen in the mepolizumab group (−54%) compared to the placebo group (−5%) 4 weeks after initiation of treatment. No further reduction of eosinophil numbers was observed in response to the two additional infusions in either group. Mepolizumab reduced tenascin C (p = 0.033) and TGF-β$_1$ (p = 0.05) expression in the esophageal epithelial layer 13 weeks after initiation of treatment. Limited improvement of clinical symptoms was seen, although a trend was seen between 4 and 13 weeks after initiating mepolizumab treatment. Mepolizumab was well tolerated and had an acceptable safety profile, even at the high 1500-mg dose level. Currently mepolizumab is being evaluated in children with EoE.

Diet containing extensively heated cows' milk and egg

Two large clinical trials investigated the tolerance of extensively heated (baked into other products) milk and egg in children with milk and egg allergy.[21,22] Previous studies have determined that children with transient egg allergy generated IgE antibodies directed primarily against conformational epitopes of ovomucoid (the major allergen in the egg white) that are destroyed during extensive heating or food processing.[6] In contrast, children with persistent egg allergy also generated IgE antibodies directed against sequential epitopes of ovomucoid that were preserved during heating or food processing. Similarly, children with persistent milk allergy generated IgE antibodies directed against specific sequential epitopes on milk major allergens.[7] Those observations suggested that at least a subset of children with less persistent milk and egg allergy might tolerate baked products containing milk and egg. In each study, over 80% of children tolerated milk or egg baked into muffins and waffles during an initial oral challenge, and

CLINICAL VIGNETTE 1

A 9-year-old girl tolerated a physician-supervised oral challenge with a muffin containing milk (~one-sixth of a cup of milk baked in an oven at 350° F for 30 minutes). She was advised to add similar extensively baked products with milk to her diet. She returned at 6 months for a feeding test with pizza and developed a mild scratchy throat and rhinorrhea within 10 minutes of 50% of the pizza serving. She continued to ingest extensively baked milk products without any problems, but reported mild facial hives and sneezing with small amounts of butter and unbaked cheese. At 12 months she tolerated the entire pizza serving without any symptoms. She added pizza to her diet up to three times per week. Twelve months later she passed an oral challenge with unheated milk and added milk and all dairy products to her diet at home.

CLINICAL VIGNETTE 2

A 7-year-old boy underwent a physician-supervised oral food challenge to a muffin containing milk. Within 10 minutes of ingesting 10% of the muffin he developed sneezing, facial flushing, diffuse urticaria, cough and mild wheezing. He was treated with intramuscular epinephrine and oral antihistamine. He was advised to strictly avoid all forms of milk in his diet. He returned for a repeat oral challenge at the age of 9 years and again reacted to a muffin. This time he developed a few hives on his face and a scratchy throat following the ingestion of 50% of the muffin. He was advised to continue strictly avoiding all forms of milk in his diet. He subsequently reported accidental ingestions of small amounts of cheese and yogurt that induced mild allergic reactions.

CLINICAL VIGNETTE 3

A 4-year-old asthmatic boy underwent a physician-supervised oral challenge to a muffin containing 1/3 of a whole egg (equivalent to 2.2 g egg white protein) baked at 350°F for 30 minutes. He tolerated the entire feeding without any symptoms and added similar extensively heated egg products to his diet at home. Three months after a challenge to baked egg, he accidentally licked a spoon with cake batter that contained raw egg. Within 5 minutes he developed facial hives, a hacking cough, difficulty breathing and wheezing. He was treated with an epinephrine autoinjector and oral antihistamine at home and then with nebulized albuterol, oxygen and intravenous methylprednisolone in the emergency department. He was discharged home after 4 hours' observation and continued to ingest extensively heated egg products while strictly avoiding unbaked egg in his diet.

added these foods to their diet at home (Clinical Vignette 1). Children were being followed every 3–6 months and tolerated the diet well; they had no increase in acute allergic reactions and no increase in the severity of underlying atopic diseases such as asthma, atopic dermatitis or eczema. There was no increase in the intestinal permeability of a carbohydrate marker over the first year on the diet, and children continued to grow well. Commercially available tests for food-specific IgE levels did not reliably identify subjects tolerant to extensively heated milk and egg, and the physician-supervised oral food challenge was necessary. However, in the milk study the majority of children who reacted to extensively heated milk had milk-specific IgE antibody levels >35 kU$_A$/L (UniCAP, Phadia), and therefore in a subsequent study subjects with milk-specific IgE antibody levels >35 kU$_A$/L were excluded. Children allergic to extensively heated milk had significantly higher basophil reactivity to stimulation with milk protein (casein) than the children tolerant to extensively heated milk.[23] Children tolerant to unheated milk had the lowest basophil reactivity to milk. In the milk study, severe reactions that required treatment with epinephrine occurred only in children who reacted to the extensively heated milk products (Clinical Vignette 2). All children who tolerated the extensively heated milk and subsequently reacted to unheated milk had mild reactions; none was treated with epinephrine. Tolerance to extensively heated milk products appears to be a marker of a mild milk allergy that is likely to be outgrown. In contrast, in the egg study there were equal proportions of children who received epinephrine during the heated and unheated egg challenges (Clinical Vignette 3).

The immunologic changes observed during the ingestion of baked goods with milk and egg included increasing food-specific IgG$_4$ antibodies, decreasing wheal sizes from skin prick tests, and a trend for decreasing food-specific IgE antibodies. There was a significantly higher percentage of proliferating allergen-specific regulatory T lymphocytes from milk protein-induced peripheral blood mononuclear cell cultures in extensively heated milk-tolerant children compared to children with allergy.[24] Control children with no history of milk allergy also had low percentages of these regulatory cells, whereas children who had outgrown their milk allergy (n = 7) had intermediate percentages. Casein-specific regulatory T cells were found to be FoxP3(+); a higher frequency of casein-specific regulatory T cells correlated with mild clinical disease and favorable prognosis.

These findings suggest that large subsets of children with milk and egg allergy may expand their diets to include extensively heated products. Furthermore, the immunologic changes induced by the diet containing baked milk and egg products parallel the changes observed during oral immunotherapy trials. Taken together, these data suggest that tolerance to extensively heated milk and egg might identify subjects with a favorable prognosis. The diet containing extensively heated milk and egg could represent a safer and more 'natural' approach to food oral immunotherapy. Follow-up studies are ongoing to establish the overall safety and efficacy of this method. Until reliable biomarkers of tolerance to extensively heated milk and egg are established, the decision to attempt the introduction of heated milk or egg needs to be carefully evaluated and introduction conducted under physician supervision.

Allergen-specific immunotherapy

Immunotherapy involves the administration of allergens with or without adjuvants that modulate the immune responses away from Th2 pro-allergic responses. In traditional allergen-specific immunotherapy, the dose escalation (also referred to as build-up phase) may by 'rushed' over one to a few days (typically done in the hospital) or may last 4–6 months (typically in an office setting). The maintenance phase begins when the highest dose has been reached. Maintenance dosing is continued for extended periods; in subcutaneous allergen immunotherapy, maintenance dosing is administered in an office setting; in oral and sublingual immunotherapy, maintenance dosing is typically administered at home. Allergen-specific immunotherapy may be carried out with native food proteins or with recombinant, engineered food proteins that have been genetically modified to reduce allergenicity.

Subcutaneous peanut immunotherapy

The evidence that immunotherapy may induce desensitization to a food allergen was provided by two controlled studies that evaluated subcutaneous immunotherapy with peanut extract. In the initial study, three treated subjects displayed a 67–100% decrease in symptoms during double-blind placebo-controlled food challenges and had a 2–5-log reduction in end-point skin prick test reactivity to peanut.[25] One placebo-treated subject completed the study and had no change in double-blind placebo-controlled oral food challenge symptoms or skin prick test sensitivity to peanut.

In a follow-up study of 12 subjects, six were treated with a maintenance dose of 0.5 mL 1 : 100 w/v peanut extract.[26] All treated subjects were able to ingest increased quantities of peanut during oral food challenges and had decreased sensitivity on titrated peanut skin prick test, whereas untreated controls experienced no similar changes. However, anaphylaxis with respiratory involvement occurred a mean of 7.7 times during 12 months of maintenance peanut immunotherapy, with an average of 9.8 epinephrine injections per study subject. Only three of six subjects were able to achieve the intended maintenance dose due to adverse events. This important study demonstrated that injected food allergens could be successfully used to induce desensitization, but the significant risk for anaphylaxis prevented this treatment from being further evaluated in clinical studies.

Birch pollen immunotherapy for the pollen–food allergy syndrome

Pollen-allergic individuals may develop oropharyngeal pruritus from the ingestion of raw plant foods (fruits, vegetables) that contain proteins homologous to the pollen proteins. The classic pollen–food allergy syndrome (PFAS or oral allergy syndrome) is due to sensitization to the birch pollen major allergen Bet v 1, resulting in local oropharyngeal symptoms from contact with the homologous apple protein Mal d 1. Subcutaneous immunotherapy (SCIT) is an established treatment for pollen-induced allergic rhinitis and theoretically could be beneficial for PFAS. An open trial of birch pollen SCIT in 49 adults with birch pollinosis and oral symptoms provoked by apple reported a significant reduction (50–95%) or complete resolution of apple-induced oral allergy symptoms (p < 0. 001) in 41 subjects (84%), compared to no controls.[27] Birch pollen immunotherapy induced a marked reduction in skin test reactivity to fresh apple in 43 subjects (88%). In a follow-up study, the duration of effect of birch pollen immunotherapy was evaluated in 30 birch pollen-allergic subjects who experienced resolution of apple-induced oral allergy symptoms and loss of skin test reactivity to fresh apple.[28] Symptoms and skin test reactivity were compared following the 12-month immunotherapy course and 30 months after immunotherapy was discontinued. Over 50% of subjects still tolerated apple at the 30-month follow-up visit, although the majority showed a return of pretreatment sensitization on skin prick testing. Subsequent clinical trials, in which oral allergy symptoms to apple were diagnosed with double-blind placebo-controlled food challenges, confirmed a beneficial effect of birch immunotherapy in some subjects.[29,30] Similar observations were reported from an observational study of 16 adults suffering from PFAS (hazelnut, walnut, lettuce, peach and cherry) and plane tree pollinosis who were treated with plane tree pollen immunotherapy.[31] The mean quantity of food necessary to provoke objective symptoms increased from 2.2 to 13.7 g (p < 0.05), and six of 11 subjects tolerated the highest amount (25 g) of the challenge food following treatment.

One explanation for the variable effects of pollen immunotherapy may relate to the fact that for many subjects with PFAS, doses of immunotherapy higher than that typically required to induce improvement in seasonal birch pollen rhinitis may be necessary to improve birch-related PFAS. The most significant effects on PFAS were observed in the studies that included adults sensitized only to birch tree pollen. An alternative explanation is that the T-cell immune responses to birch pollen cross-reactive food allergens, such as apple Mal d 1, hazelnut Cor a 1 and carrot Dau c 1, are at least in part Bet v 1 independent. In that case, vaccines based on modified recombinant food allergens might represent a superior approach to the treatment of PFAS. Of note, a few case reports have highlighted the possibility of developing allergy to cross-reactive food allergens in the course of immunotherapy for the environmental allergens, such as the development of allergic reactions to snails during immunotherapy to dust mites, or to raw fruits during immunotherapy to pollens.

Oral immunotherapy

The first successful oral immunotherapy was reported in the early 20th century in a boy with anaphylactic egg allergy.[32] Following a long hiatus, oral immunotherapy to food has been revisited and is the subject of many current research studies. The oral route of administration utilizes cells and immune pathways involved in the induction of oral tolerance. Animal studies suggest that feeding high doses of an antigen results in a state of non-responsiveness due to anergy or deletion of antigen-specific T cells, whereas continuous ingestion of antigen in low doses induces suppressive responses due to the development of regulatory T cells.[3,33] In contrast, intermittent feedings or non-oral exposures (e.g. cutaneous or inhalational) may induce IgE sensitization and allergic symptoms upon food ingestion.[34,35]

'Desensitization' is different from permanent oral 'tolerance'. In a desensitized state, the protective effect depends on daily uninterrupted exposure to the allergen, e.g. food, drug, pollen. However, when the dosing is interrupted, the protective effect may be lost or significantly decreased. In the desensitized state, factors that increase intestinal permeability, such as exercise, viral gastroenteritis, stress or menses, may result in a reaction to a previously tolerated dose, even when the maintenance dose has been achieved. Possible mechanisms responsible for oral desensitization include increased food-specific IgG_4, decreased food-specific IgE antibodies, and decreased reactivity of mast cells and basophils. In contrast, when permanent oral tolerance is established, the food may be ingested without allergic symptoms despite prolonged periods of abstinence. The mechanism of persistent tolerance probably involves the initial development of regulatory T cells and immunologic deviation away from the pro-allergic Th2 response, and later anergy. The permanence of protection may be tested with intentional interruption of dosing for at least 4–8 weeks followed by a supervised oral food challenge.

Oral immunotherapy trials

During oral immunotherapy, food is mixed in a vehicle and ingested in gradually increasing doses. The dose escalation occurs in a controlled setting; regular ingestion of tolerated doses during the build-up phase and a maintenance (or maximal tolerated) dose occurs at home. Early case series and uncontrolled trials provided evidence that a subset of food-allergic subjects could be 'desensitized' to a variety of foods, including milk, egg, fish, fruit, peanut and celery.[35–38] Those studies did not distinguish the effects of oral desensitization from the natural resolution of food allergy and did not evaluate the permanency of the desensitized state. In some subjects who ultimately tolerated a maintenance dose, even for a significant period, allergic symptoms recurred if the food was not ingested on a regular basis, highlighting a concern that permanent tolerance was not achieved.[39] In the first randomized trial of oral immunotherapy, children with challenge-proven IgE-mediated cows' milk allergy or hen's egg allergy were randomly assigned to oral immunotherapy or elimination diet as a control group.[40] The oral treatment was performed with fresh cows' milk or lyophilized hen's egg protein at home on a daily basis according to a study protocol. Children were re-evaluated by food challenge after a median of 21 months. Children in the oral immunotherapy group were subsequently placed on an elimination diet for 2 months prior to a follow-up rechallenge to determine whether oral tolerance had developed. At the follow-up challenge, nine of 25 children (36%) in the oral immunotherapy group showed permanent tolerance, three of 25 (12%) were tolerant with regular intake, and four of 25 (16%) were partial responders. In the control group, seven of 20 children (35%) also developed tolerance over the study period. Allergen-specific IgE decreased significantly in children who developed natural tolerance during the elimination diet ($p < 0.05$) and in those treated with oral immunotherapy ($p < 0.001$). Although the rate of permanent tolerance was not different between the groups, some children treated with oral immunotherapy were tolerant with regular intake and some were tolerant to a smaller maintenance dose (desensitized) and were protected from inadvertent exposures as they continued to ingest the daily dose of the food in question.

In the first randomized placebo-controlled trial of oral immunotherapy, 20 children with IgE-mediated milk allergy were randomized to milk or placebo (2:1 ratio).[41,42] Dosing occurred in three phases: the build-up in-office day (initial dose 0.4 mg of milk protein; final dose 50 mg), daily doses with eight weekly in-office dose increases to a maximum of 500 mg, and continued home daily maintenance doses for 3–4 months. Double-blind placebo-controlled food challenges, end-point titration skin prick tests and serologic studies were performed before and after oral immunotherapy. Nineteen patients, 6–17 years of age, completed the treatment, 12 in the active group and seven in the placebo group. The median milk threshold dose in both groups was 40 mg at the baseline challenge. After oral immunotherapy the median threshold dose inducing a reaction in the active treatment group was 5140 mg (range 2540–8140 mg), whereas all patients in the placebo group reacted at 40 mg ($p = 0.0003$). Among 2437 active doses and 1193 placebo doses, there were 1107 (45.4%) and 134 (11.2%) total reactions, respectively, with local symptoms being most common (see Table 17.3). Milk-specific IgE levels did not change significantly in either group. Milk-IgG levels increased significantly in the active treatment group, with a predominant increase in milk-IgG_4 level.

The safety and efficacy of oral immunotherapy for children with severe cows' milk protein-induced anaphylaxis was studied in 60 children with a history of severe milk-induced anaphylaxis and milk-specific IgE > 85 kU_A/L, who reacted to ≤0.8 mL of milk during a baseline milk challenge.[43] Thirty children were randomized to oral immunotherapy with a 10-day rush phase including three to 10 daily doses up to 20 mL of undiluted milk in the hospital and a slow dose escalation phase at home (increasing by 1 mL every second day). The remaining 30 children were randomized to continue on a milk-free diet and were followed for 1 year. After 1 year, 11 (36%) of 30 subjects in the oral immunotherapy group were able to ingest a daily dose of milk ≥150 mL, 16 (54%) were able to ingest from 5 mL to <150 mL. Three children (10%) were unable to complete the study because of the ongoing adverse reactions. In the comparison group, all 30 children reacted to less than 5 mL of milk during the repeated oral food challenge at 12 months. Adverse reactions, including systemic reactions, were common in both groups, but no child had severe anaphylaxis. During the rush phase, intramuscular epinephrine was administered four times in four children. During the home phase, two children required treatment including epinephrine in the emergency department.

Peanut oral immunotherapy

Peanut oral immunotherapy trials conducted in young children with peanut allergy have received significant attention.[44,45] In a US study, 39 subjects were enrolled (64% male), median age was 57.5 months (range 12–111 months).[43] All children completed the initial day escalation phase during which the starting dose of 0.1 mg peanut protein was doubled every 30 minutes, up to 50 mg. During the build-up phase, children ingested peanut flour with other safe foods every day. Doses were increased by 25 mg every 2 weeks until 300 mg was reached. During the maintenance phase, the dose of 300 mg was continued daily until the follow-up food challenge was performed. Following the food challenge, the daily dose was increased to 1800 mg. Children were evaluated every 4 months while on continued maintenance dosing: a total of 36 months. Ten (25%) children withdrew following the initial day escalation phase. Six discontinued for personal reasons, including transportation issues, parental anxiety, and failure to perform home dosing. These six had reactions during the initial escalation day of similar severity to the children who continued in the study. The remaining four children discontinued because of allergic reactions to the therapy that did not resolve with continued treatment or dose reduction. Three had gastrointestinal complaints and one had symptoms of asthma. Twenty-nine subjects completed all three phases of the study and peanut challenges.

During the initial day escalation, 36 patients (92%) experienced some symptoms; most common were upper respiratory symptoms, with 27 patients (69%) reporting mild sneezing/itching and mild laryngeal symptoms. No patients experienced severe upper respiratory or laryngeal symptoms. Seventeen patients (44%) reported mild to moderate nausea or abdominal pain, and eight (21%) had diarrhea/emesis. Twenty-four subjects (62%) had mild or moderate skin symptoms. Six patients (three with a history of asthma) experienced chest symptoms during the initial escalation day; four had mild wheezing and two had moderate wheezing. During the final food challenge, 27 of the 29 children who completed the protocol ingested 3.9 g peanut flour. By 6 months, titrated skin prick tests and activation of basophils had decreased significantly. Peanut-specific IgE antibody concentrations decreased by 12–18 months, whereas peanut-specific IgG_4 increased significantly. Serum factors inhibited IgE-peanut complex formation in an IgE-facilitated allergen binding assay. Secretion of the cytokines IL-10, IL-5, IFN-γ and TNF-α from peripheral blood mononuclear cells increased over a period of 6–12 months. Peanut-specific regulatory T cells increased until 12 months and decreased thereafter. In addition, T-cell microarrays showed downregulation of genes involved in the apoptotic pathways.

Safety of oral immunotherapy home dosing

During the initial escalation, the risk of mild wheezing was 18%.[44,46] The probability of any symptoms following the build-up phase dose was 46%, with a risk of 29% for upper respiratory tract and 24% for skin symptoms. The risk of an adverse reaction with any home dose was 3.5%; upper respiratory tract (1.2%) and skin (1.1%) symptoms. Treatment was given for 0.7% of home doses. Two subjects received epinephrine after one home dose each. Allergic reactions during home dosing were more common in the milk oral immunotherapy, from 2.55% to 96.4% of doses per subject in the first 3 months compared to 0–79.8% in the subsequent 3 months.[42] Local and multisystem reactions decreased, whereas all other reactions remained unchanged during the latter part of therapy. Several systemic reactions occurred at previously tolerated doses in the setting of exercise or viral illness. As highlighted by a recent paper from the Burks group, the risk of an allergic reaction to a previously tolerated dose of food is associated with physical exertion after dosing, dosing on an empty stomach, dosing during menses, concurrent febrile illness, and suboptimally controlled asthma[41,44,47] (Table 17.3).

Sublingual immunotherapy

Another approach to desensitization or possibly induction of tolerance is sublingual immunotherapy (SLIT) with food allergens. An initial case report described modified SLIT with fresh kiwi pulp extract in a 29-year-old woman with a history of kiwi-induced anaphylaxis.[48] The extract or kiwi cube was kept under the tongue for 1 minute before swallowing. There was a decrease in IgE reactivity to the major kiwi allergen Act c 1 (30 kDa) in Western blots with kiwi extract. Five years into kiwi modified SLIT, treatment was interrupted for 4 months and then resumed without any problems.[49]

Subsequently, a randomized double-blind placebo-controlled trial of SLIT was conducted for the treatment of hazelnut allergy.[50] Adults with hazelnut allergy (54.5% with a history of oral allergy symptoms) confirmed by double-blind placebo-controlled food challenge were randomly assigned to hazelnut immunotherapy (n = 12) or placebo (n = 11). Subjects kept the hazelnut extract solution in the mouth for at least 3 minutes and then spat it out. All subjects receiving hazelnut immunotherapy reached the planned maximum dose with a 4-day rush protocol, followed by a daily maintenance dose (containing 188.2 μg of Cor a 1 and 121.9 μg of Cor a 8, major hazelnut allergens). Systemic reactions were observed in 0.2% of the total doses administered, were limited to the rush build-up phase, and were treated successfully with oral antihistamines. Local reactions, mainly immediate oral pruritus, were observed in 7.4% (109 reactions/1466 doses). Four patients in the active group reported abdominal pain several hours after dosing on one occasion each, and only during the build-up phase. All local reactions during the maintenance phase were limited to oral pruritus and occurred in only one patient. After 5 months of SLIT, the mean threshold dose of ingested hazelnut provoking allergic symptoms increased from 2.3 g to 11.6 g in the active group (p = 0.02) compared to 3.5 g to 4.1 g in placebo (NS). Almost 50% of treated subjects tolerated the highest dose (20 g) of hazelnut during follow-up double-blind placebo-controlled food challenges, compared to 9% in the placebo group. Levels of serum hazelnut-specific IgG$_4$ antibody and total serum IL-10 increased only in the active group, but there were no differences in hazelnut-specific IgE antibody levels before and after immunotherapy.

Another study evaluated SLIT in eight children with cows' milk allergy.[51] One day after an initial positive oral milk challenge, children started SLIT with 0.1 mL of milk for the first 2 weeks, increasing by 0.1 mL every 15 days until 1 mL/day was given. Milk was kept in the mouth for 2 minutes and then spat out. Seven subjects completed the protocol; one withdrew because of oral symptoms. After 6 months of treatment the threshold dose of milk increased from a mean of 39 mL at baseline to 143 mL (p < 0.01).

Recently, a randomized double-blind placebo-controlled trial of SLIT with a Pru p 3 (major peach allergen) quantified peach extract was reported.[52] The efficacy of SLIT was evaluated by determining the fold increase in dose inducing local symptoms or systemic symptoms during a double-blind placebo-controlled oral peach challenge following 6 months of SLIT with a maintenance dose of 50 μg Pru p 3. In the SLIT-treated subjects (n = 37) the doses of Pru p 3 needed to induce local reactions (usually oral pruritus) were nine times higher, and to induce systemic reactions (usually transient gastrointestinal discomfort or mild rhinitis) were three times higher than pre-SLIT doses after 6 months of SLIT. In contrast, the placebo-treated subjects had no significant changes in the doses of Pru p 3 inducing symptoms at baseline and after 6 months. Specific IgE to rPru p 3 increased in both the active (p < 0.001) and the placebo (p = 0.025) groups, although the increase remained only significant at 6 months in the active group (active 4.23, p < 0.001; placebo 4.04, p = 0.079, t-test). IgG$_4$ to nPru p 3 increased significantly in the active group (p = 0.007) but not in the placebo group (p = 0.185).[48] Peach SLIT was reportedly well tolerated.

Preliminary data on oral immunotherapy and SLIT are encouraging; however, at present these treatments are considered experimental. Additional studies must answer many questions, including optimal dose, ideal duration of immunotherapy, degree of protection, efficacy for different ages, severity and type of food allergies responsive to treatment, and the need for patient protection during home administration. In view of the recent reports of reactions to the tolerated doses of oral immunotherapy at home, it may be necessary to hold doses during acute febrile illness, avoid exercise within 2 hours of dosing, and take the daily dose with a meal or snack.[47] Rhinitis and asthma should be maintained under optimal control. Finally, since a subset of children with food allergies develops tolerance spontaneously, the future studies must address diagnostic tests that would distinguish between transient and persistent food allergies to identify those who will benefit from therapy.

Epicutaneous immunotherapy (EPIT)

An alternative delivery route of IT has been explored using epicutaneous patches. A placebo-controlled double-blind trial in 37 adults allergic to grass pollen reported significantly decreased scores in nasal provocation tests in the first (p < 0.001) and second years (p = 0.003) following treatment.[53] There were no severe adverse events but local eczema under the patch applications was common. EPIT was safe and well tolerated. A proof of concept study on the efficacy of EPIT on intact skin in mice sensitized to aeroallergens or food allergens was carried out.[54] In mice sensitized to pollen, house dust mite, ovalbumin and peanut, EPIT was as efficacious as subcutaneous immunotherapy, considered as the reference immunotherapy.

In a pilot study, 18 children (mean age 3.8 years, range 10 months to 7.7 years) with cows' milk allergy were randomized 1:1 to receive active EPIT or placebo.[55] Cows' milk allergy was confirmed by a supervised oral challenge at baseline and the cumulative tolerated dose of milk was established. Children received three 48-hour applications (1 mg skimmed milk powder or 1 mg glucose as placebo) via the skin patch per week for 3 months. EPIT-treated children showed a trend toward increased cumulative tolerated dose at the follow-up oral milk challenge following 3 months of EPIT, from a mean 1.8 mL at baseline to 23.6 mL at 3 months. The mean cumulative tolerated dose in the placebo-treated group did not change. There were no significant changes in cows' milk-specific IgE levels from baseline to 3 months in either group. The most common side effects were local pruritus and eczema at the site of application. There were no severe systemic adverse reactions, but one subject in the active group had repeated episodes of diarrhea following EPIT with milk. Reports from earlier mouse studies have demonstrated increased potential for the development of IgE sensitization to peanut via the epicutaneous route compared to ingestion, raising concerns as to whether epicutaneous delivery might worsen food allergy. It is impossible to fully understand the effect of EPIT on milk allergy from this small pilot study, owing to the small sample size and the short duration of the study, as well as limited information about immunologic parameters. However, this preliminary report suggests that further investigation of the novel epicutaneous antigen delivery for food allergy immunotherapy is warranted.

Immunotherapy with modified recombinant engineered food proteins

Modification of the IgE antibody-binding sites (epitopes) that reduces IgE antibody binding to an allergen is one approach to reducing the risk of an allergic reaction during immunotherapy. Point mutations introduced by site-directed mutagenesis in the known IgE epitopes of major food allergens or polymerization of proteins result in decreased IgE binding during immunotherapy. The in vivo efficacy of engineered recombinant peanut proteins was tested in peanut-allergic mice,[56,57] which were sensitized to whole peanut and then desensitized by intranasal administration of engineered recombinant Ara h 2 (three doses per week for 4 weeks). Desensitization with the modified (engineered recombinant) Ara h 2 protein suppressed synthesis of Ara h 2-specific IgE and significantly reduced the severity of anaphylactic reactions following oral peanut challenge compared to a control group (Table 17.4). Modified food allergens were combined with heat-killed *Listeria monocytogenes* as bacterial adjuvants to further reduce food-specific IgE production.[58] In subsequent studies a nonpathogenic strain of *E. coli* was used as an adjuvant delivered orally and rectally. Oral delivery was not effective, probably due to breakdown of the peanut-containing *E. coli*. Peanut-allergic mice received 0.9 (low dose), 9 (medium dose), or 90 (high dose) μg of heat-killed *E. coli* expressing modified proteins Ara h 1–3 (HKE-MP123) per rectum, HKE-containing vector (HKE-V) alone, or vehicle alone (sham) weekly for 3 weeks.[59] Mice were challenged with peanut 2 weeks after the final vaccine dose, and then at monthly intervals for 2 more months. After the first peanut challenge, all three doses of HKE-MP123- and the HKE-V-treated groups had reduced severity of anaphylaxis ($p < 0.01$, 0.01, 0.05, 0.05, respectively) compared to the sham-treated group. However, only the medium- and high-dose HKE-MP123-treated mice remained protected for up to 10 weeks following treatment. Peanut-specific IgE levels were significantly lower in all HKE-MP123-treated groups ($p < 0.001$); they were most reduced in the high-dose HKE-MP123-treated group at the time of each challenge. Mice treated with the high-dose HKE-MP123 produced in vitro significantly less IL-4, IL-13, IL-5 and IL-10 ($p < 0.01$, 0.001, 0.001, and 0.001, respectively) upon peanut stimulation. IFN-γ and TGF-β production were significantly increased ($p < 0.001$ and 0.01, respectively) compared to sham-treated mice at the time of the last challenge. A phase I clinical safety study is currently enrolling adults with peanut allergy. In the future, probiotic bacteria might be used as adjuvants to avoid the concerns of excessive Th1 stimulation by killed pathogenic bacteria.[19]

Other approaches

Three additional immunomodulatory approaches to peanut allergy were evaluated in the animal studies but subsequently abandoned in favor of other treatments (Table 17.4). In peptide immuno-therapy, the vaccine consists of overlapping pep-tides (10–20 amino acids long) that represent the entire sequence of a specific protein. The antigen-presenting cells are provided with all possible T-cell epitopes, but mast cells are not activated because the short peptides are unable to cross-link two IgE molecules. Pretreatment with two doses of the major peanut protein Ara h 2 peptide mixture prior to peanut challenge was shown to prevent anaphy-lactic reactions in peanut-sensitized mice.[60] Peptide immunotherapy allows for the formulation of vac-cines against any food in which major allergenic proteins are known, because IgE-binding sites for each food protein do not have to be mapped. However, peptide immunotherapy is currently not feasible because the FDA requires quantification of each peptide within the mixture. It is possible that peptide immunotherapy will be revisited when the relevant epitopes for T cells on major peanut aller-gens are identified and the vaccine contains only the selected peptides that represent T-cell epitopes.

Immunization with bacterial plasmid DNA (pDNA) that encodes specific antigens can induce prolonged humoral and cellular immune Th1 responses, attributable to immunostimulatory sequences (ISSs) consisting of unmethylated cyto-sine and guanine motifs (CpG motifs) in the bacte-rial pDNA backbone. An early study found that the intramuscular immunization of naive AKR/J (H-2^K) and C3H/HeJ (H-2^K) mice with pDNA encoding Ara h 2 prior to intraperitoneal peanut sensitization had some protective effect in AKR/J mice, but induced anaphylactic reactions in C3H/HeN mice following peanut challenge.[61] In another study, oral chitosan-embedded Ara h 2 had a protective effect in AKR mice.[62] Li and colleagues (unpublished data) tested the therapeutic effect of pDNA-expressing Ara h 2 in peanut-allergic mice and found no reduction in peanut-IgE antibody levels. Taken together, these data indicate that pDNA-based immunotherapy may not be universally effective in reversing IgE-mediated hypersensitivity.

A different approach to DNA-based immunother-apy is based on the synthetic immunostimulatory oligodeoxynucleotides containing unmethylated CpG motifs (ISS). ISS-conjugated allergen adminis-tration was more effective than a mixture of antigen and ISS in the suppression of allergic airway responses, probably owing to the enhanced den-dritic cell uptake of ISS allergen. C3H/HeJ mice were immunized intradermally with ISS-linked Ara h 2, or ISS-linked major ragweed pollen allergen as a control.[63] Four weeks after immunization, mice were sensitized via the intragastric route with peanut and challenged with Ara h 2 5 weeks later. ISS-Ara h 2-treated mice did not develop symptoms and had significantly lower plasma histamine levels follow-ing oral challenge than the control-treated mice. Intradermal immunization with a mixture of ISS and β-galactosidase (β-gal), but not with ISS alone or β-gal alone, provided protection against fatal anaphylaxis induced by intraperitoneal β-gal sensi-tization and challenge, which was associated with an increase in IgG$_{2a}$/IFN-γ and a reduction in IgE/IL-4 and IL-5.[64] This effect was comparable to immu-nization with the pDNA-encoding β-gal. Therefore, antigen-ISS immunization may have a prophylactic effect against food allergy. However, the ability to reverse established food allergy remains to be determined.

Conclusions

Food allergy is an increasingly prevalent problem in westernized countries. The novel therapeutic approaches currently being evaluated in clinical trials include Chinese herbs, modified peanut vaccine, and oral and sublingual immunotherapy with peanut, milk and egg. Monoclonal anti-IgE antibody is being investigated in combination with milk oral immunotherapy. Diets containing exten-sively heated (baked) forms of milk or egg are toler-ated by about three quarters of children allergic to unheated milk or egg and might represent an alter-native approach to oral immunomodulation in food allergy.

References

1. Sicherer SH, Sampson HA. Food allergy: recent advances in pathophysiology and treatment. Annu Rev Med 2009;60:261–77.

2. Skripak JM, Sampson HA. Towards a cure for food allergy. Curr Opin Immunol 2008;20(6):690–6.

3. Scurlock AM, Burks AW, Jones SM. Oral immunotherapy for food allergy. Curr Allergy Asthma Rep 2009;9(3):186–93.

4. Shreffler WG, Beyer K, Chu TH, et al. Microarray immunoassay: association of clinical history, in vitro IgE function, and heterogeneity of allergenic peanut epitopes. J Allergy Clin Immunol 2004;113(4):776–82.

5. Flinterman AE, Knol EF, Lencer DA, et al. Peanut epitopes for IgE and IgG4 in peanut-sensitized children in relation to severity of peanut allergy. J Allergy Clin Immunol 2008;121(3):737–43.

6. Wang J, Lin J, Bardina L, et al. Correlation of IgE/IgG4 milk epitopes and affinity of milk-specific IgE antibodies with different phenotypes of clinical milk allergy. J Allergy Clin Immunol 2010;125(3):695–702.

7. Cooke SK, Sampson HA. Allergenic properties of ovomucoid in man. J Immunol 1997;159(4):2026–32.

8. Chatchatee P, Jarvinen KM, Bardina L, et al. Identification of IgE- and IgG-binding epitopes on alpha(s1)-casein: differences in patients with persistent and transient cows' milk allergy. J Allergy Clin Immunol 2001;107(2):379–83.

9. Savage JH, Matsui EC, Skripak JM, et al. The natural history of egg allergy. J Allergy Clin Immunol 2007;120(6):1413–7.

10. Skripak JM, Matsui EC, Mudd K, et al. The natural history of IgE-mediated cows' milk allergy. J Allergy Clin Immunol 2007;120(5):1172–7.

11. MacGlashan DWJ, Bochner BS, Adelman DC, et al. Down-regulation of Fc(epsilon)RI expression on human basophils during in vivo treatment of atopic patients with anti-IgE antibody. J Immunol 1997;158:1438–45.

12. Leung DY, Sampson HA, Yunginger JW, et al. Effect of anti-IgE therapy in patients with peanut allergy. N Engl J Med 2003;348(11):986–93.

13. Kuehr J, Brauburger J, Zielen S, et al. Efficacy of combination treatment with anti-IgE plus specific immunotherapy in polysensitized children and adolescents with seasonal allergic rhinitis. J Allergy Clin Immunol 2002;109(2):274–80.

14. Li XM, Zhang TF, Huang CK, et al. Food allergy herbal formula -1 (FAHF-1) blocks peanut-induced anaphylaxis in a murine model. J Allergy Clin Immunol 2001;108:639–46.

15. Srivastava KD, Kattan JD, Zou ZM, et al. The Chinese herbal medicine formula FAHF-2 completely blocks anaphylactic reactions in a murine model of peanut allergy. J Allergy Clin Immunol 2005;115(1):171–8.

16. Qu C, Srivastava K, Ko J, et al. Induction of tolerance after establishment of peanut allergy by the food allergy herbal formula-2 is associated with up-regulation of interferon-gamma. Clin Exp Allergy 2007;37(6):846–55.

17. Srivastava KD, Qu C, Zhang T, et al. Food Allergy Herbal Formula-2 silences peanut-induced anaphylaxis for a prolonged posttreatment period via IFN-gamma-producing CD8+ T cells. J Allergy Clin Immunol 2009;123(2):443–51.

18. Wang J, Patil SP, Yang N, et al. Safety, tolerability, and immunologic effects of a food allergy herbal formula in food allergic individuals: a randomized, double-blinded, placebo-controlled, dose escalation, phase 1 study. Ann Allergy Asthma Immunol 2010;105(1): 75–84.

19. Frossard CP, Steidler L, Eigenmann PA. Oral administration of an IL-10-secreting Lactococcus lactis strain prevents food-induced IgE sensitization. J Allergy Clin Immunol 2007;119(4):952–9.

20. Straumann A, Conus S, Grzonka P, et al. Anti-interleukin-5 antibody treatment (mepolizumab) in active eosinophilic oesophagitis: a randomised, placebo-controlled, double-blind trial. Gut 2010;59(1):21–30.

21. Nowak-Wegrzyn A, Bloom KA, Sicherer SH, et al. Tolerance to extensively heated milk in children with cows' milk allergy. J Allergy Clin Immunol 2008;122(2):342–7, 347.

22. Lemon-Mule H, Sampson HA, Sicherer SH, et al. Immunologic changes in children with egg allergy ingesting extensively heated egg. J Allergy Clin Immunol 2008;122(5):977–83.

23. Wanich N, Nowak-Wegrzyn A, Sampson HA, et al. Allergen-specific basophil suppression associated with clinical tolerance in patients with milk allergy. J Allergy Clin Immunol 2009;123(4):789–94.

24. Shreffler WG, Wanich N, Moloney M, et al. Association of allergen-specific regulatory T cells with the onset of clinical tolerance to milk protein. J Allergy Clin Immunol 2009;123(1):43–52.

25. Oppenheimer JJ, Nelson HS, Bock SA, et al. Treatment of peanut allergy with rush immunotherapy. J Allergy Clin Immunol 1992;90(2):256–62.

26. Nelson HS, Lahr J, Rule R, et al. Treatment of anaphylactic sensitivity to peanuts by immunotherapy with injections of aqueous peanut extract. J Allergy Clin Immunol 1997;99(6 Pt 1):744–51.

27. Asero R. Effects of birch pollen-specific immunotherapy on apple allergy in birch pollen-hypersensitive patients. Clin Exp Allergy 1998;28:1368–73.

28. Asero R. How long does the effect of birch pollen injection SIT on apple allergy last? Allergy 2003;58(5):435–8.

29. Bucher X, Pichler WJ, Dahinden CA, et al. Effect of tree pollen specific, subcutaneous immunotherapy on the oral allergy syndrome to apple and hazelnut. Allergy 2004;59(12):1272–6.

30. Bolhaar ST, Tiemessen MM, Zuidmeer L, et al. Efficacy of birch-pollen immunotherapy on cross-reactive food allergy confirmed by skin tests and double-blind food challenges. Clin Exp Allergy 2004;34(5):761–9.

31. Alonso R, Enrique E, Pineda F, et al. An observational study on outgrowing food allergy during non-birch pollen-specific, subcutaneous immunotherapy. Int Arch Allergy Immunol 2007;143(3):185–9.

32. Schofield AT. A case of egg poisoning. Lancet 1908;1:716.

33. Chehade M, Mayer L. Oral tolerance and its relation to food hypersensitivities. J Allergy Clin Immunol 2005;115(1):3–12.

34. Strid J, Hourihane J, Kimber I, et al. Epicutaneous exposure to peanut protein prevents oral tolerance and enhances allergic sensitization. Clin Exp Allergy 2005;35(6):757–66.

35. Patriarca C, Romano A, Venuti A, et al. Oral specific hyposensitization in the management of patients allergic to food. Allergol Immunopathol (Madr) 1984;12(4):275–81.

36. Patriarca G, Schiavino D, Nucera E, et al. Food allergy in children: results of a standardized protocol for oral desensitization. Hepatogastroenterology 1998; 45(19):52–8.

37. Patriarca G, Nucera E, Roncallo C, et al. Oral desensitizing treatment in food allergy: clinical and immunological results. Aliment Pharmacol Ther 2003;17(3):459–65.

38. Patriarca G, Nucera E, Pollastrini E, et al. Oral rush desensitization in peanut allergy: a case report. Dig Dis Sci 2006;51(3):471–3.

39 Rolinck-Werninghaus C, Staden U, Mehl A, et al. Specific oral tolerance induction with food in children: transient or persistent effect on food allergy? Allergy 2005;60(10):1320–2.

40. Staden U, Rolinck-Werninghaus C, Brewe F, et al. Specific oral tolerance induction in food allergy in children: efficacy and clinical patterns of reaction. Allergy 2007;62(11):1261–9.

41. Skripak JM, Nash SD, Rowley H, et al. A randomized, double-blind, placebo-controlled study of milk oral immunotherapy for cows' milk allergy. J Allergy Clin Immunol 2008;122(6):1154–60.

42. Narisety SD, Skripak JM, Steele P, et al. Open-label maintenance after milk oral immunotherapy for IgE-mediated cows' milk allergy. J Allergy Clin Immunol 2009;124(3):610–2.

43. Longo G, Barbi E, Berti I, et al. Specific oral tolerance induction in children with very severe cow's milk-induced reactions. J Allergy Clin Immunol 2008;121(2):343–7.

44. Jones SM, Pons L, Roberts JL, et al. Clinical efficacy and immune regulation with peanut oral immunotherapy. J Allergy Clin Immunol 2009;124(2):292–300.

45. Clark AT, Islam S, King Y, et al. Successful oral tolerance induction in severe peanut allergy. Allergy 2009;64(8):1218–20.

46. Hofmann AM, Scurlock AM, Jones SM, et al. Safety of a peanut oral immunotherapy protocol in children with peanut allergy. J Allergy Clin Immunol 2009;124(2): 286–91.

47. Varshney P, Steele PH, Vickery BP, et al. Adverse reactions during peanut oral immunotherapy home dosing. J Allergy Clin Immunol 2009; 124(6):1351–2.

48. Mempel M, Rakoski J, Ring J, et al. Severe anaphylaxis to kiwi fruit: Immunologic changes related to successful sublingual allergen immunotherapy. J Allergy Clin Immunol 2003;111(6):1406–9.

49. Kerzl R, Simonowa A, Ring J, et al. Life-threatening anaphylaxis to kiwi fruit: protective sublingual allergen immunotherapy effect persists even after discontinuation. J Allergy Clin Immunol 2007; 119(2):507–8.

50. Enrique E, Pineda F, Malek T, et al. Sublingual immunotherapy for hazelnut food allergy: a randomized, double-blind, placebo-controlled study with a standardized hazelnut extract. J Allergy Clin Immunol 2005;116(5):1073–9.

51. De Boissieu D, Dupont C. Sublingual immunotherapy for cows' milk protein allergy: a preliminary report. Allergy 2006;61(10):1238–9.

52. Fernandez-Rivas M, Garrido FS, Nadal JA, et al. Randomized double-blind, placebo-controlled trial of sublingual immunotherapy with a Pru p 3 quantified peach extract. Allergy 2009;64(6):876–83.

53. Senti G, Graf N, Haug S, et al. Epicutaneous allergen administration as a novel method of allergen-specific immunotherapy. J Allergy Clin Immunol 2009;124(5):997–1002.

54. Mondoulet L, Dioszeghy V, Ligouis M, et al. Epicutaneous immunotherapy on intact skin using a new delivery system in a murine model of allergy. Clin Exp Allergy 2009;40(4):659–67.

55. Dupont C, Kalach N, Soulaines P, et al. Cows' milk epicutaneous immunotherapy in children: a pilot trial of safety, acceptability, and impact on allergic reactivity. J Allergy Clin Immunol 2010;125(5):1165–7.

56. Bannon GA, Cockrell G, Connaughton C, et al. Engineering, characterization and in vitro efficacy of the major peanut allergens for use in immunotherapy. Int Arch Allergy Immunol 2001;124(1–3):70–2.

57. Srivastava KD, Li XM, King N, et al. Immunotherapy with modified peanut allergens in a murine model of peanut allergy. J Allergy Clin Immunol 2002;109:S287.

58. Li XM, Srivastava K, Huleatt JW, et al. Engineered recombinant peanut protein and heat-killed Listeria monocytogenes coadministration protects against peanut-induced anaphylaxis in a murine model. J Immunol 2003;170(6):3289–95.

59. Li XM, Srivastava K, Grishin A, et al. Persistent protective effect of heat-killed Escherichia coli producing 'engineered,' recombinant peanut proteins in a murine model of peanut allergy. J Allergy Clin Immunol 2003;112(1):159–67.

60. Li S, Li XM, Burks AW, et al. Modulation of peanut allergy by peptide-based immunotherapy. J Allergy Clin Immunol 2001;107:S233.

61. Srivastava K, Li XM, Bannon GA, et al. Investigation of the use of ISS-linked Ara h2 for the treatment of peanut-induced allergy [Abstract]. J Allergy Clin Immunol 2001;107:S233.

62. Roy K, Mao HQ, Huang SK, et al. Oral gene delivery with chitosan–DNA nanoparticles generates immunologic protection in a murine model of peanut allergy. Nat Med 1999;5(4):387–91.

63. Horner AA, Nguyen MD, Ronaghy A, et al. DNA-based vaccination reduces the risk of lethal anaphylactic hypersensitivity in mice. J Allergy Clin Immunol 2000;106(2):349–56.

64. Nguyen MD, Cinman N, Yen J, et al. DNA-based vaccination for the treatment of food allergy. Allergy 2001;56(Suppl. 67):127–30.

CHAPTER 18

Natural History and Prevention of Food Allergy

Scott H. Sicherer and Atsuo Urisu

KEY CONCEPTS

- Allergies to egg, cows' milk, wheat and soy are likely to resolve in early childhood, whereas allergies to peanuts, tree nuts, fish, crustaceans and buckwheat are likely to persist. Recurrence of peanut allergy after documented resolution has also been reported.

- Persistence of an allergy is associated with: sensitization to multiple foods, high allergen-specific IgE antibody levels, a history of anaphylaxis, comorbid conditions such as atopic dermatitis, and particular IgE-recognition patterns, such as evidence of

response to particular proteins or epitopes of specific allergens.

- Exclusively breastfeeding infants for 4–6 months is a general recommendation that may reduce atopic disease compared to using whole protein formulas.

- There are no current proven means to prevent food allergies through dietary manipulation.

- Emerging data question the efficacy of prolonged dietary allergen avoidance as a means to prevent food allergies and atopic disease.

This chapter addresses two common concerns about food allergy. First, we discuss the natural course of resolution or persistence of common food allergies and consider some of the indicators that may predict outcomes. Second, we address various early dietary strategies that have been evaluated for primary prevention of atopy and food allergy.

PART 1. NATURAL HISTORY

Introduction and pathogenesis

The prevalence of food allergy has significantly increased worldwide in the past decade. peaking at 6–8% at 1 year of age[1] and declining gradually to 2–4% in older children and adults. This decline reflects the fact that many early childhood food allergies resolve. The rate and probability of resolution varies significantly between specific foods. Generally, egg,[2] milk,[3] wheat and soy allergies resolve relatively early in life, whereas allergies to peanuts,[4] tree nuts,[5] sesame seeds,[6] fish, crustacean shellfish[7] and buckwheat are likely to persist. The estimated rates of resolution vary among studies for any specific food. Predictors of allergy persistence or resolution have been delineated in some studies, although not all confirm the identified predictors. Some identified factors are sensitization to multiple food allergens, high allergen-specific IgE antibody levels, a history of anaphylaxis, comorbid atopic diseases such as atopic dermatitis,[2] and particular IgE-binding patterns on the food allergens. Here we consider the natural history according to individual food allergens. It remains unclear why some children or adults achieve natural tolerance and others do not. However, baseline variations in the degree and type of immune response, as evidenced from studies of food-specific IgE levels and epitope binding, present some indication of the chance for an individual to become tolerant.

Clinical features

Hen's egg (Table 18.1)

Allergy to egg is one of the most common food allergies in infancy. In general, egg allergy has a good clinical prognosis and according to one study tends to resolve in 55% of patients in the first 6 years of life.[8] The cumulative tolerance probability was 16% at 1 year of follow-up, 28% at 2 years,

52% at 3 years, 57% at 4 years and 66% at 5 years.[8] In addition, this study found that specific IgE antibody level was an important prognostic marker in children who only had cutaneous symptoms. The tolerance rate increased in inverse proportion to egg white IgE antibody concentration: 76% (22/29) for egg white IgE antibody level <1.98 kU$_A$/L and 41% (12/29) for egg white IgE antibody level >1.98 kU$_A$/L.[8]

Resolution rates vary by study, probably owing to differences in patient selection. In a study of a referral population, Savage et al.[2] reported an increased persistence of egg allergy. Egg was tolerated by only 4% at 4 years of age and by 12% at 6 years of age, rates that are far lower than those reported by Boyano et al.[8]

Table 18.1 Natural history of allergies to hen's eggs, cows' milk and wheat

Allergen	Reference		n	Duration of follow-up	Rate of resolution (Age)
Hen's egg	Boyano-Martinez T	J Allergy Clin Immunol 2002; 110: 304–309	58	7–86 M	16% at 12 M of follow-up, 28% at 24 M, 52% at 36 M, 57% at 48 M, and 66% at 60 M
	Savage JH	J Allergy Clin Immunol 2007; 120: 1413–1417	881	5–285 M (median: 59 M)	4% (4 Y), 12% (6 Y), 37% (10 Y), 68% (16 Y)
	Montesinos E	Pediatr Allergy Immunol 2010; 21: 634-639	42	15–118.6 M	50% (15–77 M)
Cows' milk	Bishop JM,	J Pediatr 1990; 116: 862–867	100	5 Y	28% (2 Y), 56% (4 Y),78% (6 Y)
					Immediate: 67%, intermediate: 87%, late reactions: 83% (8 Y?)
	Høst A	Allergy 1990; 45: 587–596	39	3 Y	IgE-mediated; 43% (1 Y), 62% (2 Y),76% (3 Y)
					Non IgE-mediated: 72% (1 Y), 94% (2 Y), 100% (3 Y)
	James JM	J Pediatr 1992; 121: 371–377	29	3 Y	38% (mean: 7 Y),
	Hill DJ	Clin Exp Allergy 1993; 23: 124–131	98	6–73 M (Mean: 24 M)	IgE-mediated: 22%,
					Non-IgE mediated: 59%
	Høst A	Pediatr Allergy Immunol 2002; 13 (Suppl. 15): 23–28	39	ND	IgE-mediated: 56% (1 Y), 77% (2 Y), 87% (3 Y), 92% (5–10 Y), 97% (15 Y)
	Skripak JM	J Allergy Clin Immunol 2007; 120: 1172–1177	807	16 Y	19% (4 Y), 42% (8 Y), 64% (12 Y), 79% (16 Y)
Wheat	Keet CA	Annal Allergy Asthma Immunol 2009; 102: 410–415	103	14 Y	29% (4 Y), 56% (8 Y), 65% (12 Y), 70% (14 Y)
	Kotaniemi-Syrjänen A	Pediatr Allergy Immunol 2010; 21: e421–428	28	7 M – 14 Y (Median: 7 Y)	59% (4 Y), 69% (6 Y), 84% (10 Y), 96% (16 Y)

According to a study by Montesinos,[9] 50% of the children developed tolerance at around 4 years of age, and only 26% remained allergic at 5 years. This rate of acquiring tolerance is similar to that of Boyano.[8] Montesinos et al.[9] speculated that atopic dermatitis was associated with the persistence of an egg allergy, and different rates of this disease explained the difference in egg allergy resolution rates in previous reports.

There are a number of laboratory correlates that may predict or be associated with persistence or resolution of egg allergy. Patients who developed tolerance showed a progressive decrease in mean serum IgE antibody levels for egg white, ovalbumin and ovomucoid over the course of follow-up. A reduction was also observed in the levels of all egg protein components in the group of patients with persistent allergy. However, non-tolerant patients showed significantly higher IgE antibody levels for egg protein components.[9] Studies have also shown that children with a persistent egg allergy have significantly higher concentrations of IgE antibody for ovomucoid than those who outgrow their reactivity.[10] Additionally, subjects with high IgE-binding activity to pepsin-digested ovomucoid are unlikely to outgrow an egg white allergy,[11] and a small 4.5 kDa fragment of a pepsin-digested ovomucoid contains an IgE epitope that appears to be associated with the persistence of an egg allergy.[12] Four major IgE-binding epitopes were identified in ovomucoid at amino acid residues 1–10, 9–20, 47–56, and 113–124. IgE antibodies of all seven patients with persistent egg allergy recognized these epitopes, whereas none of 11 children who outgrew their egg allergy did so.[13] The measurement of specific IgE antibodies to these peptides or IgE epitopes yields useful information for the prediction of a persistent egg allergy that may be useful in designing future prognostic tests.

Cows' milk (Table 18.1)

Cows' milk allergy affects approximately 2–3% of infants/young children. Generally, the prognosis for developing tolerance to cows' milk is very good, similar to data on egg allergy. Like egg allergy, the rates of resolution differ according to various reports. In the study by Host et al.,[14] 76% of those with an IgE-mediated milk allergy and 100% of those with a non-IgE-mediated milk allergy were tolerant by the age of 3 years. These resolution rates are far higher than those presented in other studies.

For example, James et al.[15] reported that 11 (38%) of 29 children developed tolerance at a median age of 3 years. In those who became tolerant to milk, specific IgE and IgE/IgG ratios to both casein and β-lactoglobulin were lower initially and decreased significantly over time. In a study from Hill's group,[16] a cohort of 100 children with a challenge-confirmed milk allergy were followed for 5 years. This study showed resolution rates of 28% by age 2 years, 56% by age 4 years and 78% by age 6. They also reported that 15 (22%) of 69 with IgE-mediated disease developed tolerance, compared to 17 (59%) of the 29 with non-IgE-mediated reactions.[17]

In a referral population, Skripak et al.[3] reported much lower resolution rates than previous studies: 19% by age 4 years, 42% by age 8 years, 64% by age 12 years, and 79% by age 16. The wide differences in the rates among the studies are most likely related to the population studied; for example, the study by Skripak included subjects specifically referred for and repeatedly evaluated for food and milk allergies. Coexisting asthma and allergic rhinitis were significant predictors of persistence.

Studies on the natural course of milk allergy, like those of egg allergy, show that laboratory correlates are indicative of the potential for resolution. The peak cows' milk IgE for each patient was found to be highly predictive of outcome, with those having higher peak concentration being less likely to resolve the allergy. Casein is one of the major allergens responsible for cows' milk allergy. As the main component in cows' milk, casein constitutes 80% of the total protein. It consists of four proteins; αs1-, αs2-, β-, and κ-casein. Chatchatee et al.[18] identified IgE- and IgG-binding epitopes on these caseins and assessed the differences in recognition of the epitopes between patients with persistent and transient cows' milk allergy. They found that two IgE-binding regions (AA 69–78 and AA 173–194) on αs1-casein were recognized by all of the older children with persistent milk allergy but none of the younger children who were likely to outgrow their allergy. No differences in IgG binding between the groups was observed.[18] Six major and three minor IgE-binding epitopes, as well as eight major and one minor IgG-binding regions, were identified on β-casein. Eight major IgE-binding epitopes, as well as two major and two minor IgG-binding epitopes, were detected on κ-casein. Three of the IgE-binding regions on β-casein and six on κ-casein were recognized by the majority of patients in the older age group, but not by the younger patients.[19] These results, indicating a clear distinction in IgE-binding profiles between those with persistent or likely transient cows' milk allergy, may be useful in developing improved diagnostic and prognostic tests for milk allergy.

Newly diagnosed tolerance of milk is usually lifelong without reported recurrences. However, there is a case report worth noting concerning a patient who developed milk-dependent exercise-induced anaphylaxis after resolution of a milk allergy.[20] We need to observe the re-emergence of food allergy caused by exacerbating factors such as exercise even after resolution of milk allergy.

Peanut (Table 18.2)

An allergy to peanut is typically lifelong, often severe, and potentially fatal. For example, Bock and Atkins[21] followed 32 children aged 1–14 years who had challenge-confirmed peanut allergy, over a period of 2–14 years. They found that 24 had accidental peanut exposures and reactions, and none seemed to outgrow the allergy. However, clear evidence that a subset of children with a peanut allergy may indeed lose sensitivity was first delineated by Hourihane et al.[22] They evaluated 230 children with a peanut allergy and performed oral challenges in 120. A total of 22 children between the ages of 2 and 9 years had a negative challenge, indicating that 18% of those challenged, or 9.8% of the total group, experienced resolution. They found that a negative challenge result was associated with a smaller skin test size and fewer allergies to other foods than in those with a persistent peanut allergy.

Spergel et al.[23] reported that of 33 children between the ages of 18 months and 8 years with a convincing history of an allergy to peanuts, 14 passed an oral food challenge and were believed to have resolved their peanut allergy. They noted some risk factors for persistence. Whereas nine of 17 patients with a history of urticaria and four of 10 with a history of atopic dermatitis became tolerant, none of the five patients with a history of peanut anaphylaxis tolerated peanut. In addition, those who developed tolerance had significantly smaller skin test responses than 19 patients with persistent allergy to peanut.

Skolnick et al.[4] reported that at least 21.5% of their cohort of peanut-allergic children outgrew their allergy. The peanut-IgE antibody levels were the best predictor of a negative challenge, with 61% of those with peanut-IgE levels <5 kU$_A$/L and 67% of those with levels <2 kU$_A$/L passing the challenge. In contrast to the study by Spergel et al., the study by Skolnick et al. did not find that the initial reaction – for example anaphylaxis – was a predictive factor for resolution.

These studies reinforce the notion that peanut allergy is likely to persist for most but not all patients. These data indicate that it is prudent to periodically re-evaluate children with peanut allergy. Patients who have not had reactions in the past 1–2 years and who have a low peanut-IgE level (<5 kU$_A$/L) should be considered for an oral food challenge to peanut. If a patient is still allergic to

Table 18.2 Natural history of food allergy to peanuts, tree nuts and sesame

Allergen	Reference		n	Duration of follow-up	Rate of resolution (Age)
Peanut	Bock SA	J Allergy Clin Immunol 1989; 83: 900–904	32	2–14 Y	0% (1–14 Y)
	Skolnick HS	J Allergy Clin Immunol 2001; 107: 367–374	223	ND	21.5% (4–17.5 Y)
	Fleischer DM	J Allergy Clin Immunol 2003; 112: 183–189	84	ND	at least 50% (4–14.2 Y, peanut-IgE levels <5)
Tree nut	Fleischer DM	J Allergy Clin Immunol 2005; 116: 1087–1093	101	ND	8.9% (3–21.6 Y)
Sesame	Cohen A	Pediatr Allergy Immunol 2007; 18: 217–223	45	1.8–14 Y (Median: 6.4 Y)	20% (Median: 8.3, Range: 2.2–54.2 Y)

peanut by late childhood or adolescence, it is very unlikely that he or she will subsequently outgrow the allergy, and regular retesting may no longer be warranted.[24]

The possibility that resolved peanut allergy, confirmed by a negative oral food challenge, may recur was first noted by Busse et al.,[25] who reported several cases where children redeveloped symptoms. They estimated a recurrence rate of roughly 8–14% and also noted that these children had not routinely added peanut to their diet after they demonstrated tolerance on the oral food challenge. In a larger and more comprehensive study, Fleischer et al.[26] also demonstrated recurrence of peanut allergy and speculated that resensitization might have occurred because these patients ingested only small amounts of peanut intermittently, rather than ingesting small amounts frequently or larger amounts intermittently, doses that might better sustain tolerance.

Tree nuts (Table 18.2)

Nine tree nuts account for the majority of tree nut allergies: walnuts, almonds, hazelnuts, Brazil nuts, cashews, macadamia nuts, pecans, pine nuts and pistachios. Although most tree nut allergies develop when a patient is young, onset is generally later than that of a peanut allergy. In one study, the median age of the first reaction to a tree nut was 36 months, compared to the median age of the first reaction to peanut of 14 months.[27] Allergic reactions to tree nuts can be severe and life-threatening.[28] Like peanut allergy, allergies to tree nuts had been considered lifelong. However, recent studies show that approximately 9% of young patients outgrow tree nut allergy, including some who had previously had severe allergic reactions.[28] Patients who passed physician-supervised oral food challenges to tree nuts were significantly less likely than those who failed to have other current food allergies. Patients who had outgrown a peanut allergy were significantly more likely to outgrow a tree nut allergy than those with ongoing tree nut and peanut allergies. No recurrent tree nut allergy has been reported in the literature to date.

Wheat (Table 18.1)

The prognosis for wheat allergy is rather good. In one study, wheat was tolerated by 59%, 69%, 84% and 96%, by the ages of 4, 6, 10 and 16 years, respectively.[29] In conclusion, most children with wheat allergy can tolerate wheat by adolescence. Sensitization to gliadin is associated with a slower achievement of tolerance and an increased risk of asthma. The incidence of asthma was 64% in the gliadin-IgE-positive children, compared to 21% in the gliadin-IgE-negative children.[29] A total of 64% of the gliadin-IgE-positive children developed asthma during the follow-up, whereas only 21% of the gliadin-IgE-negative children developed asthma. In a different study by Keet et al.,[30] the rates of resolution were 29% by 4 years of age, 56% by 8 years and 65% by 12 years. In this referral population, higher wheat IgE levels were associated with an increased risk for persistence; however, many children outgrew a wheat allergy with even the highest levels of wheat IgE. Thus, both studies support the notion that wheat allergy typically resolves by adolescence.

Sesame (Table 18.2)

Studies thus far on the natural history of sesame allergy report results that are similar in pattern to peanut allergy.[4] Sesame allergy appears to present most frequently during childhood, although onset may be at any age.[31] A questionnaire-based survey in Britain suggested that sesame was responsible for a significant number of severe reactions.[32] Cohen et al.[6] reported that nine (20%) patients developed tolerance during the follow-up period of 1.8–14 years (median 6.4 years). Clinical scoring and severity of symptoms were not found to be predictive in the development of tolerance.

Several studies show that sesame food allergy appears to be persistent, similar to allergies to foods such as fish[33] and peanuts.[4] Agne et al.[34] found that three out of 14 children who 'outgrew' their sesame food allergy showed a previous drop in IgE antibody for sesame seed and a reduction in reactivity to a skin prick test.

Fish and crustacean shellfish

Allergies to fish and shellfish tend to develop after the first year of life and are often persistent. These allergies are an important cause of food-induced anaphylaxis in both children and adults.[35] One study followed 11 patients with shrimp allergy over a 2-year period and found that there were no significant changes in shrimp-specific antibody levels during that time.[36]

Other foods

Soy allergy develops in the first year of life and is likely to be outgrown in early childhood. In the studies by Sampson et al.,[7] over 50% of soy allergic children became tolerant over a 1–2-year follow-up period. Similar results of good prognosis for soy allergy were shown by Asronov et al.[37]

Adverse reactions to fruits, vegetables and cereal grains in infants are typically very short-lived[1] and may represent intolerance rather than allergy. However, some children do have severe IgE-mediated allergies to these foods that may persist over time. There have been no adequate studies on the natural history of allergy to most foods other than the previously discussed most common allergens.

Non-IgE-mediated food allergy

Food protein-induced enterocolitis syndrome (FPIES) is a non-IgE-mediated gastrointestinal food hypersensitivity disorder.[38] Cows' milk and soy are the most common offending foods, but cereal grains (rice, oat and barley), fish, poultry and vegetables may also cause FPIES. The majority of cases resolve by the age of 3 years.

Summary and recommendations

Studies on milk, egg, wheat and soy allergies generally show that these resolve during childhood. Therefore, frequent reassessment, for example yearly testing if there are no clinical reactions, may be warranted. Peanut, tree nut, fish and shellfish allergies tend to be more persistent, but some children do become tolerant. Therefore, periodic testing and re-evaluation, perhaps more often in the first few years of life, may be warranted. For older children, e.g. after age 6, with persistent allergies to these foods, evaluations may be pursued less frequently. However, there is a lack of long-term studies in adults, and the potential for an allergy to resolve spontaneously over time should be considered on a case-by-case basis.

PART 2. PREVENTION

Introduction

Although definitive proof is lacking, there are several studies indicating an increase in the prevalence of food allergies. Various theories to explain this, which appears primarily to be a problem in westernized countries, include general environmental circumstances that reduce infection and exposure to microbes, the timing of introduction of foods to infants, and the manner in which particular foods are processed and cooked.[39] For decades, investigations aimed at preventing food allergies and atopic diseases such as atopic dermatitis, asthma and allergic rhinitis focused on the possibility of altering the maternal or infant diet. Most of this research focuses on the removal of common dietary allergens, such as egg, milk, peanut, tree nuts and fish, from the maternal diet and avoidance of these allergens by the infant until a time of presumed immunologic and gastrointestinal maturity. The four primary areas of focus for dietary prevention of atopy include the maternal diet during pregnancy and lactation; the infant's early exposure to breast milk or a commercial formula, if given; the type of formula; and the timing and types of complementary foods. Although early studies supported measures emphasizing the avoidance of or delay in introducing of common allergens, various flaws in study design have limited the quality of evidence of these approaches and more recent studies present negative results. Although there is a pressing interest in preventing or delaying allergy, doing so through dietary avoidance is increasingly being questioned by emerging data.

Pathogenesis

The primary goal of a food allergy prevention strategy using dietary means is to prevent sensitization and allow tolerance to develop. The immunopathogenesis of oral tolerance to foods is incompletely understood[40] and is reviewed in Chapter 1. One view is that avoidance of an allergen will result in a lack of sensitization. This view arises from the notion that the immune system is unlikely to mount an adverse reaction if there is no exposure to an allergen, and is supported in part by early studies showing that delayed introduction of allergens such as milk and egg are associated with less milk allergy, atopic dermatitis and sensitization.[41] This view also formed the basis for recommendations to avoid specific allergens in pregnancy and lactation, and for the young infant or child. For example, the American Academy of Pediatrics in 2000[42] recommended that in a family with allergy risk factors a pregnant mother should consider avoiding peanut during pregnancy, reduce allergen ingestion during lactation, and not introduce cows' milk to the infant until age 1 year, egg until age 2 and fish, nuts and peanut until age 3. These recommendations were based largely on a study showing less milk allergy and atopic dermatitis in a group of children from mothers following this advice than in those randomized to standard feeding practices.[41] However, the study did not show a long-term effect; for example, by ages 4–7 years the treatment group and the control group had similar outcomes.

Another view is that exposure to food proteins is required to allow appropriate benign immune responsiveness, the induction of tolerance. Animal models and human data show that exposure to antigens by the oral route most often results in active immune responses that do not cause disease.[40] The general observation is that low-dose tolerance occurs with the generation of suppressive cells and high-dose tolerance with deletion of reactive immune responses. That exposure to the antigen is necessary for this process is clear, and also forms the basis of current avenues of immunotherapy where a food allergen is purposefully administered in gradually increasing doses over weeks and months. If oral exposure is needed to induce tolerance, then deliberate allergen avoidance diets could be at odds with the notion that exposure is required. However, mechanisms of oral tolerance should be active at any age or time of introduction of a new allergen, otherwise adults would routinely develop adverse reactions to any new foods. Nonetheless, there may be an early period of infancy when oral exposure may occur at a time when oral tolerance mechanisms are not mature, leading to sensitization and allergy.

A concern that ties together the opposing views that allergen avoidance may be beneficial to prevent sensitization, or detrimental in not allowing oral tolerance to develop, is the possibility that non-oral exposures may occur during a period of avoidance and in themselves be sensitizing. For example, adults may become reactive to raw fruits or vegetables based on increasing sensitization to homologous proteins in pollens to which respiratory sensitization develops over time. Similarly, skin exposure with the lack of oral exposure may be a sensitizing route. Evidence for this possibility includes animal studies showing that sensitization can occur readily through aerosolized or topically applied food proteins, but not so easily by the oral route unless various means are employed, such as neutralization of the stomach acid and use of adjuvants.[43]

Evidence that environmental food exposure may be allergy-promoting comes from a study by Fox et al.,[44] who used a questionnaire-based case–control design to evaluate maternal and household peanut consumption among 133 children with peanut allergy, 150 non-allergic children and 160 with egg but not peanut allergy. Although there was no difference in peanut consumption among the children, household peanut consumption was significantly greater in the peanut-allergic children (18.8 g) than in egg-allergic (1.9 g) or non-allergic controls (6.9 g). They found no relationship with maternal peanut ingestion, but noted a dose–response risk relationship in household (environmental) exposure to peanut. The authors further showed data to support the notion that early oral exposure may have been protective for those with increased environmental exposure. Since food allergy and atopic dermatitis are closely related, it has also been postulated that the loss of intact skin may present a route of sensitizing exposure to environmental food allergens, particularly if the food has not been ingested routinely to allow oral tolerance to develop.[45]

Additional variables may be important when considering the relative impact of dietary allergen avoidance. First, the timing of exposure may be relevant. It may be that the gastrointestinal immune system is not prepared to process whole protein antigens in the first months of life. Support for this notion comes from studies comparing atopy outcomes of infants fed whole protein infant formula compared to extensively or partially hydrolyzed ones in the first months of life.[46] Most studies support the notion that those infants at risk for atopy fed whole protein (cows' milk or soy) develop more atopy than those breastfed or fed alternative 'hypoallergenic' formulas.[47]

Another concern is that other dietary components may influence allergy outcomes. For example, in a German cohort of 2642 children followed to age 2 years, maternal consumption during pregnancy of fish containing omega-6 polyunsaturated fats, compared to consumption of omega-3 polyunsaturated fats, found for example in margarines, was associated with less atopic disease, whereas maternal consumption of allergens such as milk, nuts and egg had no influence.[48] In this respect, advice to avoid a major allergen such as fish may have contrary effects because of reduced ingestion of non-allergen components that may reduce atopy risks.

Clinical features

Most studies that have attempted to evaluate the effect of diet on atopy prevention have focused on 'high-risk' infants, typically ones with one or two first-degree relatives with a documented atopic disease. Modalities of allergen avoidance that have been evaluated include the maternal diet during pregnancy and lactation, breastfeeding, the use of one or another commercial infant formulas, and the timing and selection of complementary foods.

Maternal diet

Maternal avoidance diets during pregnancy are difficult to study, partly because outcomes measured later in an infant's or child's life will be influenced by many factors. Studies from the 1980s failed to show an impact of maternal avoidance of cows' milk or egg.[49-51] A Cochrane database analysis included four studies with a total of 334 subjects where maternal allergen avoidance during pregnancy was undertaken and concluded that there was no evidence of a protective effect on atopic dermatitis at 18 months.[52] The restricted diet was associated with a lower mean gestational weight gain. The reviewers concluded that an antigen avoidance diet aimed at women at high atopy risk is unlikely to substantially reduce her child's risk of atopic diseases, and such a diet may adversely affect maternal or fetal nutrition, or both.

Maternally ingested allergens may pass into breast milk. Concern that this represents a sensitizing exposure is the basis for studying maternal avoidance during lactation. In a long-term study of infants whose mothers avoided major allergens in the first 3 months of lactation, there was less atopic dermatitis than in control infants; however, there were no long-term differences.[53] A Cochrane meta-analysis of this topic included only one study on maternal allergen avoidance during lactation, and overall concluded that an avoidance diet during lactation may reduce the child's risk of developing atopic eczema, but this was a tentative conclusion because better trials are needed.[52] The literature on this topic includes studies where maternal avoidance was associated with increased atopy.[54]

Peanut allergy has garnered much attention because of its severity and persistence, and several studies have evaluated the role of maternal ingestion of peanut during pregnancy or lactation. Twenty-five children with IgE to peanut were compared to 18 who had positive tests to milk or egg but not peanut.[55] Maternal ingestion of peanut more than once per week during pregnancy trended towards being a risk for peanut sensitization (OR 3.97, p = 0.063). This small study was potentially biased by dietary recall, because children were up to age 3 years and their peanut allergies were known. One additional study implicated maternal ingestion of peanut as a risk factor for peanut allergy. Hourihane et al.[56] used a questionnaire to evaluate 622 individuals with peanut allergy and noted that probands under age 6 were more likely to have mothers who consumed peanut during pregnancy or breastfeeding than did older probands. The onset of peanut allergy was earlier in the younger probands and had increased in prevalence over generations, leading the authors to conclude that maternal ingestion may be a risk factor. Two population-based studies concluded that peanut consumption during pregnancy/lactation was not a risk factor for peanut allergy.[57,58] One study focusing on maternal ingestion of nuts during pregnancy showed an increased risk of wheeze when there was daily maternal nut consumption (OR 1.42; 95% CI 1.1–1.9), but the study did not show an increase risk of nut allergy or a dose-response.[59]

Breastfeeding

Breastfeeding is a general recommendation for all infants regardless of allergic disposition. Studies have addressed whether breastfeeding is protective of atopy, which generally means comparisons to formula feeding. It is not possible to randomize infants to breast versus formula feeding, and various biases in such studies would make comparisons very difficult. Meta-analyses and reviews of the available literature generally support the notion that compared to feeding with whole cows' milk, exclusive breastfeeding for 3–4 months is generally associated with a lower incidence of atopic dermatitis, asthma, and possibly cows' milk allergy,[60-63] but not all studies agree[64] and the effect on long-term outcomes of food allergy remain uncertain.[65,66] A Cochrane review included only one study that discussed blinded oral food challenges and concluded that at least 4 months of exclusive breastfeeding did not protect against food allergy at 1 year of age.[67] In these various reviews the protective effects of exclusive breastfeeding were more evident among studies of infants at risk for atopic disease. Studies focusing on food allergy outcomes in unselected cohorts have not demonstrated protective effects of breastfeeding, whereas some studies of high-risk mothers show reduced food allergies at least during short-term follow-up.[68] Although various methodological issues abound in such studies, the numerous health benefits of breastfeeding, at least for the first several months of life, generally contribute to the widespread conclusion that this is the ideal feeding for infants.

Commercial formula

Numerous studies have evaluated the role of cows' milk hydrolyzate formulas as a primary prevention for atopy.[47] Comparisons are typically made to whole protein cows' milk formula. The German Infant Nutritional Intervention (GINI) study evaluated an extensively hydrolyzed casein-based formula, a partially hydrolyzed whey formula and an extensively hydrolyzed whey formula compared to standard cows' milk formula.[46] The extensively hydrolyzed casein-based formula and the partially hydrolyzed whey-based formula were protective for atopic dermatitis and general allergy. In the intent-to-treat analysis the relative risk of a physician's diagnosis of allergic manifestations compared with cows' milk was 0.82 (95% CI 0.70–0.96) for partially hydrolyzed whey formula, 0.90 (95% CI 0.78–1.04) for extensively hydrolyzed whey formula, and 0.80 (95% CI 0.69–0.93) for extensively hydrolyzed casein formula. The corresponding results for atopic eczema were 0.79 (95% CI 0.64–0.97), 0.92 (95% CI 0.76–1.11), and 0.71 (95% CI 0.58–0.88), respectively. The study lacked power to evaluate the outcomes of cows' milk allergy. A 2006 Cochrane database review[69] concluded that there is insufficient evidence to support feeding with a hydrolyzed formula for the prevention of allergy rather than breastfeeding. However, in high-risk infants who could not be exclusively breastfed, the analysis concluded that there is limited evidence that feeding with a hydrolyzed formula rather than a cows' milk-based formula could reduce infant and childhood allergy and infant cows' milk allergy. Regarding the outcome of cows' milk allergy, studies have been inconclusive.[68]

Several studies that evaluated the role of soy formula failed to show a protective effect over cows' milk-based formula. Amino acid-based formulas have not been evaluated for their effect on atopy reduction.

Complementary foods

Early studies suggested that early introduction of solid foods, or the early introduction of more rather than fewer types of solid foods, was associated with a higher risk of eczema.[70,71] However, recent studies have failed to show that earlier introduction of foods is associated with increased atopic disease. For example, a birth cohort study from Germany following 2073 infants failed to show an effect of introducing various solids before 4 months or after 6 months on atopic dermatitis, asthma or rhinitis.[72] In fact, some cohort studies relate later introduction of wheat[73] or milk[74] to increased outcomes of atopy. However, it is often difficult to tease out the effects of reverse causation in these observational studies. That is, families may delay solids or specific allergens if they notice signs of atopy in their infants, leading to a false association between delay in introduction and increased risks of atopy.

The avoidance of introducing peanut has been targeted in prevention recommendations. In 1998–2000, the Committee on Toxicology (UK) and the American Academy of Pediatrics[42] recommended that women with infants at risk for atopy should avoid peanuts during pregnancy and lactation and not feed children peanut until age 3 years. The outcome of this advice is unclear. Hourihane et al.[75] evaluated parent–child pairs in a UK school cohort born after the avoidance advice (n = 1072). Eight mothers of 20 children with peanut allergy had reduced and one stopped peanut ingestion during pregnancy. Dean et al.[76] followed a birth cohort on the Isle of Wight, UK, born between September 2001 and August 2002, and noted that 65% of 838 children available for follow-up had avoided peanut. A total of 658 were skin tested to peanut and 13 were positive; mothers had avoided peanut in 10 of 13 cases (85% of these had a family history of atopy). The authors of both of these studies interpreted their findings to suggest that avoidance of peanut had no discernible effect.

Another study sheds doubt on the need to significantly delay the onset of introduction of peanut into the diet. In a study using a validated questionnaire, the peanut allergy rates in a school-aged cohort of Israeli Jewish children (n = 5615) was only 0.17%, compared to a cohort of Jewish children in the UK where the rate was about 10 times higher (1.85%; p < 0.001).[77] A separate survey was undertaken in general clinics using a validated food consumption questionnaire administered to 77 UK and 99 Israeli Jewish families. This additional survey found that monthly consumption of peanut at ages 8–14 months was 7.1 g in Israel compared to 0 g in the UK (p < 0.0001). Thus, these data support the notion that early oral exposure may in fact not be a risk for peanut allergy but may rather promote tolerance compared to prolonged avoidance. However, randomized studies are needed.

Alternative approaches

Rather than avoiding allergens, there is interest in active approaches to promote immune responses that are focused primarily on the use of probiotics (microbes that promote a healthy immune response), prebiotics (food ingredients that promote the growth of specific bacterial species) and synbiotics (a combination of pre- and probiotics). These approaches are based on various studies showing health benefits of these substances and the observation that atopic infants are more likely colonized with *Clostridium* species rather than bifidobacteria. These observations, in context of the 'hygiene hypothesis', would argue that providing pre- and probiotics may be a rational means to reduce atopy.

Unfortunately, studies thus far have been inconclusive, having focused primarily on outcomes of atopic dermatitis in high-risk infants rather than outcomes of food allergy. In a Cochrane review meta-analysis in 2007,[78] five studies reporting outcomes in 1477 children found a reduction in infant atopic dermatitis (RR 0.82, 95% CI 0.70–0.95); however, there was a high dropout rate in the studies, and when objective outcomes such as skin test results were included there were no significant differences. A 2008 meta-analysis by Lee et al.[79] evaluated six prevention studies and concluded that there was a reduction in pediatric atopic eczema. No studies have so far showed a reduction in specific food allergies. Variations in study results may be explained by the dosing regimens, selection of probiotics, timing of treatment, subject selection and various study design issues. Although these approaches have some promise, the lack of clear effects has so far resulted in general conclusions that these approaches are not ready for general clinical practice.[68]

Recommendations

A review through EuroPrevall assessed the infant feeding recommendations of various professional organizations and countries' government recommendations and showed a variety of discrepant conclusions.[68,80–82] However, there was wide support for exclusive breastfeeding to 6 months of age for all infants, and the use of hypoallergenic formulas for infants at higher risk of atopic disease if they are not exclusively breastfed (although the evidence remains weak). It was noted that there are no typically formal dissemination plans or monitoring of whether recommendations are followed, nor routine evaluation of outcomes. Table 18.3 summarizes the potential interventions. Because there are limited supportive data, firm conclusions cannot be often drawn and therefore variations in recommendations are not surprising. Unfortunately, it appears that many more studies will be needed to present a more solid evidence base upon which to base recommendations. This is a very difficult area of inquiry because studies must consider numerous interrelated variables of diet and environment, cannot easily randomize feeding practices, and must consider various treatment options and outcomes among other pitfalls and challenges.

CLINICAL CASE

A mother with two children who have peanut allergy is now pregnant. She wants to know what she can do to prevent peanut allergy in her next child.

Discussion

Because there are currently no clear prevention strategies, no specific dietary advice is available. Some families such as this one may exclude peanut from their home already, and so the mother may by default be avoiding ingestion of peanut. The primary suggestion would be to breastfeed her infant.

The mother mentioned above had given birth to an infant now aged 1 year. Her two older children aged 4 and 5 years remain allergic to peanut and they avoid it in their home. She wants to know if she should feed her 1-year-old peanut.

Table 18.3 Feeding recommendations for prevention of atopy/food allergy

Approach	Evidence, recommendations and comments
Exclusive breastfeeding 4–6 months	Various groups recommend 4–6 or 6 months Almost universal recommendations to breastfeed regardless of allergy risk for various health reasons
Use of partially or extensively hydrolyzed formulas	Studies with overall weak evidence of an effect compared to feeding with a whole protein based formula Effect may be more evident with higher-risk group Effect may be stronger for extensive hydrolyzate, although cost and taste is an issue Effect may vary by specific formula Most guidelines suggest use of these formulas in high-risk groups if breastfeeding is not undertaken or exclusive
Maternal diet during breastfeeding and lactation	Some evidence for allergen lactation avoidance diet reducing atopic dermatitis but maternal health is a consideration and long-term effect is unproven No clear evidence that maternal allergen avoidance during pregnancy is influential Most recommendations acknowledge a lack of evidence
Introduction of complementary foods and specific allergens	Timing is associated with duration of exclusive breastfeeding Recommendations for extensive delays in allergen introduction are generally rescinded Recommendations for solids include waiting 17 weeks, 4–6 months, or not introducing wheat before 4 months or later than 7 months to reduce risk of wheat allergy (based on one study)

Discussion

Although data currently do not support the need to wait long periods of time to add peanut to the diet, this child is at increased risk for peanut allergy because of the strong family history, and there are practical reasons to avoid feeding this infant peanut when her older siblings are avoiding it. Therefore, it may be practical to wait longer.

However, an argument can also be made to test the infant prior to introduction because there is an elevated risk of peanut allergy in a sibling.

The mother of a 6-month-old with atopic dermatitis noted that her infant developed urticaria and wheezing after a first ingestion of a milk-based formula. The infant tolerates a formula comprised of an extensive hydrolyzate of casein. The mother wishes to know if she can now introduce egg into the diet.

Discussion

Although recent studies do not support waiting long periods before adding various allergens to the infant diet, this infant already shows several signs of atopic disease and food allergy. Therefore, her current risk of egg allergy is high and testing may be warranted before adding more allergens to the diet.

References

1. Bock SA. Prospective appraisal of complaints of adverse reactions to foods in children during the first 3 years of life. Pediatrics 1987;79:683–8.
2. Savage JH, Matsui EC, Skripak JM, et al. The natural history of egg allergy. J Allergy Clin Immunol 2007;120:1413–7.
3. Skripak JM, Matsui EC, Mudd K, et al. The natural history of IgE-mediated cows' milk allergy. J Allergy Clin Immunol 2007;120:1172–7.
4. Skolnick HS, Conover-Walker MK, Barnes-Koerner C, et al. The natural history of peanut allergy. J Allergy Clin Immunol 2001;107:367–74.
5. Fleischer DM, Conover-Walker MK, Matsui EC, et al. The natural history of tree nut allergy. J Allergy Clin Immunol 2005;116:1087–93.
6. Cohen A, Goldberg M, Levy B, et al. Sesame food allergy and sensitization in children: the natural history and long-term follow-up. Pediatr Allergy Immunol 2007;18:217–23.
7. Sampson HA, Scanlon SM. Natural history of food hypersensitivity in children with atopic dermatitis. J Pediatr 1989;115:23–7.
8. Boyano MT, García-Ara C, Díaz-Pena JM, et al. Prediction of tolerance on the basis of quantification of egg white-specific IgE antibodies in children with egg allergy. J Allergy Clin Immunol 2002;110:304–9.
9. Montesinos E, Martorell A, Félix R, et al. Egg white specific IgE levels in serum as clinical reactivity predictors in the course of egg allergy follow-up. Pediatr Allergy Immunol 2009;20 [Epub ahead of print].
10. Bernhisel-Broadbent J, Dintzis RZ, Sampson HA. Allergenicity and antigenicity of chicken egg ovomucoid (Gal d I) compared with ovalbumin (Gal d II) in children with egg allergy and in mice. J Immunol 1994;93:1047–59.

11. Urisu A, Yamada K, Tokuda R, et al. Clinical significance of IgE-binding activity to enzymatic digests of ovomucoid in the diagnosis and the prediction of the outgrowing of egg white hypersensitivity. Int Arch Allergy Immunol 1999;120:192–8.

12. Takagi K, Teshima R, Okunuki H, et al. Kinetic analysis of pepsin digestion of chicken egg white ovomucoid and allergenic potential of pepsin fragments. Int Arch Allergy Immunol 2005;136:23–32.

13. Järvinen K-M, Beyer K, Vila L, et al. Specificity of IgE antibodies to sequential epitopes of hen's egg ovomucoid as a marker for persistence of egg allergy. Allergy 2007;62:758–65.

14. Host A, Halken S. A prospective study of cow milk allergy in Danish infants during the first 3 years of life. Clinical course in relation to clinical and immunological type of hypersensitivity reaction. Allergy 1990;45:587–96.

15. James JM, Sampson HA. Immunologic changes associated with the development of tolerance in children with cow milk allergy. J Pediatr 1992;121:371–7.

16. Bishop JM, Hill DJ, Hosking CS. Natural history of cow milk allergy: clinical outcome. J Pediatr 1990;116:862–7.

17. Hill DJ, Firer MA, Ball G, et al. Natural history of cows' milk allergy in children: immunological outcome over 2 years. Clin Exp Allergy 1993;23:124–31.

18. Chatchatee P, Jarvinen K-M, Bardina L, et al. Identification of IgE- and IgG-binding epitopes on αs1-casein: differences in patients with persistent and transient cows' milk allergy. J Allergy Clin Immunol 2001;107:379–83.

19. Chatchatee P, Jarvinen K-M, Bardina L, et al. Identification of IgE- and IgG-binding epitopes on β- and κ-casein in cows' milk allergic patients. Clin Exp Allergy 2001;31:1256–62.

20. Caminiti L, Passalacqua G, Vita D, et al. Food-exercise-induced anaphylaxis in a boy successfully desensitized to cow milk. Allergy 2007;62:335–6.

21. Bock SA, Atkins FM. The natural history of peanut allergy. J Allergy Clin Immunol 1989;83:900–4.

22. Hourihane JO, Roberts SA, Warner JO. Resolution of peanut allergy: case-control study. BMJ 1998;316:1271–5.

23. Spergel JM, Beausoleil JL, Pawlowski NA. Resolution of childhood peanut allergy. Ann Allergy Asthma Immunol 2000;85:473–6.

24. Fleischer DM, Conover-Walker MK, Christie L, et al. The natural progression of peanut allergy: Resolution and the possibility of recurrence. J Allergy Clin Immunol 2003;112:183–9.

25. Busse PJ, Nowak-Wegrzyn AH, Noone SA, et al. Recurrent peanut allergy. N Engl J Med 2002;347:1535–6.

26. Fleischer DM, Conover-Walker MK, Christie L, et al. Peanut allergy: Recurrence and its management. J Allergy Clin Immunol 2004;114:1195–201.

27. Sicherer SH, Furlong TJ, Muñoz-Furlong A, et al. A voluntary registry for peanut and tree nut allergy: characteristics of the first 5149 registrants. J Allergy Clin Immunol 2001 Jul;108(1):128–32.

28. Fleischer DM, Conover-Walker MK, Matsui EC, et al. The natural history of tree nut allergy. J Allergy Clin Immunol 2005;116:1087–93.

29. Kotaniemi-Syrjänen A, Palosuo K, Jartti T, et al. The prognosis of wheat hypersensitivity in children. Pediatr Allergy Immunol 2009;30 [Epub ahead of print].

30. Keet CA, Matsui EC, Dhillon G, et al. The natural history of wheat allergy. Ann Allergy Asthma Immunol 2009;102:410–5.

31. Dalal I, Binson I, Levine A, et al. The pattern of sesame sensitivity among infants and children. Pediatr Allergy Immunol 2003;14:312–6.

32. Derby CJ, Gowland MH, Hourihane JO. Sesame allergy in Britain: a questionnaire survey of members of the Anaphylaxis Campaign. Pediatric Allergy Immunol 2005;16:171–5.

33. Eigenmann PA, Sicherer SH, Borkowski TA, et al. Prevalence of IgE-mediated food allergy among children with atopic dermatitis. Pediatrics 1998;101:E8.

34. Agne PS, Bidat E, Agne PS, et al. Sesame seed allergy in children. Eur Ann Allergy Clin Immunol 2004;36:300–5.

35. Sicherer SH, Munoz-Furlong A, Sampson HA. Prevalence of seafood allergy in the United States determined by random telephone survey. J Allergy Clin Immunol 2004;114:159–65.

36. Daul CB, Morgan JE, Lehrer SB. The natural history of shrimp-specific immunity. J Allergy Clin Immunol 1990;86:88–93.

37. Asronov D, Tasher D, Levine A, et al. Natural history of food allergy in infants and children in Israel. Ann Allergy Asthma Immunol 2008;101; 637–40.

38. Nowak-Wegrzyn A, Muraro A. Food protein-induced enterocolitis syndrome. Curr Opin Allergy Clin Immunol 2009;9:371–7.

39. Sicherer SH, Sampson HA. Peanut allergy: emerging concepts and approaches for an apparent epidemic. J Allergy Clin Immunol 2007;120(3):491–503.

40. Chehade M, Mayer L. Oral tolerance and its relation to food hypersensitivities. J Allergy Clin Immunol 2005;115(1):3–12.

41. Zeiger R, Heller S. The development and prediction of atopy in high-risk children: Follow-up at seven years in a prospective randomized study of combined maternal and infant food allergen avoidance. J Allergy Clin Immunol 1995;95:1179–90.

42. American Academy of Pediatrics. Committee on Nutrition. Hypoallergenic infant formulas. Pediatrics 2000;106(2 Pt 1):346–9.

43. Li XM, Zhang TF, Huang CK, et al. Food Allergy Herbal Formula-1 (FAHF-1) blocks peanut-induced anaphylaxis in a murine model. J Allergy Clin Immunol 2001;108(4):639–46.

44. Fox AT, Sasieni P, Du TG, et al. Household peanut consumption as a risk factor for the development of peanut allergy. J Allergy Clin Immunol 2009;123(2):417–23.

45. Lack G. Epidemiologic risks for food allergy. J Allergy Clin Immunol 2008;121(6):1331–6.

46. von Berg A, Filipiak-Pittroff B, Kramer U, et al. Preventive effect of hydrolyzed infant formulas persists until age 6 years: long-term results from the German Infant Nutritional Intervention Study (GINI). J Allergy Clin Immunol 2008;121(6):1442–7.

47. Hays T, Wood RA. A systematic review of the role of hydrolyzed infant formulas in allergy prevention. Arch Pediatr Adolesc Med 2005;159(9):810–6.

48. Sausenthaler S, Koletzko S, Schaaf B, et al. Maternal diet during pregnancy in relation to eczema and allergic sensitization in the offspring at 2 y of age. Am J Clin Nutr 2007;85(2):530–7.

49. Falth-Magnusson K, Kjellman N. Development of atopic disease in babies whose mothers were receiving exclusion diets during pregnancy – a randomized study. J Allergy Clin Immunol 1987;80:868–75.

50. Falth-Magnusson K, Kjellman NI. Allergy prevention by maternal elimination diet during late pregnancy– a 5-year follow-up of a randomized study. J Allergy Clin Immunol 1992;89(3):709–13.

51. Lilja G, Dannaeus A, Foucard T, et al. Effects of maternal diet during late pregnancy and lactation on the development of atopic diseases in infants up to 18 months of age–in-vivo results. Clin Exp Allergy 1989;19(4):473–9.

52. Kramer MS, Kakuma R. Maternal dietary antigen avoidance during pregnancy or lactation, or both, for preventing or treating atopic disease in the child. Cochrane Database Syst Rev 2006;3:CD000133.

53. Hattevig G, Sigurs N, Kjellman B. Effects of maternal dietary avoidance during lactation on allergy in children at 10 years of age. Acta Paediatr 1999;88(1):7–12.

54. Pollard C, Bevin S, Little S, et al. Influence of maternal diet during lactation upon allergic manifestation in infants – tolerisation or sensitisation? J Allergy Clin Immunol 1996;97(1):240.

55. Frank L, Marian A, Visser M, et al. Exposure to peanuts in utero and in infancy and the development of sensitization to peanut allergens in young children. Pediatr Allergy Immunol 1999;10(1):27–32.

56. Hourihane JO, Dean TP, Warner JO. Peanut allergy in relation to heredity, maternal diet, and other atopic diseases: results of a questionnaire survey, skin prick testing, and food challenges. BMJ 1996;313(7056):518–21.

57. Lack G, Fox D, Northstone K, et al. Factors associated with the development of peanut allergy in childhood. N Engl J Med 2003;348(11):977–85.

58. Tariq SM, Stevens M, Matthews S, et al. Cohort study of peanut and tree nut sensitisation by age of 4 years. BMJ 1996;313(7056):514–7.

59. Willers SM, Wijga AH, Brunekreef B, et al. Maternal food consumption during pregnancy and the longitudinal development of childhood asthma. Am J Respir Crit Care Med 2008;178(2):124–31.

60. Muraro A, Dreborg S, Halken S, et al. Dietary prevention of allergic diseases in infants and small children. Part III: Critical review of published peer-reviewed observational and interventional studies and final recommendations. Pediatr Allergy Immunol 2004;15(4):291–307.

61. Gdalevich M, Mimouni D, David M, et al. Breast-feeding and the onset of atopic dermatitis in childhood: a systematic review and meta-analysis of prospective studies. J Am Acad Dermatol 2001;45(4):520–7.

62. Gdalevich M, Mimouni D, Mimouni M. Breast-feeding and the risk of bronchial asthma in childhood: a systematic review with meta-analysis of prospective studies. J Pediatr 2001;139(2):261–6.

63. van Odijk J, Kull I, Borres MP, et al. Breastfeeding and allergic disease: a multidisciplinary review of the literature (1966–2001) on the mode of early feeding in infancy and its impact on later atopic manifestations. Allergy 2003;58(9):833–43.

64. Kramer MS, Matush L, Vanilovich I, et al. Effect of prolonged and exclusive breast feeding on risk of allergy and asthma: cluster randomised trial. Br Med J 2007;335(7624):815.

65. Matheson MC, Erbas B, Balasuriya A, et al. Breast-feeding and atopic disease: a cohort study from childhood to middle age. J Allergy Clin Immunol 2007;120(5):1051–7.

66. Laubereau B, Brockow I, Zirngibl A, et al. Effect of breast-feeding on the development of atopic dermatitis during the first 3 years of life–results from the GINI-birth cohort study. J Pediatr 2004;144(5):602–7.

67. Kramer MS, Kakuma R. Optimal duration of exclusive breastfeeding. Cochrane Database Syst Rev 2002;(1):CD003517.

68. Grimshaw KE, Allen K, Edwards CA, et al. Infant feeding and allergy prevention: a review of current knowledge and recommendations. A EuroPrevall state of the art paper. Allergy 2009;64(10):1407–16.

69. Osborn DA, Sinn J. Formulas containing hydrolysed protein for prevention of allergy and food intolerance in infants. Cochrane Database Syst Rev 2006;(4):CD003664.

70. Fergusson DM, Horwood LJ, Shannon FT. Early solid feeding and recurrent eczema: a 10-year longitudinal study. Pediatrics 1990;86:541–6.

71. Kajosaari M, Saarinen UM. Prophylaxis of atopic disease by six months; total solid food elimination. Arch Paediatr Scand 1983;72:411–4.

72. Zutavern A, Brockow I, Schaaf B, et al. Timing of solid food introduction in relation to eczema, asthma, allergic rhinitis, and food and inhalant sensitization at the age of 6 years: results from the prospective birth cohort study LISA. Pediatrics 2008;121(1):e44–e52.

73. Poole JA, Barriga K, Leung DY, et al. Timing of initial exposure to cereal grains and the risk of wheat allergy. Pediatrics 2006;117(6):2175–82.

74. Snijders BE, Thijs C, van Ree R, et al. Age at first introduction of cow milk products and other food products in relation to infant atopic manifestations in the first 2 years of life: the KOALA Birth Cohort Study. Pediatrics 2008;122(1):e115–e122.

75. Hourihane JO, Aiken R, Briggs R, et al. The impact of government advice to pregnant mothers regarding peanut avoidance on the prevalence of peanut allergy in United Kingdom children at school entry. J Allergy Clin Immunol 2007;119(5): 1197–202.

76. Dean T, Venter C, Pereira B, et al. Government advice on peanut avoidance during pregnancy–is it followed correctly and what is the impact on sensitization? J Hum Nutr Diet 2007;20(2):95–9.

77. Du Toit G, Katz Y, Sasieni P, et al. Early consumption of peanuts in infancy is associated with a low prevalence of peanut allergy. J Allergy Clin Immunol 2008;122(5):984–91.

78. Osborn DA, Sinn JK. Probiotics in infants for prevention of allergic disease and food hypersensitivity. Cochrane Database Syst Rev 2007;(4):CD006475.

79. Lee J, Seto D, Bielory L. Meta-analysis of clinical trials of probiotics for prevention and treatment of pediatric atopic dermatitis. J Allergy Clin Immunol 2008;121(1):116–21.

80. Host A, Halken S, Muraro A, et al. Dietary prevention of allergic diseases in infants and small children. Pediatr Allergy Immunol 2008;19(1):1–4.

81. Agostoni C, Decsi T, Fewtrell M, et al. Complementary feeding: a commentary by the ESPGHAN Committee on Nutrition. J Pediatr Gastroenterol Nutr 2008;46(1):99–110.

82. Greer FR, Sicherer SH, Burks AW. Effects of early nutritional interventions on the development of atopic disease in infants and children: the role of maternal dietary restriction, breastfeeding, timing of introduction of complementary foods, and hydrolyzed formulas. Pediatrics 2008;121(1):183–91.

Diets and Nutrition: Cross-reacting Food Allergens

Vicki McWilliam

Introduction

To date the only treatment for food allergy is strict avoidance of the offending food and products containing that food. Cows' milk, egg, peanut, tree nuts, fish, soy and wheat cause around 95% of all food allergies in children, either as a single allergy or in combination. For example, an infant with a cows' milk allergy may also be allergic to egg, soy, wheat or peanut.[1] This chapter will explore the practical aspects of excluding some of the common food allergens from the diet and the nutritional considerations to ensure dietary adequacy. The role and process of the diagnostic exclusion or elimination diet will also be discussed.

Cross-reactivity relationships in food allergy

Reactions to multiple foods can be due to separate allergies or through cross-reactivity between certain foods, such as the 20–50% of individuals allergic to peanut also reacting to certain tree nuts, and some individuals allergic to latex also reacting to foods such as avocado, bananas and chestnut. Increased knowledge and understanding of food allergens has led to the identification of specific allergenic proteins within foods. The binding site of these proteins with antibodies within the immune system is known as an epitope. Epitopes on different allergens from different foods can have a degree of amino acid similarity or homology

that allows an antibody specific to one allergen to bind with another structurally similar allergen epitope.[2]

Homologous epitopes are responsible for the frequent cross-reactivity between different foods and also between food allergens and allergens from pollens and insects seen in conditions such as oral allergy syndrome (pollen–food syndrome). This epitope homology is more important than botanical classification in determining cross-reactivity. Cross-reactivity relationships for some key foods are outlined in Table 19.1.

Cows' milk

Cows' milk protein allergy (CMPA) is one of the most common food allergies in infants and children. Presentation is typically after the first exposure to cows' milk-based infant formula, yogurt or custard; however, milk proteins are transferrable in breast milk, so some infants have symptoms despite being exclusively breastfed.[13] Managing cows' milk protein allergy can be complex, as management can involve the maternal diet of breastfed infants, infant formula and the infant's diet. Infant formula contributes significantly to an infant's nutrition depending on age. Cows' milk and products made from cows' milk, such as yogurt, cheese and custard, provide protein, calcium, phosphorus, thiamine, riboflavin, niacin, vitamin A and D to the diet. Ensuring nutritionally equivalent alternatives is important (Table 19.2).

Table 19.1 Cross-reactivity relationships for some common allergenic foods

If allergic to	Chance of being allergic to other foods
Cows' milk protein	Soy protein 3–14% for IgE cows' milk-allergic infants and up to 40% for non-IgE cows' milk-allergic infants[3,4]
Cows' milk protein	Goat or sheeps' milk protein High degree of cross-reactivity due to over 90% sequence identification between α and β caseins from cow, goat and sheep[5]
Cows' milk protein	Beef 13–20%[6] (typically less well cooked forms of beef)
Fish	Other fish Cross-reactivity with other fish appears to be variable, but has been outlined as below: Cod: tuna, mackerel, herring, plaice, sole, bass, eel Tuna: cod, trout, salmon Salmon: sardine, mackerel, tuna Mackerel: anchovy, cod, salmon, herring, sardine, plaice Prawns: lobster, crab, crayfish Mussels: octopus, squid Shellfish: cockroach, house dust mite, snails[2]
Shellfish	Other shellfish: highly likely due to high cross-reactivity between species of shellfish[2]
Shellfish	Fish: rare[7]
Wheat	Other grains This will depend on type of grain: see Table 19.10
Peanut	Tree nuts 20–50%[8,9]
Peanut	Other legumes Soy is rare, 1–3%[10,11] Lupin more common 44%[12]
A tree nut	Other tree nuts – 45%[8]

Breastfed infants

Breast milk remains the ideal choice for the cows' milk protein-allergic infant. Although the cows' milk protein β-lactalbumin can be detected in the breast milk of 95% of lactating women, tolerance is highly variable in cows' milk-allergic infants.[14]

If CMPA symptoms are present or persist in the breastfed infant, then maternal dietary exclusion of cows' milk and cows' milk-based products is indicated. It is important to consider the adequacy of the breastfeeding mother's diet, particularly energy and calcium. Energy requirements are around 2000 kJ higher and an additional 300–500 mg of calcium are required each day during lactation.[15] Particularly for non IgE mediated reactions, replacement of cows' milk-based products with soy products in the maternal diet may exacerbate allergic symptoms in the infant. Therefore, exclusion of cows' milk and soy protein may be required. Calcium intake may only be achieved through the use of supplements. It is also important to consider the lifestyle burden maternal exclusion diets can place on the mother and the family, who are likely to be caring for an unsettled infant.

Formula-fed infants

There are several different types of infant formula available for infants and children with allergy to cows' milk (Table 19.2). Soy, extensively hydrolyzed cows' milk formulas or casein hydrolyzate formulas or amino acid-based infant formulas would be appropriate choices depending on the age, allergic syndrome and associated symptoms of the infant. Lactose-free partially hydrolyzed cows' milk formulas and goats' milk-based infant formula are not suitable for the management of CMPA. Lactose-free formulas contain cows' milk protein and are therefore not suitable. Partially hydrolyzed formulas (PHF) are based on cows' milk protein, but the protein has been hydrolyzed, resulting in reduced peptide length. These formulas are designed to be used in an allergy prevention context for infants with a family history of allergy but who are asymptomatic. Infants with established CMPA should not use PHF.[16] Other mammalian milks and infant formulas made from these milks, such as sheeps' and goats' milk, are also not suitable as β-lactoglobulin, a major protein in cows' milk, is present in all studied mammalian milks, meaning that cross-reactivity is high.[5]

Soy products

Prior to the development of extensively hydrolyzed casein and amino acid-based formulas, soy formulas were the only alternative for treatment of CMPA. This practice has now changed. There are several issues to consider in the use of soy formulas or

Table 19.2 Summary of cows' milk alternatives[16]

Product	Features	Suitability
Breast milk		Breastfeeding mother may need to be on CMP-free diet
Partially hydrolyzed infant formula		Not suitable for infants with established cows' milk protein allergy
Extensively hydrolyzed cows' milk-based infant formula (whey predominant or casein predominant)	Based on cows' milk, but contains smaller protein peptides	First treatment choice for formula-fed infants with cows' milk allergy. Not tolerated by approximately 10–20% of infants with cows' milk allergy
Non-milk based extensively hydrolyzed infant formula	Not available in Australia and New Zealand Palatability an issue	Used more in malabsorption syndromes
Amino acid-based formula	Based on synthetically derived free amino acids	Treatment choice for infants with severe cows' milk allergy who do not tolerate extensively hydrolyzed formula Includes products for infants >12 months of age with higher energy and calcium content
Soy-based infant formula		Not suitable for infants < 6 months of age or infants with non-IgE-mediated allergic reactions Reasonable first alternative for infants over 6 months of age with IgE-mediated CMPA where soy allergy has been excluded and infant refusing extensively hydrolyzed formula
Lactose-free cows' milk-based infant formula	Based on cows' milk but the carbohydrate component, lactose, has been removed	Not suitable
Other mammalian milks or infant formula, e.g. goat		Not suitable
Soy milk		May be suitable for infants >18 months to 2 years depending on nutritional adequacy of diet
Cereal-based milks such as oat or rice	Not nutritionally equivalent to cows' milk. Low in fat, protein, fat-soluble vitamins and minerals found in cows' milk Calcium-fortified brands available	Not suitable for infants under 2 years Usually well tolerated if reactions to cows' milk and soy Use with caution in children under 2 years or with slow growth

soy milk as a replacement for cows' milk-based products. It is now well recognized that cross-reactivity with soy is relatively common in infants with cows' milk allergy.[17] This is thought to be due to a 30 kDa, glycinin-like protein from the soybean that cross-reacts with cows' milk casein,[18] and appears to be more of a concern for infants with non-IgE mediated cows' milk allergy, which affects up to 40% of infants[4] compared to 3–14% of infants with IgE-mediated cows' milk allergy.[19] In addition, soy infant formula contains phytoestrogens and there are concerns regarding their effects on infants' development based on animal studies.[4]

Owing to an absence of adequate scientific research that quantifies the level of risk, many countries have formulated guidelines that advise against the use of soy formulas in young infants, particularly those less than 6 months of age.[4,20]

For children 1–2 years of age options for a cows' milk replacement product could include continuing with a suitable infant formula or a soy- or cereal-based milk replacement product. The nutritional profile of these products can vary enormously with respect to energy, protein, fat, calcium and other micronutrient levels (see Table 19.3). Careful consideration of growth and the contribution of

Table 19.3 Nutritional comparison per 100 mL of cows' milk and alternative products

Product	Energy (kJ)	Protein (g)	Fat (g)	Calcium (mg)	Iron (mg)
Breast milk	290	1.3	4	34	0.1
Cows' milk	195	3.3	3.6	125	0.1
Extensively hydrolyzed formula	280	2	3.5	54	1
Elecare	280	2	3	80	1.5
Neocate	290	2	3.5	50	1
Elecare > 1 yr	420	3.3	5	120	2
Neocate Adv	420	3	4.6	110	1.3
Soy milk	170–300	2–4	1–4	0–160*	–
Rice milk	210–270	0.6–1.5	0.8–1.3	0–120*	–
Oat milk	230–250	0.5–2.5	1.3–1.8	0–120*	–
Almond milk	380	1.1	3.7	0–120*	–

*If calcium fortified.

nutrients from the diet is important in ensuring the product recommended is nutritionally appropriate. Continuing with an infant formula provides a complete range of micronutrients not present in soy milk or cereal-based beverages; however, the formulations for infants under 12 months are lower in calcium. This could be the option for infants with very limited diets, although a calcium supplement may also be required for children over 12 months of age. Changing to an amino acid-based preparation formulated for older children provides more calcium, but significantly increases the energy contribution from formula. Volumes should be reviewed to ensure that appetites are not affected by large quantities of energy-dense formula. Cereal-based beverages, if fortified with calcium, can be an excellent source of calcium but are very low in fat and protein. These products are not recommended for children under 2 years of age and should never be used as a replacement for infant formula for infants under 12 months. Special nutritional assessment is recommended for children with poor growth, limited diets or multiple food allergies if using cereal-based beverages as a cows' milk replacement. There has also been some recent concern with high levels of arsenic in rice beverages, and the Food Standards Agency in the UK does not recommend rice beverages for children under 4.5 years.[21] Calcium-fortified oat milk is an alternative.

CLINICAL CASE 1

A 12-month-old avoiding cows' milk and soy had been breastfed plus some feeds of extensively hydrolyzed formula (EHF). The family was finding it difficult to increase the volumes of EHF. The only commercial milk replacement product available would be a cereal-based beverage, but this is not generally recommended for children under 2 years of age because of the low protein and fat content. Calcium requirements at 12 months are around 500 mg/day. To meet calcium requirements with EHF alone (around 50 mg/100 mL) the child would require a large volume, around 1000 mL/day.

Nutritional interventions may include:

1. Concentrating the EHF by 25–50% (350–420 kJ/100 mL). This would reduce target volumes to meet calcium requirements to 650–800 mL/day.

2. Incorporate some calcium-fortified cereal beverage into the diet, either in cooking, on breakfast cereal or as a custard. Fortified cereal beverages have double the amount of calcium of EHF (around 120 mg/100 mL). EHF would need to be continued as a drink where possible, as cereal beverages are low in protein and fat and generally not recommended for children under 2 years of age.

3. Calcium supplement in addition to EHF.

Practical acceptance of specialized formula

A major clinical challenge in the use of the extensively hydrolyzed and amino acid-based formulas is their palatability. The following strategies may be useful to enhance acceptability:

1. Introduce the flavor of the formula early. An infant allergic to cows' milk and soy will not usually develop tolerance until 2–3 years of age. Even if the child continues to be breastfed they will require additional calcium, energy and protein to replace the cows' milk and cows' milk-based products that would normally be present in the diet. A breastfed infant can have the formula as custard or incorporated into solids to develop familiarity with the taste.

2. Use the current formula or expressed breast milk as a carrier for the specialized formula and gradually transfer to the replacement formula. Note that some amino acid-based formulas do not mix with breast milk because of the lipase. This strategy is also not recommended if reactions to cows' milk protein have been severe.

3. If attempting to wean, have someone other than the breastfeeding mother offer the formula until taken.

4. Offer the specialized formula in a sipper cup supported in a non-feeding position such as a rocker or tilted highchair.

5. Mask the smell and flavor with a few drops of vanilla essence or golden syrup. Remove these once the formula has been accepted.

6. For older children there are flavored versions of the amino acid-based formulas or flavor modules that can be added to the standard products. Commercial milk flavoring powders or syrups are also an option. As with the vanilla essence or golden syrup, remove the flavoring once the formula has been accepted.

7. Formula powder can be added to meals. It can be useful to provide families with a scoop guide for the day. If using this strategy, ensure adequate fluid from other sources. This strategy can result in the child refusing to take solids if too much formula powder is used.

CLINICAL CASE 2

A 4-month-old had a history of reaction to cows' milk-based infant formula, confirmed by a positive skin prick test (SPT). The infant was also sensitized to egg and peanut. Soy-based formula trialed at hospital challenge based on a 3 mm SPT. Soy challenge ceased at 20 mL due to vomiting and eczema exacerbation. Advised to avoid milk, soy, egg and peanut. Although the infant is currently

exclusively breastfed, a prescription for extensively hydrolyzed formula (EHF) was provided and the family advised to trial introduction as a custard or added to solids. Advice regarding introduction of cows' milk, soy, peanut and egg-free solids was provided.

The outcome was that the infant took the EHF formula well in solids and as a custard most days in conjunction with ongoing breastfeeding.

At 12-month review SPTs were repeated with cows' milk, soy, peanut and egg; all remained positive. Advised to continue to avoid. Mother now keen to cease breastfeeding. Advised to use EHF as a drink until 24 months and target volumes provided.

Alternative management for this baby could have been at the initial appointment, providing cows' milk, soy, peanut and egg-free solids advice and continuing with breastfeeding, and at 12-month review a prescription for EHF given when the mother indicated her desire to cease breastfeeding. The likely scenario is that the infant refuses to drink the EHF and the family requires intensive assistance with EHF acceptance and achieving adequate volumes for growth and nutrition.

Comment

Most infants allergic to cows' milk and soy will not develop tolerance until 2–3 years of age. The most appropriate milk replacement is an EHF. For exclusively breastfed infants the early introduction of the flavor of the specialized formula is a very important strategy to ensure its acceptance. This can be done through the use of the formula in foods or as a custard while continuing to breastfeed.

Note: This is a fictional case scenario based on similar real-life cases.

Cows' milk avoidance

Avoidance of cows' milk in commercial food products can be problematic as it is a common base for many ingredients (Table 19.4). Cows' milk is included in mandatory labeling requirements in the European Union, Australia, New Zealand and the US.

Peanuts, legumes, seeds and tree nuts

Peanuts

Peanuts are one of the eight common foods known to cause up to 95% of all food reactions, and peanut allergy has become increasingly common, with a prevalence of between 1.3% and 1.5%. Peanuts

Table 19.4 Common sources of cows' milk and cows' milk-based ingredients in commercial food products

Cows' milk (fresh, UHT, evaporated, condensed, dried/
   powdered, fermented milk products)
Butter, butter milk, most margarines
Cream, sour cream
Cheese
Chocolate
Ice cream
Yogurt, fromage frais
Casein, caseinates, hydrolyzed casein, sodium caseinate
Curd
Ghee
Lactoglobulin
Milk solids, non-fat milk solids
Whey, hydrolyzed whey, whey powder

have been shown to be responsible for the majority of all reported food-induced fatal anaphylaxis cases.[23] Peanuts are part of the botanical family known as Fabaceae or Leguminosae and are classified as a legume. Despite being in the same family as other legumes such as peas, beans and lentils, clinically relevant allergic cross-reactivity with these foods is relatively rare. There is an association between peanut allergy and soy allergy due to epitope homology, but it does not appear to be clinically relevant, with the incidence of soy allergy in people with established peanut allergy reported as 1–3%.[23,24] In contrast, the epitope homology between peanuts and tree nuts is much more clinically relevant, as people with a peanut allergy have a 1 in 5 chance of also being allergic to tree nuts.[8,9]

Currently there are nine identified allergens in peanuts, Ara h 1 to Ara h 9. Everyone with peanut allergy is sensitized to Ara h 2, making it the allergen involved in most allergic reactions to peanut; however, it is Ara h 1 that is responsible for the most severe reactions.[25] Cooking and processing of peanuts changes the allergenicity of the proteins. Fried and boiled peanuts have been found to be less allergenic due to the reduction in Ara h 1. However, roasting peanuts increases the binding capacity of Ara h 1 and Ara h 2, making them significantly more allergenic than raw peanuts.[26]

The safety of oils for people with food allergies is often difficult to determine. Safety depends very much on the technique used to extract the oil. Refining commercial-grade or distilled peanut oils appear to remove virtually all the peanut protein and thus makes them safe for most people with

peanut allergy. Cold-pressed or gourmet peanut oils can result in peanut proteins remaining and allergic reactions have been reported. Peanut oil can be used in cosmetics and is often labeled as arachis oil.[27]

Tree nuts

Tree nuts include cashew, almond, Brazil nut, hazelnut, pistachio, pecan, walnut and macadamia. A person can be allergic to one or several tree nuts and there is high allergic cross-reactivity between peanuts and tree nuts. It has been shown that 23–50% of atopic patients are allergic to both peanuts and tree nuts, and the level of cosensitization varies with the type of tree nut.[22]

Avoidance of peanut and tree nuts

Peanuts and tree nuts are a source of protein, fatty acids and various micronutrients, but for most people these nutrients are also present in other foods in the diet, so eliminating nuts is not a nutritional issue. Vegans or children with multiple food allergies may be an exception, as nuts are a good source of protein and iron if meat and eggs are excluded from the diet.

Avoiding peanuts and tree nuts can be difficult (Table 19.5). Both are included in the mandatory labeling requirements in the European Union, Australia, New Zealand and the US; however, the specific tree nut does not need to be identified in all countries. Because of the relatively high incidence of cross-reactivity between peanuts and tree nuts, the difficulty patients have in distinguishing one nut from another,[28] and the lengthy timeframes involved in performing multiple nut challenges in many hospitals, the advice to patients is often to avoid all peanuts and tree nuts.

Further complicating peanut and tree nut avoidance is that both can be referred to by different names (Table 19.6). This is important if using imported products or travelling overseas.

Soy

Soy allergy is rare in isolation and usually occurs in combination with allergies to other foods. It has been shown that 3–14% of non-IgE-mediated cows' milk-allergic infants and up to 40% of non-IgE-mediated cows' milk allergic infants will also react to soy protein.[4,19]

Table 19.5 Avoiding peanuts and tree nuts

Sources of peanut and tree nuts	• Peanut butter • Other nut butters or pastes • Peanut and satay sauce (peanut based) • Chocolate spreads, e.g. Nutella – (hazelnut) • Nut biscuits such as amaretto, macaroons, florentines – (almond) • Crushed nuts on top of cakes, fruit buns, ice cream and desserts (can be peanut or other nuts) • Baklava, Greek pastry (walnut or peanut) • Waldorf salad (walnuts) • Nut-filled chocolates (can be peanut or other nuts) • Praline, fine nut (usually hazelnut) product added to desserts and chocolates • Marzipan icing, confectionery or cake decorations (usually almond based)
Common sources of peanut or tree nuts that should be checked carefully	• Muesli and breakfast cereal • Muesli bars and health bars • Energy mixes or trail mix • Fruit crumble mix • Christmas cakes and puddings • Fruit cake icing • Friands and flourless cakes (often contain almond meal) • Nougat and fudge • Pesto • Flavored cheeses (fruit and nut, walnut) • Worcestershire sauce • Asian-style meals (particularly Thai and Indian dishes) • Salad dressings • Textured or hydrolyzed vegetable protein • Pastries containing lupin flour
Products at high risk of being contaminated with peanuts or tree nuts	• Takeaway foods or restaurant meals • Commercial breakfast cereals • Chocolate • Asian foods • Commercial biscuits and ice creams
Non-food sources of peanut or tree nuts	• Animal and bird feeds • Cosmetics and massage oils (check for arachis oil) • Prometrium (progesterone cream derived from peanuts) • Craft activities

Table 19.6 Alternative names for peanut and tree nuts

Peanut	Peanuts, ground nuts, earth nuts, monkey nuts, arachis oil, arachis hypogaea, groundnut oil, peanut oil, peanut flavor, peanut butter
Hazelnut	Filbert, cob nut
Macadamia	Queensland nut, candle nut
Pecan	Hickory nut, mashuga

There are limited nutritional consequences of avoiding soy except for vegans; however, it is a common ingredient in many commercial food products and can appear in a broad range of food products (Table 19.7). The combination of cows' milk and soy allergy makes dairy replacement more difficult. Soy is included in mandatory labeling laws in the European Union, Australia, New Zealand and the US.

Other legumes

The botanical family Fabaceae is large and includes peanut and soy, which have been previously discussed. Other allergy relevant legumes include lupin, chickpeas, lentils and peas. Legumes can be an important source of protein in the diet and allergy to legumes seems to vary across different countries depending on the frequency of use in the diet. As with other food allergens clinical cross-reactivity is determined more by allergen structure

Table 19.7 Avoiding soy

Sources of soy that should definitely be avoided	• Soy milk • Soy-based infant formula • Soy yoghurts and custards • Soy cheese
Common sources of soy that should be checked carefully	• Non-dairy ice creams and ice confections • Soy sauce (fermentation does not destroy allergen) • Tamari • Tempeh • Textured vegetable protein • Tofu (soy bean curd) • Miso soup • Soy-based chocolate
Soy based ingredients usually tolerated	• Most regular breads contain soy flour • Many 'allergy' food products contain soy flour, e.g. wheat-free flours, bread mixes, pancake mixes etc. • Home-made bread mixes • Hydrolyzed vegetable protein • Baked goods such as biscuits, cakes and pastries • Cake and pancake mixes • Sauces and soup mixes • Baby cereals and meals • Ice creams and ice confection • Refined soy oil • Soy lecithin

than the botanical family relationships and clinical cross-reactivity within the legume family is rare. An exemption seems to be peanut and lupin which has been reported in one study to be as high as 44%.[12]

Lupin can be eaten as a legume or in the form of flour. Lupin flour has become an increasingly common addition to flour mixes owing to its high protein content. It can often be added into wheat-free flour mixes and lupin allergy appears to be increasing. As a result, lupin now falls under mandatory labeling laws in Europe, but so far not Australia, New Zealand or the US.[29,30,31]

Seeds

Allergic reactions have been reported to a variety of different seeds, including sesame, linseed (flaxseed), poppy seed, cottonseed, mustard seed, annatto seed and sunflower seed. Prevalence varies in different countries.[2] Sesame is the most common seed to cause allergic reactions, thought to be because of increased consumption both as a seed and as oil.[32]

Unlike peanut oil, which is often refined and considered safe to include for people with peanut allergy, seed oils are often cold pressed and still potentially allergenic.

Mustard seed allergy is common in Europe and included in the European Union mandatory

Table 19.8 Common food sources of seeds

Sesame	Sesame oil, tahina, halvah, hummus, vegetarian products, 'health bars', seeded breads, Asian foods
Poppy	Seeded breads, muffins, cakes, Asian meals, Indian curry pastes
Mustard	Curry powder, pickles, seeded mustard, sandwiches and smallgoods
Sunflower	Seeded breads, cooking oil, birdseed products, sunflower seed spread
Linseed	Seeded breads, linseed supplemented products

labeling requirements. Sesame seed is included in mandatory labeling laws in the US, Europe, Australia and New Zealand, but labels will often only specify seeds.

Typical food sources for seeds include breads, cakes, biscuits, muffins, 'health bars' and nut bars, breakfast cereals, trail mix and unrefined oils (Table 19.8).

CLINICAL CASE 3

A 4-month-old exclusively breastfed infant girl was assessed as having atopic dermatitis, which persisted despite appropriate use of emollients and topical steroids. The mother had an unrestricted diet.

Skin prick testing (SPT) of the child produced wheals of 4 mm to cows' milk, 3 mm to hen's egg and 2 mm to peanut. The mother was advised to avoid dairy products (but not soy), eggs, peanuts and tree nuts, and to continue standard eczema treatment of the baby. She was instructed in how to examine food labels to avoid cows' milk and cows' milk-based food products, egg and peanut. Within 2 weeks, the baby's dermatitis had dramatically improved but not completely resolved, and there was significantly less requirement for topical steroids. Recommendations were given on introducing solids, avoiding egg, nut and cows' milk products until after 12 months of age. The mother was advised to systematically challenge dairy products and egg in her diet to gauge the effect on the dermatitis.

When reassessed at 12 months, the child's dermatitis was relatively mild. Expansion of the mother's diet to include milk and egg in all forms had not had a significant effect on her skin. Inadvertent exposure to cows' milk had occurred 2 months earlier without clinical reactivity in the baby. The baby was also able to tolerate egg cooked in cake, but not uncooked egg in cake batter, which had caused facial urticaria. Repeat SPT gave the following wheal results: cows' milk, no reaction; egg, 9 mm; peanut, 5 mm. A home-based milk introduction was recommended, a formal hospital-based baked egg challenge and the continued avoidance of peanut was advised. The baked egg challenge was negative and cows' milk and baked egg were introduced successfully.

At 2 years of age, SPT wheal results were: egg, 3 mm; peanut, 1 mm; other tree nuts, no reaction. A formal hospital-based challenge to peanut was negative. A formal hospital-based raw egg challenge resulted in facial urticaria and a delayed exacerbation of dermatitis. Continued avoidance of raw egg was advised. Home-based tree nut introduction was discussed.

Comment

Cooking partially destroys the allergen in egg, and so patients with mild to moderate reactivity may tolerate egg if well cooked. The clinical significance of a reaction to egg becoming less severe over subsequent skin prick tests in the context of a history of previous clinical reaction needs to be determined by deliberate challenge. Even then, the size of the wheal does not correlate well with the severity of any reaction that occurs.

Note: This is a fictional case scenario based on similar real-life cases.

Wheat and other cereal grains

Wheat

There are a number of possible food hypersensitivity reactions to wheat, with multiple mechanisms involved. Depending on the route of allergen exposure and the underlying immunologic mechanisms, wheat allergy is classified into the following:

- IgE-mediated food allergy affecting the skin, gastrointestinal tract or respiratory tract
- Food-dependent exercise-induced anaphylaxis (FDEIA)
- Occupational asthma (baker's asthma)
- Rhinitis
- Contact urticaria
- Non-IgE- or T-cell-mediated intestinal inflammation.

Ingestion of wheat may also cause celiac disease and dermatitis herpetiformis. Wheat has also been recently implicated in irritable bowel syndrome, possibly owing to its fructan content.[33]

Wheat allergy in children seems to begin in infancy and is outgrown by 3–5 years of age, as seen with other common food allergens such as milk and egg.[1] Immediate reactions include urticaria, angioedema, nausea, abdominal pain, or in severe cases anaphylaxis. Delayed hypersensitivity symptoms appearing 24–48 hours after wheat ingestion include gastrointestinal symptoms and exacerbation of eczema. The majority of wheat-allergic children suffer from moderate to severe eczema, and sensitization to other foods such as egg and milk is common.

Wheat allergy is not common in adults and is more likely to be seen as a specific form of anaphylaxis known as food-dependent exercise-induced anaphylaxis (FDEIA) (see Chapter 9). Other presentations include reactions induced by non-ingested forms such as occupational asthma or baker's asthma, which is triggered by the inhalation of raw wheat flour, or skin symptoms such as urticaria or eczema to wheat-based ingredients in cosmetics.[34] This is reviewed in more detail in Chapter 8.

Avoiding wheat

Wheat is the most widely consumed food grain in the world. It is a major nutrient source and a base to many commercial food product ingredients (Table 19.9). A wheat-free diet may result in sub-optimal intake of thiamine, riboflavin and energy. In addition, wheat-based products such as bread and breakfast cereals may be fortified with other nutrients not naturally present in wheat as a way of fortifying a population's diet (e.g. iron, folate, iodine, calcium, omega 3 fatty acids).

Table 19.9 Food sources of wheat

Contain wheat	Likely to contain wheat
• Wheat flour	• Rissoles and sausages
• Bulgar and durum wheat	• Processed meats and sandwich meats
• Wheatgerm	• Breakfast cereals
• Wheat starch	• Soy products (wheat-based maltodextrin)
• Semolina	
• Couscous	
• Wheat pasta	• Chicken stuffing and skin seasonings
• Wheat noodles	
• Regular bread	• Dry roasted nuts
• Battered or crumbed meats	• Gravy, stock cubes and sauces
• Soups with pasta or noodles	• Canned soups
• Baked products such as biscuits, cakes, pancakes, pastry	• Soy sauce
	• Flavored crisps
	• Confectionery
• Commercial teething rusks	• Flavored milk powders, coffee creamers and whiteners
• Pretzels	
• Ice cream cones and wafers	• Icing sugar mixture

When providing advice about wheat avoidance, it is important to consider the purpose of exclusion, as dietary recommendations will vary for wheat allergy, celiac disease and non-allergic hypersensitivity reactions to wheat. The following information is relevant for wheat allergy.

Wheat has high cross-reactivity with barley, rye and oat. Rice, corn and potato are the best grain substitutes for wheat-allergic patients.[35] A summary of wheat substitutes and their suitability is given in Table 19.10.

Other grains

IgE-mediated allergic reactions to grains other than wheat seem to be rare or are less well documented. In countries where rice or corn are the main carbohydrate staple, allergic sensitization and reported allergy seems to be higher.[2] Where cereal allergy seems to be more of a clinical issue is in gastrointestinal food allergy conditions such as food protein-induced enterocolitis (FPIES) and eosinophilic esophagitis. As discussed in detail in Chapter 11, FPIES is a rare form of T-cell-mediated gastrointestinal food hypersensitivity that presents in infancy. Reactions have been reported predominantly to cows' milk and soy protein; however, multiple grains including wheat, oat, rice, barley and corn have all been implicated, either individually or in combination. Rice has been reported as the most common food involved in solid food FPIES.[36,37]

Wheat, oats, barley and rye are included in UK, US, Europe, Australia and New Zealand mandatory labeling laws. Rice and corn are not included at present. Sources of rice and corn include:

Rice: rice flour, ground rice, rice cakes and crackers, rice pudding, rice noodles.
Corn: cornflour, breakfast cereals, tortilla wraps, corn chips, taco shells, polenta, popcorn, cornstarch and corn syrup.

Egg

Egg is one of the most common food allergies in infants and young children, with a prevalence estimated at between 0.5% and 2.5%. Egg sensitization is closely associated with atopic dermatitis, particularly in infants who develop eczema in the first year of life.[38] Delayed exacerbations of eczema may occur in children without evidence of sensitization to egg, most likely due to T-cell-mediated allergic reactions. Improvement in symptoms of eczema has been demonstrated with an egg-free diet in children observed to experience exacerbation after egg ingestion.[39]

Other IgE manifestations reported to egg include urticaria, angioedema, vomiting, diarrhea and anaphylaxis. A smaller number of children with egg allergy present with gastrointestinal symptoms, including allergic proctocolitis or eosinophilic esophagitis.[38]

Clinically relevant allergens are found in both egg yolk and egg white, but egg white allergy is more commonly seen. Five major allergens have been identified, including Gal d 1–5. Egg white contains ovomucoid (Gal d 1: 11%), ovalbumin (Gal d 2: 55%), ovotransferrin (Gal d 3,12%), lysozyme (Gal d 4, 3%) and ovomucin (4%). Ovomucoid appears to be the predominant allergen and is associated with persistent egg allergy into adulthood. Egg yolk allergens include ovoflavoprotein, apovitellenins I and IV, phosvitin and α-livetin.[2]

Treatment is the avoidance of egg and egg-containing products (Table 19.11), but eggs are an important source of protein, fat, vitamin E, riboflavin, thiamine and folic acid. Dietary assessment should therefore ensure there are adequate alternative sources of these nutrients in the diet,

Table 19.10 Summary of substitutes for wheat

Grain or grain substitute	Description	Suitability
Barley	Barley is a member of the grass family. Consumed as a flour or dehulled as pearl barley in stews and soups. Contains gluten	55% cross-reactivity reported, best to avoid unless tolerated on oral challenge
Oats	Oats are members of the grass family. Consumed most commonly as milled oatmeal	High cross-reactivity with wheat, include only after negative oral challenge
Rye	Rye is a member of the grass family and is closely related to barley and wheat. Contains gluten	High cross-reactivity with wheat, include only after negative oral challenge
Tapioca/cassava	Tapioca is a starch extracted from the root of a plant commonly known as cassava. Made into flakes, sticks or pearls that are soaked in water before use. Used as a thickening agent in products or made into snack foods	Yes
Rice	Rice is a member of the grass family. It is a versatile grain that can be eaten as a whole grain or milled as flour	Yes
Corn/maize	Corn is a member of the grass family. Has a wide range of uses. It is consumed straight off the cob or popped, as a flour and manufactured into ingredients such as corn syrup and corn starch	Yes
Potato	An edible tuber. Used whole in many forms in the diet. Also processed to form flour and potato starch	Yes
Buckwheat	Buckwheat is not a cereal or a grass and is often referred to as a pseudo cereal. Milled as flour used for breads, noodles, pancakes, or as groats for porridge	Yes
Amaranth	Amaranth is a herbal plant. Its leaves are consumed as a vegetable in some countries. The seeds can be milled to a flour	Yes
Chickpea flour (besan, garbanzo)	Chickpeas are a legume that can be ground into a high-protein flour product commonly used in Indian products.	Yes
Sago	Sago is the starch extracted from the pith of sago palm stems. Can be baked or ground into a powder used as a thickener or a flour, or made into a dessert	Yes
Sorghum	A member of the grass family	Yes
Kamut	Wheat hybrid. Name is actually a US trademark	No
Lupin	Member of the legume family	Yes
Quinoa	Grain-like crop, not a member of the grass family. Can be eaten as an alternative to rice, a breakfast food or a flour	Yes
Soy flour	Member of the legume family	Yes
Triticale	Hybrid of wheat	No
Millet	Cereal or grain of the grass family. Consumed as a porridge or a flour	Yes
Spelt	Wheat hybrid used as a flour or as a bread	No
Arrowroot	Edible starch from the tuber of the arrowroot plant. Used in similar ways to tapioca and sago	Yes
Chia flour	Made from the seed of the chia plant	Yes
Gluten-free products	The definition of gluten-free varies in different countries. Countries that use *Codex alimentarius* define gluten-free as <20 ppm gluten which may still include wheat starch. Other countries use 'no detectable gluten' as per an ELISA test, and these products would be suitable	Will be variable

Table 19.11 Sources of egg (well cooked, loosely cooked, raw)

Well-cooked egg*	Slightly cooked or high egg white containing	Raw
• Cakes	• Meringues	• Fresh mousse
• Biscuits	• Pavlova	• Fresh mayonnaise
• Dried egg pasta	• Lemon curd	• Fresh ice cream
• Oven-baked meat dishes (meatloaf, meatballs, sausage rolls)	• Quiche and frittata	• Fresh sorbet
• Well-cooked fresh egg pasta	• Scrambled egg	• Horseradish sauce
• Egg glaze on pastry	• Boiled egg	• Tartar sauce
	• Fried egg	• Raw egg in cake mix
	• Omelette	• Egg flips or eggnog
	• Poached egg	
	• Egg in batter	
	• Egg in breadcrumbs: fish, schnitzels	
	• Hamburgers or rissoles	
	• Asian dishes with omelette or egg white added	
	• Hollandaise sauce	
	• Egg custard	
	• Pancakes	
	• Mud cake	

*egg protein in low dose and exposed to high temperature for prolonged periods of time

particularly for vegetarians or patients with multiple food allergies.

The degree of egg avoidance required can be variable. Maternal ingestion of egg has been shown to increase ovalbumin concentrations; however, the amounts are highly variable.[40] The need to exclude egg from the maternal diet of women breastfeeding infants with allergy symptoms should be individually assessed.

Reaction to raw or lightly cooked egg but tolerance of more extensively cooked egg such as in cakes and biscuits is commonly reported. The egg allergens ovomucoid and ovalbumin can be altered by heat and acidity, but lysozyme appears to be unaffected.[41]

Another issue to consider is whether the continued exposure to cooked egg at a level below that which induces symptoms increases IgE levels or delays the acquisition of tolerance in allergic individuals. This is an area of some controversy, and although some studies have demonstrated a decrease in IgE levels with continued exposure to egg, it is unclear how this compares to the natural resolution of egg allergy.[38] Clinical Case 4 provides a guide to the different food forms of egg.

For commercial food products, egg is included in US, European Union, Australian and New Zealand mandatory labeling laws. For home baking and cooking commercial egg replacers are available, or eggs can be replaced with fruit or vegetable puree or the use of vinegar, baking powder and water.

CLINICAL CASE 4 HIDDEN SOURCES OF NUTS AND SEEDS

A 22-year-old with peanut, multiple tree nut and sesame allergies is attending a family wedding which is catered by family friends and relatives. Issues for this person are that the food has been prepared in domestic kitchens where compliance with and communication of potential allergens is difficult to determine.

The menu consists of:

Entrée: Asian rice balls, crumbed and deep fried.

High risk: Possible source of sesame or peanut oil in rice filling or as the cooking oil.

Main meal: Fish and salad.

After discussion with the family member who prepared the dish, the patient is informed that the fish is cooked in a blended vegetable oil.

Salad dressing can be a home-made dressing of balsamic vinegar, garlic and olive oil or a commercial 'gourmet salad' dressing.

Lowest risk is the balsamic dressing. Blended vegetable oil and olive oil are not likely to contain unrefined nut or seed oils. 'Gourmet salad dressing' is more likely to contain unrefined nut oils, which can be a source of residual protein.

Dessert: Wedding cake – chocolate cake, iced with royal icing.

High risk: Chocolate cake may have almond meal as an ingredient and the royal icing may have a marzipan layer underneath.

Note: This is a fictional case scenario based on similar real-life cases.

Seafood

Seafood includes vertebrate finned fish such as cod, salmon and tuna, crustaceans such as prawns, crab and lobster, and molluscs such as squid, scallops, clams, oysters and snails. Crustaceans and molluscs are often referred to as 'shellfish'.

Adverse reactions to seafood include immunologic, such as IgE-mediated allergy triggered by ingestion or inhalation of proteins, and adverse reactions that are not immune based, caused by toxins or infectious contaminants. Allergic reactions to ingestion of seafood can include anaphylaxis, and skin contact and inhalation of vapors may cause asthma and contact dermatitis. The prevalence of seafood allergy varies around the world, but is usually higher in communities with higher seafood consumption. Seafood allergy is often lifelong, with one study[42] demonstrating that 65.5% of fish-sensitized children maintained their sensitization until school age.

Parvalbumins have been identified as the major allergen in fish species and tropomysin in crustacean and molluscs. Interspecies cross-reactivity is common; therefore people diagnosed with a fish allergy often have to avoid all fish or all shellfish.[43] Individual IgE testing is advisable before consuming other types of fish or shellfish if the person has an established seafood allergy. There appears to be no clinically relevant allergic cross-reactivity between shellfish and fish. The specific cross-reactivity relationships between seafood species seems to be variable; however, a recent food hypersensitivity text summarized this clinical issue (Table 19.12).[2]

Table 19.12 Seafood cross-reactivity relationships

Seafood	Cross-reacting species
Cod	Tuna, mackerel, herring, plaice, sole, bass, eel
Tuna	Cod, trout, salmon
Salmon	Sardine, mackerel, tuna
Mackerel	Anchovy, cod, salmon, herring, sardine, plaice
Prawns	Lobster, crayfish, crab
Mussels	Octopus, squid
Shellfish	Cockroach, house dust mite, snails

Seafood allergens respond differently to heat. Fish allergens can be degraded with very high heat; therefore, people with a salmon or tuna allergy may tolerate commercially prepared forms of canned salmon and/or tuna. Allergens from crustaceans and molluscs remain potent allergens after cooking, and there have been reported reactions from the vapors emitted while cooking shellfish. As discussed in more detail in Chapter 8, patients with seafood allergies should exercise caution to avoid cross-contamination when purchasing fresh seafood from markets or consuming seafood in restaurants where multiple types of fish or shellfish may be handled.

The consideration and exclusion of seafood poisoning as a differential diagnosis for seafood allergy is important, as seafood poisoning symptoms are often identical to food allergy symptoms.

Avoidance of seafood is relatively straightforward compared to that for other common allergens; however, anchovies can be used in many dishes to enhance flavor, and sauces such as Worcestershire and fish sauce are common ingredients in Asian dishes and condiments. Fish, crustaceans and molluscs are all included in US, European Union, Australian and New Zealand mandatory labeling laws.

Fish oil supplements may not be advisable for people who are highly sensitive to small amounts of fish as some fish proteins may still be present. The omega-3 in infant formula can be from variable sources including fish, and is considered safe for infants with fish allergy or sensitization.[2]

Fruits and vegetables

Although rare, allergic reactions to fruits and vegetables can occur as a result of primary food allergy to the protein/s present in various fruits and vegetables (Table 19.13). This form of allergy seems to be more of an issue for older children, adolescents and adults. It is often isolated to one particular food, and both raw and cooked forms will elicit reactions. The types of fruit and vegetable responsible for allergic reactions seem to vary around the world; for instance, peach allergy is common in Spain, carrot allergy in Central Europe, and celery allergy in Sweden and France. Symptoms can vary from urticaria to anaphylaxis, and reactions are usually rapid.[2]

A more common and secondary form of allergic reaction is through cross-reactivity of fruit and

Table 19.13 Summary of allergic reactions involving fruits and vegetables

		Type of reaction	
	Primary fruit and vegetable allergy	**Pollen allergy**	**Latex allergy**
Common foods involved	Kiwi Apple Peach Celery Carrot Potato	**Birch Pollen:** Apple, pear, cherry, nectarine, apricot, plum, kiwi, hazelnut, almond, celery, carrot, potato **Birch/Mugwort:** Celery, carrot, spices, sunflower, honey **Grass:** melon, watermelon, orange, tomato, potato, peanut **Ragweed:** watermelon, melon, orange, tomato, potato, peanut **Plane:** hazelnut, peach, apple, melon, kiwi, peanuts, maize, chickpeas, lettuce, green beans **Plantain:** melon, watermelon, tomato, orange, kiwi	Avocado Chestnut Banana Passionfruit Kiwi Papaya Mango Tomato Pepper Potato Celery
		70% of people with pollen allergy	40% of people with latex allergy
	One fruit or veg	Multiple fruits or vegetables	Multiple fruits or vegetables
Form of the fruit or vegetable involved in reactions	Raw and cooked	Raw	Raw

vegetable proteins with proteins in pollens, grasses or latex; this group of reactions are known as oral allergy syndrome. This form of allergy can involve multiple fruits and/or vegetables and can include nuts. Symptoms tend to be isolated to the oropharynx and include itching, tingling, swelling of the lips, palate and tongue. Latex reactions can involve anaphylaxis. Reactions tend to be with fresh rather than cooked forms of fruits and vegetables (see Chapter 7).

As with other forms of food allergy, it is the specific allergen type that determines cross-reactivity relationships, rather than botanical family.

Manufactured foods

Food labeling laws

For manufactured food products, successful allergen avoidance requires careful reading of product ingredients. This information is found in the ingredient list, where foods are listed in descending order of predominance. Mandatory labeling of the major allergens is now required in many countries (Table 19.14). Food allergens must be clearly identifiable either within the ingredient list or as a

general statement at the end of the list. As an example, the milk protein casein can be labeled in the following ways:

1. Casein (milk)
2. Milk casein
3. At the end of the ingredients list a generic statement that says 'contains milk'.

Allergenic ingredients must be identified no matter how small the amount, including their use as a processing aid, such as wheat flour dusted on food molds to prevent sticking.

Although this level of ingredient labeling has assisted consumers enormously in identifying whether an allergen is present, ultimately it is the amount and nature of the allergenic protein in the food product that will determine its safety. The current labeling laws do not exempt food ingredients derived from the common allergenic sources that contain little or no protein. Even in cases where evidence exists to indicate that the ingredient is not allergenic, its declaration may still be required. This can lead to unnecessary restriction of food products.

Examples include refined peanut oils, wheat maltodextrin, soy lecithin and wheat glucose syrup.

Table 19.14 Summary of allergen food labeling in different countries

	Country		
	US	**Europe and UK**	**Australia and New Zealand**
Mandatory Allergens	Milk Egg Fish Crustacean shellfish Tree nuts Peanuts Wheat Soybeans	Milk Egg Fish Crustacean shellfish Peanuts Soybeans Tree nuts Cereals containing gluten Celery Mustard Sesame Added sulfites *Lupin *Molluscs	Milk Egg Fish Crustacean shellfish Peanuts Soybeans Tree nuts Sesame seed Cereals containing gluten Added sulfites
Year legislation adopted	2006	2005 *added 2007	2002
Precautionary labeling details	Not regulated	Not regulated	Not regulated VITAL guidelines
Governing Organization	Food Labeling and Consumer Protection Act, regulated by FDA	European Union	Food Standards Australia and New Zealand (FSANZ)

Another issue is the lack of identification of many foods that can cause reactions, such as rice, corn, lupin and molluscs. Lupin and molluscs have been included in the European Union legislation since 2007.

Precautionary labeling

The current labeling laws relate only to intentionally added ingredients. Commercial food production can result in food allergen residues through practices such as shared manufacturing or packaging equipment. Food companies are aware of the risk this contamination can pose to highly allergic individuals, and as a result have adopted advisory labeling statements. Examples include:

1. May contain milk
2. Made on equipment that processes nuts
3. Manufactured in a facility that processes peanut.

These statements are not governed by the same regulations as the mandatory ingredient labeling and pose a significant amount of confusion for consumers and health professionals. Some of the controversies include:

- The use of precautionary labeling is voluntary; therefore, a product free from such labeling is not necessarily safer than one that includes it.
- The wording used is not standardized. One survey in the US found 25 different versions, and despite consumer perception the type of statement does not indicate varying levels of risk.[44]
- The use of precautionary labeling is becoming more common. In the US, 17% of food products were found to contain precautionary labeling,[44] and in Australia this has been reported as high as 95% for some product lines.[45]

The chances of having an allergic reaction through contamination during processing is extremely unlikely; however, studies in the US have shown that the amounts detected can be highly variable and in some instances can cause anaphylaxis.[46] The issue for consumers and the health professionals advising them is to determine the level of risk, which is very difficult. Threshold levels for reactions have been determined for milk, egg and peanut;[47] however, food companies do not routinely assay products to determine their allergen content, and individual patients are rarely aware of their threshold levels for reactions. In many circumstances ignoring precautionary labeling will pose minimal risk for allergic consumers, but highly allergic individuals should be advised against this and be encouraged to contact companies directly to explore food processing, packaging and cleaning procedures.

Nutritional issues

A detailed history is an important baseline for the nutritional management of a patient diagnosed with food allergies. Important aspects include:

- Results of medical tests such as specific IgE and skin test results
- Anthropometrics: current weight and height and growth history should be plotted on standardized growth charts
- Family history of allergic disease should be explored and documented – hayfever/rhinitis, asthma, eczema, food allergy
- Detailed diet history:
  - Known and perceived triggers for symptoms
  - Diet prior to onset of symptoms
  - Current diet
  - Infant feeding history, including duration of breastfeeding, introduction of infant formula, introduction of solids
  - Maternal diet for breastfed infants.

Monitoring growth and assessing the adequacy of overall micronutrient intake is important for children with food allergies. Poor growth is not uncommon in children with food allergies and numerous studies have demonstrated this.[48,49] Lower intakes of energy, fat, protein, calcium, riboflavin and niacin have been reported in children with cows' milk-free diets.[50]

There are many factors that can contribute to inadequate intakes:

- The presence of multiple food allergies. This is particularly relevant for children needing to exclude cows' milk or wheat, as they are important sources of energy, protein and other important nutrients in a child's diet. Milk and wheat are also a common base for many commercial food product ingredients, so exclusion from the diet can make food variety very limited.

- Slow progression with solids due to parental anxiety or fussy or difficult eating behavior.
- Use of inappropriate milk substitute products or inadequate volumes due to poor palatability can result in poor growth and micronutrient deficiencies.
- Energy deficits of severe eczema.
- Other concurrent dietary restrictions for cultural, ethical or religious purposes. For example, excluding peanut and egg from the diet because of allergies may not pose a nutritional risk to someone who has alternate sources of protein and iron in their diet such as dairy products and meat; however, for a vegan this may be an issue.

Ensuring adequate growth

It is important to monitor weight and height. If growth has faltered specialist dietetic advice is recommended. Strategies to achieve catch-up growth can include:

- High-energy formula
- Added fats and oils
- Specific advice regarding energy-dense foods and snacks
- Glucose polymer.

Ensuring adequate calcium

It may not be possible to achieve adequate calcium intakes on a cows' milk protein-free diet. Calcium intake recommendations vary slightly for different countries and with age (Table 19.15). It is important

Table 19.15 Calcium requirements summary

Age	Calcium requirement (mg/day)		
	US[52] (AI)	UK[51] (RNI)	Australia[15]
0–12 mths	210–270	525	210–270 (AI)
1–3 yrs	500	350	500 (RDI)
4–8 yrs	800	450	700 (RDI)
9–13 yrs	1300	550	1000–1300 (RDI)
14–18 yrs	1300	Male 1000 Female 800	1300 (RDI)
19+	1000	700	1000 (RDI)
Lactation		+ 550	1000 (RDI)

Table 19.16 Examples of cows' milk protein-free sources of calcium

Food product	Calcium (mg)
1 glass (200 mL) calcium fortified soy milk	240
1 glass (200 mL) calcium fortified rice or oat milk	240
50 g tofu	250
1 tub soy yogurt	100–240
75 g bony fish (if bones eaten)	250
3 dried figs	170
75 g boiled spinach and raw parsley	125
2 tablespoons red kidney beans	100
1 tablespoon white sesame seeds	80
1 tablespoon tahini	75 g
Bony fish (must eat bones)	75 g
150 g baked beans	75
1 medium orange	75
12 almonds	65
100 g other dark green vegetables	50
30 g soy cheese	50–90

to continue to reassess dietary intake to ensure adequate calcium. Non-dairy sources of calcium (Table 19.16) can be suggested, but it is often difficult for children to consume the quantities required on a regular basis.

CLINICAL CASE 5

A 14-month-old allergic to milk, soy, wheat, egg and peanut. Intake to date has included around 4–6 breastfeeds each day with meals consisting of the following:

Breakfast. oat-based porridge (unfortified), prepared with water

Lunch: rice or gluten-free pasta with a tomato-based vegetable sauce

Dinner: offered meat but not keen to eat

Good range of vegetables

Snacks: rice crackers, home-made muffins, fruit

Nutritional Issues: low energy, low calcium and low iron intake

Comments: breast milk alone is low in calcium and iron, and more bioavailable adequate calcium and iron intakes do rely on a reasonable intake of calcium and iron to be coming from food at 14 months of age

---

Strategies

Calcium

Recommended calcium intake is around 500 mg/day.

Could be met with combination of extensively hydrolyzed formula (EHF) and calcium fortified cereal beverage in cooking and on breakfast cereal.

If inadequate volumes of EHF taken, can be added to foods or made into a custard, as exclusion of cows' milk and soy results in no other calcium-rich food choices such as yogurt or custard.

Iron

For toddlers that are not keen to take meat, strategies often include use of peanut paste, egg and iron-fortified breads and cereals as alternative sources of iron. For this toddler the options are limited by the allergies.

Possible strategies include:

- Incorporating iron-fortified cereal with oat porridge
- Incorporating legumes with meals
- Use of EHF will also improve iron intake.

Energy

Cows' milk-based products such as full cream milk, cheese and yogurt contribute a significant proportion of energy and protein to a toddler's diet. Fats and oils added to meals and offering higher-protein foods at two meals a day may be necessary to ensure adequate energy intakes and growth.

Note: This is a fictional case scenario based on similar real-life cases.

Elimination/exclusion diets for diagnosis of food allergy and intolerance

Elimination or exclusion diets are a diagnostic tool used when diet seems to contribute to symptoms and there are no other diagnostic methods available or diagnostic methods seem to be incomplete. The type of diet selected, the foods excluded and the duration of exclusion will all vary depending on the age of the person, the clinical history and the symptoms present. In general the process involves three phases:

Food exclusion: The initial diet may be very restrictive, including only a few food items, or one or several specific foods may be eliminated. The type of diet used and the duration of the diet will depend on symptoms and should be formulated in consultation with the medical team responsible for the patient.

Food reintroduction/challenges (Chapter 14): If resolution of symptoms is achieved while undertaking the diet then foods should be systematically reintroduced and symptoms monitored in an attempt to identify trigger foods. A food and symptom diary is useful to document this process.

Home challenges are not recommended if there is still a strongly positive skin prick test or specific IgE result, or if there is a past history of the food causing anaphylaxis. The amount and rate of grading of the foods back into the diet will depend on the type of allergy, type of symptoms and the age of the child. Food reintroduction should be approached in consultation with the medical team responsible for the patient.

Maintenance diet: Once any trigger foods have been identified, the baseline diet should be assessed for maximum variety and to ensure nutritional adequacy. As children often outgrow their allergy, timeframes for ongoing challenges should be discussed.

References

1. Ramesh S. Food allergy overview in children. Clin Rev Allergy Immunol 2008;34:217–30.

2. Skypala I, Venter C (editors). Food Hypersensitivity: Diagnosing and Managing Food Allergies and Intolerance. Blackwell Publishing Ltd, 2009.

3. Klemona T, Vanto T, Juntunen-Backman K, et al. Allergy to soy formula and extensively hydrolyzed whey formula in infants with cows' milk allergy: a prospective, randomized study with follow-up to the age of 2 yrs. J Pediatr 2002;140:219–24.

4. Agostoni C, Axelsson I, Goulet O, et al. Soy protein infant formulae and follow-on formulae: a commentary by the ESPHGHAN Committee on Nutrition. J Pediatr Gastroenterol Nutrition 2006;42:352–61.

5. Resanti P, Berretta B, Fiocchi A, et al. Cross-reactivity between mammalian proteins. Ann Allergy Asthma and Immunol 2002;89(6 Suppl 1):11–5.

6. Jarvinen KM, Chatchatee P. Mammalian milk allergy: clinical suspicion, cross reactivities and diagnosis. Curr Opion Allergy Clin Immunol 2009;9:251–8.

7. Van Do T, Elsayed S, Florvaag E, et al. Allergy to fish parvalbumins: studies on the cross-reactivity of allergens from 9 commonly consumed fish. J Allergy Clin Immunol 2005;116:1314–20.

8. Sicherer SH, Munoz-Furlong A, Sampson HA. Prevalence of peanut and treenut allergy in the United States determined by means of random digit dial telephone survey: a 5 year follow up study. J Allergy Clin Immunol 2003;112:1203–7.

9. Ewan PW. Clinical study of peanut and nut allergy in 62 consecutive patients: new features and associations. BMJ 1996;312:1074–8.

10. Sampson HA, McCaskill CC. Food hypersensitivity and atopic dermatitis: evaluation of 113 patients. J Pediatr 1985;107:669–75.

11. Bock SA, Atkins FM. The natural history of peanut allergy. J Allergy Clin Immunol 1989;83:900–4.

12. Moneret-Vautrin D-A, Guérin L, Kanny G, et al. Cross-allergenicity of peanut and lupine: the risk of lupine allergy in patients allergic to peanuts. J Allergy Clin Immunol 1999;104:883–8.

13. Host A. Frequency of cows milk allergy in childhood. Ann Allergy Asthma Immunol 2001;12(Suppl. 14):78–84.

14. Resanti P, Gaiaschi A, Plebani A, et al. Evaluation of the presence of bovine proteins in human milk as a possible cause of allergic symptoms in breast-fed children. Ann Allergy Asthma and Immunol 2000;84:353–60.

15. Nutrient reference values for Australia and New Zealand. National Health and Medical Research Council, 2006.

16. Kemp A, Hill DJ, Allen KJ, et al. Guidelines for the use of infant formulas to treat cows milk protein allergy: an Australian consensus panel opinion. MJA 2008;188(2):109–12.

17. Klemona T, Vanto T, Juntunen-Backman K, et al. Allergy to soy formula and extensively hydrolyzed whey formula in infants with cows milk allergy: a prospective, randomized study with follow-up to the age of 2 yrs. J Pediatr 2002;140:219–24.

18. Rozenfeld P, Docena GH, Anon MC, et al. Detection and identification of a soy protein component that cross-reacts with caseins from cows milk. Clin Exp Immunol 2002;130:49–58.

19. Zeigler RS, Sampson HA, Bock SA, et al. Soy allergy in infants and children with IgE-associated cows milk allergy. J Pediatr 1999;134:614–22.

20. Australian College of Paediatrics. Position statement: soy protein formula. J Paediatr Child Health 1998;34:318–9.

21. Meharg AA, Deacon C, Campbell R, et al. Inorganic arsenic in rice milk exceeds EU and US drinking water standards. J Environ Monit 2008;10:428–31.

22. Skripak J, Wood RA. Peanut and tree nut allergy in childhood. Pediatr Allergy Immunol 2008;19:368–73.

23. Sampson HA, McCaskill CC. Food hypersensitivity and atopic dermatitis: evaluation of 113 patients. J Pediatr 1985;107:669–75.

24. Bock SA, Atkins FM. The natural history of peanut allergy. J Allergy Clin Immunol 1989;83:900–4.

25. Sicherer SH, Sampson HA. Peanut allergy: Emerging concepts and approaches. J Allergy Clin Immunol 2007;120:491–503.

26. Beyer K, Morrow E, Li XM, et al. Effects of cooking methods on peanut allergenicity. J Allergy Clin Immunol 2001;107:1077–81.

27. Hourihane JO, Bedwani SJ, Dean TP, et al. Randomised, double blind, crossover challenge study

of allergenicity of peanut oils to subjects allergic to peanuts. BMJ 1997;314:1084–8.

28. Ferdman RM, Church JA. Mixed up nuts: identification of peanuts and tree nuts by children. Ann Allergy Asthma Immunol 2006;97:73–7.

29. Hefle SL, Lemanske RF Jr, Bush RK. Adverse reaction to lupine-fortified pasta. J Allergy Clin Immunol 1994;94(2 pt 1):167–72.

30. Novembre E, Moriondo M, Bernardini R, et al. Lupin allergy in a child. J Allergy Clin Immunol 1999;103:1214–6.

31. Parisot L, Aparicio C, Moneret-Vautrin D-A, et al. Allergy to lupine flour. Allergy 2001;56:918–9.

32. Gangur V, Kelly C, Nauluri L. Sesame Allergy: A growing food allergy of global proportions. Ann Allergy Asthma Immunol 2005;95; 4–11.

33. Shepherd SJ, Gibson PR. Fructose malabsorption and symptoms of irritable bowel syndrome. Guidelines for effective dietary management. J Am Diet Assoc 2006;106:1631–9.

34. Inomata N. Wheat allergy. Curr Opin Allergy Clin Immunol 2009;9:238–43.

35. Pourpak Z, Mesdaghi M, Mansouri M, et al. Which cereal is a suitable substitute for wheat in children with wheat allergy? Pediatr Allergy Immunol 2005; 16:262–6.

36. Nowak-Wegrzyn A, Muraro, A. Food protein-induced enterocolitis syndrome. Curr Opin Allergy Clin Immunol 2009;9:371–7.

37. Pasini G, Simonato B, Curioni A, et al. IgE mediated allergy to corn: a 50 kDa protein, belonging to the reduced soluble proteins, is a major allergen. Allergy 2008;57(2):98–106.

38. Tey D, Heine RG. Egg allergy in childhood: an update. Curr opin Allergy Clin Immunol 2009;9:244–50.

39. Bath-Hextall F, Delamere FM, Williams HC. Dietary exclusions for established atopic eczema. Cochrane Database Syst Rev 2008:CD005203.

40. Palmer DJ, Gold MS, Makrides M. Effect of maternal egg consumption on breast milk ovalbumin concentration. Clin Exp Allergy 2008;38:1186–91.

41. Boyano MT, Garcia-Ara C, Diaz-Pena JM, et al. Validity of specific IgE antibodies in children with egg allergy. Clin Exp Allergy 2001;31:1464–9.

42. Priftis KN, Mermiri D, Papadopoulou A, et al. Asthma symptoms and bronchial reactivity in school children sensitised to food allergens in infancy. J Asthma 2008;45:590–5.

43. Van Do T, Elsayed S, Florvaag E, et al. Allergy to fish parvalbumins: studies on the cross-reactivity of allergens from 9 commonly consumed fish. J Allergy Clin Immunol 2005;116:1314–20.

44. Pieretti MM, Chung D, Pacenza R, et al. Audit of manufactured products: Use of allergen advisory labels and identification of labeling ambiguities. J Allergy Clin Immunol 2009;124:337–41.

45. Koplin J, Osborne N, Allen K. Prevalence of allergen avoidance advisory statements in a supermarket. Abstracts of the 19th Annual ASCIA Mtg. Int Med J 2008;38:A149-75.

46. Hefle S, Furlong T, Niemann L, et al. Consumer attitudes and risks associated with packaged foods having advisory labeling regarding the presence of peanuts. J Allergy Clin Immunol 2007;120:171–6.

47. Taylor SL, Hefle SL, Bindslev-Jensen C, et al. A consensus protocol for the determination of the threshold doses for allergenic foods: how much is too much? Clin Exp Allergy 2004;34:689–95.

48. Christie L, Hine J, Parker JG, et al. Food allergies in children affect nutrient intake and growth. J Am Diet Assoc 2002;102:1648–51.

49. Isolauri E, Siitas Y, Salo M, et al. Elimination diet in cow's milk allergy: Risk for impaired growth in young children. J Pediatr 1988;132:1004–9.

50. Henriksen C, Eggesbo M, Halvorsen R, et al. Nutrient intake among two-year old children on cows' milk restricted diets. Acta Paediatr 2000;89(3):272–8. Abstract.

51. COMA. Dietary Reference Values for Food Energy and Nutrients for the United Kingdom. Report of the Panel on Dietary Reference Values of the Committee on Medical Aspects of Food Policy. London: HMSO, 1991.

52. Food and Nutrition Board: Institute of Medicine. Dietary Reference Intakes for calcium, phosphorus, magnesium, vitamin D and fluoride. Washington DC: National Academy Press; 1997.

CHAPTER 20

Diagnostic and Therapeutic Dilemmas: Adverse Reactions to Food Additives, Pharmacologic Food Reactions, Psychological Considerations Related to Food Ingestion

John O. Warner

Introduction

Over the last 40 years the basic mechanisms underlying conventional allergic diseases, including those associated with foods, have been unraveled. This has led to improvements in both diagnosis and treatment. It has facilitated the identification of foods as a cause of a wide range of acute allergic disorders, ranging from catastrophic anaphylaxis, angioedema and urticaria through to more chronic problems such as atopic eczema and, albeit less frequently, food-induced enteropathies. However, difficulty remains when no underlying mechanism can be found to explain the association between a food, or food ingredient, and a clinical response. Under such circumstances there is no objective diagnostic test beyond dietary exclusion and controlled challenge, preferably employing a double-blind placebo-controlled strategy. The concept becomes further strained when the reaction to the food cannot be measured as a change in function but merely as a change in behavior.

Medical opinion has become polarized by the sometimes unsubstantiated claims made primarily in the lay media rather than scientific channels about debilitating and chronic symptoms of ill health coming from intolerance to certain foods.[1] The danger is that the reaction of the profession to such claims will 'throw the baby out with the bathwater' and provide no help for the patient.

Classification of reactions to foods

The best definition of food allergy and intolerance comes from Lucretius, the Roman poet and philosopher, who was driven mad by a love potion and during his moments of sanity wrote a number of books and poems. A paraphrasing of one of his statements is: 'One man's meat is another man's poison'.

There have been a number of attempts to produce a subclassification of adverse reactions to foods (Fig. 20.1). These can either be predictable or unpredictable. Within the predicted category (Fig. 20.1a), most if not all members of the population will be affected to a greater or lesser extent. There are toxins in foods which, under some circumstances, will cause symptoms that very closely mimic acute allergic responses. This is exemplified by reactions to scombroid fish such as tuna, which if badly stored accumulates large quantities of histamine.

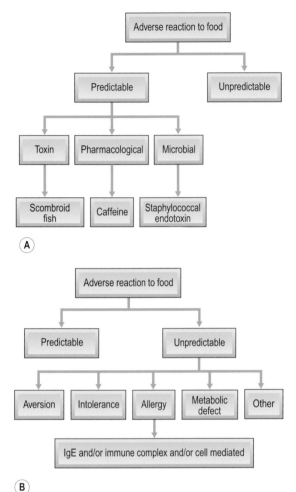

Figure 20.1 **(A)** The different categories of adverse responses to food which occur to a greater or lesser extent in all individuals who are exposed to constituents or contaminants in a food. **(B)** The classification of unpredictable adverse responses to foods which occur only in a subsection of the population, as a consequence either of psychological problems or an organic abnormality in metabolic or immune responsiveness.

CLINICAL CASE 1

JC, a boy of 14 years, was referred to the allergy clinic with a diagnosis of tuna allergy, but the general pediatrician could not explain why the skin prick test and specific IgE to tuna were negative. JC gave a history of prior exposure to tinned and freshly cooked tuna without any reaction. Recently, while eating freshly cooked tuna at a friend's house, he experienced a tingling sensation in his mouth and within minutes of finishing the dish had a generalized erythematous eruption associated with a pounding headache. The symptoms lasted for 30 minutes and then subsided without treatment. In retrospect, he stated that

the fringes of the tuna steak were rather darker than normal. All contents of the meal other than tuna he had eaten again since the event without reaction. He said that his friend had also experienced an odd sensation in his mouth when eating the tuna, but unlike him had not completed the meal. He had no history of any atopic diseases and tolerated all common other food allergens. Repeat skin and blood tests for tuna remained negative. He subsequently had no reaction to a supervised tuna challenge. The history was in any case typical of scombroid fish poisoning. Badly stored tuna has a progressively increasing histamine content sufficient to cause systemic symptoms when ingested. A challenge was necessary to exclude the 5% chance that the allergy tests were falsely negative.

Caffeine and other neuroactive constituents which can produce changes in behavior exist in many foods. Food can, of course, be contaminated with microbial factors such as staphylococcal endotoxin to produce a reaction which could be confused with allergy.

Among the unpredictable responses that only occur in subgroups of the population, food aversion must be discriminated from true reproducible intolerance (Fig. 20.1B). The former may be defined as a bodily reaction caused by a food which cannot be reproduced in a double-blind placebo-controlled food challenge (DBPCFC), whereas intolerance is a reproducible reaction to a food or food ingredient. The label intolerance makes no assumption of the mechanisms involved and could be due to enzyme defects, which can lead to failed processing of nutrients such as occurs in lactase deficiency. Food allergy is a reproducible reaction on DBPCFC associated with a hypersensitive immune response. It is often subclassified as IgE or non-IgE mediated, the latter being associated with IgG immune complexes or cellular responses involving eosinophils, neutrophils and/or lymphocytes.

There is one additional category that will challenge the allergist's skills to disentangle the diagnosis and provide effective direction for management. Patients or their carers can totally fabricate symptoms and signs masquerading as allergy. It is clear that allergy, particularly to foods, features in patients with so-called Munchhausen's and Munchhausen's-by-proxy syndromes, now known as fabricated or induced illness (FII),[2] and can result in significant nutritional compromise.[3] This can be difficult to distinguish from the genuinely worried parent whose child has non-specific and inexplicable symptoms. Complementary and alternative medicine

(CAM) practitioners have frequently been consulted in such cases. Using totally unsubstantiated and bogus tests such as 'whole blood analysis' and so-called 'vega' tests leads to fallacious diagnoses of food intolerance/allergy with recommendation of potentially nutritionally unsound exclusion diets.

CLINICAL CASE 2

SG, a boy of 6 years, was referred to the allergy clinic with a history of behavioral problems which his mother attributed to ingestion of various foods. He was described by his mother as becoming 'evil' within 30 minutes of ingesting foods or drinks labeled with an E-number (a notation for permitted food additives in Europe). His school had complained about his aggressive behavior. She had sent a sample of his hair to a CAM service, which confirmed her belief that he was allergic to artificial food colorings and preservatives. He was also supposedly allergic to milk, egg, wheat, pork, beef, fish and soy. His diet for the last year had consisted of chicken, corn, potato and grapes. His weight had dropped from the 50th to the 10th centile over that period. Additional perceived problems were recurrent infections necessitating very frequent school absences, and a range of non-specific symptoms, including diarrhea alternating with constipation, headaches, and generalized lethargy. His parents had divorced some years previously and both his mother and his 16-year-old sister were also said to be 'food allergic'. Allergy tests to common inhalants and ingestants were all negative, and his total IgE was 20 kU/mL. Serum ferritin and vitamin D were abnormally low. He was admitted for food challenges and his diet was progressively normalized without any adverse reaction. He gained 11 kg in weight over the subsequent 2 months and most of his non-specific symptoms disappeared. Even his behavior was reported to have improved.

Allergy clinics report that a high percentage of patients referred with ill-defined symptoms have consulted CAM practitioners or submitted samples of hair or blood for unsubstantiated tests, such as for IgG antibodies, and have subsequently introduced exclusion diets without any dietitian input to deal with nutritional inadequacies. The adverse consequences can sometimes be considerable, as illustrated in this case.

However, the frequency with which parents report that their children's behavior is adversely affected by certain food additives does require further scrutiny, and the concept cannot necessarily be dismissed.

Food additives

Food additives are any substances added to foods for non-nutritional purposes, for example to enhance color, taste, smell, texture, or maintain quality and lengthen shelf life. Thus, they cannot be regarded as a single group of substances to be randomly excluded from the diet. Some, such as colorings, could be omitted without compromise, whereas others serve essential purposes such as preventing bacterial and fungal contamination. There are 3–4000 flavoring substances and at least 350 antioxidants, colors, preservatives etc.[4] Some additives are naturally occurring, and even ascorbic acid when used as an antioxidant has a notation as an additive on food labels. The main concern about adverse effects, however, has focused on the azo dyes such as tartrazine.

A population study of perceived and challenge-confirmed food additive intolerance showed that 7.4% of over 18 000 respondents in the UK stated they had a problem with food additives. A wide range of symptoms were perceived to be induced by the additives, which ranged from conventional allergic symptoms through to headache, behavioral and mood changes and musculoskeletal problems. In a small subgroup who completed a double-blind placebo-controlled challenge study, only three of 81 showed a consistent positive response, suggesting that the calculated population prevalence of reaction to food additives would be 0.026% (95% confidence interval (CI) 0.003–0.049%). In other words, less than 4% of people who believe themselves to react adversely to additives actually do so on DBPCFC.[5] This was very different to the prevalence of perceived in relation to challenge proven adverse reactions to natural foods as identified by the same research team in the UK. This study found a 20.4% rate of self-reported food allergy, 19.4% of which had a positive DBPCFC[6] (Fig. 20.2). These prevalence rates have been similar in subsequent studies from other countries such as Denmark, with 16.6% of participants reporting food hypersensitivity but 2.3% responding on oral challenge. In other words, 14% who believed they had adverse reactions had a reproducible response.[7] The latter study found that even perceived additive reactions were rare, and in no child was the reaction confirmed on challenge.

The greater differences between perceived and actual responses to food additives compared with natural foods and the differences in perception between countries should be understood in the context of popular concepts. The media and branches of so-called complementary medicine have stoked public suspicion about food

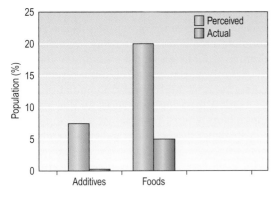

Figure 20.2 Histogram of the population prevalence of perceived versus challenge-proven food additive and natural food intolerance in the UK. Modified from Young E, Patel S, Stoneham M, et al. The prevalence of reaction to food additives in a survey population. J R Coll Physicians Lond. 1987 Oct; 21(4): 241–7 and Young E, Stoneham MD, Petruckevitch A, et al. A population study of food intolerance. Lancet. 1994 May 7; 343(8906): 1127–30.

manufacturers and regulatory authorities colluding to expose consumers to unnatural and unsafe additions in food for commercial gain. This is not a new phenomenon, and on occasions has proved to be a genuine concern.[4]

Additives and urticaria/angioedema

CLINICAL CASE 3

RB, a 7-year-old girl, had a history of recurrent bouts of urticaria for the last 18 months, occurring at least once each week and each lasting for 30–60 minutes. Treatment with regular antihistamine (chlorpheniramine) only partially prevented the problem. Her mother had perceived that some of the episodes followed shortly after the ingestion of highly colored confectionery products and fizzy drinks. Other episodes occurred after attending birthday parties and in association with exercise and/or exciting events. Placing her on an azo-coloring and benzoate preservative-free diet resulted in a significant reduction in the frequency of episodes. She was submitted to a double-blind placebo-controlled challenge with a fruit drink containing a mixture of azo-food dyes and sodium benzoate or no additives, having stopped the antihistamine medication. An urticarial reaction developed within 30 minutes after the active challenges only. Interestingly, she at the same time became very irritable and overactive. This was assumed to be due to the itching associated with the urticaria. She was recommended to maintain the dietary restriction, but as other triggers were also involved she was prescribed a more effective regular

antihistamine, cetirizine, which proved highly effective and allowed her to relax the dietary restriction.

This case illustrates that food additives can exacerbate urticaria but is unlikely to be the primary cause. The newer antihistamines are highly effective in preventing acute episodes and are likely to be preferred to avoidance diets by children.

It has long been known that certain artificial food additives can sometimes induce acute urticaria and angioedema.[8–10] A number of the references suggest an association with aspirin intolerance, though this is not clear from more recent studies. The association of food additives in relation to urticaria has been questioned in that a follow-up study in children suggested that the majority were only transient in nature, with at least 76% of children apparently losing their sensitivity over a 5-year follow-up.[11] Furthermore, it has been suggested that tartrazine-induced acute urticaria and angioedema is only rarely reproducible by oral challenge.[12]

Additives and eczema

There are variable outcomes from studies of food additives in relation to atopic eczema, some of which have shown associations.[13–15] Other studies have failed to show a relationship.[16] Randomized placebo-controlled oral challenges with food additive mixes in a population of 54 patients with allergic disease failed to show any significant dermatologic adverse reactions or aggravation of atopic eczema. However, five patients in the group had responses to the active and not the placebo, with itching, flushing or urticaria.[17]

Additives and asthma

It is clear that sulfites added to food and drinks can induce asthma, possibly by release of sulfur dioxide.[18] However, it is less clear whether other forms of food additives can genuinely aggravate asthma. Tartrazine has been shown in a selected group of children to increase bronchial hyperreactivity,[19] but considerable dispute remains over whether any of the artificial food colorings or benzoate preservatives do genuinely provoke acute asthmatic reactions.[20] There are methodological criticisms of much of the work, and if the prevalence rate is very low, as is likely, this could explain discrepancies between studies.[21]

Potential mechanisms of reactions to additives

Given that no-one has been able to demonstrate an IgE-mediated mechanism for any food additives causing an aggravation of allergic disease, and with no other obvious mechanistic explanation, there is neither an objective test to confirm or refute a diagnosis nor any agreement about the existence of a real association. However, one study has suggested that IgD may be involved.[22] Another study investigated in vitro leukocyte histamine release on exposure to azo-dyes from normal and urticarial subjects. In a minority of the subjects leukocytes released significant quantities of histamine on stimulation with levels of azo-dye that were calculated to be likely to exist in the circulation after ingestion of a standard daily intake. This response was consistent on repeat testing and was not altered by pre-incubation with anti-human IgE or calcium ionophore, suggesting a pharmacologically (non-IgE) mediated effect.[23] Following this study, challenges were conducted on normal subjects and demonstrated significant histamine release in nine of the 10 subjects challenged with a large but not small dose of tartrazine, the latter of which exceeded the maximum population estimated daily intake from the diet by a factor of 2 (Fig. 20.3).[24]

In vitro studies have shown biological activity of some food colorings related to lipid solubility,[25]
which could potentially affect neurotransmitter activity.[26] Chronic dosing of rat pups with food colors produced behavioral changes but there was no dose–response effect.[27]

Finally, our own group has recently demonstrated a potential unifying explanation for the variable clinical observations in relation to the potential non-IgE-mediated histamine release associated with exposure. We have shown in a group of children identified to have adverse behavioral reactions to a double-blind food additive challenge that polymorphisms in the histamine degradation gene histamine N-methyltransferase (HNMT) T939C and HNMT Thr105Ile moderated the effects of the additive challenge. These two polymorphisms are associated with reduced activity of the enzyme, which in turn would be expected to be associated with a slower elimination of histamine. This could explain how a food additive in moderate to large doses which can produce histamine release will only affect a subgroup of subjects who fail to eliminate the histamine appropriately, and who thereby are more likely to have either an aggravation of pre-existing allergic problems, an enhancement of bronchial hyperresponsiveness, or in some cases an aggravation of behavioral disorder. This latter phenomenon will be discussed in more detail.[28]

Additives and behavior

Feingold[29] was the first to report the potential association between behavioral disorder and dietary factors. In a group of children with learning difficulties and behavior problems, he claimed a 68% improvement with a diet eliminating artificial colors, preservatives and putative salicylate-containing fruits and vegetables. This was an uncontrolled observational study which was greeted with considerable skepticism.[30] Furthermore, many of the excluded foods contained no salicylates, whereas others that remained in the diet contained significant quantities.[31]

The main difficulty in understanding the considerable diversity in the results of subsequent studies either supporting or refuting the Feingold claims is that the definition of behavior disorders such as attention deficit hyperactivity disorder (ADHD) and conduct disorders was not consistent. The former involves overactivity, inattention and impulsivity, and is to a certain extent hereditable,[32]

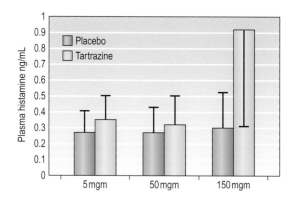

Figure 20.3 The median and ranges of plasma histamine in 10 normal adults after challenge with increasing doses of tartrazine, showing that the high dose induced significant histamine release. Redrawn with permission from Murdoch RD, Pollock I, Naeem S. Tartrazine induced histamine release in vivo in normal subjects. J R Coll Physicians Lond. 1987 Oct; 21(4): 257–61.

whereas the latter are much more a consequence of social environment and child-rearing practices.[33] Furthermore, genuine reactions to additives resulting in urticaria could be missed while at the same time the patient becomes overtly irritable as a consequence of the extreme pruritus.[8]

Estimates from the general population would suggest that behavioral problems occur in 10–15% of 3-year-olds, and this figure is consistent in a number of studies.[34] Although the definition of ADHD is relatively precise in encompassing the three components of overactivity, inattention and impulsivity, each of these occurs to a greater or lesser extent across the population, albeit varying in intensity with age. The diagnosis of ADHD is usually reserved for those children with severe symptoms and a pervasive pattern of behavior from a young age which impairs functioning and particularly educational attainment.[35] Methods used to score the degree of behavior disturbance on or off food additives have varied from study to study, and the populations from which subjects have been selected have also varied. Thus some have come from special patient populations prediagnosed with ADHD, or from those referred to allergy services. A few studies have involved attempts to characterize the problem in whole populations.

Effects of exclusion diets on behavior

Following the Feingold observations, Connors[36] conducted a rigorous study on children referred for hyperkinetic syndrome to a special clinic. Seventeen children had 4 weeks each on a controlled diet and an additive-containing diet and 15 completed the study. Only teachers' ratings of children's behavior during the use of the Feingold diet showed a statistically significant improvement, and there was the potential that the blinding of the diet was inadequate. Furthermore, in this study there was a marked order effect in that the exclusion diet was only more effective when it was followed by the placebo.[37] Subsequent studies either revealed totally negative outcomes[38] or suggested positive outcomes, although in the positive study the diet involved a far wider range of foods and a high percentage of the children included were also genuinely allergic.[39]

Additive challenge and behavior

CLINICAL CASE 4

AW, aged 9 years, had attention deficit hyperactivity disorder (ADHD) which was severely compromising his education. Because of his disruptive behavior in school he had been temporarily expelled pending assessment of his clinical and educational needs. He was of normal intelligence but from infancy had exhibited a range of behavioral problems, including poor concentration and easy distractability, with periodic aggressive outbursts. There was no evidence of atopic disease in him or his parents and four siblings, but there were appreciable psychosocial problems in the family. Treatment with methylphenidate produced a partial improvement in his behavior. His mother was convinced that 'E-numbers' aggravated abnormal behavior and avoidance led to further improvement. However, additional support was required to facilitate his assimilation back into school. His mother would not consent to him having a supervised controlled additive challenge.

This is a typical story of ADHD, which is more common in boys, and clearly psychosocial compromise is a common association. It would be very easy to dismiss the concept of food additives as an aggravating factor. Supporting the parental belief might be viewed as inappropriate collusion, but it helps empower the parents to take action themselves and improve the attention they give to their child. They are perhaps then more likely to accept the additional help and treatment that is required. However, only a DBPCFC will clarify the issue, but parents are understandably reluctant to allow this if they perceive that an intervention has produced significant improvement.

Some studies have employed a double-blind challenge protocol when children were already on an exclusion diet. Again, conflicting results can be partly explained by trial design, with some only using open challenges. In those using a double-blind challenge most only employed a single crossover design, such as the Egger study, which had a very considerable order effect. It has been argued that a minimum of three crossover challenges are required in order to reliably diagnose food intolerance in individual patients.[40]

Another problem in interpreting trial results is variation in the dose and variety of additives employed. Some have used doses well above those that would normally be expected in a child's diet, whereas others have attempted to mimic the levels of normal exposure. The way in which the challenge materials were presented also differed, with some employing incorporation into standard foods[41] and others using encapsulated forms.[42] The latter study[42] employed a prolonged series of double-blind cross-over challenges. Although the dropout rate was high, there were consistent differences on Connors scores for hyperactivity between the active and the placebo weeks. However, parents were unable to consistently identify the active and placebo periods (Fig. 20.4).

A meta-analysis of double-blind placebo-controlled trials has now been conducted and showed that there is a significant effect of artificial food colors and other additives on the behavior of children with ADHD.[43] This analysis was on 15 trials containing 219 subjects with hyperactivity. There was also a secondary analysis of 132 participants from eight studies in children who were not hyperactive. In both cases there was a significant effect. Following this publication there have been two publications further investigating the effects of artificial food colors and a benzoate preservative in a mixture from general population samples, both with larger than the accumulated numbers in the Schab and Trihn meta-analysis.[43]

The first study, conducted on the Isle of Wight, involved children selected into four subgroups defined from a whole population questionnaire administered to the parents of 1873 children in their fourth year of life. The groups were hyperactive and allergic; allergic and not hyperactive; hyperactive and not allergic; or neither allergic nor hyperactive. The children (n = 277) were placed on an elimination diet, and then over a 3-week period

subjected to a double-blind crossover challenge in random order with a drink either containing a mixture of artificial food colors and benzoate preservative at a dose that might be expected that a 4-year-old would be exposed to daily, or a placebo mix. According to parental reports there were significant reductions in hyperactive behavior during the withdrawal phase and significantly greater increases in hyperactive behavior during the active compared to the placebo challenge. However, an attempt to assess the degree of behavioral disturbance during a formal clinic visit by a psychologist failed to show any differences. Based on the parental reports there were no significant effects of prior presence or absence of hyperactivity, or indeed of allergy. In other words, the effects on parentally observed changes in behavior occurred across all groups, with equal effects. These results could not be questioned on the basis of systematic breaking of the blinding, as the materials were subject to panel testing prior to being used in the study. It could be argued that the absence of objective confirmation from a psychologist invalidated the observations. However, it is well known that parents will be much more sensitive to changes in their child's behavior during the stresses of normal life than will be observed during a very formal clinic assessment, where children tend to be on their best behavior[44] (Fig. 20.5).

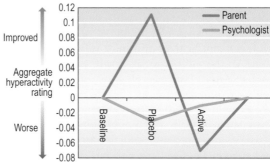

Figure 20.5 A population-based double-blind crossover challenge with a food additive and benzoate preservative mix in 3-year-old children. There were significant differences in the parental rating of behavior but not in a psychologist's formal clinical assessment. Redrawn with permission from Bateman B, Warner JO, Hutchinson E, et al. The effects of a double blind, placebo controlled, artificial food colorings and benzoate preservative challenge on hyperactivity in a general population sample of preschool children. Arch Dis Child. 2004 Jun; 89(6): 506–11.

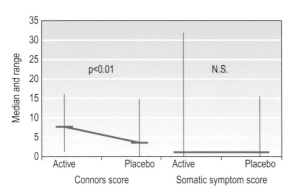

Figure 20.4 The median and ranges for Connors scores of hyperactivity and a combined physical symptoms score in children submitted to double-blind crossover challenges for 1-week periods with an encapsulated food additive mix or placebo. Redrawn with permission from Pollock I, Warner JO. Effect of artificial food colours on childhood behaviour. Arch Dis Child. 1990 Jan; 65(1): 74–7.

Given the criticisms of this latter study, the whole program was repeated on a totally separate population of 3-year-olds (n = 153) but with the addition of a group of 8-year-olds (n = 144). The children were recruited from a whole population in schools and early-years settings with no prior screening for ADHD or allergy. They were challenged in double-blind form with a placebo, with the same mixture of additives employed in the Isle of Wight study but also including a second mixture based on an updated evaluation of the additives prevalent in the diet of children at the time of the study. This study replicated the findings in 3-year-olds (Fig. 20.6a) and extended them to 8/9-year-olds (Fig. 20.6b). The effect size was equivalent to that which had been calculated in the meta-analysis by Schab and Trinh.[45]

Thus the accumulated evidence from a meta-analysis and two large subsequent studies indicates that various food additives and a benzoate preservative in a mixture do have a significant effect on children's behavior. It would appear that these effects are independent of the prior presence of ADHD and are not specifically associated with underlying allergy. The latter study has also suggested a degree of dose-related effect, at least in the 8/9-year-olds.

No study, however, has yet been able to disentangle whether the deleterious effect is a consequence of the mixture or due to individual components. However, there is a suggestion from in vitro studies that mixtures are particularly important in influencing neural development, with significant synergy observed between combinations of brilliant blue with glutamic acid, or quinoline yellow with aspartame, in the inhibition of growth of neurites in a mouse neuroblastoma cell line.[46] Further studies will be required to disentangle effects, but based on the magnitude of the effect, eliminating the additives studied from the populations' diet would result in an appreciable reduction in the prevalence of hyperkinetic disorders. This has led to the European Parliament adopting a legislative package which mandates that products containing the artificial colors should be labeled with a health warning 'may have an adverse effect on activity and attention in children'. Whereas removal of the benzoate preservative could have adverse consequences for food quality, the same is clearly not true of food colors, which could be removed without consequences for consumers. Given the accumulated evidence, this would seem to be a reasonable approach.

Results – 3 year olds

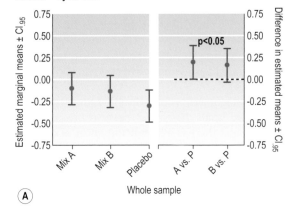

(A) Whole sample

Results – 8/9 year olds

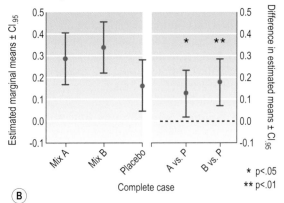

(B) Complete case

* p<.05
** p<.01

Figure 20.6 (a) The global hyperactivity aggregate during challenge with food additive mixes or placebo and the significances of difference in 3-year-old children recruited from a whole population.
Redrawn with permission from McCann D, Barrett A, Cooper A. Food additives and hyperactive behaviour in 3-year-old and 8/9-year-old children in the community: a randomised, double-blinded, placebo-controlled trial. Lancet. 2007 Nov 3; 370(9598): 1560–7.
(b) The global hyperactivity aggregate during challenge with food additive mixes or placebo and the significances of difference in 8/9-year-old children recruited from a whole population. Redrawn with permission from McCann D, Barrett A, Cooper A. Food additives and hyperactive behaviour in 3-year-old and 8/9-year-old children in the community: a randomised, double-blinded, placebo-controlled trial. Lancet. 2007 Nov 3; 370(9598): 1560–7.

Putative mechanisms of food additive effects on behavior

There is considerable evidence that genetic factors contribute to variations in the manifestation of ADHD. Thus twin studies have indicated that

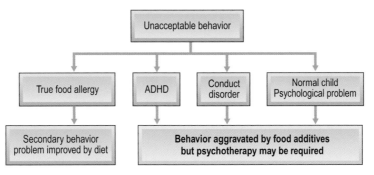

Figure 20.7 The likely relationships between food and behavior.

approximately two-thirds of the variance in ADHD can be explained by genetic differences.[47] Molecular genetic studies have identified a group of genes influencing the dopamine, serotonin and noradrenergic neurotransmitter systems, but the size of effect for each has only been small. Furthermore genome-wide association studies have failed to identify any genes with a significant effect.[48] One possible explanation for this disparity is that genetic factors will only be highlighted if they are associated with a particular environmental exposure. The observations of an enhancing effect of polymorphisms in the histamine N-methyltransferase gene in relation to behavioral responses to artificial food colors is the first study to demonstrate a gene–environment interaction affecting ADHD.[28]

HNMT polymorphisms are associated with reduced enzyme activity, which in turn impairs histamine clearance.[49] Studies have shown that food coloring challenge causes histamine release both in vitro and in vivo.[23,24] Thus the combination of challenge with coloring, leading to histamine release with impaired degradation, provides a potential mechanistic explanation for the effect. There are histamine-3 receptors in the brain.[50] Furthermore, two of the standard treatments for ADHD, methylphenidate and atomoxetine, have effects on the histamine system.[51,52]

As artificial food colors and preservatives are only one group of factors that will result in an increase in histamine release, this mechanism may explain why infections, a number of other food items and other environmental factors can aggravate ADHD.[53] It clearly also identifies a potential target for therapeutic intervention which could well focus on H3 receptors.[54]

Summary

It has become clear that certain food colors and maybe benzoate preservative can have an adverse effect on a range of allergic disorders and on behavior in children. The magnitude of the effect in relation to eczema, asthma, urticaria and angioedema is very much smaller than has perhaps been perceived in the recent past. However, the impact on childhood behavior is rather more pervasive than has been appreciated, and is unrelated to atopy (Fig. 20.7)

The mechanisms involved in generating these responses are beginning to be unraveled (Fig. 20.8). In terms of current classifications of adverse responses to foods and food ingredients, it is very difficult to place food additives. In some respects they could be considered as producing a predictable response because they will uniformly produce non-IgE-mediated histamine release from mast cells and basophils. However, the response is unpredictable in that it will only produce symptoms in a subgroup of patients who either already have allergic disease or polymorphisms in histamine degradation genes. Is this therefore a food intolerance or a non-IgE-mediated food allergy? In the final analysis it perhaps is immaterial in terms of classification. The key is to recognize when additives may be genuinely involved in aggravating problems and conduct appropriate preferably double-blind placebo-controlled food challenges to establish the diagnosis, and then provide advice on appropriate avoidance. With regard to ADHD, additives are but one of many factors that will aggravate the problem. They are not the primary

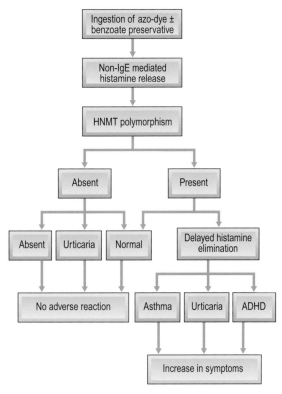

Figure 20.8 A potential mechanistic explanation for the diversity of responses to additive ingestion. This will only induce an increase in symptoms in individuals with both a polymorphism in the *N*-histamine methyltransferase (HNMT) gene, and an associated problem such as allergic disease or attention deficit hyperactivity disorder.

cause of the condition, and targeting the basic mechanisms will ultimately provide the most effective management.

References

1. Gamlin L. Cooking up a storm. New Scientist 8th July 1989; 45–9.
2. Warner JO, Hathaway MJ. Allergic form of Meadow's syndrome (Munchausen-by-proxy). Arch Dis Child 1984;59:151–6.
3. Roesler TA, Barry PC, Bock SA. Factitious food allergy and failure to thrive. Arch Pediatr Adolesc Med 1994;148:1150–5.
4. Lessof MH. Adverse reactions to food additives. J Roy Coll Phys 1987;21:237–40.
5. Young E, Patel S, Stoneham M, et al. The prevalence of reaction to food additives in a survey population. J Roy Coll Phys London 1987;21:241–7.
6. Young E, Stoneham MD, Petruckovitch A, et al. A population study of food intolerance. Lancet 1994;343:1127–30.
7. Osterballe M, Hansen TK, Mortz CG, et al. The prevalence of food hypersensitivity in an unselected population of children and adults. Pediatr Allergy Immunol 2005;16:567–73.
8. Supramaniam G, Warner JO. Artificial food additive intolerance in patients with angioedema and urticaria. Lancet 1986;2:907–9.
9. Juhlin L. Recurrent urticaria: clinical investigation of 330 patients. Brit J Derm 1981;104:369–81.
10. Juhlin L, Michaelsson G, Zetterstrom O. Urticaria and asthma induced by food and drug additives in patients with aspirin sensitivity. J Allergy Clin Immunol 1972;50:92–8.
11. Pollock I, Warner JO. A follow up study of childhood food additive intolerance. J Roy Coll Phys London 1987;21:248–50.
12. Nettis E, Colanardi MC, Ferrannini A, et al. Suspected tartrazine-induced acute urticaria / angioedema is only rarely reproducible by oral challenge. Clin Exp Allergy 2003;33:1725–9.
13. Van Bever HP, Docx M, Stevens WJ. Food and food additives in severe atopic dermatitis. Allergy 1989;44:588–94.
14. Fuglsang G, Madsen C, Halkken S, et al. Adverse reactions to food additives in children with atopic symptoms. Allergy 1994;49:31–7.
15. Worm M, Ehlers I, Sterry W, et al. Clinical relevance of food additives in adult patients with atopic dermatitis. Clin Exp Allergy 2000;30:407–14.
16. Hannuksela M, Lahti A. Peroral challenge tests with food additives in urticaria and atopic dermatitis. Int J Dermatol 1986;25:178–80.
17. Park H-W, Park C-H, Park S-H, et al. Dermatologic adverse reactions to 7 common food additives in patients with allergic diseases: a double blind placebo controlled study. J Allergy Clin Immunol 2008;121:1059–61.
18. Vally H, Carr A, El-Saleh J, et al. Wine induced asthma: a placebo controlled assessment of its pathogenesis. J Allergy Clin Immunol 1999;103:41–6.
19. Hariparsad D, Wilson N, Dixon C, et al. Oral tartrazine challenge in childhood asthma: effect on bronchial reactivity. Clin Allergy 1984;14:81–5.
20. Simon RA. Food and drug additives. Immunology and allergy clinics of North America 1995;15:489–527.
21. Madsen C. Prevalence of food additive intolerance. Hum Exp Toxicol 1994;13:393–9.
22. Weliki N, Heiner DC. Hypersensitivity to chemicals. Correlation of tartrazine hypersensitivity with characteristic serum IgD and IgE immune response patterns. Clin Allergy 1980;10:375–94.
23. Murdoch RD, Lessof MH, Pollock I, et al. Effects of food additives on leukocyte histamine release in normal and urticarious subjects. J Roy Coll Phys 1987;21:251–6.
24. Murdoch RD, Pollock I, Naeem S. Tartrazine induced histamine release in vivo in normal subjects. J Roy Coll Phys London 1987;21:257–61.
25. Levitan H. Food, drug and cosmetic dyes: Biological effects related to lipid solubility. Proc Nat Acad Sci USA 1977;74:9214–8.

26. Augustine GJ, Levitan H. Neurotransmitter release from a vertebrate neuromuscular synapse affected by a food dye. Science 2002;207:1489–90.

27. Shaywitz BA. Effects of chronic administration of food colours on activity levels and cognitive performance in developing rat pups treated with 6-hydroxydopamine. Neurobehav Toxicol 1979;1:41–7.

28. Stevenson J, Sanuga-Barke E, McCann D, et al. Polymorphisms in a histamine degradation gene and the moderation of the impact of food additives on ADHD symptoms in children. Amer J Psychia 2010;167:1108–15.

29. Feingold BF. Hyperkinesis and learning disabilities linked to artificial food flavours and colours. Am J Nurse 1975;75:797–803.

30. David T. The overworked or fraudulent diagnosis of food allergy and food intolerance in children. J Roy Soc Med 1985;78(Suppl. 5):21–31.

31. Swain AR, Dutton SP, Truswell AS. Salicylates in foods. J Am Diet Assoc 1985;85:950–60.

32. Swanson JM, Sergeant JA, Taylor E, et al. Attention-deficit hyperactivity disorder and hyperkinetic disorder. Lancet 1998;351:129–38.

33. Rutter M, Macdonald H, Le Couteur A, et al. Genetic factors in child psychiatric disorders – II Empirical findings. J Child Psychol Psychiatr 1990;31:39–83.

34. Campbell SB. Behavior problems in pre-school children: a review of recent research. J Child Psychol Psychiatr 1995;36:113–49.

35. Overmeyer S, Taylor E. Annotation: principles of treatment for hyper-kinetic disorder: practice approaches for the UK. J Child Psychol Psychiatr 1999;40:1147–57.

36. Conners CK, Goyecce CH, Southwick DA, et al. Food additives and hyper-kinesis: a controlled double-blind experiment. Pediatrics 1976;58:154–66.

37. Sprague RL. Critical review of food additive studies. Washington DC: American Psychol Association; 1976.

38. Harley JP, Matthews CG, Eischman PL. Synthetic food colors and hyperactivity in children: a double-blind challenge experiment. Pediatrics 1978;62:975–83.

39. Egger J, Carter CM, Graham PJ, et al. Controlled trial of oligoantigenic treatment in the hyper-kinetic syndrome. Lancet 1985;1:540–5.

40. Pearson DJ. Food allergy, hyper-sensitivity and intolerance. J Roy Coll Phys London 1985;19:154–62.

41. Mattes JA, Gittelman R. Effects of artificial food colorings in children with hyperactive symptoms. Arch Gen Psychiatry 1981;38:714–8.

42. Pollock I, Warner JO. Effect of artificial food colours on childhood behaviour. Arch Dis Child 1990;65:74–7.

43. Schab DW, Trinh NT. Do artificial food colours promote hyperactivity in children with hyperactive syndromes? A meta-analysis of double-blind placebo controlled trials. J Dev Behav Pediatr 2004;25:423–34.

44. Bateman E, Warner JO, Hutchinson E, et al. The effects of a double-blind placebo controlled artificial food colourings and benzoate preservative challenge on hyperactivity in a general population sample of pre-school children. Arch Dis Child 2004;89:506–11.

45. McCann D, Barrett A, Cooper A, et al. Food additives and hyperactive behaviour in 3 year olds and 8/9 year old children in the community: a randomised double-blind placebo controlled trial. Lancet 2007;370:1560–7.

46. Lau K, McLain WG, Williams DP, et al. Synergistic interactions between commonly used food additives in a developmental neurotoxicity test. Toxicol Sci 2006;90:178–87.

47. Waldman ID, Ficks C, Grizer IR. Candidate gene studies of ADHD: a meta-analytic review. Human Genet 2009;126:51–90.

48. Franke B, Neale BM, Faraone SV. Genome-wide association studies in ADHD. Human Genet 2009;126:13–50.

49. Preuss CV, Wood TC, Szumlanski CL, et al. Human histamine M methyl transferase. Pharmacogenetics: common genetic polymorphisms that alter activity. Mull Pharmacol 1998;53:708–17.

50. Sakurai E, Orelamdf L, Nishiyama S, et al. Evidence for the presence of histamine uptake into the synaptosones of rat brain. Pharmacology 2006;78:72–80.

51. Horner WE, Johnson DE, Schmidt AW, et al. Methylphenidate and atomoxetine increase histamine release in rat prefrontal cortex. Europ J Pharmacol 2007;558:96–7.

52. Liu LL, Yang J, Lei GF, et al. Atomoxetine increases histamine release and improves learning deficits in an animal model of attention deficit hyperactivity disorder: the spontaneous hypertensive rat. Basic Clin Pharmacol Toxicol 2008;102:527–32.

53. Pelsser LM, Buitelarr JK, Savelkoul HF. ADHD as a (non) allergic hypersensitivity disorder: a hypothesis. Paediatr Allergy Immunol 2009;20:107–12.

54. Gemkow MJ, Davenport AJ, Harich S, et al. The histamine H3 receptor as a therapeutic drug target for CNS disorders. Drug Discov Today 2009;14:509–15.

Index

Page numbers followed by "f" indicate figures, "t" indicate tables, and "b" indicate boxes.

A

abdominal pain, eosinophilic esophagitis, 131
Act c 1, 26
Act c 2, 90
Act d 2, 26
Act d 8, 25–26
actinidin, 26
adenosine triphosphate (ATP), 18
adolescents
  diagnosis of new allergies in, 171–172
  empowering, 232–233
  self-injectable epinephrine devices, 211
  severe reactions in, 210
Adrenaclick, 54
adrenaline see epinephrine
adults
  anaphylaxis reports in, 116, 116t–117t
  diagnosis of new allergies in, 171
  immune system, 9
adverse reactions to food, 49–60
  classification of, 285–287, 286f
  see also specific reactions/symptoms
advisory labeling, 221
  see also food labels
airborne allergens, 56
alcohol, 208, 210–211
allergen extracts, 176–177
allergen-non-specific therapy, 236–240, 236t
allergens, 2
  animal food see animal food allergens
  avoidance see dietary elimination; food avoidance
  in breast milk, 9
  carryover, 222
  classification, 16
  class II, 87t
  common, in infants, 167–168
  common properties and structural attributes of food, 16–23
  contact, avoiding, 222–225 (see also food avoidance)
  definition, 16

exposure to prevent allergies developing, 257
incomplete food, 83
inhalation see inhalation exposure
introducing potential, 12
major, 16
maternal avoidance of potential, 12
minor, 16
oral ingestion of, causing respiratory symptoms, 103
plant food see plant food allergens
predicting, 22
recombinant, 95
respiratory disease, 102–103
  see also specific allergens
allergen-specific immunotherapy, 242–243
allergic rhinitis, 56, 101
  and introduction of solid foods, 259
  prevalence, 40, 100–101
  risk factors, 104–105
almond major protein (amp), 27
almonds, 27
α-amylase inhibitors, 20
α-amylase/trypsin inhibitors, 19–20
α-conglutin, 28
α-lactalbumin, 18, 23–24
α-livetin, 24
amaranth, 275t
Amb a 4, 84
Americans with Disabilities Act (ADA), 227
amino acid based formulas, 267–268
Ana o 1, 27
Ana o 2, 27
Anapen, 125, 126t
anaphylaxis, 33–34, 113–127
  associated conditions worsening, 121, 122t
  clinical features, 120, 120f
  definition, 36, 113–115, 114t
  diagnosis, 122, 226t
  emergency room protocols, 208
  epidemiology, 115–118
  estimates of the prevalence of, 38–40
  exercise-induced, 29, 55
  fatal, 116–118, 117f
    epidemiology of, 40
    risk factors, 231, 232t
  food-dependent, exercise-induced see food-dependent, exercise-induced anaphylaxis (FDEIA)

grading of, 114, 114t, 206t
historical background, 113
identifying the causal factor, 208–210
IgE-mediated food reactions, 49–51
late-onset food-induced, 121
meat, 121
natto, 121
and oral food challenges, 196t
pathogenesis, 118
pollen-food syndrome, 85
reports in adults, 116, 116t–117t
reports on children, 115–116, 117t
respiratory symptoms, 107
symptoms, 114, 114t, 226
treatment/management, 123–125, 124f, 206–208
  comorbidities affecting, 208
  emergency room protocols, 208
  long-term, 125, 208–216
  observation period, 125
  patient education, 226
  pharmacological, 123–125
  unusual variants, 121
anemia
  dyspnea associated with in infants, 104
  food protein-induced enteropathy, 153
  food protein-induced proctocolitis, 150–151
anergy, 8
angioedema
  acute, 76
  clinical features, 78
  first 6 months of life, 168
  see also urticaria/angioedema
animal food allergens, 23–25
  cow's milk, 23–24
  egg, 24
  families, 17–19
  fish, 24–25
  shellfish and crustaceae, 25
antibodies see immunoglobulins (Igs); specific immunoglobulins
antigen-presenting cells, 3f, 4
antigens
  food see food antigens
  oral tolerance see oral tolerance
  trafficking across the epithelium, 2–4
  transport, 3f

antihistamines
  anaphylaxis, 125, 207
  choice of, 54
  emergency kit, 212
  IgE-mediated food allergy, 49–50
  minor symptoms, 226
  timing of administration, 53–54
anti-IgE, 236–239, 236t, 238f–239f
anti-interleukin 5 antibodies, 56–57, 240
antimicrobial peptides, 2
anti-ulcer medication, 43
anxiety, 230–231
Apiaceae, 89
Api g 1, 25–26, 89, 93–94
Api g 4, 89
Api g 5, 26, 89
apoptosis, 8
apple, 25–27, 90, 94–96
arachidonic acid, 118
arachin, 28
Ara h 1, 28
Ara h 2, 2, 28
Ara h 3, 28
Ara h 6, 28
Ara h 7, 28
Ara h 8, 28, 94
arginine kinases, 18, 25
arrowroot, 275t
Art v 1, 84
asparagus, 26
aspartame, 102, 292
aspirin and food-dependent, exercise-induced anaphylaxis, 77
asthma, 99
  acute, induced by food allergy, 105–106
  and anaphylaxis, 121
  in bakers, 102
  and β$_2$-agonists, 208
  epidemiology, 100
  and fatal reactions, 210–211
  filaggrin gene mutations, 64
  and food additives, 102–103, 288
  and infantile colic, 158
  inhalation of food allergens, 103
  and introduction of solid foods, 259
  lipopolysaccharide in, 11
  prevalence, 40, 100–101
  recurrent/chronic, 107–108
  risk factors, 104–105
  routine testing of food allergy, 107–108
  and wheat allergy, 255
atopic dermatitis, 29, 61–73
  clinical case, 62b
  clinical evidence supporting the link between food allergy and, 65–66

clinical features, 64–65, 65t
definition, 61
diagnosis, 68–70, 69f
environmental and dietary exposure, 67–68
epidemiology, 62
immunological evidence supporting the link between food allergy and, 66
and introduction of solid foods, 259
management, 70
natural history, 70–71, 70t
pathogenesis, 62–64, 63f
and probiotics, 260
and respiratory symptoms, 105
triggers, 65t
atopic diseases, 44, 61
  and infantile colic, 158
  see also specific diseases
atopic march, 44, 61, 168
atopy patch testing (ATP)
  atopic dermatitis, 62–63
  eosinophilic esophagitis, 134–136
  food protein-induced enterocolitis syndrome, 147–148
attention deficit hyperactivity disorder (ADHD), 289–293
auriculotemporal syndrome, 79
avocado, 26–27
avoidance *see* dietary elimination; food avoidance
axon reflex, 77
azo-dyes, 287, 289

B
bacteria, mucosal, 1
bacterial infections and anaphylaxis, 121
baker's asthma, 102
banana, 26, 84
barley, 275t
basophil activation test (BAT), 94–95
basophil histamine release assay, 182
basophils, 118
B cells, 7
beclomethasone, 136–137
beef, 134
behavior
  additive challenge and, 290–292, 291f
  changes, 285, 287
  effects of exclusion diets on, 290
  food additives and, 289–293, 291f, 293f
bell pepper, 26
benzoate preservative, 293
Ber e 1, 27
β$_2$-agonists, 124–125, 207–208
β-conglutin, 28

β-conglycinin, 28
β-lactoglobulin, 2, 18, 23–24
Bet v 1, 20–21
  cross-reactivity, 89
  in fruit, 26–27
  in legumes, 28
  pollen-food syndrome, 85, 87t, 88–89
  pollen–fruit cross-reactive allergies, 25–26
Bet v 2, 87t
bi-cupins, 21
bifidobacteria, 260
bifunctional inhibitors, 20
biphasic allergic reactions, 120
birch homologs, 2
birch pollen
  basophil activation test, 94
  immunotherapy, 237t, 242–243
  inhalation, 25
  pollen-food syndrome, 84–85, 89–90, 95–96
Bra j 1, 27
Bra o 3, 26
Brazil nuts, 27
breastfeeding
  and allergy prevention, 258–259
  and atopic dermatitis, 67–68
  avoiding allergens during *see* maternal avoidance of allergens
  and cows' milk protein allergy, 266
  and food allergy, 44
  and food protein-induced proctocolitis, 150–151
  and infantile colic, 156t–157t, 158–159
breast milk
  allergens in, 9
  composition, 9
brilliant blue, 292
bronchial hyperreactivity (BHR), 106–107
bronchospasm, 206
buckwheat allergy
  anaphylactic reactions, 116, 118
  inhalation of allergens, 103
  urticaria/angioedema, 77
buckwheat as a wheat substitute, 275t
budesonide, 136–137

C
cabbage, 26
caffeine, 286
calcium
  and cows' milk protein allergy, 266–268
  ensuring adequate, 280–281
  requirements, 280t, 281
  sources of, 281t

CAP-fluoroenzyme immunoassay (CAP-FEIA), 35–36
CAP-RAST Fluorescent Enzyme Immunoassay, 180
cardiac arrhythmia, 207
cardiovascular disease and anaphylaxis, 121
cardiovascular shock, 206
cardiovascular symptoms, 114t, 120, 124, 206t, 226t
carrot, 25–26, 26f, 85, 94
casein
    cows' milk allergy, 18, 23, 253–254
    effect of processing on, 23–24
    micelles, 18
    structure, 18f
cashew nuts, 27
Cas s 1, 26
cassava, 275t
CD30, 154
CD4+ cells, 4–5, 9
celery allergy
    allergens, 25–26
    pollen-food syndrome, 85, 89, 94
    skin tests, 93
celery root, 26, 182
celiac disease, 29, 45, 57, 273
cereal-based beverages, 267–268
cereals, 29
cesarean section, 10, 41
cetirizine, 54, 226
chamber prick test, 80
chef card template, 222, 223f
chemical defences, 2
chemokines, 118
cherry, 25–26, 93
chestnut, 26
chia flour, 275t
chick peas
    inhalation of allergens, 103
    pollen-food syndrome, 84
    as a wheat substitute, 275t
children
    allergen avoidance, 225
    anaphylaxis reports, 115–116, 117t
    empowerment, 229–231
    eosinophilic esophagitis, 130–131 (see also eosinophilic esophagitis (EE))
    food allergy in, 33
    skin prick testing, 177
    treatment plans, 227
Chinese herbal medications, 235, 239–240
Chinese restaurant syndrome, 103
chitin, 22
chitinases, class I, 22, 26
chymase, 118
chymotrypsin, 23–24

Cit s 1, 26
classification of reactions to food, 285–287, 286f
Clostridium species, 260
cocaine, 210–211
colic, 46
    infantile see infantile colic
colitis
    eosinophilic, 138
    ulcerative, 138
colorings, food, 287, 289, 292–293
community, management of food allergy, 213–216, 215f
complementary and alternative medicine (CAM), 286–288
complementary feeding see weaning
component-resolved diagnostics (CRD), 84, 91, 96, 182
conarachin, 28
conformational epitopes, 15–16
Connors scores, 290–291, 291f
Consortium of Food Allergy Research (CoFAR), 68
constipation, cows' milk protein allergy, 46
contact exposure, 222–225
continuous epitopes, 15–16
cooking of food proteins, 224
cooking oils, 10–11
Cor a 1, 89
Cor a 1.01, 27–28
Cor a 1.04, 27–28, 89
Cor a 8, 27–28
Cor a 9, 27
Cor a 11, 27
corn, 84, 274, 275t
corn proteins, 150–151
coronary heart disease, 207
corticosteroids
    anaphylaxis, 207
    emergency kit, 212
    eosinophilic colitis, 138
    eosinophilic esophagitis, 56–57, 132–133, 136–137
    eosinophilic gastroenteritis, 138
    food protein-induced enterocolitis syndrome, 148–149
cosmetics, 81
cough, 105
counseling, dietary, 70
cows' milk allergy
    allergens, 2, 23–24
    anaphylactic reactions, 115–116, 118
    atopic dermatitis, 61–62, 66–68
    caseins, 18
    clinical features, 252t, 253–254
    cross-reactivity, 171
    definition, 34
    diagnosis, 169

dyspnea associated with anemia in infants, 104
eosinophilic colitis, 138
eosinophilic esophagitis, 134
epicutaneous immunotherapy, 247
epitopes, 235
extensively heated milk, 240–242
first 6 months of life, 168
food avoidance, 167
food protein-induced enterocolitis syndrome, 143, 145–149
food protein-induced enteropathy, 152–154
food protein-induced proctocolitis, 150–151
future therapies, 235
immunotherapy, 125, 237t
    oral, 55, 243–244
    sublingual, 246
infantile colic, 155, 158–159
inhalation of allergens, 103
natural history, 253–254
non-IgE-mediated, 45
oral food challenges, 191t
positive predictive values, 187t
prevalence, 36, 37f–39f
regulatory T-cells, 182
resolution of, 70–71, 253–254
respiratory symptoms, 102, 105–106, 108
skin prick testing, 175, 177
tolerance, 253
T-regulatory function, 8
urticaria/angioedema, 78
in vitro tests, 179–180, 180t
and weaning, 169
cows' milk formula, 259
cows' milk protein allergy (CMPA), 265
    alternative products, 267t–268t
    breastfed infants, 266
    colic and, 46
    cows' milk avoidance, 269
    formula-fed infants, 266
    nutritional comparison of alternative products, 268t
    practical acceptance of specialized formula, 268–269
    presentation, 46
    proctocolitis, 46
    soy products, 266–268
cows' milk protein (CMP) enterocolitis, 169
cows' milk protein (CMP) enteropathy, 45
cows' milk protein (CMP) proctitis, 167
COXs, 118
Crohn's disease, 2, 138
cromolyn, 138

cross-contamination, 221–222, 223t
cross-reactive carbohydrate
    determinants (CCDs), 16,
    90–91
cross-reactivity, 50–51, 265, 266t
    and atopic dermatitis, 69
    Bet v 1, 89
    and eosinophilic esophagitis, 134
    lipid transfer proteins, 86–88
    and pollen-food syndrome, 85, 95
    and urticaria/angioedema, 80
    see also specific allergens
Crustacea, 17, 25
    definitions, 221t
    urticaria/angioedema, 77–78
    see also shellfish
crying episodes, infantile colic, 158
Cucurbitaceae family, 84
cupins, 21, 21f, 86t
cupin seed globulins, 27, 85
cutaneous lymphocyte-associated
    antigen (CLA), 66
cysteine (C1) papain-like proteases, 22
cytokines, 2–5, 118

D

dairy products
    eczema, 167
    introducing at weaning, 170
    see also specific dairy products
Dau c 1, 25–26, 26f, 94
Dau c 4, 94
defence system proteins, 86t
delayed-onset reactions see non-
    immunoglobulin E-mediated
    food allergy
deletion, 8
dendritic cells
    antigen sampling, 3f, 4–5
    atopic dermatitis, 62–63
    in neonates, 9
dermatitis herpetiformis, 273
dermographism, 79
desensitization, 55, 235, 243–244
development of allergy, 8–10
diagnosis, 165–173
    common allergens in infants,
        168–170
    dilemmas, 285
    elimination/exclusion diets,
        290–291
    first consultation, 165–167
    immune mechanisms causing
        problems, 167–168
    international and intercultural
        considerations, 170
    under 6 months of age, 168–169
    new allergies after infancy, 170–171
    new allergies in adolescents,
        171–172

new allergies in adults, 172
    other conditions mimicking food
        allergy, 166, 166f
    6-18 months of age, 169–170
    tests see testing for food allergy;
        specific tests
    and therapy proceeding
        simultaneously, 169
    see also specific conditions
diarrhea
    food protein-induced enterocolitis
        syndrome, 145–146
    food protein-induced enteropathy,
        153
diet
    atopic dermatitis, 67–68
    disease management see dietary
        elimination; food avoidance;
        nutritional management
    and food allergy incidence, 41
    maternal restriction see maternal
        avoidance of allergens
dietary counseling, 70, 165–166
dietary elimination, 205
    adequate/proper, 210
    atopic dermatitis, 70
    for diagnosis, 281–282
    effects on behaviour, 290
    eosinophilic esophagitis, 136
    eosinophilic gastroenteritis, 138
    food protein-induced proctocolitis,
        151
    maternal see maternal avoidance of
        allergens
    respiratory symptoms, 109
    urticaria/angioedema, 80
dietary protein-induced proctitis, 58
diphenhydramine, 54, 226
dose-dependent tolerance, 194, 200
double-blind placebo-controlled food
    challenges (DBPCFC), 34–35,
    34t, 188–190, 190t, 192
D-α-tocopherol, 10–11
D-γ-tocopherol, 10–11
dust mites, 56
dysphagia, 56–57, 131–132, 132b
dyspnea associated with anemia in
    infants, 104

E

eczema
    exacerbations, 56
    within first 6 months of life, 168
    within first two years of life,
        104–105
    food additives and, 288
    and food allergy, 44
    IgE-mediated food allergy, 44
    and infantile colic, 158
    and introduction of solid foods, 259

and maternal avoidance of
    allergens, 258
    oral food challenges, 199–200,
        199t
    prevalence, 40
    at 6-18 months of age, 169–170
    skin exposure to allergens, 10
education
    family, 212–213
    patient see patient education
    schools, 216
EF-hand motifs, 17–18
egg allergy, 274–276
    allergens, 24, 274
    anaphylactic reactions, 115–116,
        118
    atopic dermatitis, 61–64
    clinical features, 252–253, 252t
    definition, 34
    diagnosis, 171
    eczema, 167
    eosinophilic esophagitis, 134
    epitopes, 235–236
    extensively heated egg, 240–242
    food avoidance, 167
    food protein-induced enteropathy,
        153
    food protein-induced proctocolitis,
        150–151
    future therapies, 235
    immunotherapy, 125
    inhalation of allergens, 103
    likelihood ratios, 188f
    natural history, 252–253
    oral food challenges, 191t
    oral immunotherapy, 55, 243–244
    persistence, 253
    positive predictive values, 187t
    prevalence, 36, 37f–39f
    resolution of, 70–71, 252–253
    respiratory symptoms, 102,
        105–106, 108
    skin prick testing, 175, 175b, 177
    sources of egg, 276t
    tolerance, 253
    urticaria/angioedema, 78
    in vitro tests, 179–180, 180t
    and weaning, 169–170
Egger study, 290
elemental diets, eosinophilic
    esophagitis, 136
11S globulins, 21, 27
elimination diet see dietary
    elimination
emergency treatment, 53
empowerment, 219, 229–233
    see also patient education
endoscopy
    eosinophilic esophagitis, 133,
        133t

food protein-induced enterocolitis syndrome, 148
food protein-induced proctocolitis, 150, 150t
energy intake, 281
enterocolitis, cows' milk protein, 169
enteropathy, cows' milk protein, 45
environmental factors
  allergy-promoting food exposure, 257
  atopic dermatitis, 67–68
  and food allergy incidence, 41
  hygiene hypothesis, 41
enzymatic degradation of two proteins, 2
enzyme allergosorbent test (EAST), 94
eosinophilic colitis, 138
eosinophilic esophagitis (EE), 56–57, 130–134
  allergic manifestations, 134–136
  anti-IL-5 antibody, 240
  in children, 45
  clinical features, 130–132, 130t
  diagnosis, 130–132, 168
  emergence, 129
  endoscopy, 133, 133t
  epidemiology, 132
  and grains, 274
  histology, 133–134, 133t
  pathophysiology, 132
  pollen-food syndrome, 85
  radiology, 132–133, 133t
  role of allergy, 134–136
  treatment/management, 136–137
eosinophilic gastroenteritis (EOG), 137–138
eosinophilic gastrointestinal diseases (EGIDs), 129–141
  see also specific diseases
eosinophil peroxidase (EPX), 133–134
eosinophils, 129, 132
  activation, 133–134
  in eosinophilic colitis, 138
  in eosinophilic esophagitis, 133–134
  in eosinophilic gastroenteritis, 137–138
  in food protein-induced proctocolitis, 150
  in urticaria/angioedema, 77–78
epicutaneous immunotherapy (EPIT), 246–247
epidemiology of food allergy, 33–48
  atopic march, 44
  definition and measurement, 34–36, 34t
  estimates of the prevalence of anaphylaxis, 38–40
  fatal anaphylaxis, 40
  incidence, 40–44

  prevalence, 36, 37f–39f
  role of race and gender, 40
epidermal barrier dysfunction, 63–64
epigenetics, 11
epinephrine
  administration, 206–207, 207t
  anaphylaxis, 49–50, 123–125, 126t, 205, 226
  choice of, 54
  contraindications, 207
  dosage, 54–55, 207
  food-dependent, exercise-induced anaphylaxis, 123–124
  food protein-induced enterocolitis syndrome, 148–149
  interactions with, 208
  routes of administration, 207
  self-injectable, 125, 126t, 211–212
    adolescents and, 232–233
    children and, 231
    device selection, 211–212, 211t
    doses, 216
    number of devices prescribed, 212
    patient selection, 211
    risks, 212
  timing of administration, 53–54
  urticaria/angioedema, 49–50, 81
EpiPen, 54, 125, 126t
epithelium, trafficking of antigen across the, 2–4, 3f
epitopes, 15–16, 182
  cross-reactivity, 265
  modification, 247
  and severity of reactions, 235
  T-cell, 95–96
Escherichia coli, 247
esophageal food impaction, 131–132
exclusion diets *see* dietary elimination
exercise, 208, 210–211
exercise-induced anaphylaxis (EIA), 29, 55
  food-dependent *see* food-dependent, exercise-induced anaphylaxis (FDEIA)
  oral food challenges, 196t, 200–201
extensively heated cows' milk and egg, 240–242
extensively hydrolyzed casein (EHC), 67–68, 149, 259, 266
extensively hydrolyzed formulas (EHF), 268
extensively hydrolyzed whey (EHW), 67, 259

F
Fabaceae, 89
fabricated or induced illness (FII), 286–287
family education, 212–213

Fas, 154
FcRn receptor, 9
fecal flora, 10
Feingold diet, 290
fetal immune system, 9
fibrosis in eosinophilic esophagitis, 132
filaggrin, 63–64
filaggrin (FLG) gene, 44
  mutations, 63–64
first consultation, 165–167
First International Gastrointestinal Eosinophil Research Symposium, 130
fish allergy
  allergens, 24–25, 103, 277
  anaphylactic reactions, 116, 118
  avoidance of fish, 277
  clinical features, 255
  cross-reactivity, 277, 277t
  diagnosis, 171
  inhalation of allergens, 103
  international and intercultural considerations, 170
  natural history, 255
  oral food challenges, 191t
  positive predictive values, 187t
  prevalence, 37f–39f
  respiratory symptoms, 101–102, 105–106
  urticaria/angioedema, 78
  in vitro tests, 179, 180t
fish oil, 11, 277
fluid support in anaphylaxis, 124
fluticasone, 136–137
folic acid, 11
food additives, 287–288, 288f
  and asthma, 102–103, 288
  and atopic dermatitis, 69
  and behaviour, 289–293, 291f–293f
  challenges, 290–292, 291f–292f
  and eczema, 288
  potential mechanisms of reactions to, 289
  and urticaria/angioedema, 288
Food Allergen Labeling and Consumer Protection Act (FALCPA), 220–221
food allergy
  and the atopic march, 44
  definition and measurement, 34–36, 34t
  development of, 8–10
  genetics and, 11–12
  increase of incidence, 40–44
  management, 205–217
  microbial influences, 10
  natural history, 251–256
  nutritional factors, 10–11
  opportunities for prevention, 12–13

pathogenesis, 251–252
prevalence, 36, 37f–39f
role of race and gender in, 40
route of exposure, 10
Food Allergy and Anaphylaxis
    Network (FAAN), 58, 216
  chef card template, 222, 223f
food allergy herbal formula-1
    (FAHF-1), 239
food allergy herbal formula-2
    (FAHF-2), 239–240
Food And Drug Administration
    (FDA), 219, 220t
food antigens, 15–32
food avoidance, 53, 219–225
  anaphylaxis, 125
  avoiding contact, 222–225
  cross-contamination, 221–222
  first consultation, 166–167, 167t
  food protein-induced enteropathy,
    153–154
  label reading, 219–221
  to prevent allergies developing, 257
  respiratory symptoms, 109
  urticaria/angioedema, 80
  see also dietary elimination
food bans, 224–225, 225t
food challenges see oral food
    challenges
food-dependent, exercise-induced
    anaphylaxis (FDEIA), 55,
    75–76
  associated conditions worsening,
    121, 122t
  causative foods, 120t
  clinical features, 120–121, 121f
  clinical symptoms, 78
  definition, 114–115
  diagnosis, 122–123, 123f
  education, 125
  epidemiology, 118, 119t–120t, 120f
  historical background, 113
  oral food challenges, 196t, 200–201
  pathogenesis, 118
  treatment/management, 123–125
    long-term, 125
    pharmacological, 123–125
  urticaria/angioedema in, 77, 79, 81
food handlers, urticaria/angioedema
    in, 78
food intolerance, 34, 286
food labels
  laws, 278–279, 279t
  precautionary, 221, 279–280
  reading, 219–221
food protein-induced enterocolitis
    syndrome (FPIES), 143–149,
    144t–145t
  clinical features, 145–147, 147t

diagnosis, 147–148
early infancy, 169
epidemiology, 143
and grains, 274
management, 149
milk, 146–149
natural history of, 149, 256
oral food challenges, 148–149,
    148t, 196t, 200
pathogenesis, 143–145, 145t
rice, 146–147
soy, 147–149
food protein-induced enteropathy,
    144t–145t, 152–154, 152t,
    153b
  clinical features, 153
  diagnosis, 153–154
  epidemiology, 152
  pathogenesis, 152, 152t
  treatment/management, 154
food protein-induced proctocolitis,
    46, 144t–145t, 149–152, 149t,
    151b
  clinical features, 150–151
  diagnosis, 151
  early infancy, 169
  endoscopy, 150, 150t
  epidemiology, 150
  management, 151–152
  mucosal biopsy, 150, 150t
  pathogenesis, 150, 150t
food proteins
  cooking of, 224
  enzymatic degradation, 2
  exposure to prevent allergies
    developing, 257
  modified recombinant engineered,
    238t, 247
food quality, 43
formula feeding
  and allergy prevention, 259
  and atopic dermatitis, 67–68
  and cows' milk protein allergy, 266
  and food protein-induced
    proctocolitis, 150–151
  and infantile colic, 156t–157t,
    158–159
  whole protein versus hydrolyzed
    formulas, 257
FOXP3, 5–7, 6f, 12, 64
fruit, 25–27, 277–278
  allergen extracts, 178–179
  allergens, 78
  cooked, 95–96
  cross-reactivity, 277–278, 278t
  eczema in infants, 168–169
  pollen-food syndrome, 84
  urticaria/angioedema, 78
future therapies, 216–217, 235–250

G
Gad c 1, 24
Gal d 1, 24
Gal d 3, 24
Gal d 4, 24
Gal d 5, 24
Gal d 6, 24
gastric juice analysis, 149
gastric pH, 9, 43
gastroenteritis, eosinophilic see
    eosinophilic gastroenteritis
    (EOG)
gastroesophageal reflux disease
    (GERD), 45, 130–132, 168
gastrointestinal symptoms, 206t, 226t
  anaphylaxis, 114t, 120
  IgE-mediated food reactions, 50
  pollen-food syndrome, 85
gastrointestinal tract
  chemical defences, 2
  flora, 41
  infant, 8–9
  mucosa see mucosa
  permeability, 2–4
  structure and function, 2–5
gender, role in food allergy, 40
genetics, 11–12
  atopic dermatitis, 64
  attention deficit hyperactivity
    disorder, 292–293
  eosinophilic esophagitis, 132
  and food allergy incidence, 41, 44
German Infant Nutritional
    Intervention Study (GINI), 67,
    259
germin-like proteins, 26
gliadins, 29, 102, 255
glucocorticosteroids, 125
glutamic acid, 292
gluten, 20, 29, 57
gluten-free products, 275t
glutenins, 29
glycinin, 28
glycoside hydrolase family 19, 22
glycoside hydrolase family 22, 18
Gly m 1, 28
Gly m 4, 28, 85, 89, 94
Gly m 5, 28
Gly m 6, 28
Gly m Bd 30 k, 28
Gly m 28 k, 28
goats milk, 166–167
granzyme A (GrA), 154
granzyme B (GrB), 154
grape, 26, 90
grass pollen allergy, 84, 90, 94
growth assessment, 280
guanido phosphotransferases, 18
gut flora, 10

H

H₁ antagonists *see* antihistamines
hazelnut allergy, 216
    allergens, 27–28, 89
    cross-reactivity, 171
    oral food challenges, 191t
    sublingual immunotherapy,
        245–246
hazelnut pollen, 27–28
hazelnuts
    alternative names for, 271t
    epitopes, 182
    introducing at weaning, 170
    pollen-food syndrome, 84, 95–96
heartburn, 132b
Helicobacter pylori infection, 43
herbs/spices, 78
Hev b 6.02, 22
Hev b 7, 26
histamine
    in anaphylaxis, 118
    food additives and, 289
    release, 50
    scombroid poisoning, 58
    urticaria/angioedema, 77
histamine *N*-methyltransferase gene,
    292–293
histamine-releasing factors (HRFs), 66
histidine, 58
history-taking, 165
HLA-DQ2, 57
HLA-DQ8, 57
HLA typing, celiac disease, 57
House Rule and Compromise
    approach, 233
humanized monoclonal anti-IgE
    antibodies, 236–239, 236t,
    238f–239f
human leucocyte antigens, 12
humoral immune system, 9
hygiene hypothesis, 5, 10, 41, 260
hyperactive airways, 105
hyperactivity, 291, 292f
    see also attention deficit
        hyperactivity disorder (ADHD)
hyperkinetic syndrome, 290
hypersensitivity reaction
    classification, 185, 186t
    type 1, 15
hypertonia, infantile colic, 158
hypoalbuminemia
    food protein-induced enterocolitis
        syndrome, 148
    food protein-induced proctocolitis,
        150–151
hypoallergenic diets, infantile colic,
    158
hypoproteinemia, 153
hypotension, 50, 206

I

ileus, 148
immediate-onset reactions *see*
        immunoglobulin E-mediated
        food allergy
immune deviation, 5
immune system
    adult, 9
    fetal, 9
    humoral, 9
    mucosal, 1–14
    neonatal, 9
immunoassays, 179–180, 180t
ImmunoCAP, 94, 179–180, 180t
immunoglobulin A+ B cells (IgA+ B
    cells)), 4
immunoglobulin A (IgA), 4
    in breast milk, 9
    food protein-induced enteropathy,
        152, 154
immunoglobulin D (IgD), 289
immunoglobulin E (IgE), 4, 7–8
    cow's milk allergy, 23
    and cross-reactive carbohydrate
        determinants, 16
    food protein-induced enterocolitis
        syndrome, 145
    food protein-induced enteropathy,
        152
    type I hypersensitivity reaction,
        15
immunoglobulin E (IgE) tests, 179,
    180t
    atopic dermatitis, 69
    eosinophilic esophagitis, 134–135
    food-dependent, exercise-induced
        anaphylaxis, 122–123
    food-induced anaphylaxis, 122
    food protein-induced enteropathy,
        154
    food protein-induced proctocolitis,
        151
    pollen-food syndrome, 93–94
    positive predictive values, 187t
immunoglobulin E-mediated food
    allergy, 49–57
    challenge, 53
    class I, 83
    class II, 83
    clinical manifestations, 206
    definition, 34
    diagnostic criteria, 34
    distinguishing from non-IgE
        mediated, 45t
    eczema exacerbations, 56
    eosinophilic esophagitis, 56–57,
        134
    epinephrine administration,
        206–207
    food-dependent, exercise-induced
        anaphylaxis, 55
    future therapies, 235
    immune mechanisms, 167
    incidence, 41–44, 42f
    management, 206–208
    natural history, 53
    nature of reaction, 50
    pollen-food allergy syndrome, 56
    prevalence, 40
    previous treatment/response to
        treatment, 51
    relating to airborne allergens, 56
    reproducibility, 50–51
    respiratory symptoms, 100
    scoring in oral food challenges,
        196–197
    studies, 34–35, 34t
    suspect foods, 50
    testing, 51–53
        false negatives, 52–53
        false positives, 52
        positive vs negative, 52
        skin test vs RAST, 51–52
    timing, 50
    treatment, 53–55
        antihistamines, 54
        avoidance, 53
        dosage, 54–55
        emergency treatment, 53–54
        epinephrine, 54
        oral immunotherapy, 55
        previous, 51
        response to, 51
immunoglobulin G (IgG), 4
    in breast milk, 9
    food protein-induced enterocolitis
        syndrome, 145
    food protein-induced enteropathy,
        152, 154
    food tests, 58
    in vitro assays, 179
immunoglobulin G4 (IgG4), 7
immunoglobulin M (IgM), 152
immunoglobulins (Igs), 15
immunostimulatory sequences
    (ISS-ODN), 238t, 248
immunotherapy, 237t
    allergen-specific, 242–243
    birch pollen, 242–243
    epicutaneous, 246–247
    with modified recombinant
        engineered food proteins, 238t,
        247
    oral *see* oral immunotherapy
    pollen-food syndrome, 95–96
    subcutaneous peanut, 242
    sublingual, 237t, 245–246
    and T regulatory cells, 8

incomplete food allergens, 83
individualized health care plan
    (IHCP), 227, 229f–232f
infantile colic, 154–161
    causes of, 155t
    clinical features, 158
    colic-food hypersensitivity
        association, 155–158, 155b,
        156t–157t
    diagnosis, 155t, 158
    epidemiology, 154–155
    management, 158–162, 159t
    pathogenesis, 155–158
    treatment, 158, 159t
infants
    atopic march, 167
    common food allergens, 167–170
    development of allergy, 8–10
    dyspnea associated with anemia in,
        104
    eczema in, 104–105
    feeding recommendations for
        prevention of allergies, 260,
        261t
    food allergy and risk for wheezing/
        hyperactive airways in
        childhood, 105
    gastrointestinal flora, 41
    introduction of solids see weaning
    non-IgE-mediated food allergy, 57
informed consent, oral food
        challenges, 195–196
ingredients list, food labels, 220, 278
inhalation exposure
    allergens causing respiratory
        symptoms, 103
    symptoms, 77, 99
    urticaria/angioedema, 81
intercultural considerations, food
        allergy diagnosis, 170–171
interferon-γ (IFN-γ), 5
interleukin-4 (IL-4), 5
interleukin-5 (IL-5)
    eosinophilic esophagitis, 137
    eosinophilic gastroenteritis,
        137–138
interleukin-6 (IL-6), 6–7
interleukin-10 (IL-10), 6–7, 7f, 12
    Lactococcus lactis expressing, 240
interleukin-12 (IL-12), 5, 9
interleukin-13 (IL-13), 5, 12
international considerations, food
        allergy diagnosis, 170–171
intestinal colonization, 10
intestinal mast cell histamine release
        assay, 182
intradermal skin tests, 179
intravenous fluids, 208
in vitro testing, 165, 179–183
    see also specific tests

in vivo testing, 165, 179–183
    see also skin testing
IPEX (immune dysregulation,
        polyendocrinopathy,
        enteropathy, X-linked)
        syndrome, 5–7, 64
iron, 281
irritable bowel syndrome, 273
iTregs, 6–7

J
Jext, 125
Job's syndrome, 8
Jug r 1, 27
Jug r 2, 27
Jug r 3, 27–28
Jug r 4, 27

K
kamut, 275t
Kazal inhibitors, 18–19
ketotifen, 138
kissing, 224
kiwellin, 26
kiwi fruit, 25–27, 90, 245
Kosher law, 219–220, 220f
Kunitz inhibitors, 22

L
label reading, 219–221
lactase deficiency, 57
Lactococcus lactis, 240
lactoferrin, 23
lactose, 23–24
    food protein-induced enteropathy,
        153
    intolerance, 57
lactose-free formulas, 266
lamina propria, 4
Langerhans' cells, 62–63
laryngeal edema, 206
latex allergy, 25, 56, 78, 81, 86–88,
        277–278
latex-fruit cross-reactive allergy
        syndrome, 26
LEAP study (Learning about Peanut
        Allergy), 68
lectins, 22, 28
legumes, 28–29
    cross-reactivity, 271–272
    eosinophilic esophagitis, 134
legumin-like seed globulins, 28
legumins, 21
Len c 1, 28
lentils, 28, 170
lettuce, 26
leukocytes, 149
leukocytoclasis, 79
leukotriene receptor antagonists, 137
leukotrienes, 118

likelihood ratios (LR), 187, 188f
linear epitopes, 15–16, 182
linseed, 272t
lipid transfer proteins (LTPs)
    in cereals, 29
    effect of processing on, 27
    fruit and vegetable allergies, 26–27
    inhalation, 102
    non-specific (nsLTP), 85, 88
    plant food allergens, 20
    pollen-food syndrome, 83–84,
        86–88, 87t, 91–93
    tree nuts and seeds allergies, 27–28
lipocalin family, 18
lipooxygenases, 118
lipopolysaccharide, 11–12
Listeria monocytogenes, 247
lobster, 17–18
lower airway symptoms, 50
    see also respiratory tract symptoms
lumen, 2
Lup an 1, 28
lupin, 28, 209–210, 272, 275t
lymph nodes, mesenteric, 4–5
lymphocyte stimulation tests, 182
lysozyme, 24, 274
lysozyme type C, 18

M
macadamia nuts, 271t
maize, 84, 274, 275t
major basic protein (MBP), 133–134
malabsorption, 152–153
Mal d 1, 25–27, 89, 94
Mal d 2, 90
Mal d 3, 26–27
manufactured foods, 278–280
mast cell inhibitors, 137
mast cells
    degranulation, 166
    intestinal mast cell histamine
        release assay, 182
    -mediated reactions, 50
    and T-regulatory cells, 7
    urticaria/angioedema, 77–78
mastocytes, 118
mastocytosis, 208
maternal avoidance of allergens
    and atopic dermatitis, 67
    evidence, 12
    polyunsaturated fats, 257–258
    prevention of allergies, 256–258
    recommendations, 166–167
    studies/trials, 168, 258
M cells, 3f, 4
meat anaphylaxis, 121
medications
    and anaphylaxis, 121
    interfering with oral food
        challenges, 195–196, 195t

support, 208
Mediterranean diet, 10–11, 26
mepolizumab, 240
mesenteric lymph nodes, 4–5
metered dose inhalers (MDIs), 136–137
methacholine, 104–106
methemoglobinemia, 146
micronutrient intake, 280
milk allergy *see* cows' milk allergy
millet, 275t
modified recombinant engineered food proteins, 238t, 247
Mollusca, 17, 25, 221t
    see also shellfish
monoclonal anti-IgE antibodies, 236–239, 236t, 238f–239f
monoclonal anti-IL-5 antibody, 235
monosodium glutamate, 102–103
montelukast, 138
mucosa
    barrier function, 2–4
    chemical defences, 2
    immunity, 1–14
    initial contact with the mucosal immune system, 4–5
    permeability, 2–4
    structure and function, 2–5
    trafficking of antigen across the epithelium, 2–4, 3f
mucus, 2
mugwort-celery-spice syndrome, 90
mugwort pollen, 84, 86–89
Munchhausen's-by-proxy syndrome, 286–287
Munchhausen's syndrome, 286–287
Mus p 1.2, 26
mustard seeds, 27, 272, 272t

N
National Cooperative Inner City Asthma Study, 101
natto anaphylaxis, 121
natural history, 251–256
negative predictive values (NPV), 187
neonates
    gastrointestinal flora, 41
    immune system, 9
Netherton syndrome, 64
neurological symptoms, 114t, 206t, 226t
neutrophils, 77–78
N-glycans, 16, 26
NOAEL (no observed adverse effect level), 194
non-immunoglobulin E-mediated food allergy, 45–46, 57–58
    celiac disease *see* celiac disease
    definition, 34
    diagnosis, 34

dietary protein-induced proctitis, 58
distinguishing from IgE mediated, 45t
eosinophilic esophagitis, 134
IgG food tests, 58
in infancy, 57
lactose intolerance, 57
natural history, 256
oral food challenges, 198–200
respiratory symptoms, 100
scombroid poisoning, 58
non-ingestion exposure, 222–225
    see also inhalation exposure
non-sensitizing elicitors, 83
non-steroidal anti-inflammatory drugs (NSAIDs), 122–123
nsLTP (non-specific lipid transfer proteins), 85, 88
nutritional management, 280–281
    and allergy development, 10–11
    eosinophilic esophagitis, 136

O
oats, 275t
obese patients, epinephrine administration in, 207
ocular symptoms, 226t
O-glycosyl hydrolase superfamily, 18
oils, 10–11, 270, 272
old friends hypothesis, 41–43
Oleaceae, 84
Ole e 2, 84
Ole e 7, 84
oleosins, 28
O-linked glycans, 16
olive oil, 10–11
omega-3 polyunsaturated fatty acids, 11, 257–258
omega-6 polyunsaturated fatty acids, 257–258
open patch test, 80
open test, 80
oral allergy syndrome (OAS) *see* pollen-food allergy syndrome
oral exposure, 10
oral food challenges, 175, 185–204
    assessment of non-IgE-mediated reactions, 198–199
    atopic dermatitis, 69–70
    atopic eczema, 199–200, 199t
    blinded, 34–35, 34t, 188–190, 190t
    choice of food matrix, 191–192
    contra-indications, 196, 196t–197t
    design, 187–201
    determination of outcome, 196–197
    doses, 191t, 193–194
        interval between, 194
        number of, 194
        site of application of first, 195

double-blind placebo-controlled, 34–35, 34t, 188–190, 190t
    foods for, 192
exercise-induced anaphylaxis, 200–201
food additives and behavior, 290–292, 291f
food-dependent, exercise-induced anaphylaxis, 122–123, 200–201
food-induced anaphylaxis, 122
food protein-induced enterocolitis syndrome, 147–149, 148t, 200
food protein-induced enteropathy, 153–154
form of challenge food, 190–191
indications for, 185–187, 186t
logistics, 195–196
methodology, 187–201
modified, 200, 200t
open, 34–35, 34t, 188–190
open vs blinded, 188–190
outcomes, 197–198, 202, 202t–203t
placebos, 193
pollen-food syndrome, 93
prior to, 201–202
procedures, 201–202
rationale, 185
respiratory symptoms in food allergy, 109
safety, 196, 196t
scoring
    of IgE-mediated allergic reactions, 196–197, 198t
    of non-IgE-mediated allergic reactions, 199–200
single-blind, 188
urticaria/angioedema, 80
variables, 187–201, 189t
oral immunotherapy, 237t, 243
    anaphylaxis, 125
    combined with anti-IgE, 239
    peanut, 244–245
    safety of home dosing, 245
    trials, 243–245
oral tolerance
    definition, 5–8
    versus desensitization, 243
    developmental stage, 8–10
    exposure, 10
    factors that influence the development of, *versus* allergy, 8–12
    genetics and, 11–12
    immune deviation, 5
    immunopathogenesis, 256–257
    microbial influences, 10
    mucosal immune system, 1
    nutritional factors, 10–11

oral immunotherapy trials, 243–244
regulatory T cells, 5–8, 6f–7f
orange pips, 26
oriental mustard seeds, 27
otitis media, recurrent/chronic, 104
ovalbumin, 24, 274
  atopic dermatitis, 67
  respiratory symptoms, 106–107
ovomucin, 274
ovomucoid, 24, 240–241, 274
ovotransferrin, 24, 274
OX40, 7f

P

pan-allergens, 22, 26, 83–88
pancreatic enzymes, 9
paperwork, 227, 228f
paracellular spaces, 2–4
parents empowering children, 230–231
Parietaria, 84, 86–88
partially hydrolyzed formulas (PHF), 266
partially hydrolyzed whey (PHW), 67–68, 259
parvalbumin oligomers, 24
parvalbumins, 17–18, 17f, 24, 277
patatin, 26
pathogenesis-related proteins (PRs), 83–84, 88–91
patient assent, oral food challenges, 195–196
patient education, 212–213, 219–234
  avoidance, 219–225
  plans and paperwork, 227, 228f
  symptom recognition and treatment, 225–227
peach
  allergens, 25–26, 86–88
  pollen-food syndrome, 94
  sublingual immunotherapy, 246
peanut agglutinin, 28
peanut allergy, 34
  allergens, 2, 270
  anaphylactic reactions, 107, 115–118
  atopic dermatitis, 61–64, 67
  avoidance of introduction of peanuts, 259–260
  avoidance of peanuts, 270, 271t
  clinical features, 254–255
  cross-reactivity, 269–270
  diagnosis, 171
  engineered recombinant immunotherapy, 238t
  eosinophilic esophagitis, 134
  epitopes, 235
  future therapies, 247–248
  genetic factors, 12, 44

humanized monoclonal anti-IgE, 236–239
immunotherapy, 125, 237t
  oral, 55, 244–245
  subcutaneous, 242
incidence, 40
international and intercultural considerations, 170
and maternal avoidance of allergens, 258
natural history, 254–255, 254t
non-ingestion exposure, 224–225
oral food challenges, 191t, 194, 202t–203t
persistence, 254–255
pollen-food syndrome, 84, 94
positive predictive values, 187t
prevalence, 36, 37f–39f, 40–41
resolution of, 70–71, 255
respiratory symptoms, 100–102, 105–106
self-injectable epinephrine devices, 211
skin prick testing, 177–180
traditional Chinese medicine, 239–240
urticaria/angioedema, 78
in vitro tests, 179–180, 180t
and weaning, 169–170
peanuts, 28–29
  alternative names for, 271t
  epitopes, 182
  hidden sources of, 276
peas, 28
pecans, 271t
pepsin, 23–24, 84–85
peptide immunotherapy, 238t, 247–248
Pers a 1, 26–27
persistence factors, 251–252
Peyer's patches, 3f, 4
pharyngeal complaints, 50
phospholipase A2, 118
Pis s 1, 28
pistachios, 27, 84
Pis v 1, 27
Pis v 2, 27
Pis v 3, 27
placebos, oral food challenges, 193
plantain pollinosis, 84
plant food allergens, 25–29
  cereals, 29
  diversity, 16
  families, 19–22
  fresh fruits and vegetables, 25–27, 26f
  legumes, including peanut, 28–29
  tree nuts and seeds, 27–28
plasmid DNA-based immunotherapy, 238t, 248

platelets-activating factor, 118
pollen, 25, 134
pollen-food allergy syndrome, 56, 83–98, 277–278
  in adolescents, 171
  birch pollen immunotherapy, 242–243
  clinical presentation, 84–85
    anaphylaxis, 85
    gastrointestinal disorders, 85
    oral allergy syndrome, 84–85
  diagnosis, 91–95, 92f
    in vitro tests, 93–94
    in vivo tests, 91–95
  epidemiology, 84
  management, 95–96
  pan-allergens, 85–88
    lipid transfer proteins, 86–88
    prolamin superfamily, 85–86
  pathogenesis-related proteins, 88–91
pollen-food syndrome, 93
pollen-fruit allergy syndrome, 21–22
pollen-fruit cross-reactive allergy syndromes, 27–28
polyunsaturated fatty acids, 11, 257–258
poppy seeds, 272t
positive predictive values (PPV), 187, 187t
potato, 275t
prebiotics, 12–13, 260
precautionary labels, 221, 279–280
prevalence
  of anaphylaxis, 38–40
  of food allergy, 36, 37f–39f, 251–252, 256
prevention of allergies, 12–13, 256–261, 261t
  see also specific prevention strategies
prick-by-prick procedure, 79–80, 93, 134–135, 178–179
probiotics, 12–13, 240, 260
proctitis
  cows' milk protein, 169
  dietary protein-induced, 58
proctocolitis, food protein-induced see food protein-induced proctocolitis
profilins, 21–22, 21f
  in legumes, 28
  pollen-food syndrome, 83–85, 90–93
prolamins, 19–20, 19f, 85–86, 86t
prostaglandins, 118
protease inhibitors, 18–19
protein contact dermatitis, 78
proton pump inhibitors, 43, 45
Pru av 1, 25–26, 93–94
Pru av 2, 90

Pru av 3, 93
Pru av 4, 93–94
Pru p 1, 25–26
Pru p 3, 26, 94, 246
pruritus, 78, 206
psyllium, 56
puddle test *see* prick-by-prick procedure

Q
quality of life (QoL), 205
quinoa, 275t
quinoline yellow, 292

R
race, role in food allergy, 40
radioallergosorbent test (RAST), 179–180
  false negatives, 52–53
  false positives, 52
  IgE-mediated food reactions, 35–36, 51–52
  pollen-food syndrome, 94
  positive vs negative, 52
  vs skin tests, 51–52
radiology in eosinophilic esophagitis, 132–133, 133t
ragweed pollen, 134
rectal bleeding, food protein-induced proctocolitis, 151
regulatory T-cells, 5–8, 6f–7f
  iTregs, 6–7
  milk allergy, 182
  in neonates, 9
Rehabilitation Act (1973), 227
resolution rates, 251–252
respiratory tract symptoms, 99–112, 206t, 226t
  allergens, 102–103
  anaphylaxis, 114t, 120
  contributing to the severity of acute allergic reaction, 107
  diagnosis/management, 108–109
    food challenges, 109
    medical history, 108
    physical examination, 108
    testing for food allergy, 108–109
  differential diagnosis of, 103–108, 104t
  epidemiology, 100–101
  IgE-mediated food reactions, 50
  mechanisms, 102
  pathogenesis, 102–103
  prevalence, 100–101
  route of exposure, 103
  treatment, 109
restaurants, cross contamination, 222, 223f
retinoic acid, 6–7

rhinitis
  allergic *see* allergic rhinitis
  recurrent/chronic, 104
rhinorrhea, 206
rice, 146–147, 274, 275t
Rosacea fruits
  allergens, 25–26
  cross-reactivity, 95
  pollen-food syndrome, 86–89
  sensitization to, 91
  urticaria/angioedema, 78
route of exposure, 10
rye, 134, 275t

S
sago, 275t
Schatzki ring, 132–133
schools
  awareness of allergies, 213–215
  elimination of foods in, 215
  information for, 216
  medications at, 216
  treatment plans for, 227
scombroid poisoning, 58, 285
scratch test, 80
seafood *see* fish allergy; shellfish allergy
seafood poisoning, 277
seed oils, 272
seeds, 27–28, 272–273, 272t
  FDA list of, 220t
  hidden sources of, 276
  resolution of allergy, 70–71
seed storage prolamins, 20, 29
seed storage protein allergens, 27
self or parent-report allergies, 34–35, 34t
sensitization, 50–51, 257
serosal eosinophilic gastroenteritis, 137
serpins, 18–19
serum albumin, 23
sesame, 220–221
  hidden sources of, 276
  seeds, 27, 272t
sesame allergy
  clinical features, 255
  natural history, 254t, 255
Ses i 1, 27
Ses i 2, 27
Ses i 6, 27
7/8S globulins, 21, 27
SFA-8, 27
Sharon fruit, 94
shellfish, definitions, 221t
shellfish allergy
  airborne allergens, 103
  allergens, 17, 25, 103
  anaphylactic reactions, 116, 118
  avoidance of shellfish, 277

clinical features, 255
cross-reactivity, 277, 277t
diagnosis, 171
effect of cooking on shellfish, 277
natural history, 255
prevalence, 37f–39f
respiratory symptoms, 101–102
urticaria/angioedema, 78
shock, cardiovascular, 206
shrimp allergy
  allergens, 17–18, 25
  natural history, 255
  oral food challenges, 191t
  respiratory symptoms, 100
Sin a 1, 27
Sin a 2, 27
skin biopsies, urticaria/angioedema, 77–78
skin exposure to allergens, 10
skin prick testing (SPT)
  accuracy, 176–177
  adverse reactions to, 177
  atopic dermatitis, 69
  eczema in infants, 168–169
  eosinophilic esophagitis, 134–135
  false negatives, 52–53
  false positives, 52
  food-dependent, exercise-induced anaphylaxis, 122–123
  food-induced anaphylaxis, 122
  food protein-induced enterocolitis syndrome, 147–148
  food protein-induced enteropathy, 154
  IgE-mediated food reactions, 35–36, 51–52
  negative predictive accuracy, 175, 176
  open patch test, 80
  pollen-food syndrome, 91–93
  positive predictive accuracy, 177
  positive predictive values, 187t
  positive vs negative, 52
  process, 175
  versus RAST, 51–52
  sensitivity and specificity, 165
  urticaria/angioedema, 79–80
  variables, 179, 179b
skin symptoms, 226t
  anaphylaxis, 114t, 120, 120f
  grading of severity of anaphylactic reaction, 206t
  IgE-mediated food reactions, 50
skin testing, 175–179
  eosinophilic esophagitis, 134–135
  intradermal, 179
  respiratory symptoms in food allergy, 108–109
  versus in vitro testing, 179, 180b
  see also specific tests

small bowel biopsy, food protein-induced enteropathy, 153–154
solid foods introduction *see* weaning
sorghum, 275t
S-ovalbumin, 24
soy allergy
    atopic dermatitis, 61–62
    avoidance of soy, 272t
    cross-reactivity, 171, 270–271
    diagnosis, 171
    eosinophilic esophagitis, 134
    food protein-induced enterocolitis syndrome, 145–149
    food protein-induced enteropathy, 153
    food protein-induced proctocolitis, 150–151
    infantile colic, 155
    natural history, 256
    oral food challenges, 191t
    resolution of, 70–71
    skin prick testing, 179
    in vitro tests, 179–180
soybean, 28, 89, 94
soy flour, 275t
soy products
    cows' milk protein allergy, 266–268
    formula feeds, infantile colic, 158
    milk, 266
specific oral tolerance induction, 55
spelt, 275t
SPINK5, 12, 64
spontaneous basophil histamine release (SBHR), 66
squamous epithelial hyperplasia, 85
steatorrhea, 153
studies
    limitations of, 35
    link between food allergy and atopic dermatitis, 65–66
    oral immunotherapy, 243–245
    strengths and weaknesses of, 34–35, 34t
    see also specific topics
subcutaneous immunotherapy
    birch pollen, 242–243
    peanut, 242
sublingual immunotherapy, 237t, 245–246
substance P, 77
sulfites, 102
sunflower oil, 10–11
sunflower seeds, 27, 272t
support medication, 208
suppressor T cells, 5–6, 6f
sweet cherry, 90
symbols, food labeling, 219–220, 220f
symptom diaries, 78–80

symptom recognition, 225–227
    see also specific body system
synbiotics, 260

T

tacrolimus, 2–4
tapioca, 275t
tartrazine, 287
T-cell epitopes, 95–96
T cells, 3f
    in atopic dermatitis, 66
    food protein-induced enterocolitis syndrome, 143
    helper *see* T-helper cells
    proliferation, 5
    regulatory *see* regulatory T-cells
    suppressor, 5–6, 6f
testing for food allergy
    respiratory symptoms, 108–109
    routine, in recurrent/chronic asthma, 107–108
    in vitro, 165, 179–183
    in vivo, 165, 175–179 (*see also* skin testing)
    see also specific conditions; specific tests
thaumatin, 89
thaumatin-like proteins (TLPs), 22
    effect of processing on, 27
    pollen-food syndrome, 87t, 89–90
T-helper cells
    Th1, 5
        atopic dermatitis, 62–63
        effect of vitamin D on, 11
        in neonates, 9
    Th2, 5
        atopic dermatitis, 62–63
        effect of vitamin D on, 11
        in neonates, 9
    Th17, 6–8
tissue transglutaminase (TTG), 57
toll-like receptors (TLRs), 10
tomato, 26
topical steroids
    eosinophilic esophagitis, 136–137
    eosinophilic gastroenteritis, 138
traditional Chinese medicine (TCM), 235, 239–240
transferrins, 18
transforming growth factor-β (TGF-β), 6–7, 7f, 9
treatment plans, 211–212, 214f, 227, 228f
tree nut allergy
    anaphylactic reactions, 107, 115–118
    avoidance of tree nuts, 270, 271t
    clinical features, 255
    cross-reactivity, 270
    diagnosis, 171

natural history, 254t, 255
    positive predictive values, 187t
    resolution of, 70–71
    respiratory symptoms, 101–102, 105
    self-injectable epinephrine devices, 211
    skin prick testing, 179
    traditional Chinese medicine, 239–240
    urticaria/angioedema, 78
    in vitro tests, 179–180, 180t
tree nuts, 27–28
    alternative names for, 271t
    FDA list of, 220t
    hidden sources of, 276
triosephosphate isomerase (TIM), 25
triticale, 275t
tropomyosins, 17, 17f, 25, 277
trypsin, 23–24
trypsin inhibitors, 20
tryptase, 118
tuna allergy, 286
TV sign, 197
Twinject, 54, 125, 126t
2S albumins, 20, 27–28
tyrosine kinases, 118

U

ulcerative colitis, 138
urticaria
    acute, 76
    and angioedema *see* urticaria/angioedema
    cholinergic, 79
    chronic, 76
    first 6 months of life, 166
    food-dependent exercise-induced, 75–76
    IgE-mediated food reactions, 49–51
    immunological (allergic) contact, 76, 78, 80–81
    virus-induced, 166, 166f
urticaria/angioedema, 75–82
    clinical features, 78
    diagnosis, 78–80
    epidemiology, 76–77
    first 6 months of life, 168
    food additives and, 288
    pathogenesis, 77–78
    prevalence, 76–77
    treatment, 80–81

V

vasculitis, 79
vega tests, 286–287
vegetable oil, 10–11
vegetables
    allergen extracts, 178–179

allergens, 25–27, 26f, 86t
  cooked, 95–96
  cross-reactivity, 277–278, 278t
  pollen-food syndrome, 84
  urticaria/angioedema, 78
vicilin-like seed globulins, 28
viral infections and anaphylaxis, 121
vitamin A, 6–7, 11
vitamin D, 11
vitamin E, 10–11
Vit v 1, 26
vivilins, 21
vomiting
  eosinophilic esophagitis, 131
  food protein-induced enterocolitis
    syndrome, 145–146

W

wall pellitory, 84
walnuts, 27–28

weaning
  and allergy prevention, 259–260
  international and intercultural
    considerations, 170
  introduction, 169
  recommendations, 68
  timing of, 43–44
Wessel's rule of threes, 154, 155t,
  158
wheals, 77–79
wheat, 29
  food sources of, 274t
  introducing at weaning, 170
  substitutes, 275t
wheat allergy, 273–274
  anaphylactic reactions, 115–116,
    118
  and asthma, 255
  avoidance of wheat, 273–274
  clinical features, 252t, 255

  eosinophilic esophagitis, 134
  food-dependent, exercise-induced
    anaphylaxis, 122–123
  food protein-induced enterocolitis
    syndrome, 149
  food protein-induced enteropathy,
    153
  natural history, 255
  oral food challenges, 191t
  resolution of, 70–71
  respiratory symptoms, 102
  skin prick testing, 179
  urticaria/angioedema, 77
  in vitro tests, 179–180
wheezing, 105–106
whey proteins, 23–24
whole blood analysis, 286–287

Y

yellow mustard seeds, 27